Mental Health and Social Problems

A social work perspective

Edited by Nina Rovinelli Heller and Alex Gitterman

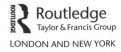
Routledge
Taylor & Francis Group

LONDON AND NEW YORK

First published 2011
by Routledge
2 Park Square, Milton Park, Abingdon, Oxon, OX14 4RN

Simultaneously published in the USA and Canada
by Routledge
270 Madison Avenue, New York, NY 10016

Routledge is an imprint of the Taylor & Francis Group, an informa business

Typeset in Baskerville
by Keystroke, Station Road, Codsall, Wolverhampton
Printed and bound in Great Britain
by CPI Antony Rowe, Chippenham, Wiltshire

British Library Cataloguing in Publication Data
A catalogue record for this book is available from the British Library

Library of Congress Cataloging in Publication Data
Mental health and social problems : a social work perspective / edited by
Nina Rovinelli Heller and Alex Gitterman.
p. cm.
Includes bibliographical references.
1. Psychiatric social work. 2. Mental illness–Etiology. 3. Social problems.
I. Heller, Nina Rovinelli. II. Gitterman, Alex, 1938–
[DNLM: 1. Mental Disorders. 2. Mental Disorders--etiology. 3. Social Problems. 4.
Social Work, Psychiatric. WM 31 M5444 2011]
HV689.M46 2011
362.2'042–dc22
2010017265

ISBN13: 978–0–415–49386–4 (hbk)
ISBN13: 978–0–415–49387–1 (pbk)
ISBN13: 978–0–203–84060–3 (ebk)

Mental Health and Social Problems

Mental Health and Social Problems is a textbook for social work students and practitioners. It explores the complicated relationship between mental conditions and societal issues as well as examining risk and protective factors for the prevalence, course, adaptation to and recovery from mental illness.

The introductory chapter presents biopsychosocial and life-modeled approaches to helping individuals and families with mental illness. The book is divided into two parts. Part I addresses specific social problems, such as poverty, oppression, racism, war, violence, and homelessness, identifying the factors which contribute to vulnerabilities and risks for the development of mental health problems, including the barriers to accessing quality services. Part II presents the most current empirical findings and practice knowledge about prevalence, diagnosis, assessment, and intervention options for a range of common mental health problems – including personality conditions, eating conditions and affective conditions.

Focusing throughout upon mental health issues for children, adolescents, adults and older adults, each chapter includes case studies and web resources. This practical book is ideal for social work students who specialize in mental health.

Nina Rovinelli Heller teaches in the masters and doctoral programs, and is the Chair of the Mental Health Substantive Area at the University of Connecticut, USA. She has provided mental health services to individuals and families for thirty years in a range of practice settings. She is the co-editor of *Integrating Psychodynamic Theory with Cognitive Behavioral Techniques* and has published in the area of social work theory and clinical practice.

Alex Gitterman is Zachs Professor of Social Work and Director of the Doctoral Program at the University of Connecticut School of Social Work. He has co-authored and co-edited a large number of books including *The Life Model of Social Work Practice, Encyclopedia of Social Work with Groups* and *The Handbook of Social Work Practice with Vulnerable and Resilient Populations*. He served as the President and on the board of the Association for the Advancement of Social Work with Groups, an international professional organization.

We dedicate this book to all people who have lived with mental health conditions.

We write with their voices in our minds and hearts.

Contents

List of contributors   ix
Preface   xi
Acknowledgements   xvii

1 **Introduction to social problems and mental health/illness**   1
   NINA ROVINELLI HELLER AND ALEX GITTERMAN

PART I
Social problems and mental health/illness   19

2 **Oppression and stigma and their effects**   21
   AMY C. WATSON AND SHAUN M. EACK

3 **Poverty and its effects**   44
   MARK R. RANK

4 **Racism and its effects**   62
   DENNIS MIEHLS

5 **War and its effects**   86
   SCOTT HARDING

6 **Homelessness and its effects**   110
   JUDITH BULA WISE

7 **Corrections and its effects**   133
   RUDOLPH ALEXANDER, JR.

8 **Immigration and its effects**   156
   GREGORY ACEVEDO AND MANNY J. GONZÁLEZ

9 **Child maltreatment and its effects**   174
   CAROLYN KNIGHT

10 **Intimate partner violence and its effects**   202
BONNIE E. CARLSON

11 **Community violence exposure and its effects**   225
VANESSA VORHIES, NEIL B. GUTERMAN, AND
MUHAMMAD M. HAJ-YAHIA

PART II
Mental health conditions   257

12 **Autism spectrum conditions**   259
JOSEPH WALSH AND JACQUELINE CORCORAN

13 **Executive function conditions and self-deficits**   282
JOSEPH PALOMBO

14 **Oppositional defiant and conduct conditions**   313
AMANDA N. BARCZYK AND DAVID W. SPRINGER

15 **Mood conditions**   331
ELLEN SMITH

16 **Anxiety conditions**   356
NINA ROVINELLI HELLER AND LISA WERKMEISTER ROZAS

17 **Eating conditions**   381
DANNA BODENHEIMER AND NINA ROVINELLI HELLER

18 **Personality conditions**   404
TERRY B. NORTHCUT

19 **Psychotic conditions**   423
ELLEN P. LUKENS AND LYDIA P. OGDEN

20 **Substance abuse**   450
MEREDITH HANSON

21 **Dementia and related problems in cognition and memory**   473
SARA SANDERS AND JOELLE K. OSTERHAUS

Index   502

Contributors

Gregory Acevedo, PhD
Associate Professor, Fordham University Graduate School of Social Services

Rudolph Alexander, Jr., PhD
Professor, Ohio State University College of Social Work

Amanda N. Barczyk, MSW
Doctoral candidate, University of Texas School of Social Policy and Practice Work at Austin

Danna Bodenheimer, DSW
Adjunct Faculty, University of Pennsylvania School of Social Policy and Practice

Bonnie E. Carlson, PhD
Professor and Associate Director, West Campus, Arizona State University School of Social Work

Jacqueline Corcoran, PhD
Professor, Virginia Commonwealth University School of Social Work

Shaun M. Eack, PhD
Assistant Professor, University of Pittsburg School of Social Work

Alex Gitterman, EdD
Zacks Professor of Social Work and Director of the Doctoral Program, University of Connecticut School of Social Work

Manny J. González, DSW
Associate Professor, Hunter College School of Social Work, The City University of New York

Neil B. Guterman, PhD
Mose and Sylvia Firestone Professor and Dean, University of Chicago School of Social Administration

Muhammad M. Haj-Yahia, PhD
Gordon Brown Chair in Social Work and Associate Professor, The Hebrew University of Jerusalem School of Social Work and Social Welfare

Meredith Hanson, DSW
Professor, Fordham University Graduate School of Social Services

Scott Harding, PhD
Associate Professor, University of Connecticut School of Social Work

Nina Rovinelli Heller, PhD
Associate Professor, University of Connecticut School of Social Work

Carolyn Knight, PhD
Professor, School of Social Work, University of Maryland Baltimore

Ellen P. Lukens, PhD
Firestone Centennial Professor of Clinical Social Work, Columbia University School of Social Work

Dennis Miehls, PhD
Associate Professor, Smith College School of Social Work

Terry B. Northcut, PhD
Associate Professor, Loyola University Chicago School of Social Work

Lydia P. Ogden, MSW
Doctoral Candidate, Columbia University School of Social Work

Joelle K. Osterhaus, MSW
Bereavement Coordinator, Barton Hospice

Joseph Palombo, MA
Founding Dean, Institute for Clinical Social Work, Chicago

Mark R. Rank, PhD
Herbert S. Hadley Professor of Social Welfare, Washington University School of Social Work in St. Louis

Sara Sanders, PhD
Assistant Professor, University of Iowa School of Social Work

Ellen Smith, PhD
Assistant Extension Professor, University of Connecticut School of Social Work

David W. Springer, PhD
University Distinguished Teaching Professor, University of Texas School of Social Work

Vanessa Vorhies, MSW
University of Chicago School of Social Administration

Joseph Walsh, PhD
Professor, Virginia Commonwealth University School of Social Work

Amy C. Watson, PhD
Assistant Professor, Jane Addams College of Social Work, University of Illinois at Chicago

Lisa Werkmeister Rozas, PhD
Associate Professor, University of Connecticut School of Social Work

Judith Bula Wise, PhD
Professor Emerita, University of Denver Graduate School of Social Work

Preface

Mental Health and Social Problems: A social work perspective is written as a textbook and reference book for social work students and practitioners. In serving as editors, we invited leading social work experts to present the state of interdisciplinary knowledge and practice wisdom about the complex bidirectional relationship between societal issues and mental health as well as about numerous mental health conditions and related life stressors. We divided the book into two parts. In Part I, we examine the societal, political and economic contexts of mental health conditions. In Part II, we examine the most current empirical findings, practice knowledge and wisdom about the major mental health conditions faced by our clients.

In Part I, our contributors examine the impact of oppression and stigma, poverty, racism, war, homelessness, corrections, immigration, childhood maltreatment, intimate partner violence, and community violence on our clients' mental health. Our contributors follow a common outline to organize their respective chapters. After introducing the contextual focus, each author discusses the societal, political, economic definitions of the social issue and its effects on mental health and mental illness. This discussion is followed by a review of the social problem's demographics, incidences and prevalence rates. The influences of race, gender, life course, sexual orientation, and ability/disability are also examined. To provide a "human face" to the empirical data, each author presents a practice illustration, and discusses relevant and salient assessment and interventions themes that emerge from the illustration. The contributions of social work and the importance of social work involvement are explicated. Chapters conclude with boxed texts consisting of web resources.

In Chapter 2, Professors Watson and Eack examine the deleterious impact of oppression and stigma on mental health. The authors begin with a discussion of the stigmatization process, which consists of five interrelated components. The first component is labeling of human differences, and attributing negative attributes to the differences. The next component is separating "us" from "them" (healthy from mentally ill). The "them" become stigmatized and the "us" become the stigmatizers. The stigmatized experience loss of social status, prejudice and discrimination. Persons suffering from mental illness are stereotyped as "dangerous, unpredictable, incompetent, irresponsible; at fault for their illness, and unlikely to recover." These negative stereotypes affect every dimension of the life of a person suffering from mental illness: education, employment, housing, health and mental health care, and interpersonal relationships.

In Chapter 3, Professor Rank analyzes the effects of poverty on mental health. He begins by describing the nature and scope of poverty in the United States. He estimates that approximately 60 million of people living in the United States live in or near poverty. At greatest risk of being poor are people with less education, who are young or old, non-white, have a disability, live in single parent families or reside in economically depressed inner cities or rural areas. Professor Rank presents a large body of research that indicates a strong association between poverty and diminished mental health. Subsequently, he raises the difficult and illusive question: how does one determine the *direction of causality* between poverty and diminished mental health? Research evidence, on the one hand, suggests that individuals with mental health problems are more likely to drift downward into poverty. Concomitantly, research evidence, on the other hand, suggests that the conditions associated with poverty decrease the quality of poor people's mental health. Professor Rank offers a trenchant observation: The direction of causality might be related to the type of mental health condition itself. The severity of schizophrenia, for example, may cause downward economic mobility that results in poverty. In contrast, poverty might trigger anxiety and mood conditions.

In Chapter 4, Professor Miehls explores the insidious effects of repeated manifestations of individual, institutional and structural and institutionalized racism on the mental health of People of Color. Those suffering from mental illness are even more likely than other People of Color to experience the devastating effects of racism, such as homelessness, unemployment, incarceration, school failure, and restricted access to health and mental health services. The concept of *"microaggressions"* is used to capture how the day-to-day experiences of being marginalized impacts the mental health of People of Color.

Professor Harding, in Chapter 5, examines the destructive effects of war and the devastating social and mental health consequences. Participating in or being exposed to military conflict exacerbates existing mental health problems and creates new ones. Harding identifies the changing face of war globally, the "new war" characterized by unconventional methods and asymmetrical warfare and the significant impact that it has had on nations, communities and individuals across the globe. He notes that there is a paucity of literature on the mental health sequelae to people who are in the midst of armed conflicts; most research focuses upon those displaced to refugee camps. Among U.S. veterans of recent wars, high levels of post-traumatic stress disorder (PTSD), depression, substance abuse and other mental health problems linked to exposure to combat have been found. The individual and family visible and invisible scars of war are evident in rising suicide rates among active duty military personnel as well as veterans.

Professor Wise, in Chapter 6, examines the association between homelessness and mental health conditions. The loss of one's living place is often precipitated by chronic mental illness and/or significant traumatic events such as loss of employment, natural or person initiated disasters, escape from a domestic violence circumstance, or a combination of simultaneously occurring life transitions and traumatic events. The author differentiates the chronically, situationally and episodically homeless, and insightfully examines the bidirectional associations among complicated conditions such as trauma, trauma responses to homelessness and mental health conditions.

In Chapter 7, Professor Alexander cites a study that estimates that 56 percent of state prisoners, 45 percent of federal prisoners, and 64 percent of jail detainees have mental health problems. Similarly, data show high numbers of incarcerated juveniles with significant mental health issues. Clearly, a certain percentage of adult and youth prisoners enter the correctional system with mental health problems. Certainly, prison life exacerbates their mental health conditions. The cumulative stress associated with confinement, violence, and lack of treatment makes worse their original condition and creates new mental problems. It is important to note that race is a critical factor in imprisonment. African American males are incarcerated at 6.6 times the rate for White males.

In Chapter 8, Professors Acevedo and González discuss the profound mental health consequences of the dislocation of "place" that immigration involves. Historically, immigration is associated with social problems, such as poverty, racial and ethnic conflict, and disenfranchisement. The profession of social work plays a critical function with the social problems and the personal, familial, and community instabilities and that are associated with immigration.

In Chapter 9, Professor Knight explores the mental health effects of childhood victimization and maltreatment. In many social work settings such as addictions, domestic violence and mental health, the majority of clients have experienced some sort of victimization in childhood. Childhood and adolescent victimization and maltreatment have serious and long-lasting consequences, particularly if sexual victimization is involved. The consequences include: mental conditions such as post-traumatic stress, depression, anxiety, dissociative identity, borderline personality, and substance abuse.

Professor Carlson, in Chapter 10, identifies a broad range of mental health symptoms and problems that have been identified as a consequence of physical, emotional, and sexual abuse, including depression, PTSD, other forms of anxiety, and substance abuse. Intimate partner violence consists of "physical violence, sexual abuse or assault, and emotional or psychological abuse that is perpetrated by partners or acquaintances, including current or former spouses, cohabiting partners, boyfriends or girlfriends, and dating partners." The devastating consequences of intimate partner violence is evident in the fact that more than half of abused women meet the diagnostic criteria for at least one mental health condition.

Community violence occurs in various settings, such as neighborhoods, streets, schools, other local institutions, stores, and playgrounds. In Chapter 11, Ms. Vorhies and Professors Guterman and Haj-Yahia offer a profound insight: "witnessing community violence or simply hearing about community violence occurring has been linked to just as serious negative mental health outcomes as direct exposure through victimization or perpetration." While youth aged 18 and younger represent approximately 25 percent of the U.S. population, they account for approximately 50 percent of the witnesses and victims of violent acts. Annually, 75 percent of African American and Latino youth are exposed to school violence and 50 percent to community violence. The authors explore the consequences of exposure to community violence.

In Part II, leading social work experts present the state of interdisciplinary knowledge and wisdom about the myriad effects and challenges of a range of mental health conditions faced by individuals and their families. The mental health conditions presented are the autism spectrum conditions; executive function conditions and self-deficits; oppositional defiant and conduct conditions; mood conditions; anxiety conditions; eating conditions; personality conditions; psychotic conditions; substance abuse; and dementia and related problems in cognition and memory. The relevant issues in helping people with mental health conditions are framed within the context of biopsychosocial and life-modeled approaches, and life course framework. In Part II, the authors also follow a common outline to organize their respective mental health conditions and associated life challenges.

The authors begin by offering political and theoretical definitions and explanations of the mental health condition and their effects on service providers and service users. An examination of the demographics, incidence and prevalence rates of the mental health condition follow the definitional analyses. Subsequently, the authors examine the developmental course and respective challenges for generational cohorts posed by the mental health condition. The assessment and diagnostic patterns and different access to mental health services according to gender, race, ethnicity, life course, sexual orientation and ability/disability are also explored.

Next the authors discuss social work programs and services: their availability, evidence of effectiveness, and the roles played by social workers. More specifically, the contributors describe and illustrate responsive professional methods and interventions. The authors conclude with an examination of social work contributions and the importance of social work involvement with the identified population. Each chapter ends with boxed texts consisting of web resources.

In Chapter 12, Professors Walsh and Corcoran discuss the severe and persistent impairments associated with the spectrum of autism. Several areas of development are reciprocally affected, including social interaction, communication skills, and a stereotypical, repetitive range of ritualized behaviors. These children demonstrate a lack of awareness of the feelings of others, a limited ability to imitate and express emotion, and to participate in social and symbolic play. Approximately 60 to 70 percent of persons dealing with autism suffer from distinct neurological abnormalities and various levels of mental retardation. The authors present creative assessment tools and evidenced-based interventions.

Professor Palombo, in Chapter 13, discusses executive function conditions and self-deficits, presents recent developments in the neurosciences and integrates them into social work practice. Certain individuals suffer from a disorganization, which interferes with their ability to successfully complete the tasks they undertake. Initiating steps to implement plans and managing time to organize resources to self-monitor and to self-regulate their actions creates complex challenges. The author discusses and illustrates distinctive assessments and interventions, which are responsive to clients with neuropsychological impairments.

In Chapter 14, Ms. Barczyk and Professor Springer focus on children who suffer from oppositional defiant and conduct conditions. These mental health conditions display similar characteristics such as breaking of societal norms, disruptive behavior, and disobedient behavior. This chapter provides an overview of these conditions, and examines the social worker's role in working with youth with these problems. Evidenced-based practices that have been utilized to help these youth, including videotape modeling parent program, problem-solving skills training, parent management training, functional family therapy, and family behavior therapy are presented and illustrated.

Professor Smith, in Chapter 15, discusses mood conditions, the leading cause of disability among people aged 15–44. The author's perspective is that the etiology of depression is complex and multi-determined. It exists on a continuum, merging from factors within the person (endogenous), as well as from the external environment (reactive). Psychological, social, environmental, and biological factors reciprocally influence one another. Significant disparities exist in terms of both accurate diagnosis and access to appropriate mental health services.

Professors Heller and Werkmeister Rozas, in Chapter 16, examine the full range of anxiety conditions which cause great distress and impaired functioning in people across the life course. They stress the importance of understanding the evolutionary history of adaptive anxiety as a means of self-preservation while understanding the multiple biological, social and cultural influences which exacerbate and mediate the experience of maladaptive anxiety. They pay particular attention to the culture bound syndromes, typically overlooked, and overrepresented among the anxiety conditions. The authors provide full discussion of the bidirectional relationship between the influences of race, ethnicity and culture with the differential manifestations and responses to anxiety. They stress the importance of cultural competency for social workers in order to understand both the meanings and functions of anxiety symptoms to both the client and their respective culture.

Dr. Bodenheimer and Professor Heller, in Chapter 17, discuss eating conditions, anorexia nervosa, bulimia nervosa, binge eating disorder, and obesity related conditions. These perplexing conditions in which physiological changes interact with social, cultural, and psychological factors are both psychiatric and social problems, and increasingly, a public health problem. Given the ample evidence that sociocultural influences are significant in the development of eating conditions and that each generational cohort appears to be at greater risk, preventive strategies are critical, social work plays a critical function with people with eating conditions.

In Chapter 18, Professor Northcut astutely describes the multiple factors that predispose, influence, create, trigger and maintain consistently rigidly dysfunctional behavior associated with personality conditions. The author cautions that people suffering from a personality disorder tend to be difficult to engage in a helping relationship. The very nature of the diagnosis requires the personality condition be of lengthy duration, pervasive in scope and rigidity of style, which "interferes with seeking out and staying with any form of treatment." The author discusses and illustrates responsive approaches that pay equal attention to intra-psychic, interpersonal and environmental forces.

In Chapter 19, Professor Lukens and Ms. Ogden present a comprehensive overview of psychotic conditions, and promising, empirically based practices for persons diagnosed with the most severe forms of psychosis. The authors examine the complex hurdles that the psychotic conditions present for persons with illness, for their families and other informal caregivers, as well as for mental health providers and policy makers. The roles for social workers in building, implementing, and advocating for recovery-oriented programs are explicated and illustrated.

Professor Hanson, in Chapter 20, views substance abuse as a biopsychosocial condition in which "personal lifestyle factors, physiological conditions, social structural arrangements and cultural practices may contribute to the emergence and development of substance abuse." Clients with other mental health conditions are likely to experience difficulties associated with the use of alcohol and other drugs. The author perceptively emphasizes that social work's ecosystem's multidimensional person-environment perspective uniquely positions the profession to be responsive to the forces that trigger the development of substance abuse and help persons suffering from its consequences.

The progression of dementia has a devastating impact on the individual, family and caregivers. Over time, the person becomes an empty shell. A sense of hopelessness and helplessness overwhelms as one observes this "disease dissolve the past memories, present lives, and future dreams." In Chapter 21, Professor Sanders and Ms. Osterhaus poignantly describe the impact of dementia on the individual and caretakers, and the diverse roles social workers assume with these clients and their significant social networks.

Our contributors present contemporary theoretical perspectives, empirical findings, and most effective social work programs and practices. Historically, the social work profession has been the primary social service provider to people (and their support networks) dealing with mental health conditions. In the current social context, providing social work services has become significantly more difficult to fulfill. For the stubborn truth is that problems have been increasing, while resources to mitigate them decrease. In our opinion, the social work profession has made heroic efforts to provide quality social work services. Through descriptions of responsive social programs and social work's contributions to them and presentation and discussion of practice illustrations, this book attempts to capture the profession's resilience and creativity.

Acknowledgements

We wish to express our appreciation to the authors for their outstanding contributions to this book, each reflecting clarity of presentation and mastery of the material.

We are very grateful to our faculty and administrative colleagues and to the support staff for making the University of Connecticut School of Social Work a special work environment. The support of our colleagues, their commitment to teaching and service and to the development and dissemination of knowledge, provide us with an exciting professional home.

Our masters and doctoral students remind us every day that to teach is to learn twice over. They are our master teachers and we write with them in mind.

We acknowledge our respective spouses, children and grandchildren. They provide richness and meaning in our lives.

Finally, we acknowledge each other. Editing this book has been a wonderful intellectual journey. We have shared ideas, explored ideas and argued ideas. Through this process, we have both grown and developed a special friendship.

Nina and Alex

1 Introduction to social problems and mental health/illness

Nina Rovinelli Heller and Alex Gitterman

The social work profession has a dual mission: "to enhance human well being and help meet the basic human needs of all people, with particular attention to the needs and empowerment of people who are vulnerable, oppressed, and living in poverty" (National Association of Social Workers (NASW), 2008). Individuals who struggle with ongoing mental health issues experience challenges in all spheres of functioning, on a daily basis. Daily life stressors and struggles can generate cumulative and chronic stress. In accordance with our profession's mission, social work practitioners help clients to restore their optimal levels of overall functioning in various domains. Because a wide range of social and personal conditions and influences promote or mitigate mental health and illness, social workers must have a clear appreciation of the power of these social and personal conditions and influences. Social work practice theory emphasizes the importance of understanding the complex relationships between people and their environments and this represents one of the distinguishing features of our profession. One of the first ecologically based practice models, the Life Model of Social Work Practice (Germain & Gitterman, 1980) provides a theoretical and practice framework for understanding the transactional and bidirectional relationships between social and personal problems and mental health and illness. The model rests upon several key concepts, including the reciprocity of person-environment exchanges; adaptedness and adaptation; human habitat and niches; vulnerability, oppression and misuse of power; social and technological pollution; the life course conception of unique pathways in human development; the importance of considerations of historical, social and individual time; life stressors and related coping tasks; resilience; the interdependence of all phenomena and ecological feminism (Gitterman & Germain, 2008, pp. 1–2). These concepts are central to our understanding of the importance of a dual perspective when assessing individual and social vulnerabilities and resiliencies, while understanding the transactional effects of living in the world with a mental health condition.

This model serves us particularly well today. Our knowledge base regarding mental health has grown exponentially since the 1980s. As we understand more about the biological determinants (genetics, brain structures and functions) of many mental health conditions we are better positioned to develop preventive and remedial strategies that can ameliorate the suffering of our clients and their families. However, there are necessary cautions in our use of this knowledge; we risk making our understanding of the human condition of mental illness unidimensional. The social work profession's strength in bringing together the understanding of biopsychosocial factors and *their relationships to each other* is critically important. We are increasingly familiar with the biological determinants of mental conditions and social workers with expertise in mental health have long contributed their understanding of psychological and environmental factors. Likewise, all social workers including micro and macro practitioners are aware of the impact of social forces and influences on our clients, their families and communities.

However, in many undergraduate and graduate schools of social work, we continue to teach mental health content as separate from other social work content, particularly from macro social issues. While we no longer tend to call these courses "Psychopathology" or "Abnormal Psychology for Social Workers," the content is tilted toward the psychological and increasingly toward the biological. Lacasse and Gomory (2003), in a survey of what they described as "psychopathology syllabi" from 58 social work schools, found a nearly exclusive focus on biological psychiatry. Fortunately, we are beginning to include more content on mental health care disparities as we begin to identify that mental health issues both affect and manifest differently among various ethnic and racial groups. While this is an important advance, we think all of the historical and contemporary social influences and problems that impact the experience of living with a mental illness must be considered.

Hurricane Katrina provides one sobering example of the importance of understanding the importance and utility of this bidirectionality between social problems and mental health conditions. We are all familiar with the difficulties in the FEMA (Federal Emergency Management Agency) response to the hurricane victims, particularly those who lacked the economic resources to flee the city before the hurricane or to resettle quickly afterwards. Many of the victims initially "housed" at the Civic Center were residents of the Ninth Ward, a predominantly African American neighborhood. While we tend to believe that natural disasters affect people without regard to race or class, this is not so (Prilleltensky, 2003). Nor is this a new observation; Spriggs (2006) reminds us of the *Titanic*, where discrepant safety planning resulted in lifeboats for first class passengers and none for those in steerage. In the case of Hurricane Katrina, Voorhees, Vick, and Perkins (2007) note that,

> it was poverty which primarily determined who lived in the most vulnerable, low-lying neighborhoods (that flooded first and emptied last), who was uninsured, who was unable to escape the storm and flood (and thus who lived and died), who had fewer choices in relocating, and who did not have the resources to return and rebuild.
>
> (Voorhees et al., 2007, p. 417)

Logan (2006) reported that indeed, preexisting disparities of race and class existed; the damaged areas were 45.8 percent African American and 29.9 percent lived under the poverty line. These represent much higher percentages than those living in the nearby, undamaged areas. These disparities put this vulnerable population at further heightened risk for many deleterious personal and social outcomes, one of which may be the mental health sequelae in the post-natural disaster period. The very issues, which place a person at greater risk for developing a particular mental condition, affect the course, outcome and experience of the illness.

In one of the first comprehensive studies of indicators of mental health conditions among the hurricane survivors, Kessler et al. (2008) used existing baseline date (pre-hurricane) from the National Comorbidity Survey Replication Study (NCRS) and did follow-up studies with survivors at 5–8 months post-hurricane and again a year later. They found that during that time, post-traumatic stress disorder (PTSD), serious mental illness, suicidal ideation, and suicide plans all increased significantly in the one-year interval. This finding is in contrast to prior ones related to natural disasters, in which post-disaster mental health problems tend to decrease with time. While the initial results suggested that adverse effects were weakly related to socio-demographic variables, one variable, low family income, consistently and significantly predicted increased prevalence of severe mental illness, PTSD and suicidal ideation. These results may not fully reflect the disparities in the incidence of post-Katrina mental health conditions because the authors note that the original (pre-hurricane) survey may have left the most marginalized segments of the population underrepresented (for example those who were unreachable by phone). Clearly, experiencing the effects of a natural disaster is not good for anyone; however, we do know that certain disadvantaged populations are at higher risk for the disaster itself, and hence for the complicated after effects. The social work response to the incidence of mental health problems in this population must consider interventions at all levels, in addition to the direct practice provisions of a range of mental health interventions and services. At the same time, we need to pay attention to the social issues and inequities, which create, promote and maintain elevated risk for a number of variables.

Consider the following practice example:

Jonya is a 16-year-old African American female who presented to a community health clinic in Houston. She was a resident of the Ninth Ward in New Orleans when Hurricane Katrina struck. She was home alone at the time of the storm; though she heard warnings to evacuate, her boyfriend told her "it would be fine." She had lived there with her mother, who was at the time tending to her own mother, who had recently been admitted to a nursing home in the next county. After spending seven days in the Civic Center without sufficient food or water, she was evacuated to Houston. She had no contact with her family during this time; when she left New Orleans she did not know whether her mother, grandmother or boyfriend had survived. Once in Houston, she lived in a makeshift shelter where her already precarious mental health deteriorated. By the time she came to the clinic, she had not spoken in several weeks. She sat quietly in the office. The social worker sat with her. She nodded her agreement, however, to come back in the following day. Over the course of the next several sessions, during which she mostly sat silent, she began to report that she was having nightmares daily and even at times when "I don't even think I was asleep." She also reported that prior to the disaster, she had been seeing a counselor at the public clinic, because her mother was concerned that she continually washed her hands (often until they bled), worried about germs, and frequently complained that she was dying and that "people were after me." These symptoms had begun six months prior to the hurricane and her mother had voiced her concerns that "you are just like your paternal grandmother; she was crazy and had to go away – no one ever saw her again." When Jonya began to talk about her experience in the immediate aftermath of the hurricane, she surprised the social worker by going on a tirade about the "black people" behaving so badly. When the social worker asked her to elaborate, Jonya described the media images and commentary that she saw on the television at the shelter. Like much of the rest of the country, she saw images of black men who were described as "looting" stores alongside images of white people, described as "securing supplies" (Voorhees et al., 2007). In her vulnerable state, Jonya began to internalize the racism inherent in that news commentary and began to express shame about herself and the people in her community. This resulted in a strong resistance to accepting any of the concrete services, which she badly needed. She then added that she "didn't like" the Civic Center and began to talk about having felt very vulnerable and frightened there – "It was dirty; I'll never be clean again."

If we consider only the "facts" of symptoms, we might conclude that Jonya has a preexisting condition, which has been exacerbated by her ordeal. We might consider a panic disorder, obsessive compulsive disorder, post-traumatic stress disorder, selective mutism. We would also note that there was a possibility of the history of schizophrenia or another psychotic condition on the paternal side (grandmother was "crazy", sent away, and never to be seen again). However, we would also need to consider Jonya in terms of her developmental stage, her gender, her race, the stigma her mother associated with her grandmother's psychiatric history, her lack of financial resources, the trauma of the disaster, her vulnerability to internalized racism, and the revictimizing experience of the delayed federal response to the disaster. We would also note that in spite of all of this, by the second or third session, Jonya was able to confide in the worker, accept services and begin to put together a coherent narrative of her harrowing experience. While Jonya might well need additional interventions, including medication evaluation, the ecological perspective and life modeled practice remind us of the interdependence of many factors as well as the resiliency of human beings under acute stress.

The experience of Hurricane Katrina is extreme but illustrates the "perfect storm" of natural, personal, social and political phenomena. We are also increasingly aware of the deleterious and complex effects of war, poverty, immigration status, oppression, racism, sexism, and all forms of violence, upon the well-being of individuals, families and communities. These pernicious influences disproportionately affect the most vulnerable (by temperament, health status or social status) among us.

Social workers tend to emphasize either the "mental health" side or the "social problems/ social justice" side of the equation. However, in doing so, we lose a great deal, the profession loses, and most importantly, our clients lose. We risk losing our appreciation of the complexity of the human condition and the ways in which the environment and social forces have the capacity to either ameliorate or advance an individual's experience with mental health and illness. We also risk assigning blame to individuals for their struggles, without considering the impact of pervasive damaging social influences. This book is a realization of our attempts to bring together both sides of our social work mission as it is reflected in our knowledge base, our practice skills and our professional values. As social workers we carry a responsibility and charge to attend to people who are suffering, triumphing, and living with both the multiple effects of mental illness and the social problems, which influence them.

Social workers and mental health

In 1985, the *New York Times* reported that there was a "quiet revolution" in the provision of therapeutic mental health services with "social workers vaulting into a leading role" (Goleman, 1985, p. 1). Today, social workers are the primary providers of mental health services for individuals with some of the most stigmatized mental illnesses (Newhill & Korr, 2004; Substance Abuse and Mental Health Services Administration, 2001, 2006). This trend has been fueled by several factors. First, social workers are now licensed, registered and/or regulated in all 50 states. This has made us eligible for third party payments through both agency and private practices. Second, the landscape has dramatically shifted for psychiatry. As our knowledge about brain based diseases of mental illness has increased, along with technological advances that allow us to "see" organic and structural changes in the brains of people with certain psychiatric conditions, the role of the psychiatrist has changed. Psychiatrists, the former primary providers of "talk therapies," have increasingly focused on biology and the roles of medication in the amelioration of psychiatric symptoms. The norm now in mental health agencies is for psychiatrists to be employed part time or on a fee for service basis, taking referrals from non-medical colleagues for medication evaluation for agency clients. Second, the utilization of mental health services increased significantly between 1994, the time of the first National Comorbidity Survey Study and the NCS-Revised, ten years later; the twelve-month utilization of services was 17 percent of the U.S. population, resulting in increased demand for additional mental health practitioners. Third, there has been an increased focus on the mental health needs of children and adolescents, a population long served by social workers in a variety of settings. Finally, the social work profession has responded to these workforce needs. Whitaker, Wilson, and Arrington (2008) in a survey of NASW members found that 37 percent worked in mental health, more than in any other single field of practice. Similarly, in a study of the NASW workforce (Center for Health Workforce Studies (CHWS), 2006) researchers surveyed national NASW members who hold state licensure (94 percent of NASW members hold licensure). They reported that of this group (BSWs and MSWs, i.e., bachelor and master's degrees in social work) 40 percent reported behavioral health as their practice area. Of that group, 37 percent identified practicing in the area of mental health, 3 percent in addictions. In the study, employment in mental health was highly correlated with the graduate degree, only 4 percent of the behavioral health social workers held only the bachelor's degree. Fully 20 percent of licensed MSWs who worked in mental health also held a license in addictions. Contrary to a perceived trend, greater numbers of social workers graduating before 1980 worked in mental health than more recent graduates (CHWS, 2006).

At the same time, social workers (and the profession) are committed to issues of social justice and diversity. Courtney and Specht in their book *Unfaithful angels: How social work has abandoned its mission* (1992) warned that the increasing identification of social workers as therapists represents an abandonment of the central social work mission. Scheyett (2005), on the other hand, argues that social workers, because we are strong advocates for social justice and equality, are particularly well suited to work with the mentally ill and to address the prejudices, which affect them. Scheyett (2005) reports that in a study of mental health social workers, she found that these social workers were clearly aware of the contemporary issues, which affected their ability to be helpful to their clients. Over half of the mental health social workers identified waiting lists for services (57 percent), increases in client eligibility requirements for services (55 percent) and decreases in services eligible for funding (53 percent) as the most significant changes in the service delivery system for their clients. One can safely assume that the recession of 2009 and subsequent federal, state and local social service budget cuts, combined with increasing need, have exacerbated these problems in the provision of services, particularly given that in 2004, 38 percent of mental health clients were Medicaid and Medicare recipients (NASW, 2008).

However, the results of a recent study raise some troubling issues about this practice area. Eack and Newhill (2008) surveyed 2,000 National Association of Social Work members about their experiences and attitudes about working with people with severe and persistent mental illness (SPMI). Previous research has consistently documented that working with people with severe and persistent mental illness is challenging (Acker, 1999; Mason et al., 2004; Reid et al., 1999), which is not surprising to practitioners. In support of their first hypothesis, they found that the frustrations that social workers experience with clients with severe and persistent mental illness would influence their attitudes toward them. However, their subsequent findings were both unexpected and disturbing. They found that social workers' attitudes toward these clients were primarily influenced by their frustrations with the clients' behaviors and treatment issues. This finding is in contrast to earlier research, which suggests that social workers' attitudes toward these clients were influenced primarily by frustrations with system-related issues (Eack & Newhill, 2008). The researchers concluded that an increased reliance upon a strength based perspective in the work with people with persistent and severe mental illness can reduce the frustrations and burnout of social workers, resulting in a reduction of large staff turnover rates in community mental health centers.

Equally troubling has been the shift toward managed care in the health and mental health care delivery systems. Managed care was initially designed as a means of controlling spiraling health care costs by placing limits on covered services and access to those services. However, in spite of requiring increasing copayments and imposing high deductibles, health care costs have continued to soar. More importantly, attention to the "bottom line" has resulted in care that is often driven by cost containment rather than by the needs of clients. Therefore, preference is given to brief models of mental health intervention and acute symptom relief with little attention to the long term and environmental factors, which may exacerbate a medical or mental health condition.

The situation is particularly dire in the provision of mental health services. When clients in an acute episode of schizophrenia for example, require hospitalization for safety and medication adjustment, only several days may be authorized. In some cases, a new medication will be tried but the client discharged before it is clear whether the medication is either effective or tolerated. Social workers experience pressures to conform to the "preferred" treatment interventions of the managed care company, risking serious sanctions for nonconformance, such as being denied "panel" status or being refused referrals. This creates disturbing dilemmas and conflicts for social workers in all mental health settings (Davidson & Davidson, 1996; Furman & Langer, 2006; Reamer, 1997). Schamess (1998, p. 24) frames the dilemma for our profession: that minimizing costs and maximizing profit impose corporate values and ideology on health and mental health agencies. These values and ideology radically differ from social welfare's commitment to human rights and provision of safety nets and buffers to our capitalist system. Furthermore, the outcome of the 2010 national health care legislation debate will have a significant impact on our clients' access to mental health care services and on the quality of those services.

Definitions of mental health, mental illness and recovery

Language matters. In the course of writing and assembling this book, we have had many spirited discussions about how language conveys values and perspectives about the profession, mental health conditions and the people affected by them. Consumers from both the mental health and disabilities movements have made great headway in demanding "person first" language and the social work profession, by and large, has incorporated this important linguistic distinction. While some may dismiss the insistence upon saying "the person with schizophrenia" rather than "the schizophrenic," this is more than a semantic issue. First, people need to have the power to define themselves. Second, all people maintain multiple identities and describing an individual by the name of their "disorder" or "condition" elevates that condition to a primary descriptor, potentially obscuring both the complexity and essence of a human being. While the major consumer advocacy group, the National Association for Mental Illness, continues to use the terminology "mental illness," some social workers prefer the term "condition" to "illness," "disorder" or "disease." While much of the practice literature and virtually all of the research literature use these latter terms, our language should be examined in light of established social work strength, empowerment and ecological perspectives. We have thus chosen to use these terms interchangeably throughout the book, in recognition of both the established nomenclature and of our awareness of the more positive and nuanced connotations associated with more neutral term, "conditions."

Language and labels in mental health can also convey a society's *social constructions, biases* and *etiological assumptions*. Conrad (1980) asserts, "Illness and diseases are human judgments on conditions that exist in the natural world" (p. 105). In this framework, illness is understood as a deviation from social norms, which can and should be "treated" and further that a society's norms and values define what constitutes an illness. For example, until 1974, the psychiatric profession classified homosexuality as a mental illness. This diagnosis was "removed" at that time in response to changing norms and values, which resulted from the gay rights and civil rights movements. That shift is about far more than language and has very real consequences for human beings. If homosexuality is a mental illness, by our shared definitions, both a treatment and a cure are required. And indeed, gay and lesbian people were often subjected to conversion therapies (Bright, 2004) by which a therapist attempted (with minimal success and a great deal of distress) to change the sexual orientation of the client.

The *social construction model* is particularly pertinent when we consider cross-cultural and global trends in "mental illness". Watters (2010) in his book *Crazy like us: The globalization of the American psyche*, documents the rapid spread of our "western symptom repertoire" across the global. Lee and Kleinman (2007) report the massive increase in individuals with eating disorders in Hong Kong and observe: "Culture shapes the way general psychopathology is going to be translated partially or completely into specific psychopathology" (p. 29). When countries import a dominant culture's conceptualization and classification systems of diagnoses and symptoms, people may "choose" to express difficulties and conflicts in ways, which reflect that influence. This may be particularly so for post-traumatic stress disorder, eating disorders, gender identity disorders and other conditions which are particularly influenced by a culture's norms and belief systems. Furthermore, evidence suggests that the course of illness varies by culture. The World Health Organization (WHO, 2007) found in studies spanning 30 years that patients outside the United States and Europe had significantly lower rates of relapse, in spite of the advanced technologies and medicines used to treat these conditions in the West. These data suggest that factors other than medical interventions (perhaps cultural attitudes, traditions, and supports) have the power to positively influence the well-being of persons dealing with a mental health condition.

Language also reflects our *biases and etiological assumptions*. In the 1950s three terms were commonly used in practice and in the research and literature. The first, "schizophreno-genic mother," was applied to the mothers of children suffering with schizophrenia. If we remember our Latin lessons, we understand this to mean, one who creates a schizophrenic. The term is laden with what we now know to be erroneous assumptions. Mothers do not create schizophrenia in their children. In fact, children who are suffering with schizophrenia provide considerable additional challenges to their parents. We now have research that clearly refutes what today seems a ludicrous etiological assumption. However, common sense should have told us the same thing; what would be the possible motivation, conscious or otherwise, for "creating" a schizophrenic child? Similarly, the mothers of children with autism were commonly referred to as "refrigerator mothers." We blamed the mothers for the brain alterations in these children, which manifest in difficulties relating to others and reading social cues, among other things. These kind of skewed etiological assumptions were extended to children with asthma as well, wherein medical problems were ascribed psychological underpinnings. The mothers of these children were commonly referred to as "smothering mothers," the irony of which is not lost on us. When mothers (who continue to be the ones who disproportionately are the ones to access health care services on behalf of their family members) brought their wheezing children to emergency rooms, they were indeed, frantic – and it's a good thing they were. In some cases, that "franticness" saved their children's lives. These mothers were "smothering" – if we can even call it that – in response to a life-threatening event; they were not the cause of that event.

The similarities among these examples are self-evident and lend themselves well to a social construction perspective for how we think about causality, psychiatric conditions and gender. In each of these examples, mothers were the common denominator. However, to fully understand how this came to be, we must understand the era in which this occurred. After World War II, women, who had both enjoyed and endured the changing roles of women in response to the needs of the nation at war, were thrust out of the workplace in order to make room for returning male veterans. Women found themselves with more constricted gender roles in relation to the family. Paradoxically, they were seen as increasingly powerful influences on their children and their mental health and functioning. As women's roles have shifted yet again, as fathers assume slowly increasing roles in the care of our children, and as we look beyond the effects of parental influence in the genesis of mental health conditions, the "mother-blaming" shifted somewhat. In fact, when we initially became aware of family systems theory, some of us acted as if the family was a closed system responsible for creating and maintaining individual disturbance such as schizophrenia and learning disability. By limiting ourselves to internal family transactions, we dismissed genetic and environmental forces, judging and blaming parents and exacerbating their stress. We progressed from blaming the cold, detached mother to blaming both parents for their double binds and ambiguous communications.

Language itself is generally embedded in culture and the western description of mental health conditions is a medicalized one. Today, the *Diagnostic and statistical manual of mental disorders* (DSM-IV-TR) of the American Psychiatric Association (2000) provides the most comprehensive and standardized description of mental health conditions. According to the DSM-IV-TR (APA, 2000), a mental disorder is "a clinically significant behavioral or psychological syndrome or pattern that occurs in an individual and that is associated with present distress . . . or disability . . . or with a significantly increased risk of suffering death, pain, disability or an important loss of freedom" (p. xxi). The manual provides criteria for each category of illness, with a focus upon the presence of particular symptoms and the degree of dysfunction associated with them. Since the advent of licensure and third party insurance payments for social work services, the social work profession has had an uneasy relationship with the DSM (Farone, 2002; Kutchins & Kirk, 1989). On the one hand, agencies and individuals depend upon insurance reimbursement, which is predicated on standardized diagnosis codes and procedural codes. These diagnostic codes are required not only by private insurance companies, but also by public programs such as Medicaid and Medicare. This practice creates problems for social workers and special challenges for social work educators. While we teach students the importance of multidimensional assessment which reflects our understanding of an ecological perspective, these same students, placed in the field, must often submit a diagnosis code on the basis of a first intake meeting with a client, in order that the agency be reimbursed for their time.

The DSM is now in its fourth incarnation and plans are in place for the fifth edition. Historically, primarily psychiatrists, with some input from psychologists and less from social workers developed the manual. The system relies on taskforce work groups who review the recent literature and survey psychiatrists. Many social workers view this process as seriously flawed and exclusionary (Kutchins & Kirk, 1989). Recent editions of the manual reflect an increasing, but insufficient attention to widening the focus of assessment by using a multiaxial diagnosis system. In addition to the first three axes which record psychiatric and medical conditions, Axis 4 assesses psychosocial stressors and Axis 5 uses a Global Assessment of Functioning Score to indicate the degree to which a client's symptoms impairs their social and occupational functioning. In practice however, these latter two axes are often not used, as they are not necessary for reimbursement. In response to concerns about the lack of attention to cultural factors, the DSM-IV-TR (2000) included an outline for cultural formulation. However, the outline was relegated to an appendix in the back of the volume and is rarely used. Interestingly, the process for a fifth edition of the manual has been opened to a wider group of stakeholders. A website has been established which lists proposed changes and the rationales for the inclusion and exclusion of various diagnoses. Practitioners from all disciplines, researchers, and people with mental health conditions and their families, were encouraged to submit via this website, their comments about the proposed changes. This process reflects a significant shift in devising the new edition but the degree to which practitioner and consumer input will influence the content of the book is as yet, unclear.

The uneasy alliance between the use of the DSM and social work has been well documented (Kirk & Kutchins, 1995; Kutchins & Kirk, 1989). Critics share concerns that use of the manual promotes labeling, substitutes social flaws with individual pathology and essentially ignores the issues of gender, social and socioeconomic factors, including culture (Bentley, 2005; López & Guarnaccia, 2005). Kirk and Kutchins (1992) went as far as to assert that the DSM is an instrument of social control, rather than a client focused aid and challenge both its validity and reliability. Kirk (2005) asserted that the DSM has led to an overreliance on psychotropic medications to sedate people rather than to address compelling social problems. Frazer et al. (2009) sampled the National Association of Social Worker's Register of Clinical Social Workers to identify why social workers use the DSM-IV; how important social workers rank the reasons for their use of it for diagnosing; and how often social workers would use it if they didn't have to. Like Kutchins and Kirk (1988) before them, they found that insurance reimbursement was the primary motivator for use of the manual. However, Frazer et al. (2009) also found that 50 percent of their sample reported that they would continue to use the manual, even if they were not required to do so and that this position held for social workers employed in both agency and private practice settings. Those social workers reported that they found the DSM-IV a useful means of assessing clients. Frazer et al. (2009) conclude with the suggestions that students be taught about the use of the DSM-IV as a *part* of assessment and about the inherent flaws and limitations of both the system itself and our overreliance upon it. They also suggest that advocacy with insurance companies regarding means for reimbursement would be helpful. These are issues that social workers can also address, particularly through legislative processes related to health care reform.

Because DSM criteria for diagnoses are so widely used, some would say entrenched, at all levels of the mental health delivery system, they are often considered to be the "truth." Most social workers suggest caution about the scope and overreliance upon the manual. However, others acknowledge that the classification system does provide a "common language" for practitioners across disciplines. For example, if a social worker refers a client suffering with paranoid schizophrenia to another worker, there will be some shared agreement about that condition and associated symptoms and vulnerabilities. The diagnosis will not convey to the worker anything about the manifestation of that condition in a particular individual or anything about the clients' strengths or transactions with family, community, or other dimensions of the environment. Clearly, the DSM cannot be a standalone assessment tool (Frazer et al., 2009). In the research community, having this shared agreement about the general characteristics of a condition is useful. If a researcher is studying the effects of a cognitive-behavioral intervention with persons with panic disorder, for example, the practitioner who relies on intervention research will understand what the researcher means by panic disorder, specifically, and will know that the findings are not generalizable to other related but distinct anxiety conditions. Overall, the DSM, with its significant shortcomings, should not "drive" social work interventions with people with mental health conditions.

Not surprisingly, a library search for definitions of mental illness produces exponentially more "hits" than a search on definitions of mental health. This reality in itself underscores our awareness of the orientation toward disease rather than wellness held by many of the professions. As maligned as Freud has become by many since the early 1980s, he is said to have believed that adult mental health could be measured by the "ability to love and work." That definition holds well now, nearly a century later. The World Health Organization asserts that,

> Mental health can be conceptualized as a state of well-being in which the individual realizes his or her own abilities, can cope with the normal stresses of life, can work productively and fruitfully, and is able to make a contribution to his or her community.
>
> (WHO, 2007)

From the WHO's constitution: "Health is a state of completed physical, mental and social well-being and not merely the absence of disease or infirmity."

Definitions of *recovery* focus upon the pathways from illness to health. White, Boyle, and Loveland (2005) write:

> recovery from mental illness must be defined as a complex, dynamic and enduring process rather than a biological end-state described by an absence of symptoms . . . Recovery is, in its essence, a lived experience of moving through and beyond the limits of one's disorder.
>
> (White et al., 2005, p. 235)

In their comprehensive view of the literature, they highlight several other characteristics of a recovery perspective: individuals must recover from illness, stigma, and at times, the iatrogenic effects of treatment (Spaniol, Gagne & Koehler, 2003); recovery exists on a continuum; there is a necessary balance between recovery debits and recovery capital (Granfield & Cloud, 1999); and there are many varieties of recovery experience. White (1996) identifies different styles of recovery: *acultural* whereby an individual has no affiliation with a community of others with similar struggles, *bicultural* whereby an individual affiliates with those within and without the community; and *culturally enmeshed styles of recovery*, wherein a person is totally immersed in a culture of recovery. Individuals in recovery may also experience critical developmental points, which heighten the likelihood of entry or acceleration into recovery (Young & Ensing, 1999). Additionally, families of persons with mental health conditions must also struggle with and adapt to both incremental and cumulative changes related to the recovery process of their loved one (Spaniol & Zipple, 1994). These principles are congruent with the best of our social work traditions; the importance of the individual: environment transactions and fit; client self-determination, and the importance of mutual aid supports. In recovery focused mental health practice, the client, rather than the worker or the intervention, may well be considered the central change agent. This is a powerful reformulating of recovery.

Demographics

The scope of mental illness nationally is staggering and can be understood through *statistics, role disability, financial burden of disease*, and notably, by the face of both *human suffering and resiliency*. The National Comorbidity Survey Replication Study (NCS-R) provides comprehensive statistics on the prevalence, severity and comorbidity (the occurrence of two or more diagnoses in an individual) of mental illness in the United States. Kessler, Chiu, Demler and Walters (2005) reported that 26.2 percent of Americans aged 18 and older suffer from a diagnosable mental disorder in a given year, which translates to nearly 60 million people. This figure pertains to the occurrence of diagnoses with various severity; they clarify that 6 percent of the population suffers from serious mental illness. However, nearly half of those with any mental health condition suffer from a second or more. These figures do not apply for children or early or middle stage adolescents, a growing subgroup of those experiencing psychiatric difficulties. By and large, the most prevalent diagnoses among the adult population are the mood conditions, which are strongly comorbid with anxiety disorders and substance abuse. Of the depressive disorders, major depression is the most prevalent and occurs nearly double the rate in women as in men (Kessler et al., 2003). Schizophrenia affects 2.4 million adults in a given year (1.1 percent of the population) (Regier et al., 1993). Anxiety disorders affect 40 million adults (18.1 percent), also have high rates of comorbidity, often with other anxiety disorders and have earlier ages of onset (Kessler et al., 2005). There has been greater attention to the incidence of post-traumatic stress disorder in the past several decades and this affects 7.7 million adults (3.5

percent) (Kessler et al., 2003). Some groups are at significantly higher risk; 19 percent of Vietnam veterans suffer PTSD at some point after serving (Dohrenwend et al., 2007).

The numbers are particularly troubling in regard to children and adolescents. The National Health and Nutrition Examination Survey (NHANES), a collaboration between the National Institute of Mental Health (NIMH) and the National Center for Health Statistics at the Centers for Disease Control (CDC), studied children ages 8–15. Thirteen percent of subjects met criteria for one of the following six disorders: attention deficit hyperactivity disorder, depression, conduct disorder, anxiety disorder or eating disorders (NIMH). Importantly, Kessler et al. (2005) found that half of all lifetime cases of mental illness begin by age 14, and three-quarters by age 24. These numbers raise critical questions about diagnosing patterns and trends, the possibility of the medicalization of normal childhood behaviors and the dramatic increase in use of psychotropic medication for children, even preschoolers.

The examination of *role disability* provides a much more nuanced understanding of both the individual and communal effects of psychiatric conditions. Merikangas et al. (2007) reported that 53 percent of adults in the United States have a mental or physical condition which interferes with either their attendance at work or conducting their usual activities for several days per year. Of that group, each experienced an average of 32 days of disability per year. Major depression was second among all conditions in disability days, at 387 million. Any of us who work with clients whose level of depression is this debilitating, understand the human costs of being unable to function as usual. While these data provide a clear picture of the economic impact of role disability, they do not reflect the personal and relational impact. For example, people with major depression are going to experience role disability in their roles as mothers and fathers, partner, relative and friend clearly affecting the well-being of families on both acute and chronic bases.

In terms of the *financial burden of disease*, Kessler et al. (2008) report that major depressive and anxiety disorders (those defined as disorders which have seriously impaired the person's ability to function for at least 30 days in the previous year) cost the nation nearly $200 billion in lost earnings. The costs are actually much higher, as the study did not include people with conditions such as schizophrenia and autism. Indirect costs, less easily computed, are also high and include the costs of treating these conditions and of providing Social Security payments for the disabled population. People are often incarcerated or are homeless as direct or indirect consequences of having a mental condition; these situations carry high financial and social costs to the nation as well. Kessler et al. (2008) also reported that there was a calculable effect on individual wage earners as well; those with serious mental illness (SMI), as defined in the study reported incomes significantly lower than those without SMI, sufficient enough to propel some individuals and families into poverty.

There is also a *human face* to the challenges and triumphs of living with a chronic mental health condition. A 37-year-old woman, Ruth, a social worker, took very seriously her professional mandate to confront social problems and injustices. In the midst of the 2009 national recession and massive budget cuts to social service and mental health agencies, she addressed a committee of a west coast state legislature. She spoke as a social worker and as a mental health consumer:

My prognosis about 15 years ago was that I would end up in a state hospital for the rest of my life. I had been in psychiatric hospitals at least six times between the ages of 12 and 19. I was in and out of short-term and long-term residential placements, partial hospital programs, a special education school and an adult group home. I have multiple psychiatric diagnoses including major depressive disorder and post-traumatic stress disorder.

When I was 12 I became involved with the Department of Mental Health (DMH). DMH provided case management support, access to resources, and continuity in my life. I was lucky to have the same case manager during my time with DMH and she knew me well and could help when it was needed. This connection has remained important throughout my life. It was through my case manager that I became involved with supported education services. Through my worker I was supported through many phases of my life. She provided so much more than meets the eye. It was through her that I was able to access important resources, navigate a daunting system, find funding, utilize state rehabilitation services and apply to schools and the list could go on. I knew I could always count on her support and she remained a guiding force throughout my schooling and beyond. It is with her support and many others that I was able to obtain an Associate's degree, a Bachelor degree in Social Work and an MSW. Without this support, I do not believe I would be where I am today. My experiences working with refugees and my studies with spiritual leaders and others provide me the support to carry on.

I feel truly lucky to have had all the support I have had in my life. I have an amazing psychiatrist and an incredible social worker. I continue to struggle with mental illness but I know that no matter what condition I am in I know I can count on the support of these professionals, family and friends. I work full time as a social worker and while that can be challenging at times, I am able to support myself. I have a wonderful supervisor who supports me and believes in me. I have had many struggles in the past months but it has been with all of this help that I have survived, prospered, and become who I am today.

I cannot stress enough the importance of having a good support system. I know that in my life and with my clients' lives this can be a guiding force in surviving mental illness. Departments of mental health have the ability to help clients with mental illness to become more than just a diagnosis. They have the ability to help clients achieve more than they thought possible. Some may say too many resources were used on me and too many resources are used on people with mental illness today. I like to think it is money well spent. In helping people to prosper, you help society as a whole. It is easy in tough economic times to cut mental health services with the thought that each service is too costly and unnecessary. I would encourage you to take a broader look at what this means for people. *It means increased hospitalizations, increased medications, and an increase in homelessness . . . and the list goes on.*

I continue to need support and know that I can count on the people in my life to provide it. It is my hope that others will be in this same position. A position where they are not only obtaining services but also helping to provide services to some of the most vulnerable in our society. I like to think that it is through my experiences that I am able to better serve clients.

Ruth speaks of the pain and the pride involved in her ongoing struggles with chronic mental health conditions. She is well aware of the social issues, which affect both the etiology and the course of the psychiatric conditions in her life. More importantly, for her as a person, a client and a social worker, she knows what social conditions favorably impact the lives of people living with mental health problems. She calls for comprehensive, ongoing, integrated services that support all areas of her life. She also warns of the social problems created when people do not have access to these services – more restrictive and costly interventions, overreliance on medication, and increased rates of homelessness and poverty. She also speaks powerfully about the importance of the helping relationships she has developed with her own social workers and other professionals. Ruth says little about her own attributes, strengths and resilience. However, they come through in her testimony and through her own work with clients.

Social work programs and social work roles

In helping people with mental health conditions, the social work function is to help clients and their families to cope with the tasks and struggles in day-to-day living, and to influence the social and physical environments to be more responsive to meeting their needs. Living with a mental health condition is often a stressful and painful experience. The stress and associated pain emerges from a perceived ecological imbalance between a person's life demands and personal and environmental resources to meet the demands. These perceived transactional imbalances create life stressors in three interrelated areas: life transitions and traumatic events, environmental pressures, and dysfunctional interpersonal processes (Gitterman & Germain, 2008).

For a person suffering from a mental heath condition, *life transitions and changes* can be particularly stressful. Transitions in life impose new demands, require new responses, and can be, therefore, often deeply distressing. Some changes in routine, some flexibility in processing new information and in problem-solving are required. For the emotionally and cognitively challenged person, these adaptive tasks place difficult demands and threaten their coping abilities. Sudden and unexpected changes are particularly stressful and debilitating. The immediacy and enormity of a *traumatic life event* often triggers deep despair, and immobilization. Helping a person with a mental health condition deal with life changes and traumatic events is a significant focus for both preventive and rehabilitative interventions.

Helping clients with mental health conditions to negotiate complex organizations and interpersonal networks is also a critical social work function. While *social and physical environments* provide resources and supports, they also serve to obstruct the tasks of daily living, and represent significant stressors. For people with mental health conditions, the social and physical environments are often overwhelming and a significant source of severe stress. Organizations such as schools, hospitals, social security, public assistance, child welfare may overpower. Interpersonal networks such as relatives, friends, workmates and neighbors may be dysfunctional, scarce and unavailable, so that clients are, in effect, socially and emotionally isolated. Interpersonal networks may also be intrusive and violate essential personal boundaries. The physical environment may be crowded, unsafe and insecure and pose overwhelming threats to our clients with mental health conditions. Helping these clients access and negotiate their social and physical environments is a distinctive social work function.

In struggling to manage life transitional and/or environmental stressors, problematic interpersonal relationships in families and groups may create and/or exacerbate existing stress. Unfulfilled mutual expectations, exploitative relationships, and blocks in communication create problems for individuals with mental health conditions as well as to their family members. Helping people with emotional and cognitive difficulties and their family members to deal with relationship and communication difficulties and to find common ground are essential social work activities.

Social workers and their clients with mental health conditions may also develop interpersonal difficulties. When social workers define the difficulties as client resistance or lack of motivation, they add to the client's overall level of stress (Gitterman, 1983, 1989; Gitterman & Nadelman,

1999; Gitterman & Schaeffer, 1972). The social work task is to define the interpersonal obstacle in transactional terms, owning our contributions to the difficulties between us.

Helping people with their life transitional, environmental and interpersonal stressors provide the social worker with a clear and distinctive professional function. We perform these functions in every aspect of service delivery to people with mental health conditions. We assume responsibilities as crisis counselors, mediators, educators, skills trainers, case managers, medication facilitators, consumer and family consultants, diagnosticians, mediators and therapists, interagency and interdisciplinary team collaborators, advocates and community organizers, program evaluators and researchers, and administrators and policy analysts (Bentley, 2002). Practice settings include formal settings such as hospitals and outpatient clinics, partial hospitalization programs, residential treatment facilities and child guidance centers. We are also offering services in schools, corrections facilities, homeless shelters, the military, and group homes. In addition, there is a promising trend, which resonates with the profession's understanding of complex environmental influences and natural support networks. There has been an increase nationwide in the use of such programs as Intensive Child and Adolescent Psychiatric Preventive Services (ICAPPS) and Assertive Community Treatment (ACT) for people with severe and persistent mental illness. Both programs utilize interdisciplinary teams, flexible professional roles and intensive, comprehensive and individualized services for individuals and their families. Developed as alternatives to more costly and restrictive levels of care such as hospitalization, these programs offer far more than cost savings. Clients served in these innovative programs typically have access to 24-hour crisis lines, a range of in-home services and a committed intervention team which includes professionals and paraprofessionals. The social work role in these programs is both flexible and responsive to the needs of individual clients at particular points of time. Most of the social worker's activity takes place in the client's natural environment, offering opportunities for more comprehensive assessment and for the mobilization of strengths in that environment. Additionally, in this kind of intervention, the willingness of the social worker to "join in" the client's life outside the agency office, offers opportunities for a working alliance that is more rooted in the client's own experience and may be more sustaining. In this role, the social worker combines the provision of concrete services and psychological support, with the shared experience of the client's day-to-day life. This can provide a powerful alliance and human connection for both the client and the worker. On a macro level, consumer alliance groups such as the National Alliance for Mental Illness (formerly the National Alliance for the Mentally Ill) have strongly endorsed a recovery model for people living with mental health conditions. Built upon the notion of "recovery" commonly associated with substance abuse treatment, and upon a commitment to patients' rights, the movement has made significant inroads from a grassroots movement to influencing federal and state policies. The Substance Abuse and Mental Health Services Administration (SAMHSA) and the Interagency Committee on Disability Research (ICDR) has worked together to develop a consensus statement (NASW, 2005) and the U.S. Department of Health and Human Services (U.S. DHHS) (2006) stated in 2005, "recovery is an individual's journey of healing and transformation to live a meaningful life in a community of his or her choice while striving to achieve maximum human potential."

As social service budgets and "entitlements" are being decimated and further stigmatized, our commitment to understanding the interdependence of mental health conditions and social problems and injustices and to our dual mission is more important than ever. We have come a long way from the days when Ruth, for example, was expected to live out her days in state hospital facilities. We have also learned from the difficulties associated with the deinstitutionalization movement of the 1970s wherein people with severe and persistent mental illness were released into communities that did not have sufficient resources for basic needs such as housing. People with mental illness can and do live fulfilling lives, develop and maintain important interpersonal relationships, love, choose partners, marry and raise children. They also study, work and give back to their communities. But, like all of us, they cannot do it alone. Social workers are in unique positions to help, advocate for, and learn from people living with mental health conditions.

Web resources

Council on Social Work Education
www.cswe.org

National Association of Social Workers
www.nasw.org

National Institute of Mental Health
www.nimh.gov

References

Acker, G.M. (1999). The impact of clients' mental illness on social workers' job satisfaction and burnout. *Health and Social Work, 24,* 112–119.

American Psychiatric Association (APA). (2000). *Diagnostic and statistical manual of mental disorders,* (4th ed., Text revision) Washington, DC: APA.

Bentley, K.J. (ed.) (2002). *Social work practice in mental health: Contemporary roles, tasks, and techniques.* Pacific Grove, CA: Brooks/Cole.

Bentley, K.J. (2005). Women, mental health, and the psychiatric enterprise: A review. *Health and Social Work, 30,* (1), 56–63.

Bright, C. (2004). Deconstructing reparative therapy: An examination of the processes involved when attempting to change sexual orientation. *Clinical Social Work Journal, 32* (4), 225–254.

Center for Health Workforce Studies (CHWS). (2006). *National study of licensed social workers.* Retrieved January 29, 2010, from www.workforce.socialworkers.org/studies/natstudy.asp

Conrad, P. (1980). On the medicalization of deviance and social control. In D. Fogarty (ed.), *The Critical psychiatry: The politics of mental health.* New York: Pantheon.

Courtney, M.E., & Specht, H. (1994). *Unfaithful angels: How social work has abandoned its mission.* New York: Free Press.

Davidson, J.R., & Davidson, T. (1996). Confidentiality and managed care: Ethical and legal concerns. *Health and Social Work, 21* (3), 208–215.

Dohrenwend, B., Turner, J., Turse, N., Adams, B., Koenen, K., & Marshall, R. (2007). Continuing controversy over the psychological risks of Vietnam for U.S. veterans. *Journal of Traumatic Stress, 20* (4), 449–465.

Eack, S.M., & Newhill, C.E. (2008). What influences social workers' attitudes toward working with clients with severe mental illness? *Families in Society: Journal of Contemporary Social Services, 89* (3), 419–428.

Farone, D.W. (2002). Mental illness, social construction, and managed care: Implications for social work. *Social Work in Mental Health, 1* (1), 99–113.

Frazer, P., Westhuis, D., Daley, J.G., & Phillips, I. (2009). How clinical social workers are using the DSM-IV: A national study. *Social Work in Mental Health, 7* (4), 325–339.

Furman, R., & Langer, C.L. (2006). Managed care and the care of the soul. *Journal of Social Work Values and Ethics, 3* (2). Retrieved January 29, 2010, from www.socialworker.com/jswve/content/blogcategory/13/46/

Germain, C.B., & Gitterman, A. (1980). *The life model of social work practice.* New York: Columbia University Press.

Gitterman, A. (1983). Uses of resistance: A transactional view. *Social Work, 28* (2), 19–23.

Gitterman, A. (1989). Testing professional authority and boundaries. *Social Casework, 70* (March), 165–171.

Gitterman, A., & Germain, C.B. (2008). *The life model of social work practice: Advances in theory and practice* (3rd ed.). New York: Columbia University Press.

Gitterman, A., & Nadelman, A. (1999). The white professional and the black client revisited. *Reflections: Narrative of Professional Helping, 5* (4), 67–79.

Gitterman, A., & Schaeffer (1972). The white professional and the black client. *Social Casework, 53* (spring), 280–291.

Goleman, D. (1985, April 30) Social workers vault into a leading role in psychotherapy. *The New York Times*, p. 1.

Granfield, R., & Cloud, W. (1999). *Coming clean: Overcoming addiction without treatment.* New York: New York University Press.

Kessler, R.C., Berglund, P., Demler, O., Jin, R., Koretz, D., Merikangas, K.R. et al. (2003). The epidemiology of major depressive disorder: Results from the National Comorbidity Survey Replication (NCS-R). *Journal of the American Medical Association, 289* (23), 3095–3105.

Kessler, R.C., Chiu, W.T., Demler, O., & Walters, E.E. (2005). Prevalence, severity, and comorbidity of twelve month DSM-IV disorders in the National Comorbidity Survey Replication (NCS-R). *Archives of General Psychiatry, 62* (6), 617–627.

Kessler, R.C., Galea, S., Gruber, M.J., Sampson, N.A., Ursano, R.J., & Wessely, S. (2008). Trends in mental illness and suicidality after Hurricane Katrina. *Molecular Psychiatry, 13* (4), 374–384.

Kirk, S.A. (ed.). (2005). *Mental disorders in the social environment: Critical perspectives.* New York: Columbia University Press.

Kirk, S.A., & Kutchins, H. (1992). *The selling of DSM: The rhetoric of science in psychiatry.* Hawthorn, NY: Aldine de Gruyter.

Kirk, S., & Kutchins, H. (1995). Should DSM be the basis for teaching social work practice in mental health? No! *Journal of Social Work Education, 31,* 159–168.

Kutchins, H., & Kirk, S.A. (1988). The business of diagnosis: DSM-III and clinical social work. *Social Work, 33,* 215–220.

Kutchins, H., & Kirk, S.A. (1989). DSM-III-R: The conflict over new psychiatric diagnoses. *Health and Social Work, 14* (2), 91–101.

Lacasse, J.R., & Gomory, T. (2003). Is graduate social work education promoting a critical approach to mental health practice? *Journal of Social Work Education, 39* (3), 383–408.

Lee, S., & Kleinman, A. (2007). Are somatoform disorders changing with time: The case of neurasthenia in China. *Psychosomatic Medicine, 69,* 846–849.

Logan, J. (2006). The impact of Katrina: Race and class in storm damaged neighborhoods. Retrieved February 12, 2010, from Brown University, www.s4.brown.edu/Katrina/report.pdf

López, S.R., & Guarnaccia, P.J. (2005). Cultural dimensions of psychopathology. In J.E. Maddux & B.A. Winstead (eds) *Psychopathology: Foundations for a contemporary understanding* (pp. 19–38). Mahwah, NJ: Lawrence Erlbaum Associates.

Mason, K., Olmos-Gallos, A., Bacon, D., McQuilken, M., Henley, A., & Fisher, S. (2004). Exploring the consumer's and provider's perspective on service quality in community mental health care. *Community Mental Health Journal, 40,* 33–46.

Merikangas, K.R., Ames, M., Cui, L., Stang, P.E., Ustun, T.B., von Korff, M., & Kessler, R.C. (2007). The impact of comorbidity of mental and physical conditions on role disability in the US adult population. *Archives of General Psychiatry, 64* (10), 632–650.

National Association of Social Workers (NASW). (2005). *Assuring the sufficiency of a frontline workforce: A national study of licensed social workers.* Washington, DC: NASW Press.

National Association of Social Workers (NASW). (2008). *Code of ethics of the National Association of Social Workers.* Washington, DC: NASW Press.

Newhill, C.E., & Korr, W.S. (2004). Practice with people with severe mental illness: Rewards, challenges, burdens. *Health & Social Work, 29* (4), 297–305.

Prilleltensky, I. (2003). Poverty and power. In S. Carr & T. Sloan (eds), *Poverty and power: From global perspective to local practice* (pp. 19–44). New York: Kluwer Academic/Plenum.

Reamer, F. (1997). Managing ethics under managed care. *Families in Society,* 78(1), 96–101.

Regier, D.A., Narrow, W.E., Rae, D.S., Manderscheid, R.W., Locked, B.Z., & Goodwin, F.K. (1993). The de facto mental and addictive disorders service system: Epidemiologic Catchment Area prospective 1-year prevalence rates of disorders and services. *Archives of General Psychiatry, 50* (2), 85–94.

Reid, Y., Johnson, S., Morant, N., Kuipers, E., Szmukler, G., Thornicroft, G. et al. (1999). Explanations for stress and satisfaction in mental health professionals: A qualitative study. *Social Psychiatry and Psychiatric Epidemiology, 34*, 301–308.

Schamess, G. (1998). Corporate values and managed mental health care. In G. Schamess and A. Lightburn (eds), *Humane managed care?* (pp. 23–35). Washington, DC: NASW Press.

Scheyett, A. (2005). The mark of madness: Stigma, serious mental illnesses, and social work. *Social Work in Mental Health, 3* (4), 79–98.

Spaniol, S., & Zipple, A.M. (1994). The family recovery process. *Journal of the California Alliance for the Mentally Ill, 5* (2), 57–59.

Spaniol, J., Gagne, C., & Koehler, M. (2003). The recovery framework in rehabilitation and mental health. In D.R. Moxley & J.R. Finch (eds), *Sourcebook of rehabilitation and mental health practice* (pp. 37–50). New York: Kluwer Academic/Plenum.

Spriggs, W.E. (2006). Poverty in America: The poor are getting poorer. *The Crisis, 13*, 14–16.

Substance Abuse and Mental Health Services Administration (SAMHSA). (2001). *Mental health, United States, 2000* (DHHS Pub. No. [SMA] 01–3537). Washington, DC: SAMHSA.

Substance Abuse and Mental Health Services Administration (SAMHSA). (2006). *Mental health, United States, 2004.* R.W. Manderscheid & J.T. Berry (eds), DHHS Pub No. (SMA) 06-4195. Rockville, MD: SAMHSA.

U.S. Department of Health and Human Services (DHHS). (2005). *National consensus statement on mental health recovery.* Rockville, MD: Substance Abuse and Mental Health Services Administration. Retrieved January 29, 2010, from www.mentalhealth.samhsa.gov/publications/allpubs/sma05-4129

Voorhees, C.C.W., Vick, J., & Perkins, D.D. (2007). "Came hell and high water": The intersection of Hurricane Katrina, the news media, race and poverty. *Journal of Community and Applied Social Psychology, 17* (6), 415–429.

Watters, E. (2010). *Crazy like us: The globalization of the American psyche.* New York: Free Press.

White, W. (1996). *Pathways from the culture of addiction to the culture of recovery.* Center City, MN: Hazelden.

White, W., Boyle, M., & Loveland, D. (2005). Recovery from addiction and mental illness: Shared and contrasting lessons. In R. Ralph & P. Corrigan (eds), *Recovery in mental illness: Broadening our understanding of wellness.* (pp. 233–258). Washington, DC: American Psychological Association.

Whitaker, T., Wilson, M., & Arrington, P. (2008). *Professional development.* NASW Membership Workforce Study. Washington, DC: National Association of Social Workers. Retrieved January 29, 2010, from www.workforce.socialworkers.org/studies/Prof.Dev.pdf

World Health Organization. (2007). Fact Sheet N220. Retrieved January 29, 2010, from www.who.int/mediacentre/en

Young, S., & Ensing, D. (1999). Exploring recovery from the perspective of people with psychiatric disabilities. *Psychiatric Rehabilitation Journal, 22* (3), 219–239.

Part I

Social problems and mental health/illness

2 Oppression and stigma and their effects

Amy C. Watson and Shaun M. Eack

People with mental illnesses face the challenge of managing an illness that at times may significantly impact their functioning and quality of life. They also face stigma and discrimination in multiple life domains that may present important, if not greater, barriers to recovery and full inclusion than the clinical features of the illness itself.[1] Fortunately, since the late 1990s, due to the growing recognition of the deleterious impact of stigma on the lives of persons with mental illness, numerous organizations and government agencies worldwide have targeted reducing mental illness stigma as a priority (Hogan, 2003; Sartorius & Schulze, 2005; U.S. Department of Health and Human Services, 1999; WHO Regional Office for Europe, 2005). More recently in the United States, the final report for the President's New Freedom Commission on Mental Health (Hogan, 2003) highlighted stigma as a major barrier to recovery for people with mental illness.

Social workers, as the primary providers of mental health services for individuals with some of the most stigmatized mental illnesses (Substance Abuse and Mental Health Services Administration, 2001), have a particularly important role to play in recognizing and reducing stigma about mental illness and its deleterious effects on clients (Scheyett, 2005). Social workers are not only expert providers, but also strong social advocates for justice, equality, and inclusion for individuals whose voices are unheard (Scheyett, 2005). People with mental illness are among the most vulnerable and marginalized by society, making them subject to oppression and injustice with few methods of recourse. Social workers can be, and frequently are, the advocates, voices, and facilitators of justice for people with mental illness. In addition, social workers uniquely focus on the biopsychosocial effects of mental disorders in their practice, which include adverse social effects, such as stigma and oppression, at multiple system and societal levels (Gitterman & Germain, 2008).

The social work profession undertakes a holistic perspective on client care. Social workers are also instruments of social justice for the underserved. Social workers must know, first, the different ways the stigma of mental illness can manifest itself; second, the serious impact stigma can have on recovery from mental illness and the improvement of quality of life; and third, the methods to prevent and reduce stigma about mental disorders at both individual and systemic levels. Above all, social workers must also know and always remember that they are not immune to developing, endorsing, or supporting social stigma about mental illness themselves. To be a social worker does not mean to be without social flaws, but rather to commit to a continuous re-examination of one's beliefs and ideology to ensure their alignment with justice and the good of the people who rely upon social work services.

In this chapter, we begin by defining stigma as a process and examine its many forms. We then review the literature on mental illness stigma, discuss its prevalence and negative impact on clients, and examine approaches to reducing stigma and ameliorating its negative consequences. We conclude with a concrete illustration of the effects of stigma on the life of a person with mental illness, and present clear methods a practitioner can use to address this problem at multiple individual and system levels.

Definitions of oppression and stigma

In his seminal work *Stigma: Notes on the management of spoiled identity*, Erving Goffman defined stigma as "an attribute that is deeply discrediting" and reduces the bearer from "a whole and usual person to a tainted discounted one" (1963, p. 3). Building on the work of Goffman (1963) as well as others (e.g. Jones, Farina, Hastorf, Markus, Miller, & Scott, 1984), Link and Phelan (2001) define stigma as a *process* consisting of five interrelated components that, when they converge, result in status loss and discrimination for members of stigmatized groups. The process begins with the labeling of human difference. Stereotyping, or attributing negative characteristics to the persons who have been labeled with a socially salient difference such as mental illness is a key example of this. Next, is the separation of "us" from "them," with "them" being the stigmatized and "us" being the stigmatizers. This results in status loss and discrimination for those who have been stigmatized. Underlying this process is the exercise of power that allows the process to unfold. Without the exercise of power, labeling, stereotyping, and separating of "us" from "them" will not produce status loss and discrimination.

Link and Phelan (2001) provide an illustrative example. Patients in a psychiatric ward may label nurses as pill pushers, attribute a number of negative stereotypes, and view the nurses as "them." The patients may even treat nurses differently and make jokes about them. The patients have labeled, stereotyped, separated and discriminated. However, the patients lack the power in the psychiatric ward context to produce negative consequences and make the nurses a stigmatized, lower status group.

Unlike the more sociological definition above, social cognitive definitions of stigma tend to limit the focus to stereotypes, prejudice and discrimination in micro level interactions. Social cognitive models view stereotypes as knowledge structures representing collectively agreed upon notions of members of groups (Hilton & von Hippel, 1996; Judd & Park, 1993). Stereotypes are particularly efficient (although many times inaccurate) tools for categorizing information and generating impressions and expectations about members of groups (Hamilton & Sherman, 1994). In other words, stereotyping is a normal cognitive process that allows us to categorize a large amount of information and figure out what to expect from other people based on group membership. It is, in a sense, a cognitive shortcut. Knowledge of stereotypes does not necessarily imply prejudice. Prejudice involves an evaluative component (generally negative) that results when stereotypes are endorsed and generate emotional reactions such as disgust, anger or fear (Devine, 1989). Prejudice, which is fundamentally a cognitive and affective response, may lead to discrimination, the behavioral reaction (Crocker, Major, & Steele, 1998). For example, a social worker working with a young man with bipolar disorder may be aware of the stereotypes that people with serious mental illnesses are incompetent and unable to work. If the social worker endorses these stereotypes as factual and experiences a negative emotional reaction (anger, less confidence in client's potential), he is prejudiced. If, as a result, the social worker discourages the young man from seeking employment, he has discriminated. This likely well-meaning social worker's discriminatory behavior may negatively impact the opportunities available to his client for recovery and full inclusion in the community.

Understanding stigma processes in the personal and interpersonal contexts such as the example described above is extremely important. However, incorporating concepts of status and power allows us to expand our focus and understand stigma's impact on the distribution of life chances and social outcomes. Thus, we as social workers can fully consider mental illness stigma and its impact from the person and environment perspective.

Oppression and stigma and mental health/illness

Mental illness is perhaps one of the most discrediting labels, as it is linked to a number of negative stereotypes. Common *stereotypes* about persons with mental illness include they are dangerous, unpredictable, incompetent, irresponsible; at fault for their illness, and unlikely to recover (Brockington, Hall, Levings, & Murphy, 1993; Corrigan et al., 2000; Hyler, Gabbard, & Schneider, 1991; Taylor & Dear, 1981; Wahl, 1995). These stereotypes persist despite evidence disputing them:

- *Dangerousness.* While research suggests a modest increase in the risk of violence associated with mental illness, the increase appears to be limited to individuals with co-occurring substance disorders or specific psychotic symptoms (Link, Andrews, & Cullen, 1992; Steadman et al., 1998). To put this in perspective, the magnitude of the increase is similar to the increase in violence risk associated with being male, young, or less educated (Link et al., 1992; Link, Phelan, Bresnahan, Stueve, & Pescosolido, 1999). When compared to individuals with the same sociodemographic characteristics from similar neighborhoods, even people with the most serious of mental illnesses are no more likely to be violent than their community counterparts (Steadman et al., 1998). People with mental illness are, however, more likely to be victims of violent crime than other people, and more likely to be victims than perpetrators of violence (Teplin, McClelland, Abram, & Weiner, 2005).
- *Incompetent and unlikely to recover.* Research indicates a wide heterogeneity of short and long-term outcomes for mental illness. While individuals may experience periods of disability, the majorities of individuals with serious mental illnesses significantly improve or recover (Harding, Zubin, & Strauss, 1992; Tsuang, Woolson, & Fleming, 1979).
- *At fault or responsible for mental illness.* The modern scientific view is that mental illnesses are caused by interplay of biological, psychological and social factors, not bad parenting, laziness or character weakness (U.S. Department of Health and Human Services, 1999).

Despite the evidence, stereotypes about mental illness are perpetuated in the media in the form of inaccurate representations of persons with mental illness as violent predators, incompetent people, or wild rebellious spirits (Hyler, Gabbard, & Schneider, 1991; Wahl, 1995). These stereotypes are reflected in laws and institutional practices that limit rights, opportunities, and social interactions that further marginalize persons with mental illness.

The good news is that public understanding of mental illness appears to be improving, at least in some ways. Replicating survey research conducted in the 1950s (Starr, 1952, 1955) Pescolsolido and colleagues (Pescolsolido, Monahan, Link, Steuve, & Kikuzawa, 1999; Phelan, Link, Stueve, & Pescosolido, 2000) found that the public's understanding of mental illness has broadened beyond stereotypical conceptions associated with psychotic disorders to include more common conditions like anxiety, personality, and substance use disorders. The more recent survey (Phelan et al., 2000) also found that people were more likely to attribute mental disorders to "chemical imbalance," "genetic factors," and "stressful life circumstances," rather than to "bad character," "the way the person was raised," or "God's will," suggesting that public understanding is consistent with current professional understanding of the causes of mental disorders.

Unfortunately, the news is not all good. Public perceptions of dangerousness related to mental illness appear to have increased since the 1950s (Phelan et al., 2000). Perhaps the most pernicious stereotype about mental illness, the belief that people with mental illness are dangerous, is associated with greater desire for social distance, defined as unwillingness to live near, socialize or work with people with psychiatric disorders, have a group home nearby, or have someone with mental illness marry into their family (Brockington et al., 1993; Cohen & Struening, 1962; Link et al., 1987; Martin, Pescosolido, & Tuch, 2000; Pescosolido et al., 1999). This means that with an increasing fear of those with mental illness, society has moved further and further away from social inclusion and community integration of these individuals. As indicated above, the increased risk of violence associated with mental illness is limited to a subset of persons with specific characteristics and similar in magnitude to the increase in violence risk associated with being male, young, or less educated (Link et al., 1992; Link et al., 1999). In addition, the largest study of violence and mental illness in the United States found that people with severe mental illness were no more likely to engage in violence than individuals living in similar sociodemographically matched neighborhoods (Steadman et al., 1998). Thus, the strong link between violence and mental illness remains one of society's most notorious myths. As a result, the public tends to grossly overestimate the risk of violence associated with mental illness, and avoids and discriminates against persons with mental illness.

Research suggests that public perceptions of persons with mental illness vary somewhat based on characteristics of the target person with mental illness. For example, a person diagnosed with depression tends to be viewed less negatively than a person diagnosed with schizophrenia (Pescosolido et al., 1999). While race and level of education of the person with mental illness have not been found to predict public attitudes, gender has, with women tending to be viewed as less dangerous than men (Schnittker, 2000). Interestingly, one study found that an employed person with mental illness elicits less stigma than an unemployed person with mental illness (Perkins, Raines, Tschopp, & Warner 2009).

Research has also found differences in stigmatizing attitudes based on the demographics of the perceiver, however findings are not always consistent. For example, several studies have found that people of color are less likely than whites to blame individuals for their illness, more likely to sympathize with them, and less likely to avoid them in social settings (Corrigan, Backs-Edwards, Green, Diwan, & Penn, 2001a; Schnittker, Freese, & Powell, 1999). People of color are also less likely to endorse genetics or family upbringing as explanations of the cause of mental illness than whites but as likely to endorse other biological and environmental causes (Schnittker et al., 1999). However, studies have also found that people of color are more likely to perceive persons with mental illness as dangerous (Corrigan & Watson, 2007) and endorse coercive treatments in segregated settings (Corrigan et al., 2001a). Additionally, they tend to have more negative perceptions of professional mental health care (Schnittker et al., 1999). Likewise, findings related to gender are not entirely consistent. While several studies have failed to find gender differences in stigmatizing attitudes, the balance of research suggests that women may be less likely to endorse negative attitudes and discriminatory behaviors than men (Corrigan & Watson, 2007).

A key personal characteristic that is associated with attitudes about mental illness is familiarity with persons with mental illness. Several studies have found that people that have more personal familiarity have less negative views and more positive affective reactions to persons with mental illness, believing them to be less dangerous and desiring less social distance from them (Arikan & Uysal, 1999; Corrigan et al., 2001a; Phelan & Link, 2004). This is true even if the "familiarity" is based on impersonal contact. Phelan and Link (2004) found that even impersonal contact, in the form of seeing people in public that appeared to have a mental illness, was associated with perceiving people with mental illness as less dangerous.

The stigma of mental illness may appear in interactions *between people and groups* (individual or public stigma), within *stigmatized persons themselves* (internalized or self-stigma), and in *institutional and social structures* (structural stigma). Individual or public stigma has been the focus of social cognitive models and researchers and advocates working to understand and reduce mental illness stigma (Corrigan, Markowitz, & Watson, 2004). This type of stigma process takes place when a person or persons with mental illness interact with members of the public who label, stereotype, and discriminate against them in some way. For example, an employer may stereotype a job applicant with mental illness as incompetent and refuse to consider the person for a job. Similarly, a college student who is accessing mental health services may not be invited to a dorm party because classmates stereotype the student as dangerous. Stigma exercised at this interpersonal level results in painful social isolation and barriers to opportunities in important life domains.

A critical life domain affected by public stigma is employment. Work provides a vehicle for social integration and a sense of self-worth and social identity. For people with mental illness, employment provides structure, social connections, goals and income – essential components of recovery (Stuart, 2006). Most people with serious mental illness are willing and able to work (Mechanic, Bilder, & McAlpine, 2002). However, their rates of unemployment are alarmingly high, ranging from 20 to 60 percent for individuals with anxiety and major depressive disorder to 80–90 percent for people with serious and persistent psychiatric disorders such as schizophrenia (Crowther, Marshall, Bond, & Huxley, 2001). While people with mental illnesses may experience periods of significant disability in which they are unable to work, there is compelling evidence that employment discrimination is a contributor to their high rates of unemployment. Many employers hold stigmatizing views of mental illness and are reluctant to hire persons with mental illness (Drehmer & Bordieri, 1985; Farina & Felner, 1973; Manning & White, 1995; Scheid, 1999; Webber & Orcutt, 1984). People with mental illness report employment related discrimination as one of their most frequent stigma experiences (Roeloffs, Sherbourne, Unutzer, Fink, Tank, & Wells, 2003; Wahl, 1999). Fear of employment related rejection may eventually lead individuals to view themselves as unemployable and to give up looking for work altogether (Stuart, 2006).

Not only employer stigma creates barriers to employment for persons with mental illness. Competitive employment has not traditionally been a focus of the mental health system (Stuart, 2006) and clinicians have discouraged individuals from considering employment for fear that the stress of employment would exacerbate the illness. The more modern recovery oriented philosophy, however, maintains that people with mental illness have the right to live and work in the community. In fact, work may be a very important recovery goal. Mental health providers may be the last group to understand that being out of work is bad for your mental health, as opposed to the other way around.

Public stigma also has consequences for persons with mental illness in other life domains, including, but not limited to, housing and health care. A safe place to live is an important goal for all of us. However, stigma creates a barrier to achieving this goal for persons with mental illnesses when landlords are hesitant to rent to persons with mental illnesses (Forchuk, Nelson, & Hall, 2006; Page, 1977) and communities resist group homes and other types of housing for persons with mental illness (Zippay, 2007). Additionally, persons with serious mental illness receive less adequate health care. One study, for example, found that people identified with comorbid psychiatric disorder were significantly less likely to undergo percutaneous transluminal coronary angioplasty after heart attack than people without a psychiatric disorder (Druss, Bradford, Rosenheck, Radford, & Krumholz, 2000). Clearly, stigma has the potential to invade and negatively impact all facets of the lives of persons with mental illnesses. Stigma processes may also occur within the individual who is stigmatized in the form of *perceived and self-stigma*. Prior to the onset and diagnosis of mental illness, most individuals are aware of and may even endorse cultural stereotypes about the group, "the mentally ill." With the onset of a mental illness, these stereotypes become relevant to the self, as individuals perceive negative reactions from others. Perceived stigma leads to a loss of self-esteem and self-efficacy and limits prospects for recovery as individuals constrict their social networks and opportunities in anticipation of rejection (Kahng & Mowbray, 2005; Link, Struening, Neese-Todd, Asmussen, & Phelan, 2001; Markowitz, 1998; Perlick et al., 2001; Sirey, Bruce, Alexopoulus, Perlick, Friedman, & Meyers, 2001). For example, college students experiencing mental illness may withdraw from academic settings for fear of loss of confidentiality and discrimination (Mowbray et al., 2006). Likewise, adults with mental illness may also choose not to pursue intimate relationships to avoid rejection due to their mental illness (Wright, Wright, Perry, & Foote-Ardah, 2007).

Perceived stigma may also prevent people who might benefit from seeking or adhering to treatment. Up to 40 percent of people with serious mental illness do not receive treatment in a given year (Regier, Narrow, Rae, Manderscheid, Locke, & Goodwin, 1993). While many factors may prevent people from obtaining services, perceived stigma plays a role. Results from the National Comorbidity Survey suggest that concerns about what others think and wanting to solve problems on one's own discourage people from seeking treatment (Kessler et al., 2001). Another study found that members of the general public who held stigmatizing attitudes about mental illness were less likely to seek care (Cooper, Corrigan, & Watson, 2003). Stigma may also affect participation once people enter treatment. Sirey et al. (2001) found that adults that perceived higher levels of public stigma where less adherent with prescribed antidepressant medication.

The impact of stigma on the self may go deeper than perceived stigma. Individuals with mental illness may also self-stigmatize (Corrigan & Watson, 2002). This occurs when they move beyond simply being aware of and actually apply the negative stereotypes they have learned about people with mental illness to themselves, feel they are different and less valuable than others and subsequently limit the social, occupational and other opportunities they allow themselves to pursue. They are not limiting the opportunities they pursue to protect themselves from negative reactions from others but instead because they feel unworthy or incapable. Obviously, this process further interferes with a person's ability to pursue life goals and maintain his or her quality of life.

Self-stigma is associated with reduced self-esteem and self-efficacy (Watson & River, 2005; Watson, Corrigan, Larson, & Sells, 2007). Research indicates that higher group identification, or seeing oneself as part of a larger group of people with mental illness, and lower perceived legitimacy of mental illness stigma and discrimination serve as protective factors that may interrupt the self-stigma process somewhere between stereotype awareness and applying stereotypes to the self. This suggests stigma resistance interventions and efforts to build self-help and social support may be useful for addressing self-stigma.

Ritsher and Phelan (2004) developed a measure of internalized stigma that incorporates components of the perceived and self-stigma. The Internalized Stigma of Mental Illness (ISMI) scale has five dimensions – Alienation, Stereotype Endorsement, Discrimination Experience, Social Withdrawal, and Stigma Resistance. In a study of outpatients with serious mental illness, they found high levels of internalized stigma and that internalized stigma (ISMI total score) predicted reduced self-esteem and depressive symptoms four months later. Participants expressing greater alienation due to their mental illness experienced the most distress. In another study using the ISMI, Lysaker, Buck, Hammoud, Taylor, and Roe (2006) found that lower internalized stigma, particularly alienation, was associated with greater hope and agency. Ritsher and Phelan (2004) suggest, "What is needed is an antidote to alienation: interpersonal engagement, such as that provided by the fellowship of self-help groups, the role recovery inherent in supported employment or the healing power of the psychotherapeutic alliance" (p. 264).

Difficult to identify but perhaps the most devastating in impact on life chances are institutional and structural discrimination (Corrigan, Markowitz, & Watson, 2004). Institutional discrimination refers to the policies of private and public institutions that intentionally restrict the rights and opportunities of members of particular groups, such as persons with mental illness

(Pincus, 1996). The effects of institutional discrimination are intentional, perhaps not by the line-level person carrying out the policy, but by the people with the power to make rules and regulations. Institutional discrimination of people with mental illness takes place in both public and private sectors. For example, a study of state laws showed approximately one-third of the 50 states restrict the rights of an individual with mental illness to hold elective office, participate on juries, and vote. Even greater limitations were evident in the family domain. About 50 percent of states restrict the child custody rights of parents with mental illness (Hemmens, Miller, Burton, & Milner, 2002). Other studies have shown similar legislative patterns for people with mental illness (Burton, 1990). Private sector institutional discrimination is apparent in organizational policies that require persons with mental illness to submit to extra screenings and examinations as a condition of employment and college and university policies that expel from student housing students who have sought mental health treatment (Bazelon Center for Mental Health Law, 2006a, 2006b; Capriccioso, 2006).

Structural discrimination refers to the set of private and public policies whose *un*intended effects limit the rights and opportunities of persons with mental illness (Pincus, 1996). Limited insurance coverage for people with serious mental illness is an example of structural discrimination. Historically, states have been responsible for the care of persons with serious mental illness. For a number of reasons, including the state sponsored mental health safety net; private insurers have typically limited coverage for mental disorders. Many people with serious mental illness do not have private insurance, and those that do quickly use up their coverage. Thus, most people with serious mental illness receive their care in the public mental health system. Salaries and benefits for clinicians tend to be better in the private health sector where people with relatively benign illnesses like adjustment disorders, relational difficulties, and phase of life problems receive care. In search of more financially rewarding positions and better working conditions, talented clinicians may opt out of the public treatment system where people with the most serious psychiatric and substance abuse disorders are served. An unintended result is that the treatment choices available for persons with serious mental illness may be limited and be of lower quality.

Another example of structural discrimination is the unintended consequences of public welfare policies that frequently stop people with mental illness from seeking paid employment. Many people with severe mental illnesses, such as schizophrenia and bipolar disorders, require some time away from work to "get back on their feet." This usually necessitates application for local and federal public assistance programs to cover the costs of expensive medications and daily living costs while working for pay is not feasible. To qualify for programs such as Supplemental Security Income (SSI), Social Security Disability Insurance (SSDI), Medicaid and Medicare, individuals must prove that they are completely disabled and unable to work. This results in people with mental illness continuously having to prove that they are ill and unable to work in order to pay for their medications and keep a roof over their head. Once individuals begin to try to go back to work (usually part-time), these necessities are in jeopardy, and entry-level jobs rarely cover the costs of living for people with mental illness. While these programs provide crucial supports and have immensely improved the lives of persons with serious mental illness (Frank & Glied, 2006), the failure of these programs to account for factors unique to mental illnesses often creates barriers to ever returning to paid employment. It should be noted that the Social Security Administration has implemented work incentives that address some of the dilemmas faced by persons with psychiatric disabilities and reduce the risks of returning to the workforce.

Social workers and allied mental health professionals often view stigma as "someone else's" problem. If only other professionals would be more responsive toward people with mental illness, they would receive more effective services. Unfortunately, social workers are not immune to harboring stigmatizing attitudes of their own about people with mental illness. In fact, as some have noted, the mental illness recovery movement has been as much about educating professionals on the significant potential of people with mental disorders, as it has been about educating clients and the general society (Farkas, Gagne, Anthony, & Chamberlin, 2005).

In a study of practicing social workers, nearly 70 percent indicated that they did not prefer to work with individuals with severe mental illness (Newhill & Korr, 2004). Additionally, in a study of mental health case managers, the investigators found that social workers and other intensive case managers were as likely to hold stigmatizing and restrictive attitudes as community members toward individuals with mental illness (Murray & Steffen, 1999). Social workers are not alone in having stigmatizing attitudes. Magliano et al. (2004) found that over 50 percent of psychiatric nurses surveyed in Europe thought that individuals with schizophrenia should not get married, and 30 percent thought that such individuals should be sent to the asylum to live. Recently, increased knowledge and interpersonal contact provided by social work education has helped to improve social workers' attitudes toward this population (Eack & Newhill, 2008).

Unwittingly, social workers and other mental health professionals perpetuate social stigma against people with mental illness. When mental health professionals embrace negative attitudes toward the clients they serve, the services they provide will considerably suffer. Professional stigma has a profound affect on clients' recovery. In inpatient treatment, for example, individuals who were subjected to particularly negative attitudes by mental health professionals had substantially worse outcomes and problem behaviors over time (Barrowclough, Haddock, Lowens, Connor, Pidliswyj, & Tracey, 2001). Similarly, in group homes for people with mental illness, negative residential staff attitudes predicted greater levels of psychiatric symptomatology and poorer quality of life among the residents (Snyder, Wallace, Moe, & Liberman, 1994). In general, negative staff attitudes and beliefs significantly impact quality of care and recovery outcomes (for a review, see Van Audenhove & Van Humbeeck, 2003). Social work educators, administrators and practitioners must pay serious attention to this phenomenon and address stigma within the discipline if we are to work effectively in partnership with persons with mental illnesses (Scheyett, 2005).

Advocacy groups, government agencies and professional associations have made stigma reduction a priority, launching campaigns aimed at the public and the media. These campaigns have used a variety of strategies, targeting various audiences and components of stigma. While limited evidence exists of the effectiveness of these campaigns for reducing mental illness stigma, a rich body of literature is available in social psychology on strategies to improve intergroup attitudes related to race and ethnicity. Corrigan and Penn (1999) reviewed this literature and grouped the various approaches to challenging stigma into three processes: protest, education, and contact.

Protest strategies identify specific instances of stigma and discrimination and highlight the injustice. The strategy attempts to shame those responsible for the injustice (Watson & Corrigan, 2005). On an individual level, a person may alert a colleague that a comment he or she made was stigmatizing, and urges the person to discontinue making such comments. On a group level, an advocacy organization may identify that a television program perpetuates a stigmatizing image of mental illness, organize a letter writing campaign to the media outlet and boycott the program's advertisers. While such protests may be effective for eliminating the offensive behavior, they may not improve attitudes. Protest approaches risk producing rebound effects with the consequence that prejudices about a group remain unchanged or possibly, even worse (Corrigan et al., 2001b; Macrae, Bodenhausen, Milne, & Jetten, 1994; Penn & Corrigan, 2002).

Despite the potential for attitude rebound, protest strategies may be useful for changing behaviors. Though largely anecdotal, there is evidence that protest can be effective (Wahl, 1995). For example, NAMI StigmaBusters is an email alert system that notifies members about stigmatizing representations of persons with mental illness in the media and provides instructions on how to contact the offending organization and its sponsors (National Alliance on Mental Illness, 2009a). In 2000, StigmaBusters played a prominent role in ABC's cancelling the program "Wonderland," which portrayed persons with mental illness as dangerous and unpredictable. In the first ten minutes of the first episode, a person with mental illness shot several police officers and stabbed a pregnant psychiatrist in the abdomen with a hypodermic needle. StigmaBusters' efforts not only targeted the show's producers and several management levels of ABC, but also encouraged communication with commercial sponsors including the CEOs of Mitsubishi, Sears, and the Scott Company. Several years later, StigmaBusters took on the Vermont Teddy Bear Company when it advertised a Valentine's Day bear dressed in a straight jacket with the caption "Crazy for You." After a letter writing campaign and meetings with company executives, Vermont Teddy Bear agreed to discontinue this particular bear. These experiences suggest that organized protest has the potential to be a useful strategy for preventing television networks and other media outlets from producing stigmatizing programs, advertisements, and articles. Protest approaches can be useful on a local level as well. In the fall of 2008, for example, a large bronze plaque was erected in front of the Neuropsychiatric Institute (NPI) on the University of Illinois Medical Campus to memorialize the site where the Chicago Cubs first played. The plaque also celebrated the location where the expression "way out in left field" originated:

> The phrase "Way out in left field" originated at West Side grounds, due to the location of a psychiatric hospital behind the ballpark's left field fence, where players and fans could hear patients making odd and strange remarks during games.

> Sponsored by the Way Out in Left Field Society, Illinois Medical district, Illinois State Historical Society, and the University of Illinois at Chicago

> September 2008

The first author's student was placed at NPI when the plaque was ceremoniously erected. She was particularly concerned about the impact of the insensitive statements on the many clients who daily walked past the sign entering the building for mental health services. In fact, several clients voiced distress about the sign. Social work students and staff of NPI launched an impromptu email campaign to the members of the University and Medical Center Administration and to the Chancellor's Council on the Status of Persons with Disabilities, expressing concern about the plaque and its blatant insensitivity. Within two days, the plaque was removed. Months later, the plaque was replaced with a sign without the "way out in left field" reference. The email focused on how the message was harmful on many levels to persons with mental illnesses and to those who care about them.

Educational approaches to stigma reduction aim to challenge inaccurate stereotypes about mental illness and replace these stereotypes with factual information. Public service announcements, books, flyers, movies, videos and other audio visual aids are utilized to dispel myths about mental illness and replace them with facts (National Mental Health Campaign, 2002; Pate, 1988). People with a better understanding of mental illness are less likely to endorse stigma and discrimination (Brockington et al., 1993; Corrigan et al., 2001b; Corrigan et al., 2002; Holmes, Corrigan, Williams, Canar, & Kubiak, 1999; Keane, 1991; Morrison & Teta, 1980; Penn, Guynan, Daily, Spaulding, Garbin, & Sullivan, 1994; Penn, Kommana, Mansfield, &

Link, 1999). Unfortunately, the magnitude and duration of these improvements is quite limited (Corrigan & McCracken, 1997) and the impact on subsequent behaviors questionable.

The limited impact of educational approaches is illuminated by research on strategies targeting race and other minority group stereotypes. (Devine, 1995; Pruegger & Rogers, 1994). Stereotypes provide a template for encoding subsequent information that may disconfirm them. Thus, if a person endorses the stereotype that people with mental illness are dangerous, they will be more attentive to the latest news story linking a violent crime to mental illness than to information that persons with mental illnesses are generally not any more dangerous than anyone else. Essentially, stereotypes are resistant to change based on new information alone (Fyock & Stangor, 1994; Stangor & McMillan, 1992). Educational approaches are certainly not without merit. They do also increase awareness and understanding of mental health issues and available services. However, education approaches by themselves have limited effects on the pernicious stereotypes about mental illness.

Interpersonal contact is the most promising approach to challenging mental illness stigma. Contact has long been considered an effective means for reducing intergroup prejudice (Allport, 1954; Pettigrew & Tropp, 2000). In formalizing the "contact" hypothesis, Allport (1954) contended, and more recent research supports (Cook, 1985; Gaertner, Dovidio, & Bachman, 1996; Pettigrew & Tropp, 2000) that "optimal" contact interventions must contain four elements:

1   Equal status between groups. In the contact situation, neither the minority nor the majority group members occupy a higher status. Neither group is in charge. This differs from the type of contact certain power groups typically have with persons with mental illness (e.g., doctor/patient, landlord/resident, employer/employee).
2   Common goals. Both groups should be working toward the same ends. Some studies of "optimal" contact have used contrived tasks such as completing a puzzle (Desforges et al., 1991). In more natural settings, this might include working together on a community project or solving a neighborhood problem.
3   No competition. The tone of the contact should be a joint effort, not a competitive one.
4   Authority sanction for the contact. This might mean the contact intervention is sponsored or endorsed by management of an employment organization, or by particular community organizations (e.g., the Board of Education, Better Business Bureau).

Contact conditions that more closely approximate the four "optimal" conditions appear to produce the largest reductions in stigmatizing attitudes (Pettigrew & Tropp, 2000). However, even brief, less interactive contact strategies have produced promising results. For example, Corrigan et al. (2001b) randomized community college students to contact, protest, education and control conditions. The contact condition involved listening to a person with mental illness tell his or her story followed by a brief opportunity to ask questions. The authors found that the contact condition produced greater improvements in attitudes than protest, education, and control conditions. In a subsequent study, contact again produced greater improvements than education and control conditions (this study did not include a protest condition) in attitudes and behavior in the form of participant donations to NAMI (Corrigan et al., 2002). While significant but smaller improvements were observed for participants in the education condition, only the contact condition improvements were maintained at the one-week follow-up. While most of the research to date has been conducted with adults, there is evidence that contact is also effective for improving attitudes among school-aged children (Pinfold, Huxley, Thornicroft, Farmer, Toulmin, & Graham, 2002).

Contact approaches can be delivered in a variety of ways. The National Alliance on Mental Illness (NAMI) developed a contact-based anti-stigma program called *In Our Own Voice: Living with Mental Illness* (IOOV). Persons in recovery from mental illness who share their personal stories and interact with their audience in a structured format deliver the program. The IOOV program has been provided to law enforcement, schools, businesses, and other community groups. As of spring 2007, the IOOV program was active in 38 states and had been provided to over 200,000 people (National Alliance on Mental Illness, 2009b). The two studies of IOOV published to date suggest that it is effective for reducing stigma and improving knowledge about mental illness (Rusch, Kanter, Angelone, & Ridley, 2008; Wood & Wahl, 2006). Additional research is needed to determine the longer-term effects of this brief structured contact intervention.

Contact can also be incorporated into professional training programs. For example, the Chicago Police Department offers a 40-hour Crisis Intervention Team (CIT) in-service training designed to improve officers' knowledge and skills for responding to mental health crises. Instead of using professional actors for the role-play portion of the training, Chicago's CIT program has employed mental health consumer/actors from a local provider, Thresholds Psychiatric Rehabilitation Centers. The actors have personal experience with mental illness and have trained and performed with the Thresholds Theatre Arts Project. They participate in role-play scenarios of mental health crises and provide feedback to the officers. This contact approach is consistent with all four "optimal conditions": first, in the training setting, actors and officers are of equal status and both are getting paid to be there; second, actors and officers are working toward the common goal of improving officers' ability to safely and effectively respond to mental health crises; third, the groups are not competing; and fourth, the Chicago Police Department supports the contact. While this program has yet to be studied, anecdotally it has been a very powerful training and stigma reduction approach for the officers and the actors. The model has potential for training a variety of professionals that work with persons with mental illnesses.

Similar to the contact model used with police officers, Scheyett and Kim (2004) used a facilitated dialogue model that brought together persons with mental illnesses and social work students to discuss effective social worker/client partnerships. The evaluation of the intervention indicated that students' attitudes improved, they developed greater empathy, and they planned to make changes in their practice following the intervention. The participating consumers also benefited from the intervention and reported feeling positive about being valued and helping others.

Each of the above approaches has certain benefits and limitations for dealing with public stigma. Protest may be particularly effective for targeting a specific behavior, such as a stigmatizing representation of mental illness in the media or a particularly discriminatory practice of an organization. This approach, however, would be inappropriate for the goal of improving attitudes about mental illness. Educational approaches are relatively easy to disseminate via print or electronic media or even lectures to large groups and have been shown to improve attitudes and knowledge about mental illness. However, the effects of educational campaigns on attitudes do not seem to be particularly durable over time. Contact appears to be the most promising approach for improving attitudes and behaviors in the long term. However, contact is less exportable than other approaches. Formalized contact interventions require more resources and time to disseminate and pose some personal risk to the individuals who disclose their illness.

Many anti-stigma campaigns, including the examples above, incorporate elements of several strategies. For example, NAMI's StigmaBusters attempts to educate their targets about mental illness and the struggles of individuals and families that are affected by it. Many educational approaches are presented by persons with mental illness who share their own stories of recovery along with more general information about mental illness. Likewise, many people who disclose their own experiences with mental illness in contact interventions (or simply in their everyday lives) must educate their audience about mental illness.

A majority of the existing anti-stigma campaigns utilize an educational approach, either by itself or in conjunction with protest or contact. In an effort to reduce the blame associated with mental illness, many of these campaigns have focused on the biological model of mental illness. Educating the public that mental illnesses are biological diseases has been a popular approach. For example, NAMI launched its "Mental Illness is a Brain Disease" campaign in which it distributed posters, buttons, and literature that provided information about the biological basis of serious mental illness. "Brain disease," "illness like any other" and "genetic" messages seem to reduce blame for psychiatric illness (Corrigan et al., 2002; Farina, Fisher, Getter, & Fischer, 1978; Fisher & Farina, 1979, Lincoln, Arens, Berger, & Rief, 2008; Phelan, 2002). However, framing mental illness solely in biological terms may inadvertently exacerbate other components of stigma (Lincoln et al., 2008; Mehta & Farina, 1997; Phelan, 2002; Read & Law, 1999; Read, Haslam, Sayce, & Davies, 2006). For example, genetic or disease-based explanations of mental illnesses have been shown to increase perceptions of unpredictability and dangerousness, increase desire for social distance, and invoke harsher treatment (Lincoln et al., 2008; Mehta & Farina, 1997; Phelan, 2002; Read & Law, 1999; Read et al., 2006). Biological explanations may further promote the idea that persons with mental illnesses are fundamentally different from everyone else (Hinshaw & Stier, 2008), solidifying the distinction between "us" and "them" – a key component in the stigma process (Link & Phelan, 2001).

Biological explanations of mental illness may also yield unintended consequences by supporting the benevolence stigma; namely, the belief that persons with mental illness are innocent and childlike and, as such, must be taken care of and supervised by a more responsible party (Brockington et al., 1993). While well intentioned, this type of stigma can be disempowering, causing persons with mental illness (and others) to view themselves as different from other people, less competent, and less able to recover and fully participate in the community. Biological explanations may also imply that persons with mental illness have no control over their behavior, and therefore are unpredictable and violent (Read & Law, 1999).

In contrast to biological messages, several studies have found that psychosocial explanations of mental illness can be effective for increasing positive images of persons with mental illness and reducing fear. Psychosocial explanations of mental illness focus on environmental stressors and trauma as causal factors. The idea is to normalize psychiatric symptoms as understandable reactions to difficult life events (Read & Law, 1999). Psychosocial messages have been shown to be effective for improving attitudes with students and health professionals (Morrison, 1980; Morrison & Teta, 1979, 1980; Morrison, Becker, & Bourgeois, 1979) particularly those attitudes related to dangerousness and unpredictability (Read & Law, 1999). Framing mental illness as a disorder with both biological and psychosocial components exacerbated by stressful life events from which people can and do recover seems most effective. Such a combined approach more accurately reflects our current understanding of mental illness and has potential to address multiple components of public stigma. The particular balance of information should be tailored to the specific component(s) of stigma, behavior(s) and group(s) being targeted (Byrne, 2001).

These approaches for dealing with the public are also applicable for institutional and structural discrimination. By definition, institutional discrimination is the intentional result of policies and practices that aim to restrict the rights and opportunities of persons with mental illnesses (Pincus, 1996). Once the individuals with the power to change the targeted policies and practices are identified (not always an easy task), a specific strategy(s) and message can be developed. Often combined or multiple parallel or serial approaches are required.

If the targeted discriminatory practices violate anti-discrimination laws such as the Americans with Disabilities Act (ADA) or the Fair Housing Amendments Act of 1988, legal strategies may be useful. For example, the Bazelon Center for Mental Health Law and two private attorneys filed a lawsuit claiming George Washington University violated the rights of a student who voluntarily admitted himself for inpatient psychiatric treatment (Bazelon Center for Mental Health Law, 2006b). The next day, the student was informed that he was barred from returning to campus and, subsequently, he was suspended and charged with a disciplinary violation. The lawsuit was settled and George Washington University agreed to review and revise its policies. The Bazelon Center has successfully represented other students in similar situations and is currently developing guidelines and model policies to assist schools in responding to mental health needs of students in compliance with the ADA. Legal rulings in these cases along with other stigma-fighting strategies may allow students with mental health problems to stay in college and receive the treatment that they need. This could create informal contact opportunities within the university setting that further reduce public stigma.

Structural discrimination may be more complicated to address, as the specific problematic policies or structures do not intentionally restrict the rights and opportunities of persons with mental illness. Thus, the first step is to highlight the unintended consequence of a policy or practice for persons with mental illness. The next step involves convincing the people with the power to change the policy or practice that whatever benefits the policy has, they are not worth the cost or unintended negative effects for persons with mental illness. The task sounds daunting. However, working for social justice is what social workers do.

The emerging literature on *internalized and self-stigma* provides some direction for amelioration strategies. As previously discussed, alienation is the component most predictive of distress (Ritsher & Phelan, 2004). Conversely, lower alienation is associated with greater hope (Lysaker et al., 2006). Strategies that support people in rejecting stigmatized views of mental illness and help them build their social networks may be useful for reducing the negative consequences of internalized and self-stigma.

Hayward and Bright (1997) suggest three elements in an approach to reducing self-stigma: using cognitive approaches to assess and combat specific stigmatizing beliefs; promoting a holistic biopsychosocial conception of mental illness; and emphasizing mental health and illness as a continuum. Strategies incorporating cognitive-behavioral elements have shown promise (Knight, Wykes, & Hayward, 2006; Macinnes & Lewis, 2008). In one study, a six-week group intervention that combined cognitive techniques emphasizing the concept of unconditional self-acceptance with psycho-education was used with persons with serious mental illness (Macinnes & Lewis, 2008). While no control group was used, the results indicated reductions in self-stigma and improvements in self-esteem and general psychological health. Similarly, Knight et al. (2006) found a group-based CBT intervention yielded improvements in self-esteem, symptoms and general psychopathology. Working with people with substance use disorders, Luoma, Kohlenberg, Hayes, Bunting, and Rye (2008) found support for a six-hour intervention based on Acceptance and Commitment Therapy (ACT), another cognitive approach, in reducing levels of internalized stigma. While these studies are limited by small samples and lack of control or comparison groups, combined, they suggest that internalized/self-stigma can be changed and that cognitive and empowerment based approaches show promise.

Based on the emerging literature on self/internalized stigma and the needs they observed in the clinical populations they served, a team based out of the University of Maryland-Baltimore and the Department of Veterans Affairs Mental Illness Research, Education and Clinical Center (VISN-5 MIRECC) and the San Francisco VA, designed a nine session course, Resisting Internalized Stigma (RIS), for veterans receiving mental health services (Lucksted et al., 2009). RIS is a manualized group intervention that incorporates cognitive-behavioral theory and empowerment and recovery oriented principles. The goal is to help participants learn coping skills and strategies to counter internalized stigma. Topics covered in the intervention include: stigma and stereotypes, internalized stigma and automatic thoughts, strengthening the positive aspects of one's self-image to resist internalized stigma, dealing with discriminatory behavior, and increasing sense of belonging through positive social connections with others. Each session is structured to combine didactic lectures with cognitive and skill building techniques and interaction discussion. Two co-leaders facilitate small groups of between four and six veterans. Preliminary results of a pilot study of RIS are promising (Calmes, 2009). The RIS team is planning to conduct a randomized controlled trial of the intervention.

Illustration and discussion

Social workers practice with a variety of individuals, groups, and systems that experience stigmatization and oppression, including individuals with psychiatric disabilities. Throughout this chapter we have provided examples of situations where people with mental health conditions were stigmatized, and the effects this had on their quality of life. Social workers have the power to tackle the issue of stigma across multiple levels. An illustration follows of the multilevel effects of stigma against a person with schizophrenia. The authors illustrate and discuss how a social worker helped to empower this individual to deal with some of the problems he experienced due to social injustice and stigma related to housing.

John is an African American male who has been living with paranoid schizophrenia for the past 20 years. He was originally diagnosed with schizophrenia when he was 21, and has, with only limited success, spent years trying to stabilize his condition. To this day, John continues to hear voices that tell him people are out to get him. Due to his history of homelessness and minor non-violent criminal record, John is well known by the community. He also comes from a prominent family in the city, who continue to remain actively involved in his life and care.

Recently, John has been receiving services from a community mental health agency where social workers have been helping him cope with his psychiatric symptoms, access community resources, and gain skills needed for independent living. Currently residing in one of the agency-operated group homes, John has shown significant progress in cooking for himself, remembering to take his medication, and maintaining his personal hygiene. In fact, his family has visited the group home on a number of occasions, and John has cooked simple meals for them and the rest of the residents. They have remarked that he is doing better than they have ever seen in the past.

The social workers attributed John's progress to his desire to live independently in his own apartment. For many years John was homeless, and one of his greatest dreams is to have a place to call his own. He has consistently demonstrated the ability to live independently, with periodic support from mental health professionals and independent living specialists. The agency social worker worked with John to create a transition plan to facilitate his move to his own apartment. A critical component of this plan was John deciding where to live. He has been fortunate enough to receive a voucher for assistance with housing that is not tied to any single apartment complex. When traveling to look at different apartments, John found one that was perfect for him and located on a quiet, upscale neighborhood close to shopping, parks, and an elementary school. The building has been well taken care of over the years, its grounds beautifully manicured, and the apartments spacious and furnished. John immediately fell in love with the apartment complex. Fortunately, they had an opening for a one-bedroom apartment that he was able to afford with his housing voucher. All that seemed to be needed was to help John fill out the application for housing at the complex. After returning to the mental health center, the worker assisted John in completing and mailing the housing application.

Several weeks went by without any word from the apartment complex. The social worker suggested that John call their business office during the day to check on the status of his application. When he called the complex, the receptionist indicated that they had no application from him. Frustrated, but persistent, John bused to the apartment complex and requested another housing application. The business office personnel indicated that apartment applications were unavailable; although several apartments were vacant in the building. The worker suspected prejudice and discrimination. With John's permission, the social worker called the apartment complex, requesting to speak to a supervisor.

After some prodding, the social worker finally reached a supervisor who informed her that while apartments were available, she had been pressured by the tenant's board at the complex, as well as the neighborhood homeowners association, about John's potential move to the area. Apparently, when visiting the apartment complex, a number of residents recognized John, and stated that they did not want a "homeless schizo" living in their building. The neighborhood homeowners banded together, expressing concerns about John living so close to where many of their children attend elementary school. They pointed out that, they had recently read a news report where a person with schizophrenia was caught attempting to kidnap a child from an elementary school. Knowing that legally they cannot refuse John housing because of his disability, the supervisor stated that living in this neighborhood would be difficult for John. The tenants all know him, as do many of the neighborhood residents, and they would make it very difficult for him.

After the phone conversation ended, the social worker considered her options. Should she share with John the supervisor's warning and suggest he consider finding someplace else to live? Or, should she simply ignore the supervisor's warning, obtain an application, and hope for the best? The social worker decided to share the supervisor's warning with John and explore their options. She realized that would be a very painful conversation, as John has experienced years of ridicule on the streets of downtown. The worker enlisted John's family for support and called a meeting with John and his family to discuss the current situation. She shared the entire scenario and informed John and his family that many people were misinformed about mental illness and acted unduly negatively toward people with mental difficulty. John became visibly upset and anxious. The worker reached for his reactions. He responded that he has always been afraid of groups of people being out to get him, and that it was unfair. Now that he was doing so well, he had hoped that he would not have to worry about this as much. John remained adamant about wanting to live in the apartment complex. John's family fully supported his goals. The social worker connected John to a local peer support and advocacy group. This group had experienced numerous successes in advocating in behalf of mentally disabled clients. After meeting John and discussing the prejudice and discrimination he experienced, group members leant a great deal of support, and agreed to advocate for him. John, a few group members, the social worker and a lawyer visited the apartment complex and successfully obtained an apartment. Group members spend several evenings a week with John at his new apartment to provide companionship and assist him with the transition toward independent living. John was grateful for the support and practical assistance.

While the social worker is very pleased about the positive outcome, she felt her job to be incomplete and engaged John in developing strategies to deal with community attitudes. She suggested several indirect interventions that would educate the apartment complex and local neighborhood residents about mental illness. They discussed the agency's outreach program, which educates the community on mental illness and stigma. John willingly supported the outreach efforts. The agency partnered with the National Alliance on Mental Illness (NAMI) and arranged to be involved in the local community's homeowners association meeting as well as a community meeting held at the elementary school for parents whose children live in the neighborhood. At these meetings, staff presented information that dispelled common inaccurate beliefs about mental illness. Mentally ill members of the support group who successfully lived in their own apartment presented their own stories on how living independently positively affected their lives, and engaged the community constituents in an open dialog about their concerns. While John was not ready to participate, he attentively attended these meetings and offered his future participation. NAMI also placed information fliers on mental illness in the mailboxes of all the residents at the apartment complex. While these interventions did not eliminate all misperceptions about mental illness, they began a process of reeducation of community members and reduction of some of the stigma John was likely to experience.

Knowing that the transition would be difficult for John, the social worker put in place a continued monitoring and assessment plan to ensure that John was able to maintain his independent living skills. John accepted that would need help and realized that ongoing support and monitoring were an essential part of his first steps toward living on his own. While John appreciated the ongoing support and monitoring for the first six months, he looked forward to being able to live on his own. The family and group members continued to represent major sources of support.

John's housing experience illustrates a relatively common problem that occurs in the lives of many people with mental illness. When communities learn of the prospect of an individual or group of individuals with a serious mental illness moving into their neighborhood, they resist. People fear violence, poor care of residences, and negative changes to the community.

Throughout the case illustration, the social worker continually demonstrated critical practice skills. Although the situation could have been resolved by referring John to another housing complex, the social worker responded to John's desires and goals. Realizing that people with mental illness often feel disempowered and stigmatized, she was committed to personal, interpersonal and structural empowerment. She always kept John at the center of the decision-making process, making sure that she herself did not contribute to the disempowerment John experienced.

The social workers' assessments and interventions moved across multiple levels, beginning with John, his family, support group and progressively toward the community. She went from John, "the case" to all the people with mental illness living in this community, "the cause." The social work professional realizes that mental illnesses and the associated stereotypes are not problems isolated to individuals, but profoundly affects the family, community, and larger society in critical ways that require for multilevel interventions. While prejudice and social stigma ultimately affect the individual, they represent societal problems, and, therefore, calls for community and societal-level interventions.

In summary, this practice illustration demonstrates the multilevel effects of stigma on individuals with mental illness, their families, and society. These effects call for multilevel interventions that should not be limited to either the individual or society, but should systematically address the effects of stigma across multiple levels and systems. In all assessment and intervention practices, the social worker must remain acutely aware of his/her own stereotypes that can severely disempower clients. By empowering the client and working across multiple system levels, the social worker has the potential to influence society's views, and ultimately improve the lives of people with mental illnesses.

Conclusion

In this chapter, we defined mental illness stigma as a process that results in the oppression and marginalization of persons with mental illness. Recent research suggests that mental illness stigma persists and impacts the lives of people on several levels and in multiple life domains. Public and structural stigma deprives people with mental illness of social and economic opportunities, and creates significant barriers to building a fulfilling and productive life in the community. Self and internalized stigma undermines the self-worth and self-efficacy needed to pursue a quality life.

Fortunately, there is hope. Some aspects of public attitudes are improving and we are learning more about effective strategies for reducing stigma and discrimination and helping people resist and cope when faced with it. Protest, education and contact can all play significant roles in combating both specific instances of stigma and discrimination as well as more general societal misconceptions and discriminatory practices. Strategies incorporating cognitive-behavioral techniques and peer support show particular promise for strengthening stigma resistance and coping skills. Whatever levels, domains and instances of stigma and discrimination we choose to deal with, and whichever approaches and strategies we select, we must do this in partnership with the people whose lives we hope to improve.

Social work professional values and training position us well to confront mental illness stigma and discrimination at multiple levels of practice. Whether we are working with individual, families, groups, communities or organizations, we have the opportunity and responsibility to reduce mental illness stigma and discrimination and promote opportunities for fulfilling and productive lives for persons with mental illnesses. The first step is to examine one's own biases. Social workers are not immune to being prejudiced and it may not be possible to completely eliminate stigmatizing thoughts and feelings. However, we can self-monitor and deal with our own prejudices and strive to minimize their impact on our practice. The next step involves determining the type and targets of our stigma efforts. Then we can select a strategy or strategies. This will vary depending on the type of stigma; specific stereotypes, behaviors, or structures; and target audience. Finally, we must evaluate our practice to determine if our intervention has been effective or if modifications are in order.

Note

1   Note that some groups reject the term "stigma" based on the implications that the "mark" is viewed as residing in or owned by the stigmatized person. This could direct attention and blame away from the stigmatizers. Our use of the term stigma does not intend to imply the recipients of stigmatization own the problem. Rather, the definition above defines stigma as a process owned by those with the power to stigmatize and the social structures they perpetuate.

Web resources

Judge David L. Bazelon Center for Mental Health Law
www.bazelon.org

Mental Health America
www.nmha.org/

National Alliance on Mental Illness
www.nami.org/

NAMI StigmaBusters
www.nami.org/template.cfm?section=Fight_Stigma

SAMHSA's Resource Center to Promote Acceptance, Dignity and Social Inclusion Associated with Mental Health (ADS Center)
www.stopstigma.samhsa.gov/

World Psychiatric Association – Open the Doors Global Program
www.open-the-doors.com/english/01_01.html

References

Allport, G. (1954). *The nature of prejudice*. Cambridge, MA: Addison Wesley.

Arikan, K., & Uysal, O. (1999). Emotional reactions to the mentally ill are positively influenced by personal acquaintance. *Israel Journal of Psychiatry and Related Sciences, 36* (2), 100–104.

Barrowclough, C., Haddock, G., Lowens, I., Connor, A., Pidliswyj, J., & Tracey, N. (2001). Staff expressed emotion and causal attributions for client problems on a low security unit: An exploratory study. *Schizophrenia Bulletin, 27* (3), 517–526.

Bazelon Center for Mental Health Law. (2006a). *Student punished for getting help*. Retrieved May 13, 2009, from www.bazelon.org/newsroom/archive/2006/3-13-06-Nott.html

Bazelon Center for Mental Health Law. (2006b). *Student and university settle lawsuit on mental health issues*. Retrieved May 22, 2009, from www.bazelon.org/newsroom/archive/2006/10-3006NottSettle.html

Brockington, I.F., Hall, P., Levings, J., & Murphy, C. (1993). The community's tolerance of the mentally ill. *British Journal of Psychiatry, 162*, 93–99.

Burton, V.S. (1990). The consequences of official labels: A research note on rights lost by the mentally ill, mentally incompetent, and convicted felons. *Community Mental Health Journal, 26* (3), 267–276.

Byrne, P. (2001). Psychiatric stigma. *British Journal of Psychiatry, 178*, 281–284.

Calmes, C. (2009). Resisting internalized stigma intervention. *MIRECC Matters, 10* (2), 1–2.

Capriccioso, R. (2006). *Counseling crisis: Inside higher ed*. Retrieved May 13, 2009, from www.inside highered.com/news/2006/03/13/counseling

Cohen, J., & Struening, E. (1962). Opinions about mental illness in the personnel of two large mental hospitals. *Journal of Abnormal Psychology, 64*, 349–360.

Cook, S.W. (1985). Experimenting on social issues: The case of school desegregation. *American Psychologist, 40*, 452–460.

Cooper, A., Corrigan, P.W., & Watson, A.C. (2003). Mental illness stigma and care seeking. *Journal of Nervous and Mental Disease, 191*, 339–341.

Corrigan, P.W., & McCracken, S.G. (1997). Intervention research: Integrating practice guidelines with dissemination strategies – A rejoinder to Paul, Stuve, and Cross. *Applied & Preventive Psychology, 6*, 205–209.

Corrigan, P.W., & Penn, D.L. (1999). Lessons from social psychology on discrediting psychiatric stigma. *American Psychologist, 54*, 765–776.

Corrigan, P.W., & Watson, A.C. (2002). The paradox of self-stigma and mental illness. *Clinical Psychology: Science and Practice, 9*, 35–53.

Corrigan, P.W., & Watson, A.C. (2007). The stigma of psychiatric disorders and the gender, ethnicity and education of the perceiver. *Community Mental Health Journal, 43*, 439–458.

Corrigan, P.W., River, L.P., Lundin, R.K., Wasowski, K.U., Campion, J., Mathisen, J. et al. (2000). Stigmatizing attributions about mental illness. *Journal of Community Psychology, 28* (1), 91–102.

Corrigan, P.W., Backs-Edwards, A., Green, A., Diwan, S.E., & Penn, D.L. (2001a). Prejudice, social distance, and familiarity with mental illness. *Schizophrenia Bulletin, 27*, 219–226.

Corrigan, P.W., River, L., Lundin, R.K., Penn, D.L., Uphoff-Wasowski, K., Campion, J. et al. (2001b). Three strategies for changing attributions about severe mental illness. *Schizophrenia Bulletin, 27*, 187–195.

Corrigan, P.W., Rowan, D., Green, A., Lundin, R., River, P., Uphoff-Wasowski, K. et al. (2002). Challenging two mental illness stigmas: Personal responsibility and dangerousness. *Schizophrenia Bulletin, 28*, 293–310.

Corrigan, P.W, Markowitz, F.E., & Watson, A.C. (2004). Structural levels of mental illness stigma and discrimination. *Schizophrenia Bulletin, 30*, 187–195.

Crocker, J., Major, B., & Steele, C. (1998). Social stigma. In D. Gilbert, S.T. Fiske, & G. Lindzey (eds), *The handbook of social psychology, Vol. 2* (4th ed., pp. 504–553). New York: McGraw-Hill.

Crowther, R.E., Marshall, M., Bond, G.R., & Huxley, P. (2001). Helping people with severe mental illness to obtain work: Systematic review. *British Medical Journal, 322*, 204–208.

Desforges, D.M., Lord, C.G., Ramsey, S.L., Mason, J.A., Van Leeuwen, M.D., West, S.C. et al. (1991). Effects of structured cooperative contact on changing negative attitudes toward stigmatized social groups. *Journal of Personality and Social Psychology, 60*, 531–544.

Devine, P.G. (1989). Stereotypes and prejudice: Their automatic and controlled components. *Journal of Personality and Social Psychology, 56*, 5–18.

Devine, P.G. (1995). Prejudice and out-group perception. In A. Tessor (ed.), *Advanced social psychology* (pp. 467–524). New York: McGraw-Hill.

Drehmer, D., & Bordieri, J. (1985). Hiring decisions for disabled workers: The hidden bias. *Rehabilitation Psychology, 30*, 157–164.

Druss, B.G., Bradford, D.W., Rosenheck, R.A., Radford, M.J., & Krumholz, H.M. (2000). Mental disorders and use of cardiovascular procedures after myocardial infarction. *JAMA: Journal of the American Medical Association, 283*, 506–511.

Eack, S.M., & Newhill, C.E. (2008). An investigation of the relations between student knowledge, personal contact, and attitudes toward individuals with schizophrenia. *Journal of Social Work Education, 44* (3), 77–95.

Farina, A., & Felner, R.D. (1973). Employment interviewer reactions to former mental patients. *Journal of Abnormal Psychology, 82*, 268–272.

Farina, A., Fisher, J.D., Getter, H., & Fischer, E.H. (1978). Some consequences of changing people's views regarding the nature of mental illness. *Journal of Abnormal Psychology, 87*, 272–279.

Farkas, M., Gagne, C., Anthony, W., & Chamberlin, J. (2005). Implementing recovery oriented evidence based programs: Identifying the critical dimensions. *Community Mental Health Journal, 41* (2), 141–158.

Fisher, J.D., & Farina, A. (1979). Consequences of beliefs about the nature of mental disorders. *Journal of Abnormal Psychology, 88* (3), 320–327.

Forchuk, C., Nelson, N., & Hall, G.B. (2006). "It's important to be proud of the place you live in." Housing problems and preferences of psychiatric survivors. *Perspectives in Psychiatric Care, 42* (1), 42–52.

Frank, R.G., & Glied, S.A. (2006). *Better but not well: Mental health policy in the United States since 1950.* Baltimore, MD: Johns Hopkins University Press.

Fyock, J., & Stangor, C. (1994). The role of memory biases in stereotype maintenance. *British Journal of Social Psychology, 33*, 331–344.

Gaertner, S.L., Dovidio, J.F., & Bachman, B.A. (1996). Revisiting the contact hypothesis: The induction of a common ingroup identity. *International Journal of Intercultural Relations, 20*, 271–290.

Gitterman, A., & Germain, C.B. (2008). *The life model of social work practice: Advances in theory and practice* (3rd ed.). New York: Columbia University Press.

Goffman, E. (1963). *Stigma: Notes on the management of spoiled identity.* New York: Simon & Schuster.

Hamilton, D.L., & Sherman, J.W. (1994). Stereotypes. In R.S. Wyer & T.K. Srull (eds), *Handbook of social cognition, Vol. 2* (2nd ed., pp. 1–68). Hillsdale, NJ: Lawrence Erlbaum Associates.

Harding, C.M., Zubin, J., & Strauss, J.S. (1992). Chronicity in schizophrenia: Revisited. *British Journal of Psychiatry, 18*, 27–37

Hayward, P., & Bright, J.A. (1997). Stigma and mental illness: A review and critique. *Journal of Mental Health, 6*, 345–354.

Hemmens, C., Miller, M., Burton, V.S., & Milner, S. (2002). The consequences of official labels: An examination of the rights lost by the mentally ill and the mentally incompetent ten years later. *Community Mental Health Journal, 38* (2), 129–140.

Hilton, J.L., & von Hippel, W. (1996). Stereotypes. *Annual Review of Psychology, 47*, 237–271.

Hinshaw, S.P., & Stier, A. (2008). Stigma as related to mental disorders. *Annual Review of Clinical Psychology, 4*, 367–393.

Hogan, M.F. (2003). New Freedom Commission Report: The President's New Freedom Commission – Recommendations to transform mental health care in America. *Psychiatric Services, 54*, 1467–1474.

Holmes, E., Corrigan, P.W., Williams, P., Canar, J., & Kubiak, M.A. (1999). Changing attitudes about schizophrenia. *Schizophrenia Bulletin, 25*, 447–456.

Hyler, S.E., Gabbard, G.O., & Schneider, I. (1991). Homicidal maniacs and narcissistic parasites: Stigmatization of mentally ill persons in the movies. *Hospital and Community Psychiatry, 42*, 1044–1048.

Jones, E.E., Farina, A., Hastorf, A.H., Markus, H., Miller, D.T., & Scott, R.A. (1984). *Social stigma: The psychology of marked relationships.* New York: Freeman.

Judd, C.M., & Park, B. (1993). Definition and assessment of accuracy in social stereotypes. *Psychological Review, 100*, 109–128.

Kahng, S., & Mowbray, C.T. (2005). Psychological traits and behavioral coping of psychiatric consumers: The mediating role of self-esteem. *Health and Social Work, 30* (2), 87–97.

Keane, M.C. (1991). Acceptance vs. rejection: Nursing students' attitudes about mental illness. *Perspectives in Psychiatric Care, 27*, 13–18.

Kessler, R.C., Berglund, P.A., Bruce, M.L., Koch, J.R., Laska, E.M., Leaf, P.J. et al. (2001). The prevalence and correlates of untreated serious mental illness. *Health Services Research, 36* (6, pt 1), 987–1007.

Knight, M.T.D., Wykes, T., & Hayward, P. (2006). Group treatment of perceived stigma and self-esteem in schizophrenia: A waiting list trial of efficacy. *Behavioural and Cognitive Psychotherapy, 34* (3), 305–318.

Lincoln, T.M., Arens, E., Berger, C., & Rief, W. (2008). Can antistigma campaigns be improved? A test of the impact of biogenetic vs. psychosocial causal explanations on implicit and explicit attitudes to schizophrenia. *Schizophrenia Bulletin, 34*, 984–994.

Link, B.G., & Phelan, J.C. (2001). Conceptualizing stigma. *Annual Review of Sociology, 27*, 363–385.

Link, B.G., Cullen, F.T., Frank, J., & Wozniak, J.F. (1987). The social rejection of former mental patients: Understanding why labels matter. *American Journal of Sociology, 92*, 1461–1500.

Link, B.G., Andrews, H., & Cullen, F.T. (1992). The violent and illegal behavior of mental patients reconsidered. *American Sociological Review, 52*, 96–112.

Link, B.G., Phelan, J.C., Bresnahan, M., Stueve, A., & Pescosolido, B.A. (1999). Public conceptions of mental illness: Labels, causes, dangerousness, and social distance. *American Journal of Public Health, 89*, 1328–1333.

Link, B.G., Struening, E., Neese-Todd, S., Asmussen, S., & Phelan, J. (2001). Stigma as a barrier to recovery: The consequences of stigma for the self-esteem of people with mental illnesses. *Psychiatric Services, 52*, 1621–1626.

Lucksted, A., Drapalski, A., Boyd, J., DeForge, B., Calmes, C., Forbes, C. et al. (2009). *Resisting Internalized Stigma: A nine session class for individuals receiving mental health services.* VA VISN-5 MIRECC. Baltimore, MD. For more information contact aluckste@psych.umaryland.edu

Luoma, J.B., Kohlenberg, B.S., Hayes, S.C., Bunting, K., & Rye, A.K. (2008). Reducing self-stigma in substance abuse through acceptance and commitment therapy: Model, manual development and pilot outcomes. *Addiction Research and Theory, 16* (2), 149–165.

Lysaker, P.H., Buck, K.D., Hammoud, K., Taylor, A.C., & Roe, D. (2006). Associations of symptoms, psychosocial function and hope with qualities of self-experience in schizophrenia: Comparisons of objective and subjective indicators of health. *Schizophrenia Research, 82* (2–3), 241–249.

Macinnes, D.L., & Lewis, M. (2008). Evaluation of a short group programme to reduce self stigma in people with serious and enduring mental health problems. *Journal of Psychiatric and Mental Health Nursing, 15*, 59–65.

Macrae, C., Bodenhausen, G.V., Milne, A.B., & Jetten, J. (1994). Out of mind but back in sight: Stereotypes on the rebound. *Journal of Personality and Social Psychology, 67*, 808–817.

Magliano, L., De Rosa, C., Fiorillo, A., Malangone, C., Guarneri, M., Marasco, C. et al. (2004). Beliefs of psychiatric nurses about schizophrenia: A comparison with patients' relatives and psychiatrists. *International Journal of Social Psychiatry, 50* (4), 319–330.

Manning, C., & White, P.D. (1995). Attitudes of employers to the mentally ill. *Psychiatric Bulletin, 19*, 541–543.

Markowitz, F.E. (1998). The effects of stigma on the psychological well-being and life satisfaction of persons with mental illness. *Journal of Health and Social Behavior, 39* (4), 335–347.

Martin, J.K., Pescosolido, B.A., & Tuch, S.A. (2000). Of fear and loathing: The role of "disturbing behavior," labels, and causal attributions in shaping public attitudes toward people with mental illness. *Journal of Health and Social Behavior, 41*, 208–223.

Mechanic, D., Bilder, S., & McAlpine, D.D. (2002). Employing persons with serious mental illness. *Health Affairs, 21* (5), 242–253.

Mehta, S., & Farina, A. (1997). Is being "sick" really better? Effect of the disease view of mental disorder on stigma. *Journal of Social and Clinical Psychology, 16*, 405–419.

Morrison, J.K. (1980). The public's current beliefs about mental illness: Serious obstacle to effective community psychology. *American Journal of Community Psychology, 8*, 697–707.

Morrison, J.K., & Teta, D.C. (1979). Impact of a humanistic approach on students' attitudes, attributions, and ethical conflicts. *Psychological Reports, 45,* 863–866.

Morrison, J.K., & Teta, D.C. (1980). Reducing students' fear of mental illness by means of seminar-induced belief change. *Journal of Clinical Psychology, 36,* 275–276.

Morrison, J.K., Becker, R.E., & Bourgeois, C.A. (1979). Decreasing adolescents' fear of mental patients by means of demythologizing. *Psychological Reports, 44,* 855–859.

Mowbray, C.T., Megivern, D., Mandiberg, J.M., Strauss S., Stein, C.H., Collins, K. et al., (2006). Campus mental health services: Recommendations for change. *American Journal of Orthopsychiatry, 76* (2), 226–237.

Murray, M.G., & Steffen, J.J. (1999). Attitudes of case managers toward people with serious mental illness. *Community Mental Health Journal, 35* (6), 505–514.

National Alliance on Mental Illness (NAMI). (2009a). *NAMI StigmaBusters.* Retrieved June 1, 2009, from www.nami.org/template.cfm?section=fight_stigma

National Alliance on Mental Illness (NAMI). (2009b). *In our own Voice: Living with mental illness.* Retrieved June 1, 2009, from www.namiorg/Template.cfm?Section=In_Our_Own_Voice&Template=/Content Management/ContentDisplay.cfm&ContentID=48516

National Mental Health Campaign. (2002). Retrieved May, 2002 from www.nostigma.org.

Newhill, C.E., & Korr, W.S. (2004). Practice with people with severe mental illness: Rewards, challenges, burdens. *Health and Social Work, 29* (4), 297–305.

Page, S. (1977). Effects of the mental illness label in attempts to obtain accommodation. *Canadian Journal of Behavioral Science, 9,* 85–90.

Pate, G.S. (1988). Research on reducing prejudice. *Social Education, 52,* 287–289.

Penn, D.L., & Corrigan, P.W. (2002). The effects of stereotype suppression on psychiatric stigma. *Schizophrenia Research, 55,* 269–276.

Penn, D.L., Guynan, K., Daily, T., Spaulding, W.D., Garbin, C.P., & Sullivan, M. (1994). Dispelling the stigma of schizophrenia: What sort of information is best? *Schizophrenia Bulletin, 20,* 567–578.

Penn, D.L., Kommana, S., Mansfield, M., & Link, B.G. (1999). Dispelling the stigma of schizophrenia: II. The impact of information on dangerousness. *Schizophrenia Bulletin, 25,* 437–446.

Perkins, D.V., Raines, J.A., Tschopp, M.K., & Warner, T.C. (2009). Gainful employment reduces stigma toward people recovering from schizophrenia. *Community Mental Health Journal, 45* (3), 158–162.

Perlick, D.A., Rosenheck, R.A., Clarkin, J.F., Sirey, J.O., Salahi, J., Struening, E.L. et al. (2001). Stigma as a barrier to recovery: Adverse effects of perceived stigma on social adaptation of persons diagnosed with bipolar affective disorder. *Psychiatric Services, 52,* 1627–1632.

Pescosolido, B.A., Monahan, J., Link, B.G., Steuve, A., & Kikuzawa, S. (1999). The public's view of the competence, dangerousness, and need for legal coercion of persons with mental health problems. *American Journal of Public Health, 89,* 1339–1345.

Pettigrew, T.F., & Tropp, L.R. (2000). Does intergroup contact reduce prejudice: Recent meta-analytic findings. In S. Oskamp (ed.), *Reducing Prejudice and Discrimination* (pp. 93–114). Mahwah, NJ: Lawrence Erlbaum Associates.

Phelan, J.C. (2002). Genetic bases of mental illness: A cure for stigma? *Trends in Neurosciences, 25* (8), 430–431.

Phelan, J.C., & Link, B.G. (2004). Fear of people with mental illnesses: the role of personal and impersonal contact and exposure to threat or harm. *Journal of Health and Social Behavior, 45,* 68–80.

Phelan, J.C., Link, B.G., Stueve, A., & Pescosolido, B.A. (2000). Public conceptions of mental illness in 1950 and 1996: What is mental illness and is it to be feared? *Journal of Health & Social Behavior, 41,* 188–207.

Pincus, F.L. (1996). Discrimination comes in many forms: Individual, institutional and structural. *American Behavioral Scientist, 40* (2), 186–194.

Pinfold, V., Huxley, P., Thornicroft, G., Farmer, P., Toulmin, H., & Graham, T. (2002). Reducing psychiatric stigma and discrimination: Evaluating an educational intervention with the police force in England. Unpublished manuscript.

Pruegger, V.J., & Rogers, T.B. (1994). Cross-cultural sensitivity training: Methods and Assessment. *International Journal of Intercultural Relations, 18,* 369–387.

Read, J., & Law, A. (1999). The relationship of causal beliefs and contact with users of mental health services to attitudes to the "Mentally Ill". *International Journal of Social Psychiatry, 45*, 216–229.

Read, J., Haslam, N., Sayce, L., & Davies, E. (2006). Prejudice and schizophrenia: A review of the "mental illness is an illness like any other" approach. *Acta Psychiatrica Scandinavica, 114*, 303–318.

Regier, D.A., Narrow, W.E., Rae, D.S., Manderscheid, R.W., Locke, B.Z., & Goodwin, F.K. (1993). The de facto U.S. mental and addictive disorders service system: Epidemiological catchment area prospective 1-year prevalence rates of disorders and services. *Archives of General Psychiatry, 50*, 85–94

Ritsher, J.B., & Phelan, J.C. (2004). Internalized stigma predicts erosion of morale among psychiatric outpatients. *Psychiatry Research, 129* (3), 257–265.

Roeloffs, C., Sherbourne, C., Unutzer, J., Fink, A., Tang, L., & Wells, K.B. (2003). Stigma and depression among primary care patients. *General Hospital Psychiatry, 25* (5), 311–315.

Rusch, L.C., Kanter, J.W., Angelone, A.F., & Ridley, R.C. (2008). The impact of In Our Own Voice on stigma. *American Journal of Psychiatric Rehabilitation, 11*(4), 373–389.

Sartorius, N., & Schulze, H. (2005). *Reducing the stigma of mental illness: A report from a Global Programme of the World Psychiatric Association.* Cambridge: Cambridge University Press.

Scheid, T.L. (1999). Employment of individuals with mental disabilities: Business response to the ADA's challenge. *Behavioral Sciences and the Law, 17* (1), 73–91.

Scheyett, A. (2005). The mark of madness: Stigma, serious mental illnesses and social work. *Social Work in Mental Health, 3* (4), 79–97.

Scheyett, A., & Kim, M. (2004). Can we talk? Using facilitated dialogue to positively change student attitudes toward persons with mental illness. *Journal of Teaching in Social Work, 24* (1), 39–54.

Schnittker, J. (2000). Gender and reactions to the mentally ill: An examination of social tolerance and perceived dangerousness. *Journal of Health and Social Behavior, 41* (2), 234–240.

Schnittker, J., Freese, J., & Powell, B. (1999). Nature, nurture, neither, nor: Black-White differences in beliefs about the cause and appropriate treatment of mental illness. *Social Forces, 78*, 1101–1132.

Sirey, J.A., Bruce, M.L., Alexopoulos, G.S., Perlick, D.A., Friedman, S.J., & Meyers, B.S. (2001). Stigma as a barrier to recovery: Perceived stigma and patient-rated severity of illness as predictors of antidepressant drug adherence. *Psychiatric Services, 52* (12), 1615–1620.

Snyder, K.S., Wallace, C.J., Moe, K., & Liberman, R.P. (1994). Expressed emotion by residential care operators and residents' symptoms and quality of life. *Hospital and Community Psychiatry, 45* (11), 1141–1143.

Stangor, C., & McMillan, D. (1992). Memory for expectancy-congruent and expectancy-incongruent information: A review of the social and social developmental literatures. *Psychological Bulletin, 111*, 42–61.

Star, S.A. (1952). *What the public thinks about mental health and mental illness.* Paper presented at the annual meeting of the National Association of Mental Health, Indianapolis.

Star, S.A. (1955). *The public's ideas about mental illness.* Chicago, IL: National Opinion Research Center.

Steadman, H.J., Mulvey, E.P., Monahan, J., Robbins, P.C., Appelbaum, P.S., Grisso, T. et al. (1998). Violence by people discharged from acute psychiatric inpatient facilities and by others in the same neighborhoods. *Archives of General Psychiatry, 55* (5), 393–401.

Stuart, H. (2006). Mental illness and employment discrimination. *Current Opinion in Psychiatry, 19* (5), 522–526.

Substance Abuse and Mental Health Services Administration (SAMHSA). (2001). *Mental health, United States: 2000.* Washington, DC: SAMHSA.

Taylor, S., & Dear, M.J. (1981). Scaling community attitudes toward the mentally ill. *Schizophrenia Bulletin, 7*, 225–240.

Teplin, L.A., McClelland, G.A., Abram, K.A., & Weiner, D.A. (2005). Crime victimization in adults with severe mental illness: Comparison with the national crime victimization survey. *Archives of General Psychiatry, 62* (8), 911–921.

Tsuang, M.T., Woolson, R.F., & Fleming, J.A. (1979). Long-term outcome of major psychoses. *Archives of General Psychiatry, 36*, 1295–1301.

U.S. Department of Health and Human Services. (1999). *Mental health: A report of the Surgeon General – executive summary.* Rockville, MD: U.S. Department of Health and Human Services, Substance Abuse and Mental Health Services Administration, Center for Mental Health Services, National Institutes of Health, National Institute of Mental Health.

Van Audenhove, C., & Van Humbeeck, G. (2003). Expressed emotion in professional relationships. *Current Opinion in Psychiatry, 16* (4), 431–435.

Van Dorn, R.A., Swanson, J.W., Elbogen, E.B., & Swartz, M.S. (2005). A comparison of stigmatizing attitudes toward persons with schizophrenia in four stakeholder groups: Perceived likelihood of violence and desire for social distance. *Psychiatry: Interpersonal and Biological Processes, 68* (2), 152–163.

Wahl, O. F. (1995). *Media madness: Public images of mental illness.* New Brunswick, NJ: Rutgers University Press.

Wahl, O.F. (1999). *Telling is risky business: The experience of mental illness stigma.* New Brunswick, NJ: Rutgers University Press.

Watson, A.C., & Corrigan, P.W. (2005). Changing public stigma: A targeted approach. In P.W. Corrigan (ed.), *A comprehensive review of the stigma of mental illness: Implications for research and social change* (pp. 281–295). Washington, DC: American Psychological Association.

Watson, A.C., & River, L.P. (2005). From self stigma to empowerment. In P.W. Corrigan (ed.), *A comprehensive review of the stigma of mental illness: Implications for research and social change* (pp. 145–164). Washington, DC: American Psychological Association.

Watson, A.C., Corrigan, P.W., Larson, J.E., & Sells, M. (2007). Self stigma in people with mental illness. *Schizophrenia Bulletin, 33* (6), 1312–1318.

Webber, A., & Orcutt, J.D. (1984). Employer's relations to racial and psychiatric stigmata: A field experiment. *Deviant Behavior, 5*, 327–336.

WHO Regional Office for Europe. (2005). *Mental health: Facing the challenges, building solutions.* Report from the WHO European Ministerial Conference. EURO Nonserial Publication. Geneva: WHO.

Wood, A.L., & Wahl, O.F. (2006). Evaluating the effectiveness of a consumer-provided mental health recovery education presentation. *Psychiatric Rehabilitation Journal, 30* (1), 46–53.

Wright, E.R., Wright, D.E., Perry, B.L., & Foote-Ardah, C.E. (2007). Stigma and the sexual isolation of people with serious mental illness. *Social Problems, 54* (1), 78–98.

Zippay A. (2007). Psychiatric residences: Notification, NIMBY, and neighborhood relations. *Psychiatric Services, 58*, 109–113.

3 Poverty and its effects

Mark R. Rank

Poverty is a fundamentally important issue for the practice of social work. It underlies many of the social problems that social workers encounter on a daily basis. One such area is the quality of an individual's mental health. This chapter is divided into three sections. First, the nature and scope of poverty in the United States are discussed. This includes ways of measuring and conceptualizing poverty, and an overview of the likelihood and prevalence of poverty in the United States. We then turn to a discussion of the relationship between poverty and mental health. The strength of the association between the two is first reviewed. Next, we take up the question of causality, that is, to what extent does poverty lead to a decline in mental health, and to what extent does compromised mental health lead to poverty? Finally, we explore some of the intrinsic aspects of poverty that are related to a deterioration of mental health.

The third section of the chapter provides a case example that illustrates the relationship between poverty and mental health. It is taken from an interview with a single mother in poverty, and was one of a number of interviews that were conducted for an earlier book focusing on the conditions and circumstances of surviving on public assistance in the United States (Rank, 1994a). Throughout the chapter, the focus is primarily on poverty and mental health within an American context.

Definitions of poverty

Poverty has been *conceptualized and measured* in a number of different ways. Over 200 years ago, Adam Smith in his landmark treatise, *Wealth of Nations* (1776), defined poverty as a lack of those necessities that "the custom of the country renders it indecent for creditable people, even of the lowest order, to be without." This type of definition is what is known as an absolute approach to defining poverty. A minimum threshold for basic living conditions is determined, and individuals falling below such a threshold are considered poor. An example of this approach is the manner in which the official poverty line is currently drawn in the United States (Blank, 2008; Citro & Michael, 1995). The U.S. poverty line is calculated by estimating the income needed for different sizes of households to obtain what is considered a minimally adequate basket of goods and services for the year. In 2008, a family of four was considered in poverty if their total income fell below $22,025 (U.S. Census Bureau, 2009). Much of the research reviewed in this chapter uses the official poverty line (or a variation of the line) as a working definition of poverty.

Alternatively, poverty can be constructed in a relative rather than an absolute sense (Brady, 2003). A frequently used relative measure is one that defines the poor as being in households whose incomes fall below 50 percent of a population's median household income. This measure is often found within a European context, as well as in comparative analyses across industrialized countries.

A third type of poverty measure attempts to go beyond low income by factoring in additional aspects of deprivation such as illiteracy, high mortality rates, chronic unemployment, and so on. The focus here is often on the concept of social exclusion or "the inability to participate in the activities of normal living" (Glennerster, 2002, p. 89). As the *Human development report* notes:

> Poverty involves much more than the restrictions imposed by lack of income. It also entails lack of basic capabilities to lead full, creative lives – as when people suffer from poor health, are excluded from participating in the decisions that affect their communities or have no right to guide the course of their lives. Such deprivations distinguish human poverty from income poverty.
>
> (United Nations Development Programme, 2003, p. 27)

This type of measure has been used by the United Nations in their construction of a human poverty index for both the developing and developed nations, and has been discussed most notably in the work of Amartya Sen (1992).

Poverty and mental health/illness

How widespread is poverty within the United States? There are several different ways of analyzing the likelihood and prevalence of poverty within a population. The dimension of time and space are fundamental in examining how these patterns vary. Specifically, the occurrence of poverty in America can be understood within a cross-sectional, longitudinal, and life course context, as well as within a neighborhood context.

A representative sample of approximately 50,000 to 60,000 U.S. households is included each year in the U.S. Census Bureau's Current Population Survey. One of its purposes is to gather information regarding individual and household income. From these data, government analysts estimate the annual official poverty rates in the United States, as well as the yearly changes in the poverty rate.

The poverty rate in 2008 stood at 13.2 percent, which represented 39.8 million individuals, or approximately one out of every seven to eight Americans (U.S. Census Bureau, 2009). The percentage of the population falling into poverty or near poverty (125 percent of the poverty line) was 17.9 percent (or 53.8 million Americans), whereas 5.7 percent of the population (or 17.1 million Americans) experienced extreme poverty (falling below 50 percent of the poverty line). Of those who fell into poverty in 2008, 43 percent were living below 50 percent of the poverty line (U.S. Census Bureau, 2009). Consequently, a significant proportion of the poor in the United States are experiencing extreme poverty.

In addition, data from the Census Bureau indicates that certain characteristics tend to put individuals at a greater risk of experiencing cross-sectional poverty. These include having less education, being young or old, living in single parent families, non-whites, those residing in economically depressed inner cities or rural areas, and individuals with a disability (U.S. Census Bureau, 2009). In combination, these characteristics can substantially raise the risk of poverty. For example, black children who were under the age of five and residing in a female-headed household had an overall poverty rate of 60.2 percent in 2008 (U.S. Census Bureau, 2009).

Cross-sectional poverty rates have also been analyzed from a comparative perspective. The Luxembourg Income Study (LIS) has gathered income and demographic information on households in approximately 30 industrialized nations from 1967 to the present. Variables have been standardized across the various national data sets, allowing researchers to conduct cross-national analyses regarding poverty and income inequality.

This body of research has shown that the rates of poverty in the United States tend to be among the highest within the developed world. Whether one looks at relative or absolute poverty among working age adults, children, or elderly people, the story is much the same (Gornick & Jäntti, 2009; Smeeding, 2005). In addition to poverty, analyses of the LIS data have also shown that levels of income inequality tend to be the most extreme with the United States. Consequently, the United States is an outlier among the developed countries in the extent and depth of its poverty.

As an example, in a study of international poverty rates among children, the United States ranked second highest among 27 other industrialized countries with a poverty rate of 21.9 percent (poverty was measured as falling below one-half of the country's median income). The only country with a higher rate of poverty among children was Mexico at 27.7 percent. In contrast, the poverty rate for children in Denmark stood at 2.4 percent (UNICEF, 2005). For American children in married couple families, single parent families, or cohabiting families, the results are similar – a much greater percentage of American children are at risk of poverty compared to their counterparts in nearly all other developed countries (Heuveline & Weinshenker, 2008).

Two reasons stand out as to why Americans at the lower end of the economic distribution do so badly when compared to their counterparts in other countries. First, the social safety net in the United States is considerably weaker than in other Western industrialized countries, resulting in more households falling into poverty (Alesina & Glaeser, 2004; Brady, 2009). Second, the United States has been plagued since the early 1980s by relatively low wages at the bottom of the income distribution scale compared to other developed countries (Fligstein & Shin, 2004; Schiller, 2008). These factors contribute to both the relative and absolute depths of U.S. poverty in comparison with other industrialized nations.

Beginning in the 1970s, researchers have increasingly sought to uncover the *longitudinal* dynamics of poverty. The focus has been on understanding the extent of turnover in the poverty population from year to year and determining the length of poverty spells. These studies have relied on several nationally representative panel data sets including the Panel Study of Income Dynamics (PSID), the National Longitudinal Survey of Youth (NLSY), and the Survey of Income and Program Participation (SIPP). Results from these longitudinal analyses have shed considerable light on understanding the patterns of U.S. poverty. Several broad conclusions can be drawn from this body of work.

First, most spells of poverty in the United States are fairly short. The typical pattern is that households are impoverished for one or two years and then manage to get out of poverty (Bane & Ellwood, 1986; Blank, 1997; Cellini, McKernan, & Ratcliffe, 2008; Duncan, 1984; Walker, 1994). They may stay there for a period of time, only to experience an additional fall into poverty at some point (Stevens, 1999).

Since their economic distance above the poverty line is often not that far, a detrimental economic event can easily throw a family back below the poverty line (McKernan & Ratcliffe, 2005). Longitudinal research has shown that events leading households into poverty include the loss of jobs or cutbacks in earnings, family dissolution, and/or medical problems (Blank, 1997; Duncan et al., 1995; Iceland, 2006).

Analysts that have looked at monthly levels of poverty have found even greater fluctuation in poverty spell dynamics. For example, Iceland (2006) examined the monthly fluctuations in and out of poverty from 1996 to 1999 and found that 34 percent of Americans experienced poverty for at least two months during this time period, while half of all poverty spells were over within four months, and four-fifths were completed at the end of one year.

On the other hand, this body of work has also shown that there is a small percentage of households that do indeed experience chronic poverty for years at a time. Typically they have characteristics that put them at a severe disadvantage vis-à-vis the labor market (e.g. individuals with serious work disabilities, female-headed families with large numbers of children, racial minorities living in economically depressed inner city areas). Their prospects for getting out of poverty for any significant period of time are greatly diminished (Devine & Wright, 1993; Wilson, 1996).

Finally, research into the dynamics of poverty has shown that many households who encounter poverty will re-experience poverty at some point in their future. Using annual estimates of poverty from the PSID data, Stevens (1994) calculated that of all persons who had managed to get themselves above the poverty line, over half would return to poverty within five years.

The picture of poverty that is drawn from this body of research is thus characterized by fluidity. Individuals and households tend to weave their way in and out of poverty, depending upon the occurrence or nonoccurrence of particular detrimental events (e.g., job loss, family disruption, ill health). Similar findings have been found with respect to the longitudinal patterns of welfare use (Bane & Ellwood, 1994; Blank, 1997; Duncan, 1984; Rank, 1994a).

A third approach for assessing the scope of poverty has been to analyze poverty as a *life course event*. Specifically, how likely and how often will an American experience poverty during his or her lifetime? Life course research has shown that the risk of poverty and the use of welfare across the American life course is sizeable. For example, Rank and Hirschl (1999a) found that between the ages of 20 and 75, 58 percent of Americans will experience at least one year of impoverishment, while 68 percent of Americans will encounter poverty or near poverty (125 percent below the official poverty line). The odds of encountering poverty across adulthood are significantly increased for African Americans and those with lower levels of education – 91 percent of blacks will encounter poverty between the ages of 20 and 75 versus 53 percent of whites, while 75 percent of those with less than 12 years of education will experience at least a year of poverty compared with 48 percent for those with 12 or more years of education (Rank, 2004; Rank & Hirschl, 1999a).

Consistent with earlier work on poverty dynamics, individuals experiencing poverty often do so for only one or two consecutive years. However, once an individual experiences poverty, they are quite likely to encounter poverty again (Rank & Hirschl, 2001a, 2001b).

Rank and Hirschl's analyses (1999b, 1999c) also indicate that poverty is prevalent during the periods of childhood and old age. Between the time of birth and age 17, 34 percent of American children will have spent at least one year below the poverty line, while 40 percent will have experienced poverty or near poverty (125 percent of the poverty line). Similarly, 40 percent of elderly people will encounter at least one year of poverty between the ages of 60 and 90, while 48 percent will encounter poverty at the 125 percent level (Rank & Hirschl, 1999c; Rank & Williams, in press).

The risk of using a social safety net program is also exceedingly high: 65 percent of all Americans between the ages of 20 and 65 will at some point reside in a household that receives a means-tested welfare program (such as food stamps or Medicaid). Furthermore, 40 percent of the American population will use a welfare program in five or more years (although spaced out at different points across the life course). As with the life course patterns of poverty, the typical pattern of welfare use is that of short spells. Consequently, only 15.9 percent of Americans will reside in a household that receives a welfare program in five or more consecutive years (Rank, 2004; Rank & Hirschl, 2002).

One program that has a particularly wide reach is the Food Stamp Program (recently renamed the Supplemental Nutrition Assistance Program). Slightly over half (50.8 percent) of all Americans between the ages of 20 and 65 years will at some point reside in a household that receives food stamps (Rank & Hirschl, 2005), while for children between the ages of 1 and 20, the figure is 49.2 percent (Rank & Hirschl, 2009).

For the majority of Americans, it would appear that the question is not if they will encounter poverty, but rather, when they will encounter poverty. In addition, the life course risk of poverty has been shown to be rising since the late 1970s (Sandoval, Rank, & Hirschl, 2009). The experience of poverty can thus be viewed as a normative economic risk within the American life course (Rank & Hirschl, 2001a).

Yet another way of measuring the extent of poverty is to conceptualize it in terms of a spatial construct – specifically, the amount of poverty within a *neighborhood*. Since the late 1980s, a number of researchers have focused on the neighborhoods that individuals reside in as another way in which to describe and understand the nature of American poverty. The argument here is that neighborhoods mired in poverty detrimentally affect all who reside in such communities, and are particularly harmful to children. For example, Jargowsky (2003) poses the question, "Why should we be concerned with the spatial organization of poverty?" His answer is the following:

> The concentration of poor families and children in high-poverty ghettos, barrios, and slums magnifies the problems faced by the poor. Concentrations of poor people lead to a concentration of the social ills that cause or are caused by poverty. Poor children in these neighborhoods not only lack basic necessities in their own homes, but also they must contend with a hostile environment that holds many temptations and few positive role models. Equally important, school districts and attendance zones are generally organized geographically, so that the residential concentration of the poor frequently results in low-performing schools.
>
> (Jargowsky, 2003, p. 2)

Research has indicated that even after controlling for individual income and race, children's well-being in high poverty neighborhoods suffers in many ways (Brooks-Gunn, Duncan, & Aber, 1997; Evans, 2004, 2006; Leventhal & Brooks-Gunn, 2000). For example, Turner and Kaye (2006) found that independent of individual characteristics,

> as a neighborhood's poverty rate rises, so too does the likelihood of negative behavior among young children, of being expelled from school, of negative school engagement, of lack of involvement in activities, of not being read to or taken on outings, of living in a family with no full-time workers, and of having a caretaker who is aggravated or in poor mental health.
>
> (Turner & Kaye, 2006, p. 20)

This neighborhood context of poverty has been particularly important in the seminal work of William Julius Wilson (Wilson, 1987, 1996, 2009), Douglas Massey (Massey, 2007; Massey and Denton, 1993), and Robert Sampson (Sampson & Morenoff, 2006; Sampson, Raudenbush, & Earls, 1997). Their research has shown that children growing up in high poverty neighborhoods suffer from many disadvantages as a result of geographical residence. In addition, the children impacted by these negative effects are often children of color due to the long established patterns of residential racial segregation in American cities (Charles, 2003; Farley, 2008; Fischer, 2003).

Demographic research has estimated the percentage of the overall population as well as the poverty population that fall into high poverty neighborhoods (Bishaw, 2005; Jargowsky, 1997, 2003; Kingsley & Pettit, 2003, 2007). This body of work has often defined high poverty neighborhoods as census tracts in which 40 percent or more of its residents fall below the poverty line (Jargowsky, 2003). Using this metric, Kingsley and Pettit (2003) report that 3 percent of the U.S. metropolitan population lived within such neighborhoods in 1980, 5 percent in 1990, and 3 percent in 2000. The percentage of the poor living in high poverty neighborhoods was 13 percent in 1980, 17 percent in 1990, and 12 percent in 2000 (Kingsley & Pettit, 2003). Other research has also shown that while concentrated neighborhood poverty increased from the 1970s through the 1980s, it fell during the 1990s (Jargowsky, 2003).

With respect to children, Timberlake (2007) estimates that in 2000, 1.3 percent of white children, 7.3 percent of Hispanic children, and 10.8 percent of black children were living in metropolitan census tracts with 40 percent or more overall poverty. Using an alternative measure of neighborhood poverty which looked at the percentage of children living in neighborhoods where 40 percent of more of children of the same race were in poverty, Drake and Rank (2009) estimated that while only 3 percent of white children lived in such neighborhoods in 2000, the percentage for black children was 37.3 percent, and for Latino children, it was 24.6 percent.

Evidence indicates that mobility out of such neighborhoods, particularly for racial minorities, is limited. For example, Quillian (2003) has shown that for black residents living in high poverty census tracts (40 percent or more poverty), nearly 50 percent were still residing in a high poverty census tract ten years later. Even more disturbing, Sharkey (2008) has found that 72 percent of black children who grew up in the poorest quarter of American neighborhoods remained in the poorest quarter of neighborhoods as adults. Consequently, the effects of neighborhood poverty upon children of color are typically prolonged and long lasting.

Given the high prevalence and likelihood of poverty in the American population, understanding the *association between poverty and mental health* takes on added importance. A substantial body of research has shown a strong relationship between the quality of overall physical health and socioeconomic status (SES) – the lower an individual's socioeconomic status, the more likely they are to encounter a wide range of health problems. These effects are particularly pronounced for those falling into poverty. Poverty is associated with a host of health risks such as elevated rates of heart disease, diabetes, hypertension, cancer, infant mortality, undernutrition, lead poisoning, asthma, and dental problems (Rank, 2004).

This section explores the relationship of poverty to mental health. We examine the strength of the association between poverty and mental health disorders, the question of causality, and the intrinsic characteristics of poverty that lead to mental health problems.

Just as poverty can be defined in various ways (discussed earlier), so too can mental health be defined in a number of ways (for example, see Chapter 1 in this volume). In general, the absence of mental health disorders and illnesses is often the standard for determining the quality of one's mental health. Consequently, individuals displaying mental health problems are considered having diminished or compromised mental health. In the research reviewed in this section, a variety of mental health disorders have been analyzed in connection to poverty, including depression, anxiety disorders, overall psychological distress, conduct disorders, and schizophrenia.

As with physical health, a large body of research has found a *strong relationship* between lower socioeconomic status (and in particular, poverty) and diminished mental health. As Hudson (2005) notes:

> One of the most consistently replicated findings in the social sciences has been the negative relationship of socioeconomic status (SES) with mental illness: The lower the SES of an individual is, the higher is his or her risk of mental illness.
>
> (Hudson, 2005, p. 3)

One of the earliest studies to explore this relationship was that of Faris and Dunham (1939), who detected much higher rates of mental illness in poor neighborhoods of Chicago than in more affluent neighborhoods. Research by Hollingshead and Redlich (1958) in New Haven, Connecticut, and the Midtown Manhattan study (Srole et al., 1977) were two seminal studies that followed. Both found a strong relationship between socioeconomic status and mental health.

Since these earlier landmark studies, various dimensions of mental health have been examined in relation to lower SES and poverty. Low SES has been associated with a greater prevelence of schizophrenia (Dohrenwend, 1990; Ortega and Corzine, 1990), depression among adults as well as children and adolescents (Goodman, Huang, Wade, & Kahn, 2003; Hirschfeld & Cross, 1982; Kubik, Lytle, Birnbaum, Murray, & Perry, 2003; Lorant, Deliège, Eaton, Robert, Philippot, & Ansseau, 2003; Wade, 2001), overall psychological distress (Belle, 1990; Bradley and Corwyn, 2002), and conduct disorders among children (Costello, Compton, Keeler, & Angold, 2003; Lipman, Offord, & Boyle, 1994).

In particular, the amount of time exposed to poverty, and the severity of poverty, have both been shown to be important in detrimentally affecting an individual's overall mental health. Longitudinal research has indicated that longer spells of poverty and encountering more severe levels of poverty have detrimental impacts upon the quality of one's mental health (Duncan et al., 1994; Evans & Kim, 2007; Goosby, 2007; McDonough & Berglund, 2003; McLeod & Shanahan, 1996). For example, in a study examining the impact of duration of poverty upon children's mental health, McLeod and Shanahan (1993) found that the

> length of time spent in poverty is an important predictor of children's mental health, even after current poverty status is taken into account. As the length of time spent in poverty increases, so too do children's feelings of unhappiness, anxiety, and dependence.
>
> (McLeod and Shanahan, 1993, p. 360)

Similarly, longer durations of poverty experienced during the transition to adulthood were shown to be important in predicting depressive symptoms among blacks and Hispanics, independent of present socioeconomic status and family background (Mossakowski, 2008).

Taken as whole, the research evidence indicates a strong relationship between poverty and diminished mental health. However, the more vexing question is determining the *direction of causality* between the two. On the one hand, it could be argued that individuals experiencing mental health problems are more likely to drift downward into poverty. This may occur because such individuals have increasing difficulty securing and keeping decent paying jobs, they tend to have larger medical expenses, and so on. As a result, such economic problems increase the chances that individuals with mental health disorders will drift downward into poverty.

On the other hand, it could be argued that the direction of causality runs the other way. That is, the condition of poverty leads to a decrease in the quality of one's mental health. This could result from the economic and psychological stress and strain that individuals routinely face when living in poverty. In addition, impoverished individuals are less likely to have the resources necessary to access the health care system in order to treat a mental health disorder, which may further exacerbate their condition.

The direction of causality could also depend on the type of mental illness itself. For example, in the case of schizophrenia, the severity of the illness may be more likely to cause downward economic mobility, resulting in poverty (Dohrenwend et al., 1992). Other conditions, such as anxiety disorders, depression, or conduct disorders, may be triggered as a result of poverty itself (Hudson, 2005).

While there is research evidence to indicate that both directions of causality are in operation (Hudson, 2005), several studies have provided strong evidence demonstrating that the condition of poverty is an important causal factor leading to mental health disorders. Three studies are of particular importance in establishing this connection.

The first examined the effect that the Moving to Opportunity (MTO) program had upon the mental health of parents and children in New York City (Leventhal, 2003). The MTO program was administered by the U.S. Department of Housing and Urban Development (HUD) in five sites across the country, and was intended to provide a means for impoverished families to relocate to more livable environments.

Leventhal (2003) examined the impact upon the mental health of parents and children who relocated from public housing in high poverty neighborhoods to private housing in less poor neighborhoods. Families were randomly assigned to an experimental group (those families who moved to lower poverty neighborhoods) and to a control group (those families who remained in high poverty neighborhoods). The authors found that:

> The most significant benefits of the MTO program were noneconomic. Experimental parents who moved to low-poverty neighborhoods displayed superior mental health, as evidence by their reporting fewer distress and depressive symptoms than in-place control parents who remained in high poverty neighborhoods.
>
> (Leventhal, 2003, p. 1580)

Furthermore, the mental health impact of moving from high poverty to low poverty neighborhoods was particularly profound for children. Children moving to low poverty neighborhoods reported significantly less anxious/depressive problems than those children who remained in high poverty neighborhoods. The effects were greatest for children aged 8 to 13, as well as for boys.

The results from this study can be seen as particularly robust because of the experimental design of the study. They indicate a direct causal relationship between moving out of a high poverty neighborhood and, as a result, reducing the extent of mental health disorders.

A second key empirical study relied on an unusual natural experimental design in order to estimate the causal impact of poverty upon mental health. The Great Smoky Mountains Study employed a longitudinal research design to look at the need for mental health services and the development of psychiatric disorders in rural and urban youth (Costello et al., 2003). The study took place between 1993 and 2000 in 11 counties located in western North Carolina, and included children from the Eastern Band of Cherokee Indians who were living on a federal reservation. Midway through the study (in 1996), a casino opened on the reservation that gave every American Indian an annual supplement of approximately $6,000. Consequently, some American Indian children were pulled out of poverty as a result of the casino income, while others remained in poverty. In addition, non-Indian children were also examined in the study across the time period.

Costello et al. (2003) were therefore able to observe the impact that an infusion of household income had on mental health for a population that remained largely in the same physical location. They found that:

> (1) Moving out of poverty was associated with a decrease in frequency of psychiatric symptoms over the ensuing 4 years: by the fourth year the symptom level was the same in children who moved out of poverty as in children who were never poor. (2) Adding to the income of never-poor families had no effect on frequency of psychiatric symptoms. (3) The effect of poverty was strongest for behavioral symptoms (those included in the DSM-IV diagnoses of conduct and oppositional disorder). Little effect of moving out of poverty on emotional symptoms (DSM-IV anxiety and depression) was observed. (4) The effect of relieving poverty was mediated by 1 stressor: level of parental supervision. (5) The same models run using the non-Indian participants showed similar results.
>
> (Costello et al., 2003, p. 2028)

Consequently, the authors conclude that their findings displayed strong support for a direct causal relationship of poverty upon symptoms of conduct and oppositional defiant disorders in children. As a result of the increased income provided by the casino proceeds, parents were able to provide closer supervision for their children, leading to a decrease in behavioral problems.

A third study that has shed light on the causal direction of poverty and mental health was conducted by Hudson (2005). The author examined approximately 34,000 patients in Massachusetts who had undergone an acute psychiatric hospitalization between 1994 and 2000. He found that while 4 percent of those in affluent communities had mental illnesses leading to repeat hospitalization, over 12 percent of those in poor communities had repeated hospitalizations.

Furthermore, because of the longitudinal design of the study, Hudson (2005) was able to follow study participants in order to examine whether mental illness was leading to downward economic mobility. Hudson detected little downward drift of those with mental health problems into impoverished communities. Rather, the direction of causality was that the condition of poverty appeared to be exasperating mental health problems. As Hudson notes:

> The current study reveals a remarkably strong and consistent negative correlation between socioeconomic conditions and mental illness, one that supports the role of social causation in mental illness and cannot be accounted for by geographic or economic downward mobility. The statewide database used in this study leaves little doubt, at least in Massachusetts, the poorer one's socioeconomic conditions are, the higher one's risk is for mental disability and psychiatric hospitalization . . . Of the various social causation hypotheses tested, the idea that the impact of SES on mental illness is mediated by economic stress received the strongest support, with this model substantially fitting the data.
>
> (Hudson, 2005, pp. 16–17)

Each of these three studies provide strong methodological and empirical support to indicate that poverty exerts a significant and negative influence on the quality of an individual's mental health. We now turn to a discussion for why poverty has such an effect.

Poverty increases mental health problems   What is it about the nature of poverty that results in an increase in mental health problems? Conroy (2009) provides an insightful observation with respect to this question:

> For the impoverished segment of society among us, daily existence is a continuous uphill battle to meet the daily demands of attaining food and shelter. The issues associated with poverty go far beyond the financial implications of destitution, and affect every singular aspect of existence, but perhaps none more negatively than in the area of mental health. The balance in lifestyle that ensures stability and enjoyment are severely lacking in those facing poverty, while the stresses of merely surviving on a day to day basis is magnified with no relief or outlet in sight. Added to this is the pressure of viewing family and children suffer the indignities of indigence, and the situation is ripe for a decline in overall mental health.
>
> (Conroy, 2009, p. 1)

There are at least three elements of poverty that have been shown to increase the risk of mental health disorders. The first is the lack of resources associated with poverty. The second is the stress resulting from trying to survive in poverty. And the third is the environmental impact of living in impoverished neighborhoods. Each is discussed below.

Lack of resources   By its very definition, poverty represents a lack or absence of essential resources. This often involves having to cut back on basic resources such as food, clothing, shelter, health care, and transportation. For example, living in poverty often means having to do without a sufficiently balanced diet and adequate intake of calories (Rank & Hirschl, 2009). Several large-scale studies have indicated that those in poverty routinely have bouts of hunger, undernutrition, and/or a detrimental altering of the diet at some point during the month (Nord, Andrews, & Carlson, 2009). Not having an adequate diet can detrimentally affect one's physical and mental health.

Perhaps the best known juggling act is what has been called the "heat-or-eat" dilemma. As heating bills climb in the winter, impoverished families may be forced into the hard decision of choosing between purchasing food and paying for heat. Bhattacharya, DeLeire, Haider, and Currie (2003) have empirically documented that poor families do indeed lower their food expenditures during cold-weather periods.

This financial strain caused by the ongoing lack of resources has been shown to be associated with mental health problems. For example, Weich and Lewis (1998) demonstrated that poverty and unemployment were directly related to mental health disorders, such as anxiety and depression. They note that, "Financial strain was strongly associated with both onset and maintenance of common mental disorders and was neither confounded nor modified by more objective risk factors" (Weich & Lewis, 1998, p. 118).

A lack of financial resources can also magnify mental health problems in that individuals may not be able to access the health care system in order to treat a mental health disorder, which in turn, may further exacerbate the condition. Indeed, as Link and Phelan (1995) point out, socio-economic status ensures an unequal allocation of resources for health, including knowledge, power, money, assets, and social networks. These, in turn, reduce the likelihood of the poverty stricken receiving adequate treatment for mental health disorders (Gonzalez, 2005).

A consequence of the economic struggles described above is that impoverishment puts a heavy weight upon the shoulders of most who walk in its ranks. In essence, poverty acts to *amplify the stress* found in everyday life and its relationships. The daily struggle of having to juggle and balance expenses, worries, and concerns places a stressful burden upon the poverty-stricken and their families.

In addition, the events that often precipitate a fall into poverty are themselves highly stress producing. As noted earlier, poverty spells are often the result of the loss of a job, the breaking up of a family, and/or a serious medical problem. All of these life events have been shown to produce extreme levels of stress in individuals and families (Rank, 2004). When coupled with the economic pressures and constraints of living in poverty, the combination can produce a toxic effect upon mental health.

Various research studies have shown that stress detrimentally impacts the quality of mental health among the impoverished (Lupien, King, Meaney, & McEwen, 2001; Marmot & Feeney, 2000; Steptoe, 2000; Turner, 2007). For example, Evans and English (2002) examined the cumulative impact that various physical and psychological stressors had upon the mental well-being of poor white children in rural areas. They found that low income children were exposed to a much greater frequency of such stressors than non-poor children, and that the negative correlation of poverty to mental health could be partially explained by children's exposure to multiple-stressors. These patterns have been found among inner-city, ethnic minority children as well (Schaefer-McDaniel, 2009).

A third element important to understanding the negative relationship between poverty and mental health is the *environmental and community context*. A large body of research has demonstrated that socioeconomic status is strongly related to overall environmental quality. Those in poverty are more likely to be exposed to a variety of environmental hazards. In summarizing this body of work, Evans and Kantrowitz (2002) note that two overall conclusions can be drawn. First, income, and particularly poverty, are directly related to environmental quality. And second, environmental quality is inversely related to multiple physical and psychological health outcomes.

Those living in high poverty neighborhoods are at a heightened risk of being exposed to environmental hazards. As discussed earlier, poverty can be measured not only in terms of household income, but also in terms of the extent of poverty within the community where one resides. Researchers have frequently defined high poverty neighborhoods as those in which 40 percent or more of residents in a community are living below the poverty line.

Substantial research has shown that individuals and families living in high poverty neighborhoods are much more likely to be exposed to a wide array of environmental risks. These include increased exposure to toxic pollutants, crime, neighborhood disorder, substandard housing, lack of public services, inferior schooling, and many others (Evans, 2004; Sampson, Morenoff, & Gannon-Rowley, 2002). These, in turn, increase the levels of stress among residents of such communities, resulting in an increase in mental health disorders (Evans & English, 2002; Ross, 2000; Schaefer-McDaniel, 2009; Schulz, Zenk, Israel, Mentz, Stokes, & Galea, 2008). The cumulative effect of experiencing these environmental hazards on a daily basis takes its toll both physically and mentally. Evans (2004) summarizes this effect in the following way:

> Poverty is harmful to the physical, socio-emotional, and cognitive well-being of children, youths, and their families. A potent explanation for this relation is cumulative, environmental risk exposure. Compared with middle- and high-income children, low-income children are disproportionately exposed to more adverse social and physical environmental conditions.
>
> (Evans, 2004: 88)

In addition, because of the embedded patterns of racial residential segregation, blacks and Hispanics are much more likely to be exposed to the ill effects of residing in high poverty communities than are whites (Drake & Rank, 2009; Wilson, 2009).

Illustration and discussion

> I waited. I waited until the very last minute, until I probably was just about down and out. I think I probably called 'em up two or three times before I really wanted to go down there. And when I did, the guy on the phone told me that I'd better get down in a hurry. Because he knew the situation. And he knew that at that time I was tryin' to make it on the support I was getting for the children, that was only two hundred and twenty dollars a month. And that was pretty darn rough. It was just about impossible. I held out as long as I could. But you can only hold on so long. Then you gotta go down.

These were the words of Mary Summers, who described her experiences of having to apply for welfare in order to make ends meet. She was one of dozens of individuals interviewed for an earlier book entitled, *Living on the edge: The realities of welfare in America* (Rank, 1994a). During the interviews, individuals expressed their frustrations and difficulties in trying to survive under the conditions of poverty. They described various problems and constraints, and how these difficulties carried over into their everyday relationships, families, and overall mental well-being.

Mary Summers was typical of many of those interviewed. A 51-year-old divorced mother with two teenage daughters, Mary turned to the welfare system because she had been unable to find work for two years (this in spite of a rigorous search for a bookkeeping or accountant's position, jobs she had held in the past). The economic struggles she was facing, combined with the frustration of not being able to find a job, were taking a toll upon her psychological health, as was apparent throughout the interview. She comments:

> This is probably about the lowest point in my life, and I hope I never reach it again. Because this is where you're just up against a wall. You can't make a move. You can't buy anything that you want for your home. You can't go on a vacation. You can't take a weekend off and go and see things because it costs too much. And it's just such a waste of life.

After paying her rent for a small, two-bedroom apartment, Mary had a remaining $370 from welfare assistance for her and her daughters to live on. This came out to approximately $12 a day, or $4 per family member. While this may seem like an implausibly small income for any household to survive on, it is quite typical of the assistance that those on welfare receive.

As a result, numerous sacrifices had to be made. For example, in order to find an inexpensive apartment to rent, Mary and her family lived in a crime-stricken neighborhood. As she describes:

> The territory is horrible. Across the street is the place that's been hitting the news lately. And it's really bad, 'cause you go away, on weekends, we go down to my older son sometimes. And you really don't know that you're gonna have left when you come back. Because the apartment next door has been broken into twice. And it's bad. You can never be comfortable at night 'cause ya can never leave your windows open. You have to lock everything up, because you never know. But I guess if you want reasonable, cheap rent, you have to.

This, in turn, placed a constant psychological strain and worry on Mary and her family. Mary is but one of many everyday examples illustrating how the conditions of poverty increase the mental and emotional stress upon the poverty stricken.

For Mary, another source of mental strain came from the growing sense of isolation that she was experiencing as a result of her long bout in poverty and without work. She notes:

> Well, actually, I enjoy working. I mean, this is just driving me up a wall, sitting around here and trying to find something to do.

She later explained:

> I really miss it [work]. I miss the paychecks, naturally, that comes first. But I also miss the time not being into the mainstream. Not having people to talk to, just everything involved. I mean people that are working everyday probably think it's a drag. But when you're not in there, it's a drag staying home . . . After two years it gets to the point where you can just about start pulling out your hair. Because there is so much that you want to do, and you see your kids growing up around you, and you can't do a damn thing to help 'em up. And, ooohh, it really drives you nuts.

This growing sense of isolation also carried over in terms of Mary's interactions with her extended family. She was asked if her relatives expressed any feelings about her economic situation:

> They don't talk about it. In fact, I like to stay away from some of the relatives until I go back to work. I mean, it's just a situation that you don't even wanna get into. Let it blow over, and when you get back on your feet and have a little dignity again, well, then you can go back.

This sense of shame is another aspect of poverty that can take its toll upon the psychological well-being of individuals and families. In the United States, poverty and the use of a social safety net are highly stigmatized behaviors. Frequently the public perception is often that individuals in poverty are economic and personal failures (Brady, 2009). Those in poverty are generally quite aware of this overall perception, and as such, it creates an additional psychological burden (Rank, 1994b). Mary's comment about not having dignity while being in poverty exemplifies this sentiment.

Throughout the interview, Mary repeatedly discussed the effect that not working and living in poverty were having on her mental health. She described what she felt were the long-term psychological effects of poverty and welfare on those experiencing such conditions:

> I wouldn't use the word lazy. I would probably use the word discouraged or depressed. When you take a human being and you take away their money, their livelihood, and you make them live on something that is just the cost of living with no luxuries and no benefits, just the drab cost of living and nothing else, you're going to have depression and you're going to have discouragement. And I think with depression there always comes a form of . . . tiredness. 'Cause you give up and you want to lie down and go to sleep. Not necessarily meaning that you're lazy, and you can't get out there. It's just that they give up hope.

When asked about her state of mind, Mary paused for a moment, and then answered.

Mary: My state of mind . . . As long as you keep busy, and as long as you keep in contact with somebody and have something out there . . . a resume, a phone call, or something . . . and you know that you have something going for you, you can retain your senses and your sanity. But I think if everything stopped, I don't know what would happen. Because there'd be . . . there'd be nothing to look forward to; they'd be just dead zone. It's just, it's a . . . it's a horrible thought. As long as you keep trying, and you keep something going for you, I think there's always . . . you keep your morale built up and your hopes high, and . . . (pause).

Q: So, in terms of being say, hopeful or depressed or angry, you'd put yourself more towards . . . ?

Mary: Well, I try to keep something going so I don't get to the depression stage and to the point where you just give up. Because you can't . . . you can't do that. You just gotta figure out some kind of a new angle so you don't.

The example of Mary Summers illustrates the profound impact that living in poverty can have upon the overall quality of mental health. Poverty represents a series of frustrations, constraints, isolation, and stigma, all of which can increase the level of stress experienced. This, in turn, has the potential to damage one's mental health. As such, it is no wonder that poverty has been shown to empirically exert a sizeable negative effect upon the overall quality of mental health.

Conclusion

The relationship of poverty to mental health has been explored in this chapter. We began with the prevalence of poverty in the United States. The likelihood of an American experiencing some amount of time in poverty is surprisingly high. For example, three-quarters of adults between the ages of 20 and 75 will encounter at least one year in poverty or near poverty. As such, the relationship of poverty upon the quality of mental health becomes particularly pertinent.

The association between poverty and mental health was then explored. Research indicates a strong correlation between socioeconomic status in general (and poverty in particular) and a range of mental health disorders. These include depression, anxieties, overall psychological distress, conduct disorders, and schizophrenia. Although there is evidence to suggest that the causal relationship between poverty and mental health disorders can run in both directions, we reviewed several studies that provided strong evidence demonstrating the direct impact of poverty upon the quality of mental health. Factors that were discussed behind this effect included the lack of resources, overall stress, and the neighborhood quality.

The third section of the chapter provided a case example intended to illustrate and provide insights into the influence of poverty upon mental health. A single parent with two teenage children described her frustrations and constraints while living in poverty. These difficulties led to a considerable degree of psychological and emotional stress in her life, which in turn, exerted a detrimental impact upon the overall well-being of her mental health.

Web resources

Health Affairs
www.content.healthaffairs.gov

Institute for Research on Poverty
www.irp.wisc.edu/

Poverty Facts – National Poverty Center, University of Michigan
www.npc.umich.edu/medpoverty/

References

Alesina, A., & Glaeser, E.L. (2004). *Fighting poverty in the US and Europe: A world of difference*. New York: Oxford University Press.

Bane, M.J., & Ellwood, D.T. (1986). Slipping into and out of poverty: The dynamics of spells. *Journal of Human Resources, 21*, 1–23.

Bane, M.J., & Ellwood, D.T. (1994). *Welfare realities: From rhetoric to reform*. Cambridge, MA: Harvard University Press.

Belle, D. (1990). Poverty and women's mental health. *American Psychologist, 45*, 385–389.

Bhattacharya, J., DeLeire, T., Haider, S., & Currie, J. (2003). Heat or eat? Cold-weather chocks and nutrition in poor American families. *American Journal of Public Health, 93*, 1149–1154.

Bishaw, A. (2005). *Areas with concentrated poverty: 1999. Census 2000: Special reports*. Washington, DC: U.S. Government Printing Office.

Blank, R.M. (1997). *It takes a nation: A new agenda for fighting poverty*. Princeton, NJ: Princeton University Press.

Blank, R.M. (2008). Presidential address: How to improve poverty measurement in the United States. *Journal of Policy Analysis and Management, 27*, 233–254.

Bradley, R.H. and Corwyn, R.F. (2002). Socioeconomic status and child development. *Annual Review of Psychology, 53*, 371–399.

Brady, D. (2003). Rethinking the sociological measurement of poverty. *Social Forces, 81*, 715–751.

Brady, D. (2009). *Rich democracies, poor people: How politics explain poverty*. New York: Oxford University Press.

Brooks-Gunn, J., Duncan, G.J., & Aber, J.L. (1997). *Neighborhood poverty: Context and consequences for children*. New York: Russell Sage Foundation.

Cellini, S.R., McKernan, S.M., & Ratcliffe, C. (2008). The dynamics of poverty in the United States: A review of data, methods, and findings. *Journal of Policy Analysis and Management, 27*, 577–605.

Charles, C.Z. (2003). The dynamics of racial residential segregation. *Annual Review of Sociology, 29*, 167–207.

Citro, C.F., & Michael, R.T. (1995). *Measuring poverty: A new approach*. Washington, DC: National Academies Press.

Conroy, T.W. (2009). Links between poverty and mental health. *Associated Content*, June 4.

Costello, E.J., Compton, S.N., Keeler, G., & Angold, A. (2003). Relationships between poverty and psychopathology: A natural experiment. *JAMA: Journal of the American Medical Association, 290*, 2023–2029.

Devine, J.A. and Wright, J.D. (1993). *The greatest of evils: Urban poverty and the American underclass*. New York: Aldine de Gruyter.

Dohrenwend, B. (1990). Socieconomic status (SES) and psychiatric disorders. *Social Psychiatry Psychiatric Epidemiology, 25*, 41–47.

Dohrenwend, B.P., Levav, I., Shrout, P.E., Schwartz, S., Naveh, G., Link, B.G. et al. (1992). Socioeconomic status and psychiatric disorders: The causation-selection issue. *Science, 255* (1047), 946–952.

Drake, B., & Rank, M.R. (2009). The racial divide among American children in poverty: Reassessing the importance of neighborhood. *Children and Youth Services Review, 31*, 1264–1271.

Duncan, G.J. (1984). *Years of poverty, years of plenty: The changing economic fortunes of American workers and families*. Ann Arbor, MI: Institute for Social Research.

Duncan, G.J., Brooks-Gunn, J., & Klebanov, P.K. (1994). Economic deprivation and early-childhood development. *Child Development, 65*, 296–318.

Duncan, G.J., Gustafsson, B., Hauser, J.R., Schmaus, G., Jenkins, S., Messinger, H. et al. (1995). Poverty and social-assistance dynamics in the United States, Canada, and Europe. In K. McFate, R. Lawson, & W.J. Wilson (eds), *Poverty, inequality and the future of social policy: Western states in the new world order* (pp. 109–151). New York: Russell Sage Foundation.

Evans, G.W. (2004). The environment of childhood poverty. *American Psychologist, 59*, 77–92.

Evans, G.W. (2006). Child development and the physical environment. *Annual Review of Psychology, 57*, 423–451.

Evans, G.W., & English, K. (2002). The environment of poverty: Multiple stressor exposure, psychophysiological stress, and socioemotional adjustment. *Child Development, 73*, 1238–1248.

Evans, G.W., & Kantrowitz, E. (2002). Socioeconomic status and health: The potential role of environmental risk exposure. *Annual Review of Public Health, 23*, 303–331.

Evans, G.W., & Kim, P. (2007). Childhood poverty and health: Cumulative risk exposure and stress dysregulation. *Psychological Science, 18*, 953–957.

Farley, J.E. (2008). Even whiter than we thought: What median residential exposure indices reveal about white neighborhood contact with African Americans in US metropolitan areas. *Social Science Research, 37*, 604–623.

Farris, R.E., & Dunham, H.W. (1939). *Mental Disorders in Urban Areas*. Chicago, IL: University of Chicago Press.

Fischer, M.J. (2003). The relative importance of income and race in determining residential outcomes in U.S. urban areas, 1970–2000. *Urban Affairs Review, 38*, 669–696.

Fligstein, N., & Shin, T.J. (2004). The shareholder value society: A review of the changes in working conditions and inequality in the United States, 1976 to 2000. In K.M. Neckerman (ed.), *Social Inequality* (pp. 401–432). New York: Russell Sage Foundation.

Glennerster, H. (2002). United States poverty studies and poverty measurement: The past twenty-five years. *Social Service Review, 76*, 83–107.

Gonzalez, M.J. (2005). Access to mental health services: The struggle of poverty affected urban children of color. *Child and Adolescent Social Work Journal, 22*, 245–256.

Goodman, E., Huang, B., Wade, T.J., & Kahn, R.S. (2003). A multilevel analysis of the relation of socioeconomic status to adolescent depressive symptoms: Does school context matter? *Journal of Pediatrics, 143*, 451–456.

Goosby, B.J. (2007). Poverty duration, maternal psychological resources, and adolescent socioeconomic outcomes. *Journal of Family Issues, 28*, 1113–1134.

Gornick, J.C., & Jäntti, M. (2009). Child poverty in upper-income countries: Lessons from the Luxembourg Income Study. *Luxembourg Income Study Working Paper Series*, no. 509, Maxwell School of Citizenship and Public Affairs, Syracuse University, Syracuse, New York.

Heuveline, P., & Weinshenker, M. (2008). The international child poverty gap: Does demography matter? *Demography, 45*, 173–191.

Hirschfeld, R.M., & Cross, C.K. (1982). Epidemiology of affective disorders: Psychosocial risk factors. *Archives of General Psychiatry, 39*, 35–46.

Hollingshead, A.B., & Redlich, F. (1958). *Social class and mental illness*. New York: John Wiley & Sons.

Hudson, C.G. (2005). Socioeconomic status and mental illness: Test of the social causation and selection hypotheses. *American Journal of Orthopsychiatry, 75*, 3–18.

Iceland, J. (2006). *Poverty in America: A handbook*. Berkeley, CA: University of California Press.

Jargowsky, P.A. (1997). *Poverty and place: Ghettos, barrios, and the American city*. New York: Russell Sage Foundation.

Jargowsky, P.A. (2003). Stunning progress, hidden problems: The dramatic decline of concentrated poverty in the 1990s. *The Living Cities Census Series*, May. Washington, DC: Brookings Institution.

Kingsley, G.T., & Pettit, L.S. (2003). Concentrated poverty: A change in course. *Neighborhood Change in Urban America Series*, May. Washington, DC: Urban Institute.

Kingsley, G.T., & Pettit, L.S. (2007). Concentrated poverty: Dynamics of change. *Neighborhood Change in Urban America Series*, August. Washington, DC: Urban Institute.

Kubik, M.Y., Lytle, L.A., Birnbaum, A.S., Murray, D.M., & Perry, C.L. (2003). Prevalence and correlates of depressive Symptoms in young adolescents. *American Journal of Health Behavior, 27*, 546–553.

Leventhal, T., & Brooks-Gunn, J. (2000). The neighborhoods they live in: The effects of neighborhood residence on child and adolescent outcomes. *Psychological Bulletin, 126*, 309–337.

Leventhal, T. (2003). Moving to opportunity: An experimental study of neighborhood effects on mental health. *American Journal of Public Health, 93*, 1576–1582.

Link, B.G., & Phelan, J. (1995). Social conditions as fundamental causes of disease. *Journal of Health and Social Behavior, 35*, 80–94.

Lipman, E.L., Offord, D., & Boyle, M.H. (1994). Economic disadvantage and child psychosocial morbidity. *Canadian Medical Association Journal, 151*, 431–437.

Lorant V., Deliège, D., Eaton, W., Robert, A., Philippot, P., & Ansseau, M. (2003). Socioeconomic inequalities in depression: A meta-analysis. *American Journal of Epidemiology, 157*, 98–112.

Lupien, S.J., King, S., Meaney, M.J., & McEwen, B.S. (2001). Can poverty get under your skin? Basal cortisol levels and cognitive function in children from low and high socioeconomic status. *Development and Psychopathology, 13*, 653–676.

Marmot, M., & Feeney, A. (2000). Health and socioeconomic status. In G. Fink (ed.), *The Encyclopedia of Stress*, (pp. 313–322). New York: Academic Press.

Massey, D.S. (2007). *Categorically unequal: The American stratification system*. New York: Russell Sage Foundation.

Massey, D.S., & Denton, N.A. (1993). *American apartheid: Segregation and the making of the underclass*. Cambridge, MA: Harvard University Press.

McDonough, P., & Berglund, P. (2003). Histories of poverty and self-related health trajectories. *Journal of Health and Social Behavior, 44* (2), 198–214.

McKernan, S.M., & Ratcliffe, C. (2005). Events that trigger poverty entries and exits. *Social Science Quarterly, 86*, 1146–1169.

McLeod, J.D., & Shanahan, M.J. (1993). Poverty, parenting and children's mental health. *American Sociological Review, 58* (3), 351–366.

McLeod, J.D., & Shanahan, M.J. (1996). Trajectories of poverty and children's mental health. *Journal of Health and Social Behavior, 37*, 207–220.

Mossakowski, K.N. (2008). Dissecting the influence of race, ethnicity, and socioeconomic status on mental health in young adulthood. *Research on Aging, 30*, 649–671.

Nord, M., Andrews, M., & Carlson, S. (2009). Household food security in the United States, 2008. Economic Research Report No. 83, Food Assistance and Nutrition Research Program, United States Department of Agriculture.

Ortega, S.T., & Corzine, J. (1990). Socioeconomic status and mental disorders. *Residential Community Mental Health, 6*, 149–182.

Quillian, L. (2003). How long are exposures to poor neighborhoods? The long-term dynamics of entry and exit from poor neighborhoods. *Population Research and Policy Review, 22*, 221–249.

Rank, M.R. (1994a). *Living on the edge: The realities of welfare in America*. New York: Columbia University Press.

Rank, M.R. (1994b). A view from the inside out: Recipients' perceptions of welfare. *Journal of Sociology and Social Welfare, 21*, 27–47.

Rank, M.R. (2004). *One nation, underprivileged: Why American poverty affects us all*. New York: Oxford University Press.

Rank, M.R., & Hirschl T.A. (1999a). The economic risk of childhood in America: Estimating the probability of poverty across the formative years. *Journal of Marriage and the Family, 61*, 1058–1067.

Rank, M.R., & Hirschl T.A. (1999b). The likelihood of poverty across the American adult lifespan. *Social Work, 44*, 201–216.

Rank, M.R., & Hirschl T.A. (1999c). Estimating the proportion of Americans ever experiencing poverty during their elderly years. *Journal of Gerontology: Social Sciences, 54B*, S184–S193.

Rank, M.R., & Hirschl T.A. (2001a). The occurrence of poverty across the life cycle: Evidence from the PSID. *Journal of Policy Analysis and Management, 20*, 737–755.

Rank, M.R., & Hirschl T.A. (2001b). Rags or riches? Estimating the probabilities of poverty and affluence across the adult American life span. *Social Science Quarterly, 82*, 651–669.

Rank, M.R., & Hirschl, T.A. (2002). Welfare use as a life course event: Toward a new understanding of the U.S. safety net. *Social Work, 47*, 237–248.

Rank, M.R., & Hirschl, T.A. (2005). Likelihood of using food stamps during the adulthood years. *Journal of Nutrition Education and Behavior, 37*, 137–146.

Rank, M.R., & Hirschl, T.A. (2009). Estimating the risk of food stamp use and impoverishment during childhood. *Archives of Pediatrics and Adolescent Medicine, 163*, 994–999.

Rank, M.R., & Williams, J.H. (in press). A life course approach towards understanding poverty among older American adults. Forthcoming in *Families in Society*.

Ross, C.E. (2000). Neighborhood disadvantage and adult depression. *Journal of Health and Social Behavior, 41*, 177–187.

Sampson, R.J., & Morenoff, J.D. (2006). Spatial dynamics, social processes, and the persistence of poverty in Chicago neighborhoods. In S. Bowles, S.N. Durlauf, & K. Hoff (eds) *Poverty Traps* (pp. 176–203). New York: Russell Sage Foundation.

Sampson, R.J., Raudenbush, S.W., & Earls, F. (1997). Neighborhoods and violent crime: A multilevel study of collective efficacy. *Science, 227*, 918–924.

Sampson, R.J., Morenoff, J.D., & Gannon-Rowley, T. (2002). Assessing "neighborhood effects": Processes and new directions in research. *Annual Review of Sociology, 28*, 443–478.

Sandoval, D.A., Rank, M.R., & Hirschl, T.A. (2009). The increasing risk of poverty across the American life course. *Demography, 46*, 717–737.

Schaefer-McDaniel, N. (2009). Neighborhood stressors, perceived neighborhood quality, and child mental health in New York City. *Health and Place, 15*, 148–155.

Schiller, B.R. (2008). *The economics of poverty and discrimination.* Upper Saddle River, NJ: Prentice Hall.

Schulz, A.J., Zenk, S.N., Israel, B.A., Mentz, G., Stokes, C., & Galea, S. (2008). Do neighborhood economic characteristics, racial composition, and residential stability predict perceptions of stress associated with the physical and social environment? Findings from a multilevel analysis in Detroit. *Journal of Urban Health: Bulletin of the New York Academy of Medicine, 85*, 642–661.

Sen, A. (1992). *Inequality reexamined.* New York: Russell Sage Foundation.

Sharkey, P. (2008). The intergenerational transmission of context. *American Journal of Sociology, 113*, 931–969.

Smeeding, T.M. (2005). Public policy, economic inequality, and poverty: The United States in comparative perspective. *Social Science Quarterly, 86*, 955–983.

Smith, A. (1776). *An inquiry into the nature and causes of wealth of nations.* London: W. Strahan & T. Cadell.

Srole, L., Langner, T.S., Michael, S.T., Kirkpatrick, P., Opler, M., & Rennie, T.A.C. (1977). *Mental health in the metropolis: The midtown Manhattan study.* New York: Harper & Row.

Steptoe, A. (2000). Health behavior and stress. In G. Fink (ed.), *The encyclopedia of stress* (pp. 323–326). New York: Academic Press.

Stevens, A.H. (1994). The dynamics of poverty spells: Updating Bane and Ellwood. *Journal of Human Resources, 34*, 557–588.

Stevens, A.H. (1999). Climbing out of poverty, falling back in: Measuring the persistence of poverty over multiple spells. *Journal of Human Resources, 34*, 557–588.

Timberlake, J.M. (2007). Racial and ethnic inequality in the duration of children's exposure to neighborhood poverty and affluence. *Social Problems, 54*, 319–342.

Turner, H.A. (2007). The significance of employment for chronic stress and psychological distress among rural single mothers. *American Journal of Community Psychology, 40*, 181–193.

Turner, J.A., & Kaye, D.R. (2006). How does family well-being vary across different types of neighborhoods? *Low-Income Working Families Series*, Paper 6. Washington, DC: Urban Institute.

United Nations Development Programme. (2003). *Human development report 2003*. New York: Oxford University Press.

UNICEF. (2005). Child poverty in rich countries. *Innocenti Report Card*, No. 6.

U.S. Census Bureau. (2009). *Income, poverty and health insurance coverage in the United States: 2008*. Current Population Reports, Series P60-236. Washington, DC: U.S. Government Printing Office.

Wade, T.J. (2001). Delinquency and health among adolescents: Multiple outcomes of a similar social and structural process. *International Journal of Law and Psychiatry, 24*, 447–467.

Walker, R. (1994). *Poverty dynamics: Issues and examples*. Aldershot, UK: Avebury.

Weich, S., & Lewis, G. (1998). Poverty, unemployment, and common mental disorder: Population based cohort study. *British Medical Journal, 317*, 115–119.

Wilson, W.J. (1987). *The truly disadvantaged: The inner city, the underclass, and public policy*. Chicago, IL: University of Chicago Press.

Wilson, W.J. (1996). *When work disappears: The world of the new urban poor*. New York: Alfred A. Knopf.

Wilson, W.J. (2009). *More than just race: Being black and poor in the inner city*. New York: W.W. Norton.

4   Racism and its effects

Dennis Miehls

This chapter elaborates the bidirectional relationship between the many manifestations of racism and mental health diagnosis, prevalence and disparities in service delivery. The concept of "microaggressions" is utilized to understand the insidious effects of repeated manifestations of individual, institutional and structural and institutionalized racism on the well-being, including mental health, of People of Color.[1] Social factors such as housing discrimination, poverty and employment opportunities which all interface with racism to exacerbate the conditions of chronic mental illness are also considered. Psychological factors include the impact of racism on the emergent identity and mental health of People of Color. Though the discussion and case examples focus primarily on the experiences of racism of African American individuals, racism affects all racial and minority groups in similar, yet distinct ways. While evidence shows the experience of racial discrimination can influence the manifestations of many psychiatric disorders, we focus here on depression, post-traumatic stress disorder and schizophrenia, three conditions that tend to be both chronic and socially debilitating. Finally, the specific impact of various forms of racism on mental health is explored through the use of three case examples.

A number of working assumptions are critical in understanding the approach to this content. First, many African American, Latino, Asian, and other minorities have developed sound, strong networks in order to buffer some experiences of racism. So, it is clear that not all People of Color necessarily develop emotionally based psychological symptoms as a result of living in a racist society. Franklin, Boyd-Franklin, and Kelly (2006) state:

> It is also important to recognize the impact of protective factors such as family and extended kinship networks, religion and spirituality, strong cultural values and racial identity, and personal strength and resiliency that may allow many People of Color to rise above the debilitating, ongoing trauma of racism.
>
> (Franklin et al., 2006, p. 18)

Recognizing the resilience of many People of Color does not, however, diminish the impact of structural and institutional racism that is manifest in myriad ways (Miller & Garran, 2008).[2]

Second, racism in the United States continues to be a dominant factor that shapes multi-leveled interactions of individuals, groups, communities and organizations. People from the dominant white culture experience privilege and power in contemporary society. White individuals consciously or unconsciously position People of Color as an "other" who is inferior to White individuals. Positioning others as inferior enables White individuals to shore up their own identities, perhaps felt as necessary as a result of being threatened by multiple internal and external factors, including, for example, the current economic recession of 2009. Institutional and structural racism, indicates systemic, societal, durable racism that is embedded in institutions, organizations, laws, customs, and social practices . . . It leads to a cumulative effect in which groups that are racially targeted are excluded from living in certain neighborhoods and working in numerous jobs and professions, have less access to social assets such as quality schools, and have greater health risks and other negative consequences and outcomes because of a variety of interacting legal, illegal, direct, and indirect practices.

(Miller & Garran, 2008, p. 29)

Further, Leonard Pitts (2009) suggests that in spite of the election of Barack Obama (a Black man) to the Presidency of the United States, "post-racial America" has not yet arrived. To accept the discourse that racism has become absent in contemporary U.S. society seems a somewhat naive response that is fueled by denial of the lived experiences of many People of Color in the United States. Indeed, Turner (1999) noted that White and Black Americans hold different views on the extent of change in race relations. Miehls (2001) comments on Turner's ideas, writing:

African Americans believe, he purported, that racial bias has changed only modestly over time . . . in all aspects, including racial bias, discrimination, opportunities. He reported that some Whites react with shocked indignation or disbelief at the notion that Blacks might still consider themselves at all disadvantaged.

(Miehls, 2001, p. 234)

Citing Shipler (1997), Miller and Garran (2008) suggest:

To be sure, many white people are well aware of the persistence of racism in the United States. Still, whites and people of color show marked differences in their beliefs about the extent of racism today, and these disparities indicate a significant perceptual racial divide in this country.

(Miller & Garran, 2008, p. 62)

They suggest that many Whites think that the United States has moved to a colorblind society, implying that skin color has no impact on the lived experiences of People of Color. Scruggs (2009) also purports that colorblindness is a "new" form of racism. She suggests that privileged individuals who say they don't see color in people are not promoting racial harmony (as they imagine) but rather are contributing to tension within People of Color who are very aware of the benefits of white privilege. Citing Bobo (2001), Miller and Garran (2008) discuss the different perceptions of white people and people of color when they note:

African Americans and Hispanics overwhelmingly believe that there is occupational discrimination in favor of whites, while less than a fourth of whites agree; and people of color view racism as a deeply entrenched, institutional phenomenon, while many whites see it as a question of attitudes and behaviors.

(Miller & Garran, 2008, p. 62)

Definitions of racism

Biologists who created three categories of individuals – Mongoloid, Caucasoid, and Negroid – first defined race (Atkinson, 2004). These categories were based upon what these "scientists" considered to be distinguishing characteristics such as skin color, hair, and facial features (Howard-Hamilton & Frazier, 2005). However, contemporary theorists suggest that these biological categories are ill-founded and not tenable in terms of accuracy. Marsiglia and Kulis (2009) suggest, "The persistence of racial distinctions in social life is remarkable given the fact that race, as a biological concept, has not survived the test of scientific scrutiny" (p. 9). These authors further suggest, "Humans cannot be categorized reliably based on phenotypical characteristics, such as those aspects of physical appearance like skin color, hair texture, and bone structure that are often thought to be markers of one's racial background" (p. 9).

Most contemporary authors suggest that race, as a "designation," is a social construction that privileges certain individuals while putting others at a disadvantage (Constantine, 2007; Franklin et al., 2006; Marsiglia & Kulis, 2009; Miehls, 2001, 2005; Miller & Garran, 2008; Tatum, 2000). Franklin et al. (2006) suggest that "Racism is complex and . . . based on erroneous principles of racial superiority, it bestows power and privilege on those who define, enforce, and establish the institutional mechanisms that maintain it" (p. 10). In other words, racism is a systematic implementation of stereotypes and discrimination and that privileges White individuals at the expense of People of Color who are marginalized and who do not have full access to the educational, financial, or employment opportunities that American society offers. Marsiglia and Kulis (2009) suggest that "The prime purpose of racial formation is to establish a hierarchy and target certain groups for discrimination" (p. 9). Even middle class Black Americans are open to discrimination – for example, being denied access to a certain apartment/neighborhood in spite of its clear availability (Pattillo-McCoy, 2007).

Tatum (2000) views racism not only as a manifestation of racial prejudice but also as more a system of practices that limits the opportunities of People of Color. Discrimination takes place at individual, institutional, and structural levels (Pincus, 2000). Oppression is manifest by targeted individuals systematically being exploited in myriad ways marginalized in society, having a sense of powerlessness, being subject to cultural imperialism (being made invisible by dominant society), and, last, by being victims of violence at a disproportionate level to individuals from the dominant culture (Young, 2000).

At the interpersonal level, many People of Color experience ongoing interactions with people from the dominant culture in which they have an experience of "being othered." This term implies that People of Color are often objectified and positioned as "lesser-than" or "inferior" persons than their White counterparts. While there is no universal experience among Black individuals as they navigate the terrain of being "othered," this practice has a long history for African Americans. Cushman (1995) describes the historical function of Negro Minstrelsy during the nineteenth century when Black men were often characterized as grotesque or clownish. This form of entertainment became extremely popular and the White audiences relied on these caricatures to frame their views of black individuals who were slaves or who were no longer legally held as slaves after the civil war. Often referred to as the Jim Crow era, this practice originated when a White minstrel performer, Thomas (Daddy) Rice, blackened his face and danced a ridiculous jig while singing the song "Jump Jim Crow" (Del Carmen, 2008). White America latched onto this imagery and began to create a discriminatory icon of African American "folks." Cushman (1995) says:

> The primary African-American character the White audience saw was a comic, foolish, empty-headed idiot: the Sambo of white folklore. Each act was framed by the taken-for-granted understanding that the White race was inherently superior, intellectually and morally, to the Black race.

> (Cushman, 1995, p. 43)

In addition, the minstrel performances were filled with self-denigrating comments about African Americans and their physical appearance; skin color, nappy hair, and pejorative name calling often were used as punchlines in a joke or dialogue among the actors. Cushman (1995) also notes that "Female African Americans were portrayed as slow-witted, lazy, ugly, vain, unclean, crude, and very sexual. They also ate prodigious amounts of ice cream and drank their dates under the table" (p. 47). These gross stereotypes laid the foundation for more contemporary stereotypes of African Americans. Though the forms of stereotyping in contemporary society might be somewhat more subtle, they still exist and are replicated in individual interactions and are enacted in various ways between white people and people of color.

In fact, Shome (1999) contends that one's body has become the site of racist attitudes and discriminatory practices in contemporary interactions in the United States. She shares the experience with other women of color when she suggests that upon entering a room mostly populated by white people

> there is that *thing in their look* . . . they welcome you, but then the way they look at you makes you feel as though your whole body is up for examination and scrutiny . . . it almost feels as though they hunt my body for differences . . . it's such a systemic thing, they don't even realize half the time that they do it.
>
> (Shome, 1999, p. 121, italics in original)

hooks (1992) attributes this practice of "white gaze" to the historical era of slavery during which black individuals were punished if they looked directly at their white superiors. She contends that many whites still have the same working assumption that being that "people of color are bold, aggressive, and out of line if the gaze is returned" (Miehls, 2001, p. 234).

Historical experiences of racism become embedded in institutional racism, which Miller and Garran (2008) suggest is "manifested through laws, policies, and formal and informal practices" (p. 63). They write that there are at least nine types of institutional racism that include "residential, educational, employment, accumulation of wealth and upward mobility, environmental and health, mental health, criminal justice, political, and media" (p. 63). The person with mental illness is more likely than others to experience deleterious effects from the impact of racism, particularly related to housing, education, employment, criminal justice, and the access to health and mental health services.

Social workers, who are often employed by the agencies that have inadvertently developed institutional practices of racism, face the challenges of both identifying and eradicating those practices, on behalf of their clients. At the same time, they must understand and intervene with those clients on a micro level. For example, African American clients who experience discriminatory practices such as "racial microaggressions" (Constantine, 2007; Miller & Garran, 2008; Sue, Capodilupo, & Holder, 2008a; Sue, Capodilupo, Nadal, & Torino, 2008b) often experience an erosion of their self-esteem which leads to a complex sense of self that may include some aspects of internalized racism. For the person with mental illness, the internalized racism may manifest in a variety of ways which may give rise to or exacerbate psychological symptoms.

Racism and mental health/illness

In addition to categorizing hundreds of psychiatric disorders, the *Diagnostic and statistical manual of mental disorders* (DSM-IV-TR: American Psychiatric Association (APA), 2000) documents the prevalence rates of these disorders in the U.S. population. This manual tends to minimize racial differences in prevalence rates of most of the descriptions of mental disorders; other research points to racial differences in the prevalence of mental illness. Below are summarized prevalence and inpatient hospitalization rates for three mental conditions – schizophrenia, major depressive disorder, and post-traumatic stress disorder.

The American Psychiatric Association's DSM-IV-TR (2000) manual suggests that the national prevalence rate of *schizophrenia* ranges between 1.5 percent and 5 percent of the general population. The manual minimizes the differences of diagnosis across race suggesting, "Studies in the United Kingdom and the United States suggest that schizophrenia may be diagnosed more often in individuals who are African American and Asian American than in other racial groups (p. 307). However, whether these findings represent true differences among racial groups or whether they are the result of clinician bias or cultural insensitivity" is unclear. Other research notes discrepant findings. Citing Zeber's research, Vedantam (2005) notes that Blacks were more than four times as likely to be diagnosed with schizophrenia as Whites. Hispanics were more than three times as likely to be diagnosed with schizophrenia as Whites. Davis (1997) points out differences in rates of admission to state hospitals between 1980 and 1992. He notes:

- Rate of admission for all persons was 163.6 per 100,000
- Rate of admission for Whites was 136 per 100,000
- Rate of admission for Native Americans and Asians was 142 per 100,000
- Rate of admission for African Americans was 364.2 per 100,000
- Rate of admission for all persons to V.A. (veterans') Hospitals was 70.4 per 100,000
- Rate of admission for African Americans to V.A. Hospitals was 118.2 per 100,000.

He goes on to say:

> Admissions of Blacks to state mental hospitals showed that 56 percent of these individuals received a primary diagnosis of schizophrenia, while only 38 percent of all individuals admitted received a similar diagnosis. Hispanics, too, received a disproportionately high (44 percent) rate of severe mental illness diagnosis on admission to state mental health institutions.
>
> (Davis, 1997, p. 630)

DSM-IV (APA, 2000) reports that "The lifetime risk for *major depressive disorder* in community samples has varied from 10 to 25 percent for women and from 5 percent to 12 percent for men" (p. 372) and further that "The prevalence rates for major depressive disorder appear to be unrelated to ethnicity, education, income, or marital status" (p. 372). However, Riolo, Nguyen, Greden, and King (2005) found that:

- Prevalence of major depressive disorder differed significantly by race
- Highest prevalence was found in White participants
- Age of onset of disorder was significantly earlier for White and Mexican American participants in contrast to African American subjects
- Persons living in poverty had nearly 1.5 times the prevalence of major depressive disorder
- For Mexican American participants, lack of education was significantly associated with prevalence of major depressive disorder.

Cultural relativity is acknowledged in the DSM-IV manual for the *post-traumatic stress disorder* diagnosis, which has a lifetime prevalence rate of "approximately 8 percent of the adult population in the United States" (APA, 2000, p. 466). The manual also notes:

> Studies of at-risk individuals (i.e., groups exposed to specific traumatic incidents) yield variable findings, with the highest rates (ranging between one-third and more than half of those

exposed) found among survivors of rape, military combat and captivity, and ethnically or politically motivated internment and genocide.

(APA, 2000, p. 466)

Later in the chapter, the interface of post-traumatic stress disorder with the lived experiences of People of Color is more fully explored. A main argument suggests that People of Color develop symptoms of PTSD and complex post-traumatic stress syndrome in response to a number of societal and institutional experiences of racism. The lack of awareness of cultural influences in the development of mental illness, the manifestation of symptoms and the life course, is only one of the limitations of our attention to race and mental illness. Many authors also suggest that People of Color have *restricted access to health and mental health services* (Johnson & Cameron, 2001; Leong, 2001; Leong & Lau, 2001; Miller & Garran, 2008; Ojeda & McGuire, 2006; Snowden, 2001, 2005; Stone, 2002; Swartz, Wagner, Swanson, Burns, George, & Padgett, 1998). In 1999, the Surgeon General of the United States (Dr. David Satcher) commissioned a report to examine mental health service delivery in the United States. Mrs. Tipper Gore, wife of the then Vice-President, Al Gore, was an ardent advocate of promoting mental health services for all Americans. Entitled *Mental health: A report of the Surgeon General* (Department of Health and Human Services (DHHS), 1999) the document was the product of a collaboration of two federal agencies – the Substance Abuse and Mental Health Services Administration and the National Institutes of Health. While this report was commissioned to examine the mental health needs of all Americans, it clearly exposed the reality that the needs of racial and ethnic minority populations were not being met adequately. In response to this information, the Department of Health and Human Services brought together myriad mental health experts to study the issues at hand and these individuals provided a supplement to the Surgeon General's report of mental health services that was entitled *Mental health: Culture, race, and ethnicity* (Department of Health and Human Services, 2001). The supplemental information describes how culture interfaces with mental health issues across minority populations. Moreover, it also contains detailed information about mental health care for four distinct groups – African Americans, American Indians and Alaska Natives, Asian Americans and Pacific Islanders, and Hispanic Americans. At the time, the document spawned a great deal of interest in mental health disparities (Lopez, 2003; Manson, 2003).

A main working assumption of the Surgeon General's (DHHS, 1999) report was that society should no longer view mental health as separate from an individual's general health. This assumption attempted to legitimize mental health treatment as an essential part of the overall health care service delivery. It was reported that the research literature reveals that mental health treatment works for a range of mental disorders. The efficacy of treatment strategies for mental health issues is correlated with a reduction of stigma of mentally ill people – in other words, if properly treated, individuals with mental illness are not necessarily ostracized or stigmatized by others. The main recommendation of the report to the American people was to seek help if you think you have symptoms of a mental disorder or if you have any mental health issues. This simple directive was an attempt to make services more available, without stigma. However, the report recognized that the mental health service delivery system is complex; therefore, differences in service delivery of public and private sectors affects the accessibility of mental health services. The influence of managed care companies limits the availability of services to all in the United States. In addition, an interface of other state and federal agencies (social welfare, housing, criminal justice, and education) with mental health service delivery puts impoverished People of Color at higher risk of not receiving adequate mental health services or indeed perhaps not receiving any mental health services.

Findings in the report that are related to African Americans who are overrepresented in high-need populations and are at particular risk for mental illness, are particularly relevant for social work. The Surgeon General's report (DHHS 1999) identifies the following at-risk groups:

- Homeless people – While 12 percent of the U.S. population was homeless at that time, African Americans make up 40 percent of that population.
- Incarcerated people – Nearly half of all prisoners in state and federal jurisdictions and almost 40 percent of juveniles in legal custody are African Americans.
- Child welfare – African American children constitute about 45 percent of children in public foster care and more than half of all children waiting to be adopted.
- People exposed to violence – African Americans of all ages are more likely to witness violence or be the victim of violence than are White individuals.
- Insurance – Nearly 25 percent of African Americans are uninsured (16 percent of the general population are uninsured).
- Medicaid covers nearly 21 percent of African Americans.
- Use of Mental Health Services – Only one-third of all Americans with mental illness receive care; however, the percentage of African Americans receiving needed care is only half that of Whites.
- African Americans of all ages are underrepresented in outpatient treatment but over-represented in inpatient treatment.
- African Americans tend to be diagnosed more frequently with schizophrenia and less frequently with affective disorders.

These are staggering figures. As the United States makes its way through the significant economic downturn that began in 2009, we can expect that these vulnerable populations will be further affected and marginalized. Even at the time, the Surgeon General, taking into account these disparities, brought together many experts to complete further research about the inequities of mental health care delivery to People of Color. Lopez (2003) sates that in his report to the American Psychological Association's annual meeting in 2001, Dr. Stacher, the Surgeon General, stated that "culture counts" and that this assumption "should echo through the corridors and communities of the nation" (p. 419). Lopez (2003) notes:

At that point, the large overflowing audience became still. They understood the signifi-cance of his words. Our nation's leading health professional recognized that the mental health status of our country's largest "minority" groups is most important to the welfare of the nation. Furthermore, the Surgeon General underscored the importance of culture by identifying key issues for four groups of People of Color – African Americans, Asian Americans and Pacific Islanders, American Indians and Alaska Natives, and Hispanic Americans. An executive summary of the report reported why "culture counts" in the following ways.

- The culture of racial and ethnic minorities influences aspects of mental illness, including how symptoms are manifest, how individuals cope with symptoms, and willingness to seek treatment.
- People of Color face social environments of inequality that includes greater exposure to racism, discrimination, violence and poverty.
- People in the lowest socioeconomic status group are two to three times more likely to

have a mental illness diagnosis (in contrast to those in the highest socioeconomic status group).
- People of Color often mistrust White institutions that provide mental health services.

Other authors also suggest difficulties in the mental health service delivery to People of Color. For example, People of Color may be misdiagnosed when mental health clinicians are unaware or insensitive to the cultural relativity of psychiatric symptomatology and thus assigning a more serious diagnosis more often to People of Color in contrast to White clients (Whaley, 1997).

In spite of the heightened consciousness of the disparities of service delivery to minority populations raised in the Surgeon General's Report (DHHS, 1999) and the Supplement to this report (DHHS, 2001), numerous studies continue to point out that discrepancies still exist. For example, Ghods, Roter, Ford, Larson, Arbelaez, and Cooper (2008) report that physicians did not assess for depression symptoms in Black individuals as much as they did with White clients. There were discrepancies even when physicians did discuss depressive phenomenology. They report "even when depression communication did occur, physicians recognized only two thirds of African Americans, but more than 90 percent of White patients, as having emotional distress" (p. 605). Similarly, DeCoster (1999) found that physicians tended to pay more attention to the "emotions" of White females and males more than they did with People of Color. This suggests a bias among the physicians who may consider Black individuals to be "overly emotional" and that their emotionality does not warrant any treatment.

Anglin, Alberti, Link, and Phelan (2008) suggest that "members of racial/ethnic minority groups are less likely than Caucasians to access mental health services despite recent evidence of more favorable attitudes regarding treatment effectiveness" (p. 17). They report that even though African Americans believe that mental health clinicians are able to assist individuals with major depression and schizophrenia, "they were also more likely to believe mental health problems would improve on their own" (p. 17). Ojeda and McGuire (2006) reported that Latinas and African American women and men exhibited lower use of substance abuse services and outpatient mental health services than did their White counterparts (p. 211). They suggest "Though efforts are being made to increase the detection of depression in minorities, systematic approaches in primary care settings where minorities are more likely to obtain care could prove helpful in eliminating race/ethnic gaps in service use" (p. 219). They speculate that "Minorities fear adverse consequences in the workplace or are embarrassed about discussing their problems with others, thus resulting in delayed or forgone care" (p. 219).

In certain instances, People of Color receive differential treatment for symptoms of their mental illness. Van Dorn, Swanson, Swartz, and Elbogen (2005) investigated prescriber's utilization patterns of a new generation of antipsychotic medication (widely known to be more expensive than previous medications) in a racially mixed group of individuals with schizophrenia. They wondered how race and/or involvement in a criminal justice system interacted with the utilization of the newer, more expensive drugs. The study revealed that "minority racial status (being African American) and arrest history both appear to play a significant role in determining which patients are least likely to receive atypical antipsychotics" (p. 130). They postulated that preconceived ideas about Black individuals may contribute to this discrepancy. For example, citing Garb (1997), they say "clinicians often rate black patients as being at higher risk than white patients for hospital readmission" (Van Dorn et al., 2005, p. 130), even though there is no real data to support this supposition. They acknowledge that the differences found in their study may be attributed to a range of factors including poverty or patients' attitudes about treatment, as examples, but they also suggest that differences are possibly related to "clinicians' subtle biases about which patients are most likely to benefit from atypical antipsychotics" (p. 131).

Barnes (2004) examined the correlation of race and admission rates to psychiatric hospitals with particular reference to individuals diagnosed with schizophrenia. He cites some historical data with regards to the percentage of African Americans who were hospitalized with a diagnosis of schizophrenia. Citing Thompson, Belcher, DeForge, Myers, and Rosenstein (1993), he suggests that the percentage of African Americans given the diagnosis of schizophrenia increased from 33 percent to 50 percent during the time period between 1970 and 1986. Regarding the influence of race in this process he writes, "research on the prevalence of mental disorders in the general population has found that there is no significant difference in the rate of schizophrenia between African Americans and Whites when socio-economic status is controlled" (Barnes, 2004, p. 242, citing Keith, Regier, & Rae, 1991). So, the economically disadvantaged African American client is likely being over-diagnosed as schizophrenic. Barnes (2004) suggests a number of factors that may be associated with this discrepancy. "Some of these factors are diagnostic bias of clinicians, lack of cultural understanding between clinicians and minority clients, and racial differences in the presentation of psychiatric symptoms" (p. 242).

Greenberg and Rosenheck (2003) question how managed care practices affect the accessibility and quality of mental health interventions with U.S. minorities. They note, "Managed care has typically introduced practices, such as utilization review, treatment guidelines, and disease management, which often constrain the delivery of services" (p. 32). They cite Provan and Carle (2000) and Scholle and Kellehar (2000), who suggested that "the introduction of managed care into mental health settings has been perceived by minorities to create barriers to care that were not experienced in fee-for-service systems" (Greenberg & Rosenheck, 2003, p. 41). One of Greenberg and Rosenheck's main findings (examining change in mental health service delivery in the Department of Veterans Affairs, nationally) was that Hispanic veterans demonstrated a declining access to outpatient care relative to their White counterparts (p. 40).

Children from minority populations are not immune to the patterns of poor accessibility and utilization of mental health services. Wood, Yeh, Pan, Lambros, McCabe, and Hough (2005) studied the relationship between race/ethnicity and at what age children use either school-based mental health services or specialty mental health care. They cite Kataoka, Zhang, and Wells (2002) when they state that their study

> provided the first nationally representative assessment of child mental health use and reported that of their sample of children and adolescents who met criteria for needing services, almost 80 percent had not received mental health care in a 1-year period. This study found that, even when researchers controlled for other factors, Latino and uninsured youth were particularly unlikely to receive needed mental health services.
>
> (Wood et al., 2005, p. 186)

Wood et al. (2005) found "that non-Hispanic White children were more likely to receive school-based services as compared to African American, Asian-Pacific Islander, and Latino children, and to begin use at an earlier age than the latter two groups" (p. 193).

There are numerous macro issues that contribute to racism in the United States. As noted, Miller and Garran (2008) refer to these factors as a web of institutional racism and these issues serve as the context for the individual experiences of many People of Color. Interpersonal racism can be as pervasive, entrenched and damaging. For example, the tendency for people from the dominant culture to deny any ill intentionality in cross-race interactions often leads to a sense of unreality within the African American individual. It is often difficult for African American individuals to hold onto a coherent sense of self when one is often told something like "Oh, I didn't mean that," "You must have misunderstood," and "You are exaggerating this."

This sort of invalidating experience can lead to confusion about one's own responses, especially if one receives this sort of message in a repetitive manner and from someone who has been legitimized in society with power and privilege. This is similar to Linehan's (1993) description of invalidating environments that people suffering with borderline personality experience when their parents disavow or reformulate interpersonal interactions. In that circumstance, parents often suggest that the child is misinterpreting anger that is actually being played out by the parent. These parents often question the feelings of the child or they may suggest to the child that her feeling of sadness is really anger, for example, and that she has no right to feel that way toward the parent.

For the Person of Color, this insistence that one is exaggerating or confusing one's own response can contribute to a subtle and insidious erosion of confidence and healthy ego ideal. This may be particularly true when individuals have internalized racism that has unconsciously but powerfully infiltrated the Person of Color's internal world. African American individuals may unfortunately internalize aspects of self-denigration if they adopt the stance and attitude of those of the dominant culture. Internalized racism can be understood as a manifestation of the notion that Whites exert more power in social relations and People of Color are subject to this unfair valence of influence, authority, and credibility. Foucault (1979) suggests that power cannot be minimized or removed from any social relationship. For Foucault, power is exercised "everywhere in a continuous way" (Foucault, 1979, p. 80). As such, African American individuals may question their own "sense of reality," colluding with the notion that "of course, the white (powerful) individual must have the corner on truth when it comes to interpersonal interactions between the two." In her article entitled "Surviving hating and being hated," Kathleen Progue White (2002) describes an incident that she experienced as dismissive, devaluing, and confusing. Progue White, a young black student who had been taught to read by her older sister, volunteered to read in her class that was being taught by a nun in her school. She writes:

> I raised my hand with enthusiasm. "I can read!" The nun said, "Don't you tell a lie, you can't possibly be able to read." "Oh, Yes I can, too!" "Here, read this," she said. I read it. She said, "That's not reading; you're not reading it right, that is not the way to read. That's why *you people* never amount to anything. You make up lies when you don't know how to do things the right way! I'll have to teach you to read proper."
>
> (Progue White, 2002, p. 404, italics in original)

This is a poignant example of how young Black children have to find ways to negotiate the mixed messages that they often receive while not denying their own sense of reality. This little girl knew she could read yet her sense of self was being contested by the powerful, authoritative, White adult. Progue White (2002) goes on to suggest that this sort of disavowal has a profound effect on one's view of oneself, causing confusion and perhaps self-hatred, at the extreme.

This author witnessed a similar dismissal of the voice of a woman of color who was being interviewed by a White student in a graduate social work class (reported previously in Moffatt & Miehls, 1999). In this instance a woman of color was trying to explain to her White colleague that she had experienced discrimination in her high-school setting when she was inappropriately assigned to basic (remedial) classes when she and her family first immigrated to Canada. In telling this to the White student, the student of color gave up on her own narrative in order to fit the appraisal of the White student. The student of color had said that she was told that she would have to take basic level courses in her program of studies. The author observed the following exchange between the two, when the White student was in the role of social worker, in a role-play exchange:

In responding to the student of color's use of the word basic, the White student said, "Oh, you mean general courses." The Latina student seemed confused and replied, "No, basic." Again, the interviewer said, "So, they wanted you to take general courses." The Latina student once again conveyed that the guidance counselor had positioned her in a class for vocational students and said, "No, it was basic." The interviewer ignored the Latina student and replied, "did you talk to the principal about this?"

(Moffatt & Miehls, 1999, p. 68)

Recognizing that the White student was altering the meaning of the narrative for the student of color, the classroom instructor attempted to have them reconstruct the dialogue. The following ensued:

The interviewer attributed the difficulty in the interaction to the Latina woman's inabilities to communicate in English. The interviewer explained that she knew that the Latina woman was using the "wrong" terminology. The apologetic Latina student commented by saying, "I am sorry, maybe I am not a right client." The interviewer said: "Don't worry, I know that I am a good interviewer."

(Moffatt & Miehls, 1999, p. 68)

This example demonstrates that the woman of color began to internalize the voice of the White student when she said, "maybe I am not a right client." The White student demonstrated a sense of arrogance and did not have any empathy for her colleague. Rather, she exercised her role as an "expert" when she gave advice to the student of color about how she should have proceeded. Questioning "did you talk to the principal," she implied that the student of color had done something wrong or perhaps had not acted on her own behalf – indeed People of Color often report that they do not act on their own behalf as they worry that articulating their concerns to a White person may add further conflict to a dialogue that is already experienced as troubling and undermining. Foucault (1980) would suggest that this sort of experience of systematically altering and devaluing the voice of the Person of Color represents an exercise of power strategies employed by the White individual. The White student fuels her sense of superiority in the exchange and leaves feeling righteous and "smart" – all at the expense of the student of color.

The interactions of being "othered" (as described above) or having one's own narrative questioned or altered occur for many reasons. Certainly the stereotypes of African American people that have been illustrated have long traditions in the United States, dating back to slavery and beyond. Levy and Karafantis (2008) suggest that all individuals are subject to and influenced by "lay theories" about individuals, groups, and institutions. Lay theories are culturally shaped and have far-reaching consequences in terms of interactions and views of interactions. Levy and Karafantis (2008) suggest that:

"Conceptions of the world" or "naïve" theories are often referred to as "lay theories," since they are used in everyday life. These lay theories may be captured by proverbs such as "Anyone can pull themselves up by their bootstraps" (J.S. proverb; refers to the Protestant work ethic).

(Levy & Karafantis, 2008, p. 111)

Lay theories have a profound impact in the development of prejudice since these common-place theories filter social information and become "short-cuts" to casting judgment on others. They suggest "that when a lay theory is relevant in a given situation, people rely on that theory to support their either socially tolerant or prejudicial attitudes and behaviors" (p. 112).

The concept of *"microaggressions"* describes how the day-to-day experiences of being marginalized affects African American individuals. Sue et al. (2008a) suggest that the term racial microaggressions describes "the brief, commonplace, and daily verbal, behavioral, and environmental slights and indignities directed toward Black Americans, often automatically and unintentionally" (p. 330). Referring to these interactions as "microinsults," Jackson (2000) suggests that "The subtle and indirect nature of these insults may result in feelings of powerlessness because of the incongruent experience between the individual's feeling state and her perception of the event" (p. 7).

Microaggressions are similar but different to experiences of racial profiling (Del Carmen, 2008) that many African American individuals experience as well. Racial profiling is a term that describes the investigation and/or charges made against People of Color by police or other authorities in disproportionate numbers than White individuals. Targeted as a result of their race, African American individuals are stopped in automobiles to be investigated, as one example. Del Carmen says that racial profiling is

> the selective targeting of individuals based on their race, ethnicity, or religious affiliation. Although the concept is often used to describe police-initiated behavior, it also pertains to individuals who are in a position to target others based on their racial, ethnic, or religious background.
>
> (Del Carmen, 2008, p. xi)

Airport security personnel may also fall into racial profiling in doing security checks. The author has heard from a number of African American clients that they are often subjected to racial profiling. For the most part, these experiences contribute to a sense of anger and frustration within the client. However, these individuals seem to readily identify the injustice in these events and while angering, these sorts of experiences do not seem to infiltrate their internal worlds in the same manner as other microaggressions.

Sue et al. (2008a) reported the results of a qualitative study that they completed using focus groups to capture the "everyday" experience of individuals who self-identified as Black or African American. Four major themes emerged from their thematic analysis – healthy paranoia, sanity check, empowering and validating self, and rescuing offenders – which they described as forming a reaction domain (p. 329). Many of their participants identified that they needed to often question whether behavior of others was fueled by racist attitudes. They thought that a certain suspiciousness of the motivations of their White counterparts was a healthy adaptation to their perception of events. This defensive posture is more favorable than internalizing attitudes of inferiority in the face of such exchanges as, "Oh, I think this customer was ahead of you in the line" (waiting for service in a coffee-shop with White customers).

The participants noted that "checking out" their perceptions with other Black friends or family members was important. African American co-workers, for example, may non-verbally, but quickly, check out their response to comments made in a meeting or in the lunch-room of their business. Similarly, some participants suggested that they keep their responses "healthy" when they locate the site of the difficulty within the person from the dominant culture, leading to an empowered and validated sense of self for the African American. Last, these participants often responded by attempting to "rescue" the offender so as to minimize the impact of the microaggression or interaction. One participant reported his behavior by actually changing his physical behavior in the presence of a White woman. He noted, "Inside an elevator, a closed space being very conscious if there is a White woman, whether or not she's afraid, or just sort of noticing me, trying to relax myself around her so she's not afraid" (Sue et al., 2008a, p. 333). The participants interpreted the microaggressions in a number of ways, including receiving the messages that you do not belong here, you are abnormal in some way, you are intellectually inferior, or you are not trustworthy. These participants seemed to come to this particular study with an awareness of how race dynamics shaped their interactions with a range of individuals from the dominant culture. As such, they were able to articulate some defensive strategies as noted above. And, even then, there was agreement that these sort of interactions take a toll on the African American individual as he/she needs to continuously be making decisions about how much to try and deconstruct these interactions. In this deconstructing, one can either question the attitudes of the White individuals or recognize the exchanges for what they are and attempt to move along, psychologically unscathed.

African American individuals, unsurprisingly, sometimes decide to minimize conflict-laden interpersonal interactions with White individuals as opposed to trying to have some resolution about the communication or microaggression. Many White individuals deny the existence of any racial transgression and think that the African American individual is exaggerating his response if he questions the White individual about an exchange. This dynamic of denial happens at an individual level and it also operates within the academy, at the professional level. Sue et al. (2008b) published an article entitled, "Racial microaggressions and the power to define reality" in response to some of the critique of their published work. For example, Thomas (2008) published an article entitled "Macrononsense in multiculturalism" suggesting that examples used by Sue et al. (2007) are exaggerated. He dismisses the idea that microaggressions would contribute to emotional distress and he says that "such stereotypes may be inappropriate, but they hardly necessitate the hand-wringing reactions described by Sue et al. (2007)." He further describes that Sue and his colleagues ought to see the *whole* person, not just race or ethnicity, when deconstructing points of miscommunication. This argument has been long used by White individuals and it serves the function of suggesting that they "don't see color" as all people are human beings, first, and a Person of Color only secondarily. Similarly, Harris (2008) in his "Racial microaggression? How do you know?" also questioned Sue's experiences. In his article, he questions the perception of Sue when he was asked to move to the back of an airplane. Sue had articulated his hypothesis that this series of events were examples of microaggressions (Sue et al., 2007).

These two articles are striking examples of the reaction that African Americans may engender when they confront others with their experience of racial microaggression in an interpersonal interaction. The author does not know the race or ethnicity of either Thomas or Harris but has heard a number of examples from his clients and students when they suggest that they did not "bother" raising any racialized issue as they did not have the "energy" to attempt to "educate" the aggressor in the microaggression experience. African American students are regularly reluctant to try and problem-solve difficult classroom situations that have components of race at the origin with colleagues and professors (Miehls, 2001). Dealing with racial microaggressions is difficult for any academic or student or individual; for the Person of Color who is experiencing problems with mental illness, this struggle may be overwhelming and defeating.

Franklin et al. (2006) suggest that the insidious and repetitive nature of race-related stress and emotional abuse that leads to an experience of psychological trauma often contributes to a state that they term "the invisibility syndrome." These authors suggest: "Symptoms of the syndrome are an outcome of the psychological conditions produced when a person perceives that his or her talents and identity are not seen because of the dominance of preconceived attitudes and stereotypes" (p. 13). They suggest that African American children and adults often are managing confusion or other unsettled feelings when they are systematically being ignored or invalidated. Being rendered invisible is being rendered powerless and without a sense of agency. These authors also suggest that a normative response to these sorts of ongoing interactions is anger and that the African American individual has the additional burden of finding ways to modulate and manage the anger that is precipitated as a result of these unfair, repetitive and frequent microaggressions.

However, African Americans are continuously positioned in a double-bind experience when it comes to managing their anger. Anyone experiencing so many ongoing slights would naturally feel anger. And, many White individuals carry a stereotype that Black individuals (especially Black men) are filled with anger and rage. This stereotype is another example of a residual effect of slavery with White people continuously trying to "stamp out the (life) anger" of the enslaved individuals. The notion that Black men are dangerous, angry, and explosive fueled and legitimized practices in which people from the dominant culture suppressed the anger of African Americans; African Americans were severely punished and/or killed if they showed any anger towards Whites. One of the author's young adolescent African American clients, Michael, described his dismay and frustration when others are fearful of him when he is simply walking down the street. He recounted many instances when he and his father witnessed White people crossing the street, in an attempt to avoid any direct face-to-face interaction. With some hesitation, Michael told the social worker that he and his father occasionally "played a game" during these interactions. Michael reported that he and his father developed a non-verbal signal with each other and that in some instances they would cue each other to also cross to the other side of the street, after observing White individuals doing this. Michael acknowledged that this was somewhat "mean-spirited" and he somewhat woefully said, "What do these fools expect? We get tired of constantly being thought of as muggers or 'angry black men'."

Michael's disclosure was illustrative in many ways. He spoke of the complexity of having to manage one's responses to the racism of others. Not only was his experience to be confused and hurt, but also he was angry at the frequency of these types of interactions. He also recognized that these experiences were fueled by racism and he spoke of his adaptation to these experiences. Michael had the benefit, in this "game", of his father's validation of his experience. While some might argue that he and his father were further fueling the stereotype of the angry Black men (when they playfully would also cross the street), the author understood this as a coping strategy that they sometimes employed so as to maintain some psychological equilibrium in the face of ongoing experiences of racism. Shortly, the chapter discusses the interface of race, trauma, and complex PTSD but first the specifics of how these sorts of microaggression affect the identity of African American adolescents, a particularly vulnerable population, is illustrated.

Illustration and discussion

The following cases illustrate how various forms of discrimination and/or stereotypes influenced the psychological well-being and hence, mental health, of an African American individual. In the first, Michael, an adolescent, struggles with depression. Charles, a middle-aged recovering substance abuser, struggles with the effects of multi-determined PTSD, and Lashonda, a biracial young adult, presents with an eating disorder.

The ongoing experience of racism can be particularly challenging for the adolescent. Michael (mentioned earlier) is an 18-year-old African American young man who was referred for therapy as a result of his worsening depressive symptoms. His parents became concerned about his increasingly poor academic performance, his withdrawal from friends and family and his suicidal thoughts. The social worker had been working with Michael for approximately six months and had a fairly solid therapeutic alliance, when in one session, Michael seemed despondent and withdrawn. The social worker noted his observation to Michael and he simply shrugged his shoulders in response, saying he really didn't want to be in the session today. The social worker agreed that it can be tough sometimes to talk about one's painful experiences. Michael agreed and said, "Yeah, especially when you don't hear what I am saying." The worker encouraged Michael to say more. Michael was encouraged to go on and he was reassured that this was exactly what he needed to do in order for the worker-client dyad to get back on track. Michael became somewhat tearful and told the social worker that he could never understand what he went through. He reported that the worker kept asking him about his relationship with his father (which the therapist had formulated as being conflict-laden) and that Michael didn't want to talk about this. He went on to say that he felt disloyal to his father when he discussed their relationship. He then said, "You never ask me about why my boss at work thinks I am lazy, or why my teachers only show interest in my athletic abilities, or why White people cross to the other side of the street when they see me approaching them."

Even though the clinician had asked Michael in a general way how he experienced living in a predominantly White community as a young Black man, the youngster had mostly denied any overt racism in his interactions with others. In this moment, he let the social worker know that his family wasn't the only source of tension for him but rather he experienced stressors on a day-to-day basis from a myriad of people. Rather than saying that he had not told the clinician about these experiences before (which would have been likely perceived as chastising and/or disbelieving) the therapist simply said that he was sorry that Michael had to be the object of such discrimination and "stupidity" at the hands of so many White individuals. Michael latched on to the word "stupidity" and said, "You haven't heard anything yet – but, yeah, he could talk about stupidity!" The clinician acknowledged this statement. They then went on to discuss, in a more authentic way, the client's lived experiences of being targeted as a young Black man in a predominantly White community. His depressive symptoms started to lessen over the next few weeks as he told the clinician about many examples of being misunderstood, being reduced to a stereotype, and being the recipient of discrimination, based upon race.

In fact, Cooper, McLoyd, Wood, and Hardaway (2008) suggest that "African American adolescents are more likely to report experiences with racial discrimination than other ethnic minority adolescents" (p. 281). These authors suggest that adolescents who perceive racial discrimination and also worry about race-related interactions "are predictive of several negative indicators of psychological functioning among African American adolescents" (p. 284). These authors cite the work of many others to support this claim. They cite references that substantiate that African American adolescents experience lowered self-esteem (Fisher, Wallace, & Fenton, 2000; Wong, Eccles, & Sameroff, 2003), increased depressive phenomenology (Simons, Murry, McLoyd, Link, Cutrona, & Conger, 2002; Wong et al., 2003), psychological distress (Fisher et al., 2000), feelings of hopelessness (Nyborg & Curry, 2003), anxiety (Gibbons, Gerard, Cleveland, Wills, & Brody, 2004), and lower life satisfaction (Brown, Wallace, & Williams, 2001).

In recent years, there has been considerable discussion in the literature that about the use of a "trauma" diagnosis for individuals who experience racism. Franklin et al. (2006) cite a number of clinicians, scholars, and researchers who have argued for an expansion in the definition of PTSD as a result of racism directed towards People of Color (I. Allen, 1996; Butts, 2002; Root, 1992; Sanchez-Hucles, 1998). However, the American Psychiatric Association (2000), in its DSM-IV-TR manual, suggests that a diagnosis of PTSD can be used only if:

> The person has been exposed to a traumatic event in which both of the following are present: (1) the person experienced, witnessed, or was confronted with an event or events that involved actual or threatened death or serious injury, or a threat to the physical integrity of self or others and (2) the person's response involved intense fear, helplessness, or horror.
>
> (APA, 2000, p. 467)

The following clinical example typifies the experience of an African American man who experienced symptoms of PTSD as a result of experiencing many traumatic events in his childhood and adult environments. Charles and his wife, Deborah, were being seen for couple therapy as a result of having numerous difficulties in the relationship that were characterized by an inability to problem-solve any conflict, no sexual relationship, and Charles' experience of many symptoms of PTSD including night terrors, flashbacks, and rage storms. These manifestations of PTSD affected the stability of the couple's day-to-day living. He had a very difficult time regulating his affect, especially any angry affect. Charles was currently on a medical leave of absence from his janitorial job in a large office complex and Deborah worked as a nursing assistant in a senior retirement housing complex. Charles had been born and raised in a housing project in Boston, Massachusetts in the early 1960s. He was raised in poverty and he withdrew from school when he was in the eighth grade. At that time, he moved out of his grandmother's home, where he had been living, and became part of a large gang that supplied drugs in the greater Boston neighborhood. He disclosed a series of traumatic events that included being physically abused by his alcoholic stepfather, witnessing his brother's death by gunshot, and being forced to prostitute himself as a gay hustler to earn money to support his own drug habit.

Desperate to leave this situation, he enlisted in the army when he was a young adult and he recounted that he experienced a great deal of racism at the hands of his senior officers and also his peers in his unit. His experiences in boot camp contributed to his first experiences of PTSD symptoms and he eventually received a medical discharge from the army for mental health issues. Charles and Deborah had met at a twelve-step meeting a number of years ago and each had achieved sobriety from alcohol and drugs for six years. Charles started to attend Alcoholics Anonymous after he experienced a number of episodes of black-outs when he was putting himself in life-threatening situations, including driving while intoxicated. He credited his beginning sobriety to a young social work intern who worked with him in an inpatient mental health unit in a V.A. hospital – he found her compassion and empathy for him to be genuine and he made an internal pledge to stay sober. In spite of this pledge, he often relapsed and had an ongoing struggle to stay employed or in any long-term relationship. He had a series of girlfriends and considered himself to be lucky to have found his current wife, Deborah, who seemed committed to him and the long-term nature of the relationship.

As noted above, and in spite of his six-year sobriety, Charles continued to show many symptoms of PTSD and the current social worker was able to assist him to begin to deal with his traumatic history. As part of the couple therapy, Charles began to eventually understand and re-narrate his trauma history. This long-term work was fundamental in Charles moving away from the legacies of his childhood and adolescent traumas. The phase-oriented couple work (Karusaitis Basham & Miehls, 2004) assisted him to deal with the many traumatic events that he had experienced. Most recently, Charles disclosed to the therapist that he also experienced racism in his workplace and that this had contributed to his need for a medical leave of absence, due to life stressors (Gitterman & Germain, 2008).

Charles clearly had symptoms of PTSD and he also fit the diagnostic category of complex post-traumatic stress syndrome as described by Herman (1992).[3] The diagnosis of PTSD of the DSM-IV-TR captures some of the responses of Black individuals experiencing ongoing racism; however, the exclusionary criteria of experiencing a "life-threatening experience" or experiencing a "threat to the physical integrity of self" does not always accurately capture the experience of traumatic experiences, based on racism. Charles certainly fit these diagnostic criteria but not all African Americans do fit these criteria. Rather, their experiences of microaggressions are insidious and long term in nature. This chapter suggests that the concept of complex post-traumatic stress syndrome, described by Herman (1992) more closely describes the experiences of African American people when they experience ongoing microaggressions in their day-to-day lives. Herman championed the need for a broader, more inclusive diagnosis concerning trauma, especially as related to survivors of childhood (physical or sexual) abuse. She developed her argument by suggesting that a key residual component of survivors of childhood trauma was the tendency of these individuals to have persistent difficulties in maintaining a positive sense of self and/or identity. She explained that many survivors of childhood trauma often blamed themselves for their abusive histories and that this insidious process affected their ability to form completely healthy self-concepts.

Lenore Terr (1991) suggested that individuals who experience a discrete traumatic event such as a natural disaster or sexual assault experience what she referred to as a Type I trauma. These discrete events often lead to an appropriate use of the DSM-IV-TR diagnosis of PTSD. She also describes Type II traumas in which the survivor of childhood trauma was subjected to ongoing, persistent, and repetitive traumatic relationships. For example, this would be the description of a young child who was sexually abused, over a number of years, by the same perpetrator. The after effects of this sort of trauma are more persistent and likely far-reaching. It is very likely that these repetitive childhood traumas lead to symptoms more consistent with Herman's (1992) description of complex post-traumatic stress syndrome. Here the sense of self is eroded and a shattered identity becomes intertwined with a range of complex defensive structures that often lead to myriad mental health symptoms.

The chapter's hypothesis is that African American individuals often experience repetitive experiences of racism which sometimes lead to an erosion of self-confidence that may lead to a confused and perhaps shaky identity. So, in addition to the development of myriad mental health symptoms that have been described in this chapter and elsewhere (Pierre, Mahalik & Woodland, 2001; Utsey, 1997; Utsey & Payne, 2000) it is likely that the core of one's "personhood" can be challenged when living with repeated and chronic situations of being "othered," of being invalidated through "microaggressions" and other racialized interpersonal interactions. In her contribution, "The courage to hear: African American women's memories of racial trauma," Jessica Daniel (2000) discusses the many ways that African American women experience trauma. The author now offers a clinical illustration that will highlight the process of this young woman's identity being challenged on many levels as a biracial Black woman. Daniel's (2000) contribution is cited, where relevant to the clinical material.

Lashonda, a 25-year-old biracial woman (African American father and White mother) was referred to the clinician by a colleague from a mid-western city. Lashonda had been in therapy for two years with another therapist when she was an undergraduate student. She moved to Western Massachusetts to attend a graduate program and she was anxious to continue her therapy. She had had a favorable experience with her previous therapist. Lashonda identified as Black and she reported that most people viewed her as Black, in spite of her biracial identity. Her stated goals at the time of the therapy were to continue to work on her issues of anxiety, depression, and uncertainty about her future career goals.

Her family history revealed that she was the only child born to professional parents. She reported that her parents had high expectations of her and that she had a difficult time pleasing them. Her father, a prominent physician in their home community, encouraged her to be proud of her African American heritage. Her mother, also a professional, experienced problems with depression throughout her adult life. She had disclosed a sexual abuse history to Lashonda who reported to the social worker that her mother had been in therapy "forever." Lashonda quipped that this was perhaps her fate as well – that being, a lifelong therapy client. This "tongue-in-cheek" self-description, however, was played out in numerous ways in her work with the social worker.

The social worker viewed Lashonda's self-description as a "lifelong client" as reflective of her belief in an impoverished sense of self that is complex, troubled, and complicated by her racial identity. Lashonda and the worker developed a strong alliance, agreeing to keep focused on her racial identity as one source of information about her strengths and her difficulties in a number of areas in her interpersonal relationships. Early in the work, Lashonda shamefully reported to the therapist that she was a binge eater and that she purged. She had had a long history of bulimic activity but had not disclosed this to her previous therapist. Lashonda recounted the painful history of her interactions with her mother when she was an adolescent. She reported that her mother was obsessed with diet regimes and imposed these on Lashonda. Her mother also noted to Lashonda that her task to stay attractive to men would be especially difficult, especially since she inherited many of her father's physical characteristics. Jessica Daniel (2000) refers to the plight of African American women in terms of appearance. She notes the image distortion of Black women in popular culture and how challenging it is for a Black woman to disavow her wish to be the American icon of womanhood – that being a White, thin, blond, and sexually appealing woman. Lashonda's identity was particularly confused as her mother was white. Lashonda told the social worker about her shame about her weight (she did not appear overweight) and that she could never get her hair to look right – she went on to describe her shame about her "frizzy" hair. She shared many examples of being teased as a child by other children when her hair would go "really frizzy" on rainy days.

Her concern about her appearance clearly marks a shaky identity and her many experiences of microaggressions enacted on her by her mother, her school chums and her potential boy-friends made her particularly vulnerable to developing a shamed sense of self. The social worker understood this sense of herself as being related to a form of complex post-traumatic stress syndrome – she experienced ongoing, insidious, and repetitive insults about her appearance and this profoundly shaped how she views herself as a Black woman in a predominantly White geographic area. This theme was played out consistently in terms of her comfort level in meeting and dating men. Daniel (2000) discusses the fears that African American women carry with regards to sexual assault. This young client often talks about how she feels scrutinized sexually by many men and she feels low-level anxiety about being the object of a sexual assault, on a regular basis (recall Shome, 1999, discussed above).

Daniel also discusses the notion that African American women experience trauma in edu-cational institutions. Here too, Lashonda had much to discuss and to work through. She attended a primarily White elementary school and she was often taunted, being called names that denounced her biracial status and her appearance as a Black child. High school was somewhat better as she was in a more heterogeneous mix but again, she shares the experiences of other People of Color. She did not have many teachers with whom to identify and/or who encouraged her to excel acade-mically. Her father was a gentle and firm supporter of her talents and abilities to do well educa-tionally. Her relationship with her father has set the tone for her to have a positive transference relationship towards her current therapist. She was able to use her therapy relationship to discuss her apprehensions about her school performance and her interactions with professors with whom she suspects some racial bias against her.

In summary, her therapy appeared to work well in spite of the many legacies that she has had to withstand in order to re-shape a sense of herself as a strong, vibrant, resilient woman who has had to modulate her reactions to what seems like a never-ending "assault" to her personhood on many levels. She most recently described to the clinician that she had the unfortunate experience of going to a "walk-in, emergency" medical clinic to secure treatment of a decidedly uncomfortable skin rash of poison ivy. She unhappily reported that she was there for over three hours and that she had had to ask the White receptionist why other White clients were being processed before her. She is able to be assertive but she reports to me how much energy it takes and how she wishes she could just "blend in" like everyone else. Again, the reader can hear the resilience of Lashonda and can empathize with the injustices that she faces on a regular basis.

Conclusion

People of Color experience racism at the institutional and interpersonal level. Racism has both direct and insidious effects on the quality of their lives. The web of institutional racism described by Miller and Garran (2008) clearly demonstrates the extent of racism in contemporary U.S. society. Social workers have a responsibility to attempt to dismantle racism and this must happen both systematically and also in micro-practice settings as well. In the broadest sense, social workers follow a Code of Ethics that directly challenges oppressive practices of any sort. The Council on Social Work Education, which accredits Schools of Social Work across the United States, also mandates that social work curriculum in required Human Behavior and Practice courses integrates content concerning issues of diversity and racism; in addition, many Schools of Social Work offer courses related to how to combat discrimination and racism.

While clearly institutional practices contribute to racism and barriers exist for People of Color in accessing useful services, some authors make suggestions for strategies that will reduce disparities in mental health service utilization. For example, Copeland (2006) suggests that disparities may lessen if mental health providers become more knowledgeable about the sociocultural environments and interpersonal barriers to treatment of African American youth. She specifically suggested that services could be enhanced if providers better understood the complex racial identity process of African American adolescents. Miranda, Bernal, Lau, Kohn, Hwang, & LaFromboise (2005) also suggest that cultural sensitivity of linguistic adaptations of providers may decrease disparities in service delivery with ethnic populations.

All social workers must assume responsibility for being culturally responsive and competent clinicians. Increasingly, authors are addressing issues of developing expertise in cross-cultural interventions (Altman, 1995, 2000; Holmes, 1992; Jackson, 2000; Leary, 1995, 1997, 2000; Perez-Foster, 1996; Ringel, 2005; Roland, 1998; Sue & Sue, 1990). Culturally responsive clinicians accept, as a given, that one's culture, ethnicity and/or race fundamentally shapes one's view of oneself and that any assessment or social work intervention needs to fully integrate the social identities of the client. This integration of cultural factors aids the social worker to initiate relationships that are accepting of differences for a range of individuals and families. In other words, the notion that there is a "right" or "normal" cultural background (read White middle-class America) is continuously challenged by the culturally competent social worker. Rather, the customs, the belief systems, and the strengths of any particular ethnic group or race are honored by the social worker so that the client is free to fully express her own value system. While this seems to be an obvious stance that social workers would adopt with clients – that is, starting where the client is, and respecting the strengths of the client, it is only since the late 1990s that matters of cultural competence have been fully articulated in social work and psychotherapeutic literature.

As noted above, it is important for social workers to be aware of racial identity development models in order to better understand the complexity of their clients' identities. A number of authors (Cross, 1991; Helms, 1990; Tatum, 1992) have suggested that People of Color experience a developmental pathway in terms of racial identity and social workers need this knowledge base in order to be effective practitioners with a diverse client caseload. Social workers who are aware of racial identity developmental theory have a better appreciation of the various responses that People of Color might have in response to White institutions, as an example. Helms (1990) also suggests that White individuals also develop a racial identity as people from the dominant culture and it is vitally important that White practitioners approach their clients with an attitude of reflexivity – that being, approaching clients with a great deal of self-awareness so as to not abuse the inherent power imbalance that may be set up between social worker and client. Miehls and Moffatt (2000) suggest that reflexive practitioners are open to self-examination and also value the differences found in diverse populations.

In conclusion, racism continues to be a major social problem in the United States. Regardless of one's role(s) in the social work profession, all have a responsibility of enacting the Code of Ethics to try to dismantle racism at every level. Social workers can do this in their interpersonal interactions with each other. If one identifies as White, one can keep a dialogue open with colleagues and friends of color so as to initiate conversations about race and the insidious impact of race on People of Color. One can trust that colleagues of color are not exaggerating their experiences when they tell about systemic racism and about their experiences of micro-aggressions. Social workers can and should initiate conversations about race in their clinical work. Perhaps, their most important task as White individuals is to truly be open to self-examination about their white privilege so they can better become an ally with others to challenge racist practices in their families, groups, organizations, and communities.

Notes

1 It is suggested that this generic term implies homogeneity among "all" People of Color whereas in fact, there is great heterogeneity among different ethnic groups that are discussed. These differences will be noted, as appropriate, throughout the chapter. The term People of Color is utilized to denote any individual who self-identifies as a non-White person.
2 Miller and Garran (2008) recognize that racism intersects with other social oppression in the United States (for example, sexism, heterosexism or classism) but their focus is on what still needs to be accomplished in the United States to dismantle institutional racism.
3 Numerous resources describe complex post-traumatic stress syndrome. For examples, see Allen (2001) and Karusaitis Basham and Miehls (2004).

Web resources

Antiracism.com: Deconstructing Racism, Reconstructing our Humanity
www.antiracism.com

Anti-Racism Resources
www.hopesite.ca/rekindle/links/racism_hrights.html

Anti-Racist Alliance
www.antiracistalliance.com

Health and Human Services
www.raceandhealth.hhs.gov

Health Statistics
www.phpartners.org/health.stats

National Center for Children in Poverty
www.nccp.org

National Mental Health Association
www.nmha.org

White Privilege and Anti-Racism
www.edchange.org/multicutlural/sites/white.html

References

Allen, I.M. (1996). PTSD among African Americans. In A.J. Marsella, M.J. Friedman, E.T. Gerrity, & R.M. Scurfield (eds), *Ethnocultural aspects of post-traumatic stress disorder: Issues, research and clinical applications* (pp. 209–238). Washington, DC: American Psychological Association.
Allen, J. (2001). *Traumatic relationships and serious mental disorders*. New York: John Wiley & Sons.

Altman, N. (1995). *The analyst in the inner city: Race, class and culture through a psychoanalytic lens.* Hillsdale, NJ: Analytic Press.

Altman, N. (2000). Black and white thinking. *Psychoanalytic Dialogues, 10,* 589–605.

American Psychiatric Association (APA). (2000). *Diagnostic and statistical manual of mental disorders* (4th ed., text revision). Washington, DC: APA.

Anglin, D., Alberti, P., Link, B., & Phelan, J. (2008). Racial differences in beliefs about the effectiveness and necessity of mental health treatment. *American Journal of Community Psychology, 42,* 17–24.

Atkinson, D. (2004). *Counseling American minorities* (6th ed.). New York: McGraw-Hill.

Barnes, A. (2004). Race, schizophrenia, and admission to state psychiatric hospitals. *Administration and Policy in Mental Health, 31* (3), 241–252.

Bobo, L.D. (2001). Racial attitudes and relations at the close of the twentieth century. In N.J. Smelter, W.J. Wilson, & F. Mitchell (eds), *American becoming: Racial trends and their consequences* (Vol. I, pp. 265–275). New York: Routledge.

Brown, T.N., Wallace, J.M., & Williams, D.R. (2001). Race-related correlates of young adults' subjective well-being. *Social Indicators Research, 53* (1), 97–116.

Butts, H.G. (2002). The Black mask of humanity: Racial/ethnic discrimination and post-traumatic stress disorder. *Journal of the American Academy of Psychiatry and the Law, 30,* 336–339.

Constantine, M.G. (2007). Racial microaggressions against African American clients in cross-racial counseling relationships. *Journal of Counseling Psychology, 54* (1), 1–16.

Cooper, S., McLoyd, V., Wood, D., & Hardaway, C. (2008). Racial discrimination and the mental health of African American adolescents. In S. Quintana & C. McKown (eds), *Handbook of race, racism, and the developing child* (pp. 278–312). New York: John Wiley & Sons.

Copeland, V. (2006). Disparities in mental health service utilization among low-income African American adolescents: Closing the gap by enhancing practitioner's competence. *Child and Adolescent Social Work Journal, 23* (4), 407–431.

Cross, W. (1991). *Shades of black.* Philadelphia, PA: Temple University Press.

Cushman, P. (1995). *Constructing the self, constructing America: A cultural history of psychotherapy.* Reading, MA: Addison-Wesley.

Daniel, J. (2000). The courage to hear: African American women's memories of racial trauma. In L. Jackson & B. Greene (eds), *Psychotherapy with African American women: Innovations in psychodynamic perspectives and practice* (pp. 126–144). New York: Guilford Press.

Davis, K. (1997). Managed care, mental illness and African Americans: A prospective analysis of managed care policy in the United States. *Smith College Studies in Social Work, 67* (3), 623–641.

DeCoster, V.A. (1999). The effects of gender and race on physician treatment of patient emotion. *Journal of Gender, Culture, and Health, 4* (3), 215–237.

Del Carmen, A. (2008). *Racial profiling in America.* Upper Saddle River, NJ: Pearson/Prentice Hall.

Department of Health and Human Services. (1999). *Mental health: A report of the Surgeon General.* Rockville, MD: U.S. Department of Health and Human Services, Substance Abuse and Mental Health Services Administration, Center for Mental Health Services, National Institutes of Health, National Institute of Mental Health.

Department of Health and Human Services (2001). *Mental health: Culture, race and ethnicity* (A supplement to *Mental health: A report of the Surgeon General*). Rockville, MD: U.S. Department of Health and Human Services, Substance Abuse and Mental Health Services Administration, Center for Mental Health Services.

Fisher, C.B., Wallace, S.A., & Fenton, R.E. (2000). Discrimination distress during adolescence. *Journal of Youth and Adolescence, 29* (6), 679–695.

Foucault, M. (1979). *Discipline and punish: The birth of the prison.* A. Sheridan (Trans.). New York: Vintage.

Foucault, M. (1980). Truth and power. In C. Gordon (ed.), *Power/knowledge: Selected interviews and other writings* (pp. 229–259). New York: Pantheon.

Franklin, A., Boyd-Franklin, N., & Kelly, S. (2006). Racism and invisibility: Race-related stress, emotion abuse and psychological trauma for people of color. *Journal of Emotional Abuse, 6* (2–3), 9–30.

Garb, H.N. (1997). Race bias, social class bias, and gender bias in clinical judgment. *Clinical Psychology: Science and Practice, 4* (2). 99–120.

Ghods, B., Roter, D., Ford, D., Larson, S., Arbelaez, J., & Cooper, L. (2008). Patient-physician communication in the primary care visits of African Americans and Whites with depression. *Journal of General Internal Medicine, 23* (5), 600–606.

Gibbons, F.X., Gerard, M., Cleveland, M.J., Wills, T.A., & Brody, G. (2004). Perceived discrimination and substance use in African American parents and their children: A panel study. *Journal of Personality and Social Psychology, 86* (4), 517–529.

Gitterman, A., & Germain, C.B. (2008). *The life model of social work practice: Advances in theory and practice.* New York: Columbia University Press.

Greenberg, G., & Rosenheck, R. (2003). Change in mental health service delivery among Blacks, Whites, and Hispanics in the Department of Veterans Affairs. *Administration and Policy in Mental Health, 31* (1), 31–43.

Harris, R. (2008). Racial microaggression? How do you know? *American Psychologist, 63* (4), 275–276.

Helms, J. (1990). *Black and White racial identity: Theory, research and practice.* New York: Greenwood Press.

Herman, J. (1992). *Trauma and recovery.* New York: Basic Books.

Holmes, C. (1992). Race and transference in psychoanalysis and psychotherapy. *International Journal of Psychoanalysis, 73* (1), 1–11.

hooks, b. (1992). Representations of whiteness in the black imagination. In L. Grossberg, P. Treichler, & C. Nelson (eds), *Cultural studies* (pp. 338–346). New York: Routledge.

Howard-Hamilton, M., & Frazier, K. (2005). Identity development and the convergence of race, ethnicity, and gender. In D. Comstock (ed.), *Diversity and development: Critical contexts that shape our lives and relationships* (pp. 67–90). Belmont, CA: Thomson/Brooks/Cole.

Jackson, L. (2000). The new multiculturalism and psychodynamic theory: Psychodynamic psychotherapy and African American women. In L. Jackson & B. Greene (eds), *Psychotherapy with African American women: Innovations in psychodynamic perspectives and practice* (pp. 1–14). New York: Guilford Press.

Johnson, J., & Cameron, M. (2001). Barriers to providing effective mental health services to American Indians. *Mental Health Services Research, 3* (4), 215–223.

Karusaitis Basham, K., & Miehls, D. (2004). *Transforming the legacy: Couple therapy with survivors of childhood trauma.* New York: Columbia University Press.

Kataoka, S.H., Zhang, L., & Wells, K.B. (2002). Unmet need for mental health care among U.S. children: Variation by ethnicity and insurance status. *American Journal of Psychiatry, 159,* 1548–1555.

Keith, S.J., Regier, D.A., & Rae, D.S. (1991). Schizophrenic disorders. In L.N. Robins & D.A. Regier (eds), *The epidemiologic catchment area study* (pp. 33–52). New York: Free Press.

Leary, K. (1995). Interpreting in the dark. *Psychoanalytic Psychology, 12,* 127–140.

Leary, K. (1997). Race, self disclosure and "forbidden talk": Race and ethnicity in contemporary clinical practice. *Psychoanalytic Quarterly, 66,* 163–189.

Leary, K. (2000). Racial enactments in dynamic treatment. *Psychoanalytic Dialogues, 10,* 639–653.

Leong, F. (2001). Guest editor's introduction to a special issue: Barriers to providing effective mental health services to racial and ethnic minorities in the United States. *Mental Health Services Research, 3* (4), 179–180.

Leong, F., & Lau, A. (2001). Barriers to providing effective mental health services to Asian Americans. *Mental Health Services Research, 3* (4), 201–214.

Levy, S., & Karafantis, D. (2008). Lay theories and intergroup relations. In S. Quintana & C. McKown (eds), *Handbook of race, racism, and the developing child* (pp. 111–131). Hoboken, NJ: John Wiley & Sons.

Linehan, M. (1993). *Cognitive-behavioral treatment of borderline personality disorder.* New York: Guilford Press.

Lopez, S. (2003). Reflections on the Surgeon General's report on mental health, culture, race and ethnicity. *Culture, medicine and psychiatry, 27,* 419–434.

Manson, S. (2003). Extending the boundaries, bridging the gaps: Crafting mental health – Culture, race and ethnicity. A supplement to the Surgeon General's report on mental health. *Culture, Medicine and Psychiatry, 27,* 395–408.

Marsiglia, F., & Kulis, S. (2009). *Diversity, oppression, and change.* Chicago, IL: Lyceum.

Miehls, D. (2001). The interface of racial identity development with identity complexity in clinical social work student practitioners. *Clinical Social Work Journal, 29* (3), 229–244.

Miehls, D. (2005). Couples counseling and psychotherapy in racial-cultural psychology. In R. Carter (ed.), *Handbook of racial-cultural psychology and counseling: Training and practice, vol. 2* (pp. 379–391). New York: John Wiley & Sons.

Miehls, D. & Moffatt, K. (2000). Constructing social work identity based on the reflexive self. *British Journal of Social Work, 30*, 339–348.

Miller, J., & Garran, A.M. (2008). *Racism in the United States: Implications for the helping professions.* New York: Thomson/Brooks/Cole.

Miranda, J., Bernal, G., Lau, A., Kohn, L., Hwang, W., & LaFromboise, T. (2005). State of the science on psychosocial interventions for ethnic minorities. *Annual Review of Psychology, 1*, 113–142.

Moffatt, K., & Miehls, D. (1999). Development of student identity: Evolution from neutrality to subjectivity. *Journal of Teaching in Social Work, 19* (1–2), 65–76.

Nyborg, V.M., & Curry, J.F. (2003). The impact of perceived racism: Psychological symptoms among African American boys. *Journal of Clinical Child and Adolescent Psychology, 32* (2), 258–266.

Ojeda, V., & McGuire, T. (2006). Gender and racial/ethnic differences in use of outpatient mental health and substance use services by depressed adults. *Psychiatric Quarterly, 77*, 211–222.

Pattillo-McCoy, M. (2007). Black picket fences: Privilege and peril among the Black middle class. In M. Andersen & P. Hill Collins (eds), *Race, class and gender: An anthology* (6th ed.). Belmont, CA: Thomson Wadsworth.

Perez-Foster, R. (1996). What is a multicultural perspective for psychoanalysis? In R. Perez-Foster, M. Moskowitz, & R.A. Javier (eds), *Reaching across boundaries of culture and class: Widening the scope of psychotherapy* (pp. 3–20). Northvale, NJ: Jason Aronson.

Pierre, M., Mahalik, J., & Woodland, M. (2001). The effects of racism, African self-consciousness and psychological functioning on Black masculinity: A historical and social adaptation framework. *Journal of African American Studies, 6* (2), 19–39.

Pincus, F. (2000). Discrimination comes in many forms: Individual, institutional, and structural. In M. Adams, W. Blumenfield, R. Castanenda, H. Hackman, M. Peters, & X. Zuniga (eds), *Readings for diversity and social justice* (pp. 31–35). New York: Routledge.

Pitts, L. (2009). Commentary: "Post-racial" America isn't here yet. Retrieved March 31, 2009, from www.cnn.com/2009/POLITICS/03/28/pitts.black.american/index.html

Progue White, K. (2002). Surviving hating and being hated: Some personal thoughts about racism from a psychoanalytic perspective. *Contemporary Psychoanalysis, 38* (3), 401–422.

Provan, K.G., & Carle, N. (2000). *A guide to behavioral health management care of Native Americans.* Tuscon, AZ: Center for Native American Health, University of Arizona.

Ringel, S. (2005). Therapeutic dilemmas in cross-cultural practice with Asian American adolescents. *Child and Adolescent Social Work Journal, 29*, 53–63.

Riolo, S., Nguyen, T., Greden, J., & King, C. (2005). Prevalence of depression by race/ethnicity: Findings from the National Health and Nutrition Examination Survey III. *American Journal of Public Health, 95* (6), 998–1000.

Roland, A. (1998). *Cultural pluralism and psychoanalysis.* New York: Routledge.

Root, M.P.P. (1992). Reconstructing the impact of trauma on personality. In M. Ballou & L. Brown (eds), *Theories of personality and psychopathology: Feminist reappraisal* (pp. 229–265). New York: Guilford Press.

Sanchez-Hucles, J.V. (1998). Racism: Emotional abusiveness and psychological trauma for ethnic minorities. *Journal of Emotional Abuse, 1*, 69–87.

Scholle, S., & Kellehar, K. (2000). Managed care for seriously emotionally disturbed children. Paper presented at a Substance Abuse and Mental Health Services Administration Managed Care Seminar, Washington, DC.

Snowden, L. (2001). Barriers to effective mental health services for African Americans. *Mental Health Services Research, 3* (4), 181–187.

Snowden, L. (2005). Racial, cultural and ethnic disparities in health and mental health: Toward theory and research at community levels. *American Journal of Community Psychology, 35* (1–2), 1–8.

Scruggs, A. (2009). Colorblindness: The new racism? Retrieved September 28, 2009, from www.tolerance.org/magazine/number-36-fall-2009-colorblindness-new-racism

Shipler, D. (1997). *A country of strangers: Blacks and whites in America.* New York: Knopf.

Shome, R. (1999). Whiteness and the politics of location: Postcolonial reflections. In T. Nakayama & J. Martin (eds), *Whiteness: The communication of social identity.* Thousand Oaks, CA: Sage.

Simons, R.L., Murry, V., McLoyd, V.C., Link K., Cutrona, C., & Conger, R.D. (2002). Discrimination, crime, ethnic identity, and parenting as correlates of depressive symptoms among African American children: A multilevel analysis. *Development and Psychopathology, 14* (2), 371–393.

Stone, J. (2002). Race and health care disparities: Overcoming vulnerability. *Theoretical Medicine, 23*, 499–518.

Sue, D., & Sue, D. (1990). *Counseling the culturally different: Theory and practice* (2nd ed.). New York: John Wiley & Sons.

Sue, D.W., Capodilupo, C.M., Torino, G.C., Bucceri, J.M., Holder, A.M.B., Nadal, K.L., & Esquilin, M. (2007). Racial microaggressions in everyday life: Implications for clinical practice. *American Psychologist, 62*, 271–286.

Sue, D.W., Capodilupo, C.M., & Holder, A.M. (2008a). Racial microaggressions in the life experience of Black Americans. *Professional psychology: Research and practice, 39* (3), 329–336.

Sue, D.W., Capodilupo, C.M., Nadal, K.L., & Torino, G.C. (2008b). Racial microaggressions and the power to define reality. *American Psychologist, 63* (4), 277–279.

Swartz, M., Wagner, H., Swanson, J., Burns, B., George, L., & Padgett, D. (1998). Administrative update: Utilization of services. I. Comparing use of public and private mental health services: The enduring barriers of race and age. *Community Mental Health Journal, 34* (2), 133–144.

Tatum, B. (1992). Talking about race, learning about racism: The application of racial identity developmental theory in the classroom. *Harvard Educational Review, 62* (1), 1–24.

Tatum, B. (2000). Defining racism: "Can we talk?". In M. Adams, W. Blumenfeld, R. Sastaneda, H. Hackman, M. Peters, & X. Zuniga (eds), *Readings for diversity and social justice* (pp. 79–82). New York: Routledge.

Terr, L.C. (1991). Childhood traumas: An outline and overview. *American Journal of Psychiatry, 148*, 10–20.

Thomas, K.R. (2008). Macrononsense in multiculturalism. *American Psychologist, 63* (4), 274–275.

Thompson, J.W., Belcher, J.R., DeForge, B.R., Myers, C.P., & Rosenstein, M.J. (1993). Changing characteristics of schizophrenic patients admitted to state hospitals. *Hospital and Community Psychiatry, 44* (3), 231–235.

Turner, C. (1999). Racial problems in society and in the classroom. Paper delivered at Smith College School for Social Work, March.

Utsey, S. (1997). Racism and the psychological well-being of African American men. *Journal of African American Studies, 3* (1), 69–87.

Utsey, S., & Payne, Y. (2000). Psychological impacts of racism in a clinical versus normal sample of African American men. *Journal of African American Studies, 5* (1), 57–72.

Van Dorn, R., Swanson, J., Swartz, M., & Elbogen, E. (2005). The effects of race and criminal justice involvement on access to atypical antipsychotic medications among persons with schizophrenia. *Mental Health Services Research, 7* (2), 123–134.

Vedantam, S. (2005). Racial disparities found in pinpointing mental illness. Retrieved September 28, 2009, from www.washingtonpost.com/wp-dyn/content/articale/2005/06/27/Ar2005062701496.

Whaley, A. (1997). Ethnicity/race, paranoia, and psychiatric diagnoses: Clinician bias versus sociocultural differences. *Journal of Psychopathology and Behavioral Assessment, 19* (1), 1–20.

Wong, C.A., Eccles, J.S., & Sameroff, A. (2003). The influence of ethnic discrimination and ethnic identification on African American adolescents' school and socio-emotional adjustment. *Journal of Personality, 71* (6), 1197–1232.

Wood, P., Yeh, M., Pan, D., Lambros, K., McCabe, K., & Hough, R. (2005). Exploring the relationship between race/ethnicity, age of first school-based services utilization, and age of first specialty mental health care for at-risk youth. *Mental Health Services Research, 7* (3), 185–196.

Young, I. (2000). Five faces of oppression. In M. Adams, W. Blumenfeld, R. Castaneda, H. Hackman, M. Peters, & X. Zuniga (eds), *Readings for diversity and social justice* (pp. 35–49). New York: Routledge.

5 War and its effects

Scott Harding

This chapter analyzes war and armed conflict as a widespread social phenomenon with a range of harmful consequences for individuals and communities. War is increasingly viewed as a significant public health problem that compromises human rights and undermines sustainable social development (Pilisuk, 2008). The increased use of "dirty war" tactics (Hicks & Spagat, 2008) and the targeting of civilians and social infrastructure have served to amplify the destructive effects of organized armed violence. These outcomes are especially pronounced in poor and developing countries, the setting of a majority of global conflicts in recent decades.

An examination of the multiple aspects of war reveals the differing vulnerabilities and risks for mental health and psychosocial problems faced by different populations. Many of these negative psychological outcomes, as with declines in overall community health, may linger or become exacerbated well after the cessation of fighting, undermining productive communal and individual social functioning. Thus the most common mental disorders associated with conflict situations – post-traumatic stress disorder (PTSD), anxiety, and depression – can require sustained and multiple levels of intervention in order to adequately address the emotional wounds produced by war. A growing body of research indicates that exposure to war-related violence and the destabilization of community functioning from armed conflict affect levels of domestic abuse, lead to increased stress, depression and other psychological troubles, undermine a sense of self-efficacy, and increases the incidence of other social problems (Jansen, 2006).

Disruption to community functioning and social networks is a principal outcome of armed conflict, underscoring the challenges to improved mental health beyond targeting at the individual level. Indeed, while limited research exists, the United Nations and leading non-governmental organizations (NGOs) note the centrality of an approach to healing war trauma that emphasizes social integration of groups and individuals affected by war. Such methods are increasingly viewed as a more feasible and culturally appropriate intervention than direct and/or sustained mental health counseling and services for individuals. Overall, this suggests a need to understand both the individual and community-level consequences of exposure to war, and the reality of resilience as a common outcome of war trauma (Krippner & McIntyre, 2003). Indeed, the World Health Organization (WHO, 2002) notes that an emphasis on the medical model "may fail to take account of the variety and complexity of human responses to stressful events," including the critical role of rebuilding social networks and community institutions as a tool to promote post-conflict healing (p. 224).

Definitions of war

While war and armed conflict are viewed as negative experiences that create widespread destruction for individuals and communities, such practices remain a fundamental reality of modern society. In spite of diminished conflict between the world's major industrial powers in the second half of the twentieth century, military violence dominates much of the conduct of international affairs. Pilisuk (2008) finds that in the 60-year period after World War II, some 250 "major" wars occurred "taking over 50 million lives and leaving tens of millions home-less" (p. 2).

Global economic and political changes during this period have increasingly challenged conventional understanding of war as being only large-scale conflict between the armed forces of nation-states. Indeed, the end of the Cold War has underscored the prevalence of "new wars" that defy easy categorization (Kaldor, 1999). Rather than a contest between nations to utilize conventional military tactics to capture or control territory, a new form of organized violence – often involving non-state actors – has become the norm. Thus as war is no longer the exclusive domain of modern states, "new wars" increasingly reflect the impact of globalization in terms of conflict over access to resources, the use of new technology, and dependence on external actors for support. Global conflict involving non-traditional actors and "unconventional" methods is viewed as "asymmetrical warfare," reflecting disparities in the size of military forces and in access to resources among those involved in armed violence (Pilisuk, 2008).

Kaldor (1999) suggests that these new forms of conflict involve a blurring of previous dis-tinctions between traditional armed violence, organized crime, and human rights violations. Most often depicted as "civil war" among competing political forces, mass media coverage of contemporary war and armed violence has also emphasized "identity politics," the rise of ethnic conflicts, and genocide (in developing countries) in recent years. Indeed, the increasing "ethnicization" of global conflict should be seen as a critical factor in terms of those most at-risk for experiencing psychological distress from organized violence. Other types of social identities – gender, religion, age – are also important variables in assessing multiple types of vulnerability during wartime.

While recognizing the inherent *political* nature of modern warfare, Kaldor (1999) rejects the notion that these events only involve local actors (as internal conflict or civil wars). Rather, she finds that the "new wars"

> involve a myriad of transnational connections so that the distinction between internal and external, between aggression (attacks from beyond) and repression (attacks from inside the country), or even between local and global, are difficult to sustain.
>
> (Kaldor, 1999, p. 2)

Such distinctions are important. Rather than viewing wars as events that occur with little warning or as phenomena that can be traced largely to internal strife or ethnic hostility, such "complex emergencies" should be seen as deliberate acts with their own politics, functions, and benefits (Keen, 2008). In this view, *global and local* interests are distinctly intertwined in war and other types of human-created disasters (Calhoun, 2004). The reality that war and global violence serve political uses and provide benefits to transnational forces, state actors and local elites challenges the notion of western indifference and impotence in the face of numerous global conflicts in the developing world.

Although the "new wars" dominate the international arena, conflict between nation-states and between nation-states and non-state actors still occurs though on different terms. Nations increasingly have utilized low-level (or "low-intensity") conflict, as well as the "covert" use of force to achieve political aims and minimize their own military casualties during war. Such was the case with Russia in its military intervention in Chechnya, and the United States in its conflict with Iraq between 1991 (the end of the Gulf War) and 2003 (the invasion of Iraq). Member states of NATO also fought against Yugoslavia (which was accused of fomenting ethnic cleansing) using conventional means in 1999. The United States has also conducted a global "war on terror" following the terrorist attacks of September 11, 2001.

Understanding different forms of war, the location where violent conflict typically occurs, and those who engage in such conduct is essential to a better appreciation of the myriad impacts that result from armed conflict. War is usually not an episodic and limited phenomenon; it is more often a long-term, structural process with multiple stages, some more evident than others. In recent decades many developing nations have been engaged in long-running armed conflicts with lethal consequences, for example, Congo, Sri Lanka, Darfur, and Colombia. Thus the different (mental health) effects of short-term versus chronic conflict bear consideration, as do the differing capacities of nations and/or local communities to deal with the physical and social disruption and trauma caused by war.

As important, the rising prevalence of civil wars and non-traditional conflict – the use of insurgency and guerilla warfare tactics – has resulted in greater casualties among civilian populations (Pilisuk, 2008). Indeed, many contemporary conflicts are marked by the targeting of non-combatants as an integral war "tactic" designed to instill terror among domestic populations. In particular, various armed groups commonly target professionals, such as doctors and educators, as a weapon of war to destabilize local communities (MedAct, 2008). As a result, the *political control* of local populations is increasingly predicated on the use of terrorism, mass killings and forced displacement of civilians (Kaldor, 1999). In addition, the increased blurring of lines between combatants and "civilians" has resulted in a greater willingness to disrupt key economic infrastructure: power grids, water supplies, food production and distribution networks, and hospitals are seen by some armed groups as legitimate targets of warfare.

This reality contrasts markedly with international efforts to regulate war and the use of armed force. In the twentieth century ideas of "just war" emerged based on meeting a series of internationally recognized criteria. This led to an emphasis on formal "laws," usually enacted by international bodies like the United Nations (UN), governing the when and how of warfare between nation-states (Byers, 2005). The aim of such global norms has been to provide and retain a plausible moral framework for engaging in war. Overall, the evolution of international law related to warfare has emphasized the principle that unilateral aggression is illegitimate. In particular, "just war" theory is predicated on a nation-state having a "just cause" to engage in armed conflict – typically seen as the idea of war as a last resort and/or the use of force to defend a country against external aggression. In addition, just war is predicated on the concept of "proportionality" in terms of the means used to wage conflict and prohibits targeting civilians (Fiala, 2008).

With the advent of increasingly lethal weapons in the twentieth century, these global norms took on added importance. Thus the Geneva Conventions were codified following World War II to strengthen civilian protections as well as to make war a more humane phenomenon for combatants. In spite of widespread global adherence to these principles, in effect laws governing the use of force are routinely violated, both by nation-states and by irregular forces (guerilla armies, terrorist groups, insurgents). The International Committee of the Red Cross (ICRC, 2009) has noted that either through deliberate targeting or a failure to distinguish civilians from combatants, millions of civilians continue to bear the burden of global conflicts. Such practices are highlighted in the "new wars," as paramilitary units, guerilla armies, mercenaries and other "rogue" forces routinely seek to inflict psychological damage in armed conflict as a primary goal through the targeting of civilians. In recent years the same claims have been leveled against countries like the United States, Russia, Israel, Colombia and Sri Lanka and in other contemporary conflicts involving more traditional armed forces.

The increased use of economic sanctions should also be recognized as an important yet overlooked conception of conflict. Sanctions are viewed by some as a useful tool that falls between diplomacy and the resort to armed force; their use is often justified as a way to "negotiate" hostilities between states without actual combat (Cortright & Lopez, 1999). Of note, sanctions avoid the traditional limits of warfare: selecting military targets, avoiding civilian casualties, creating obligations of belligerent states to local populations (Garfield, 2002). Thus, sanctions are typically carried out to achieve political goals, and are most often imposed by strong states or the international community against smaller, weaker nations (often depicted as "rouge" or "outlaw" states). Sanctions have been widely used in the post-Cold War era, both by the UN and the United States, purportedly as a tool to prevent violence, protect human rights, and promote democracy. Since the late 1980s, they have been employed against Iraq, North Korea, Cuba, Sudan, Somalia, former Yugoslavia, and Myanmar (Burma), among other countries. In their use by the United States, sanctions retain significant bipartisan political support, and are often seen as a "cheap" way to engage in conflict with perceived American adversaries largely out of the media spotlight and public scrutiny.

What are the different *impacts* of war and militarization? How does violent conflict disrupt local communities and other critical social functions? Armed conflict usually creates long-term disruption to social and health systems, more so in developing countries. By disrupting water and sanitation systems, for example, war significantly increases the likelihood of a decline in public health. Gupta, Clements, Bhattacharya, and Chakravarti (2002) found that reductions in infant mortality, which occur during direct conflict, continue during the post-conflict period. In an analysis of the post-conflict consequences on major diseases and health conditions, civil wars were found to "greatly raise the subsequent risk of death and disability from many infectious diseases, including malaria, tuberculosis, and other respiratory diseases" (Ghobarah, Huth, & Russett, 2004, p. 881). Using a formula that assessed "the life years lost" and "disabilities incurred from conditions contracted in earlier years when a civil war was active" (p. 870), researchers found that post-conflict situations were more lethal than the actual direct impacts of civil war.

Civil war and internal strife, the majority of contemporary armed conflicts, "typically triggers a prolonged reversal of economic and social development that often results in poverty continuing from one generation to the next" (UNICEF, 2004, pp. 40–41). In addition, the vulnerabilities produced by armed conflict make civilian populations more susceptible to disruptions caused by natural disasters or global economic crisis, multiplying the adverse effects (ICRC, 2009). Violent conflict also typically displaces civilian populations, most notably women, children, the elderly, and persons with disabilities. From 1990 to 2003, tens of millions of people were displaced or made refugees from 59 different armed conflicts in 48 separate locations, including more than one million children (UNICEF, 2004).

Armed conflict and war often provoke a disruption of the agricultural and health care sectors, education and other key infrastructure, creating long-term effects that perpetuate conditions that undermine economic and social development. With global conflicts increasingly marked by the use of "terror" tactics, the targeting of food production and distribution networks has often exacerbated access to food and conditions of malnutrition, especially among low-income groups. Amartya Sen (1984) has argued that famine typically occurs in weak and/or authoritarian states and reflects failures in the distribution of food via existing networks, as well as a lack of public efforts to relieve the consequences, factors which are often caused or amplified by armed conflict.

War may gradually induce or contribute to environmental destruction, jeopardizing food production, health and water quality. This often creates long-term conditions of starvation and disease, especially in developing countries, and may harm more people indirectly than who die from direct fighting (Krause & Mutimer, 2005). More generally, militarization – especially military production and the presence of military bases – are seen as creating widespread ecological threats and public health risks to the military and public alike (Gould, 2007).

While intended to force political change in target countries, economic sanctions are seen as violating human rights, as they typically produce a range of negative conditions beyond their stated (political) goals (Garfield, 2002). Their impact typically falls on civilian populations, rather than the political leadership or other ostensibly targeted groups. By undermining the economy of already vulnerable states, sanctions create rapid economic dislocation and food shortages, especially among the poor, unemployed, and other vulnerable groups. In addition, sanctions often generate adverse impacts on the agricultural and health care sectors and other key infrastructure of a country, creating long-lasting effects that threaten fundamental access to basic goods and services. Such conditions often continue well after sanctions have been eliminated. For these reasons sanctions are seen by some as "a form of collective punishment – an approach that is rebuked by all the tenants of Western legal practice" (Garfield, 2002, p. 97).

The case of Iraq, which experienced international trade sanctions from 1990 until 2004, offers an instructive example of the widespread economic and social costs caused by this policy tool. Sanctions played a key role in the decline of Iraq's infrastructure, public health, and social development. The impact of sanctions fell most heavily on Iraqi civilians, especially children and other vulnerable groups (Garfield, 1999; UNICEF, 1998). This included an abrupt increase in maternal mortality, along with a doubling of death rates for children under age five. Sanctions contributed to malnutrition, a public health problem new to Iraq. Along with increased rates of pneumonia and diarrhea (linked to declining access to clean water and adequate health care), this produced thousands of preventable deaths among children (Abergavenny, 2000). Despite controversy about the effects of sanctions, reliable public health research linked sanctions to the "excess deaths" of 300,000–500,000 infants and children in Iraq during the 1990s (Garfield & Leu, 2000). By 2003, the state of social development in Iraq contrasted sharply with its status before the imposition of sanctions. Until the mid-1980s, Iraq was "fast approaching standards comparable to those of developed countries" in terms of social development (United Nations Development Program (UNDP), 2002, p. 11). By 1990 Iraq was ranked second highest in human development in the Middle East (Pedersen, 2007). Yet 12 years after their imposition, the UN found that sanctions caused Iraq to experience "a shift from relative affluence to massive poverty" (UNDP, 2002, p. 12).

As this discussion shows, war produces direct and indirect adverse effects on individuals, communities and nation-states. While physical destruction and casualties are the more obvious result of armed conflict, other negative outcomes are notable. War, armed conflict, and militarization often skew economic production (and local distribution networks) by emphasizing the production and/or acquisition of military goods (Oakes & Lucas, 2001). This is especially problematic for poor and developing nations already struggling to meet key human development standards: increased military spending in response to conflict typically continues after fighting ends, reducing spending on vital activities like education and health care (Gupta et al., 2002). Over time, such trends contribute to the poverty and underdevelopment that prevails in much of the developing world with especially harmful outcomes for children (Carlton-Ford, 2004).

An imbalance in resources devoted to war and military production, while not as pronounced, is also a feature of many of the leading developed states. In the United States, in particular, militarism remains a basic feature of most aspects of society. This is linked to assumptions about the "right" of the United States to assume the role of global superpower and to wage war whenever deemed necessary to "protect" American interests. Thus, 20 years after the end of the Cold War, the United States maintains a "permanent war economy" (Melman, 1974) based on a shared consensus about its perceived economic benefits, the centrality of foreign weapons sales as a part of the economy, as well as a reliance on military force to resolve political conflict. Efforts to cut weapons systems or to limit military spending in the United States typically provoke a bipartisan political reaction aimed at preserving military-related jobs at all costs. These social norms have been reinforced since September 11, 2001, as the United States has waged a "war on terror" and fought concurrent wars in Iraq and Afghanistan. While the economic costs and the tradeoffs in terms of lost investment that result from allegiance to a military industrial complex have been challenged (Hossein-Zadeh, 2007), some argue that a perpetual state of war preparedness in the United States has also exacted a domestic toll – largely unexamined – on the civilian population (Lutz, 2002). The effects of living in a state of "para-war" and the constant threat of external violence generated through war preparedness have received limited research attention (Piachaud, 2008).

Disruptions to a range of "macro" level social structures and institutions are one aspect of the consequences imposed by violent conflict. Social work and other disciplines have increasingly addressed the *individual* effects caused by war and the myriad other ways in which armed conflict undermines the health of communities and social systems. In particular, the mental health outcomes associated with the trauma of war bear special consideration. These effects vary significantly across different populations. While greater attention has been paid to the relationship between mental health problems and war in recent decades (Krippner & McIntyre, 2003), understanding of these processes remains uneven. Much scholarship that exists has focused on treating refugees in third countries, rather than those living in (active or former) conflict zones. This underscores a need for analysis of community-based interventions that seek to stabilize local communities and promote social capital in the wake of armed conflict. That significant research gaps exist illuminates the uneven nature of mental health promotion and services worldwide. It further suggests the lack of a global commitment to fully appreciate some of the most significant "costs" of war.

War and mental health/illness

Research on the health consequences of war has led to growing recognition that the mental health effects linked to armed conflict are significant (Levy & Sidel, 2008). In part this reflects a consensus, embraced by the World Health Organization, that the conception of health should include "physical, mental, and social well-being, and not merely the absence of disease or infirmity" (Declaration of Alma-Ata, 1978, para. 2). While this represents an evolution in the promotion of public health, it also highlights the necessity of education and investment to ensure adequate mental health services in a global context. Given the lack of capacity to both assess and treat mental health symptoms in many countries experiencing conflict, greater awareness and creativity in dealing with this phenomenon must occur (Ghosh, Mohit, & Murthy, 2004). This is critical since with adequate diagnosis and quality intervention, most mental health problems are treatable.

Recent attention has focused on the psychological effects of war and related traumatic events on soldiers and their varied mental health needs (Englehard, Huijding, van den Hout, & de Jong, 2007; Paulson & Krippner, 2007). Among U.S. veterans of the wars in Iraq and Afghanistan, for example, high levels of depression, post-traumatic stress disorder, and other mental health problems linked to exposure to combat have been found. Hoge, Auchterlonie, and Milliken (2006) cited a high prevalence of mental health problem linked to active combat duty in these two conflicts, along with a relatively high level of mental health care utilization upon return to the United States. A report by the RAND Corporation found that more than 30 percent of returning veterans from Iraq and Afghanistan met the criteria for PTSD or major depression (Tanielian & Jaycock, 2008). Given the prolonged deployments of U.S. military personnel in these wars, and the high rate of traumatic brain injury – a "signature wound" of these conflicts – there is a strong likelihood that recognition of the *invisible* wounds of war will increase in future years. Such developments will likely place added strain on soldiers, their families, and continue to burden mental health care systems.

In a further sign of the human toll exacted by war, rising suicide rates among active duty military personnel have been reported in recent years, reaching a nearly 30-year high, while suicide among U.S. veterans has also risen (Kuehn, 2009). Of note, in 2008 the suicide rate among the military exceeded the civilian rate ("Evidence-based prevention . . .", 2009). Researchers found that large numbers of troops serving in Iraq and Afghanistan sustained serious injuries or developed psychiatric conditions during their deployment that have increased the risk of suicide (Tanielian & Jaycock, 2008). Strains on military families and increased incidence of child maltreatment during periods when soldier-parents were deployed have also been linked to participation in these wars (Gibbs, Martin, Kupper, & Johnson, 2007). The Army Center for Health Promotion and Preventive Medicine found that members of one Army unit that served in Iraq were accused of numerous murders and violent assaults after returning to the United States (U.S. Army Center for Health Promotion and Preventive Medicine (USACHPPM), 2009). In light of recent efforts to address mental health needs among U.S. troops serving in combat situations, these findings suggest continued stigma about reporting depression and other mental health problems within the military.

Addressing the varied forms of trauma experienced by soldiers should be of concern to mental health practitioners, especially given the lack of adequate psychological services for U.S. veterans. Among those experiencing a traumatic brain injury or suffering PTSD or other mental health conditions from deployment in Iraq and Afghanistan, only about one-half have sought psychiatric treatment and overall levels of mental health care are uneven (Tanielian & Jaycock, 2008). The growing strains placed on military families and the well-documented instability caused by mental health problems – lost work and low productivity, family disruption, and heightened probability of developing other disorders – underscore the need for an integrated system of care for military veterans. Ultimately, Wheeler and Bragin (2007) suggest a need for greater social work engagement on mental health issues for returning U.S. veterans and their families. They find that current services tend to pathologize returning veterans (based on use of a medical model to treat PTSD and other conditions) and are inadequate to promote integration of soldiers into local communities.

While the issues affecting soldiers are significant, given the extensive literature on the community level impacts of armed conflict, the focus of this chapter is on the health and mental health consequences of war for *civilians* worldwide. In light of the growing disruption of community functioning and increased rates of civilian casualties linked to armed conflict, this emphasis seems essential. How does war and exposure to armed conflict produce different mental health impacts? Who is affected, and what are the key risk factors for elevated symptoms of depression, anxiety, and other psychiatric disorders? What forms of intervention can be developed to grapple with the disintegration of social and family networks? What indigenous or local forms of coping and healing from trauma which are culturally relevant and accessible currently exist?

Krippner and McIntyre (2003) identify both *war stress* and *war trauma* as distinct phenomenon produced by armed conflict that impact individuals and communities. They describe war stress as a range of stressors that people are exposed to in war – psychological, biological, social, cultural – either directly or indirectly. War trauma is seen as an "extreme" stressor resulting from the effects of war that has both individual and collective dimensions. War stress includes physical or psychosocial consequences, like depression and anxiety, and PTSD, although PTSD is relatively uncommon. Other typical manifestations of stress resulting from armed conflict include increased rates of substance abuse, social isolation, and suicidal behavior (World Health Organization, 2002), all of which can impede successful coping and social functioning.

Secondary effects associated with war include increased domestic and gender-based violence, child abuse, and other acts of violence (Satcher, Friel, & Bell, 2007; Watts, Siddiqi, Shukrullah, Karim, & Serag, 2007).

At the group and communal level war trauma addresses "all the health, social, economic, cultural, and political consequences of war stress" (Krippner & McIntyre, 2003, p. 7). Psychological stresses resulting from armed conflict typically stem from physical displacement (both "voluntary" and forced), the loss of community and a need to adjust to a new environment, social isolation, loss and grief, reduced social standing within a community, or a loss of family (World Health Organization, 2002). These effects are often pronounced for refugees, who typically face prolonged periods of family separation, displacement, and a loss of status and personal identity (Lacroix, 2006).

The prevalence of mental disorders has been found to increase during warfare and in post-conflict settings, affecting significant portions of local populations. The mental health effects of war are likely to be exhibited in numerous symptoms, many of which go undiagnosed and/or untreated in conflict settings (especially in developing countries). In addition, for a variety of reasons including the stigma associated with mental illness and treatment, limited diagnostic capacity, or a lack of understanding of psychological distress, these conditions often go unrecognized. Thus in different cultural contexts, psychological problems may actually present themselves as a variety of *physical* problems (headaches, gastrointestinal symptoms, heart or chest pain, backaches) that are addressed by "easier," more typical forms of treatment.

While a lack of consistent baseline data limits much research, most of those who develop diagnosable disorders from war trauma are thought to have little or no prior mental health problems. Chronic conflict in Africa and the Middle East, for example, has had a significant effect on mental health. In the first national level study in Lebanon of the effect of war on mental disorders during the lifespan of individuals, more than one-fourth of those surveyed had at least one DSM-IV disorder in their lifetime (Karam et al., 2008). This figure rose to one in three Lebanese by the age of 75, with major depression and anxiety disorders being most common. In a country that has experienced chronic conflict for decades, "there was a cumulative effect of war exposure increasing the likelihood" of developing various psychiatric disorders for the first time (p. 583). Eight years after a genocide that took the lives of at least 10 percent of Rwandan citizens, a survey of adults in four communities found that one in four met the symptom criteria for PTSD, a rate that was higher among women. More than 90 percent reported exposure to at least one traumatic event. Ethnicity, age and gender, cumulative traumatic exposure, and geographic proximity to specific events were statistically significant predictors of PTSD symptoms (Pham, Weinstein, & Longman, 2004).

Two multi-cluster population-based surveys of the mental health impact of war in Afghanistan (Lopes Cardozo et al., 2004; Scholte et al., 2004) found high levels of anxiety, depression, and PTSD. Exposure to trauma and gender – being female – were found to increase the risk of developing mental health symptoms. The impact of trauma was also found to increase feelings of hatred and attitudes toward revenge in Afghanistan (Lopes Cardozo et al., 2004), as well as in previous research among war victims in Kosovo (Lopes Cardozo, Kaiser, Gotway Crawford, & Againi, 2003).

Despite prohibitions on the targeting of non-combatants, the majority of casualties of modern warfare are civilians; this population is increasingly victimized through both physical and psychological violence. In part this reflects the increase in "civil wars, with enemies consisting of groups within the same population. This type of warfare focuses on civilians as targets" and seeks to disrupt the larger social environment (Oakes & Lucas, 2001, p. 143). One study that sought to measure levels of prohibited or undesirable outcomes inflicted during armed conflict – so called "dirty war" tactics like torture and civilian death – found that the targeting of civilians was used by illegal paramilitaries, as well as government troops and (more traditional) guerrilla forces (Hicks & Spagat, 2008).

Given the rise in attacks on civilians and the disruption of social institutions and networks, those groups seen as most at risk in war zones are women, elderly people, children, people with disabilities, low-income populations, and ethnic and religious minorities. The targeting of key community figures is increasingly common in war and internal armed conflict as well. Thus educators, medical professionals, union leaders, religious figures, neighborhood leaders, and public officials are frequently victims of assassination, kidnappings, or threatened with violence (either directly or toward their family), undermining social networks and community relations. The rise in the targeting of civilians in war has been marked by a corresponding focus on the psychological impact of armed conflict on civilian populations (Krippner & McIntyre, 2003).

As basic community structures like places of worship, public spaces, and employment opportunities are increasingly targeted in armed conflict, public health and well-being suffer. The loss of key community and social supports interacts to produce distinct forms of trauma and psychological suffering among different civilian groups, though this may often manifest itself in ways that appear unrelated to armed conflict. If children cannot attend school on a regular basis, if women can no longer shop or be in the public sphere safely, as basic social networks become fractured, the varied mental health effects linked to armed conflict are compounded. Community disruption linked to war thus plays out at the individual level in terms of increased social isolation, distrust and fear, a heightened sense of uncertainty about everyday life, and the loss of the ability to engage in routine forms of social interaction and community functions.

A lack of research on the *long-term* psychological effects of exposure to war and armed conflict challenges efforts to ensure adequate mental health treatment. What is clear, however, is the need for a return to basic social functioning and integration after armed conflict ends – access to schooling, work, and key social institutions, and the maintenance of family and social networks among those displaced by conflict and who are able to return to their community.

Existing *gendered power differentials* are amplified in conditions of war, as women are typically more vulnerable to and disproportionately affected by the harmful effects of armed conflict (Jansen, 2006). Women's roles as neighborhood leaders, caregivers, and homemakers serve to heighten community vulnerability to disruption in wartime as women are increasingly targeted by violence (Ross-Sheriff, 2006). A rupture in existing social networks and relationships that depend upon the participation and leadership of women thus produces a ripple effect that weakens other social supports within local communities. Forced migration and the loss of male household contributions often increases women's caretaking duties, and the added strains of health, nutrition, and security concerns places added stress on the mental health status of women. Yet for many women in conflict situations the "effects of war trauma and the violation of dignity and rights are often unrecognized and untreated" (Jansen, 2006, p. 141).

Historically, women have been subjected to the physical harm and psychological trauma of rape and other forms of violence in wartime (Milillo, 2006). The targeting of women has been seen as a normal aspect of armed conflict, especially the use of rape as a "spoil" of war, furthering the subordinate status of women (Snyder, Gabbard, Dean May, & Zulcic, 2006; Watts et al., 2007). The use of rape, often in a systematic manner, received significant attention in the 1990s during civil war in the former Yugoslavia. In that conflict, so-called rape camps were discovered and the scope of violence against women in war was highlighted through mass media coverage (Kozaric-Kovacic, Folnegovic-Smalc, Skrinjaric, Szajnberg, & Marusic, 1995).

Attention to the targeting of women and girls in war has highlighted the use of rape and sexual violence, in particular its function in undermining local culture and household relations (Farwell, 2004), as well as in disrupting women's sense of safety and personal control (Watts et al., 2007). While rape in war is sometimes used against men and boys, it is largely a tactic employed against women and girls. For Jansen (2006), "in war, women's bodies become a battleground – rapes, forced pregnancies, kidnappings, and sexual servitude are common" (p. 136). With its growing use as a "deliberate, strategic, and political tactic" (PLoS Medicine Editors, 2009, p. 1), sexual violence in war is clearly designed to terrorize women and girls, disrupt family structure, and undermine local community functioning.

> Psychologically the effects are no less devastating. Traumatized by the event, women are often unable to care for their children or households, fear leaving their homes, can become socially ostracized and isolated, and may be rejected by their husbands, families, or communities.
>
> (PLoS Medicine Editors, 2009, p. 1)

Advocacy about the status of women in war led to the adoption of two United Nations Security Council resolutions in recent years: a 2000 decree called for equal participation by women in conflict resolution efforts, and a 2008 declaration identified the specific obligations of individual states and UN bodies to prevent and punish the use of sexual violence against women when used as a weapon of war. Despite interest in the status of women in conflict settings, war rape in particular continues to be a hallmark of contemporary armed violence. Chronic conflict in the Congo, for example, has been marked by human rights violations of civilian groups and pervasive sexual violence targeting women and girls. The UN Development Fund for Women (UNIFEM, 2008) found that a lack of political action on gender violence by member states has hampered efforts to protect women in war zones. The inability to realize greater progress on this issue has led some groups to call for creation of a UN coordinator focused on the broad issue of women and armed conflict (Human Rights Watch, 2008).

Mortality rates in wartime for *children* are among the highest of any group; an estimated two million children have been killed and six million wounded or permanently disabled from wars since 1990 (United Nations Security Council, 2008). Armed conflict extracts a toll on children in other ways, highlighting the "social contexts that lead to war and produce low levels of life chances" among this population (Carlton-Ford, 2004, p. 185). In particular, as young children react quickly to major changes in their social environment, their vulnerability to the impact of war is heightened. Children in countries experiencing war are more likely to suffer malnutrition than other groups, and are more susceptible to death and health problems from poor sanitation and lack of access to clean water. Carlton-Ford (2004) examined conflicts in Iraq, Liberia, and the Congo, finding significantly increased child mortality rates related to war in each location at a time when global child mortality decreased markedly.

Research documenting the psychological effects of conflict on children is less robust than findings related to children's overall health stemming from war (Attanayake, McKay, Joffres, Singh, Burkle, & Mills, 2009). The *political* response to the psychosocial needs of children affected by war has also lagged (McIntyre & Ventura, 2003), despite the prevalence of children as war victims. The relationship between public health and individual mental health in children due to armed conflict is nonetheless noteworthy. Whether by hearing family or friends discuss adverse events related to war, being directly exposed to violence, or experiencing physical displacement, children appear more prone to display the adverse psychological effects linked to war. These can be short term, as in anxiety, displays of anger, the loss of sleep, and submissiveness, or they may be longer term behavioral changes like depression and even PTSD (Santa Barbara, 2000). As with research on other groups, the cumulative impact of exposure to traumatic events among children appears to increase the incidence of such behaviors.

In a meta-analysis of research about mental disorders in children exposed to war, researchers found that symptoms of PTSD occurred within every study; elevated anxiety disorders and depression were reported in one-fourth of the examined literature (Attanayake et al., 2009). A study of Angolan adolescents, many of whom had grown up in a context of constant war, periodic famine, and widespread social disorganization, found a high prevalence of PTSD among those still living in Angola compared to refugee youth living in another country (McIntyre & Ventura, 2003). Key differences among the three groups in behavioral adjustment, anxiety and depression, and other psychological problems related to their direct exposure to war suggest "a global negative effect of war trauma on these adolescents' development" (p. 44).

Displacement from armed conflict appears to be key risk factor for the prevalence of mental disorders in children, as does the actual timing of exposure to traumatic events (Attanayake et al., 2009). The loss of one or both parents in war creates profound turmoil in the emotional and physical well-being of children, adding to economic instability, jeopardizing the right to an education, and increasing the risk of exploitation (UNICEF, 2004). Parental loss may not occur solely through mortality linked to war; family separation, often for prolonged periods, is common in wartime as different family members are forced to flee local communities as refugees or internally displaced persons.

The growing use of child soldiers in armed conflict, typically through forced recruitment, represents another way that human development is undermined and children's life chances are severely compromised in war (Kimmel & Roby, 2007). While the use of children under age 18 by paramilitaries, armed political groups and tribal militias has received most attention, more than ten countries utilized child soldiers in their regular armed forces since 2000. Boys are most often forced or recruited into soldering, yet increasingly girls are utilized as fighters and helpers; but in either instance girls face routine sexual assault and rape by other soldiers (Coalition to Stop the Use of Child Soldiers, 2004).

An analysis of former child soldiers in Nepal found higher levels of mental health problems compared with Nepalese children who were not conscripted (Kohert et al., 2008). All study participants experienced at least one type of trauma and "both groups displayed a substantial burden of mental health and psychosocial problems" (p. 700). However, the cumulative exposure to traumatic events was thought to explain child soldiers' worse mental health outcomes, a finding similar to other research. Kimmel and Roby (2007) note that as child soldiers are denied the ability to engage in typical childhood and adolescent experiences, they are susceptible to psychological problems and an inability to engage in normal social functioning, effects that are often long term.

The rise in the number of *internally displaced persons* (IDPs) *and refugees* fleeing war illustrates multiple ways that armed conflict causes disruption of basic community functioning and family life. The United Nations High Commissioner for Refugees (UNHCR) reported that in 2008 the highest number of IDPs ever recorded – more than 14 million – received direct assistance from the UN, and that nearly 12 million others had to survive on their own or rely on other forms of assistance (UNHCR, 2009). A significant literature has emerged on the relationship between exposure to war and community violence and psychological well-being among refugees. This research not only illustrates the effects of armed conflict on mental health, but also suggests the relevance of individual and community interventions and services that promote resilience and the healing of trauma.

Long-term displacement, especially as refugees in camps, can lead to diminished health status, induce a range of mental health conditions, and undermine educational opportunities and daily routines that are critical for child development. Yet the lack of psychosocial and mental health services for refugee women and children in Africa (Sossou, 2006) suggests an inability to adequately address war trauma among this population. Despite some shared events in conflict settings and/or in the process of becoming a refugee, there are key differences in the experiences and health and mental health outcomes affecting those uprooted by war, illustrating the importance of the social context of trauma (Kett, 2005). For some refugees, mental health symptoms may intensify throughout their experience, and even those who successfully resettle to third countries "may continue to have psychological distress and difficulty adapting and adjusting" (Kroll, 2003, p. 669).

Another challenge is in addressing the mental health needs of refugees dispersed into urban settings. This is the case with most Iraqi refugees fleeing conflict and violence following the 2003 U.S. invasion of Iraq. A high percentage of Iraqi families in Jordan and Lebanon are experiencing "a period of serious emotional and psychosocial threats. These threats create widespread distress in (the) living environment of displaced Iraqis" (International Organization of Migration (IOM), 2008, p. 14). In Syria refugees reported "a high exposure to distressing and traumatic events" in Iraq, such as being a victim of violence, kidnappings, and torture. In addition, "high incidences of domestic violence as well as anxiety and depression" have been reported among this population (International Catholic Migration Commission (ICMC), 2008, p. 8). Outreach to Iraqi refugees to assess their psychosocial needs remains problematic due to their illegal status in these countries and their fear of being monitored while accessing existing services. Thus, international and local organizations have been hampered in their efforts to design and implement effective mental health programming.

Importantly, many of these mental health effects may be long lasting. One study of Mexican and Latin American refugees and immigrants living in the United States, on average for more than 14 years, found that those exposed to "political violence" in their country of origin had high levels of depression, PTSD, and other mental health disorders (Eisenman, Gelberg, Liu, & Shapiro, 2003). Those reporting exposure to political violence also suffered significantly poorer quality of health, including chronic pain and impaired physical functioning. Only 3 percent of this population had ever reported these traumatic experiences to a physician, and few were receiving mental health services.

A significant proportion of refugees are thought to experience torture, yet treatment of torture victims and research examining the efficacy of such interventions is relatively new. Common symptoms of those subjected to torture are depression and PTSD, though significant variation is common:

> risk factors for a greater severity of symptoms include longer duration and greater intensity of torture, a history of abuse during childhood (before the torture), an absence of social support after the torture, young age at the time of torture (children are particularly vulnerable), and any history of mental illness.
>
> (McCullough-Zander & Larson, 2004, p. 57)

Efforts to understand successful *responses to the stress and trauma* produced by armed conflict must include recognition of the relevance of cultural factors in different contexts. In addition, given the scale of war trauma and stress, traditional mental health interventions targeting individuals are usually "not suitable to respond quickly and efficiently to the needs of large groups of civilians in a war or postwar situation" (Krippner & McIntyre, 2003, p. 107). Increasingly, a psychosocial approach to addressing the impact of war-related trauma is aimed at promoting community building efforts, especially those that facilitate self-help, community mobilization, and integrate cultural, spiritual and religious healing practices (Inter-Agency Standing Committee (IASC), 2007). Thus community-based approaches that recognize social context and can address the psychosocial needs of large numbers of persons appear as relevant as mental health care for those with severe psychological responses to war trauma.

Witmer and Culver (2001) describe the research emphasis on individual mental health problems and intervention among Bosnian refugees, and a corresponding lack of attention to resilience, adaptation, and key family and community supports. Yet even individualized services for those affected by armed conflict that integrate cultural and social factors appear most effective (World Health Organization, 2002). Nonetheless, Piachaud (2008) notes that those with pre-existing conditions of severe mental illness are among the most vulnerable populations in post-conflict settings. He warns that the "focus on 'post-conflict mental health,' on 'trauma' and on the 'psychosocial' might detract from services for those with long-standing and enduring mental illness" (p. 325). The use of learning theory and cognitive behavioral therapy, especially with refugees, may provide significant opportunities for addressing depression and a greater sense of self-control for those dealing with war trauma (Paulson, 2003). Such approaches, however, may fail to adequately address deep-seated emotional wounds.

Individual and family-based therapy is often required for specific cases of torture. Yet training of helping professionals, including social workers, to treat torture survivors is in its infancy in the United States and other countries, which accept large numbers of refugees (Engstrom & Okamura, 2004). Interventions vary depending on the severity of victims' experiences; psychotherapy using a cognitive behavioral approach and "talk" therapy appear as dominant forms of intervention in Europe and the United States (McCullough-Zander & Larson, 2004).

The U.S.-based Center for Victims of Torture (CVT) is one of several international organizations that work with torture survivors, offering evaluation, psychological services, and other forms of assistance. They operate from the premise that survivors can recover, particularly with a multifaceted treatment approach. Recognizing that many survivors of torture do not seek help, CVT works with service providers, community-based organizations, and local leaders to provide training on recognizing the effects of war trauma and torture and implementing culturally relevant responses.

Research examining key protective factors that can moderate the effects of exposure to armed conflict is undeveloped, yet suggests several important methods to promote resiliency. Berthold (2000) notes the importance of social supports in addressing war trauma among refugee youth and its role in helping improve educational and social outcomes. Creating a space for survivors to share their experiences has been shown to produce positive effects for victims of extreme trauma (Oakes & Lucas, 2001). Thus, Bosnian refugee children who demonstrated significant war stress were shown to benefit from opportunities to discuss their war-related experiences (Angel, Hjern, & Ingleby, 2001). Argentinean victims who suffered trauma from political repression and torture also experienced gains from the use of reflection groups to process shared experiences (Edelman, Kersner, Kordon, & Lagos, 2003). Aside from access to relevant social services and culturally competent social workers, Nash, Wong, and Trlin (2006) cite the importance of social integration for successful resettlement experiences among refugees. The role of humanitarian and social service agencies in facilitating integration for Albanian Kosovar refugees has also been noted (Pittman, Drumm, & Perry, 2001).

Processes of transitional justice and reconciliation represent another key element of community-based efforts to address war trauma. The use of traditional community-based methods of resolving disputes was adapted in Rwanda to promote judicial and reconciliation efforts following the 1994 genocide (Pham, Weinstein, & Longman, 2004). The *gacaca* trials, used for those accused of less serious crimes during the genocide, involve the use of locally elected committees of lay judges. Yet researchers note that the process of promoting and *achieving* reconciliation emerges as a difficult task in post-conflict settings, especially when utilizing an approach based on norms of justice:

Reconciliation is a complex process that entails difficult tasks such as the reforging of societal linkages and the rebuilding of communities. Whether judicial responses are capable of contributing substantially to this process has not been empirically tested.

(Pham et al., 2004, p. 603)

In this case, "reconciliation" was defined as a community-based process that developed a shared sense of community, promoted the establishment of mutual ties and obligations, recognized individual rights, and emphasized non-violence. Among more than 2,000 study participants, approximately three-fourths had been forced to flee their home, had their property destroyed, or had a close family member killed. One in four met the symptom criteria for PTSD. The highest percentage of participants favored the use of local (*gacaca*) tribunals (compared other forms of legal justice), with nearly two-thirds reporting an ability to be interdependent with other ethnic groups and supportive of the process of achieving social justice. However, among those with symptoms of PTSD there was less support for independence and a belief in community (Pham et al., 2004). As can be seen from this example, repairing and rebuilding communities fractured by war must be seen as a long-term process that requires considerable investment on the part of community leaders, professionals, and local government.

Research has shown the important role played by women in establishing social networks for survival during wartime and post-conflict recovery. In an assessment of Afghan refugees, Ross-Sheriff (2006) found that the significant responsibilities afforded women in the home and within local communities provided a strategic opportunity to help nurture community healing in post-conflict settings. Her research emphasizes the ways in which resilience among those directly affected by war is linked to the ability to maintain social networks and key cultural and/or religious practices. The ability to utilize religion and traditional (tribal) values was also found to moderate the impact of war on the developmental and psychological status of Angolan youth, as were other social supports like intact families (McIntyre & Ventura, 2003). In the first nationally representative mental health survey performed in Afghanistan, key coping strategies that modified high prevalence rates of symptoms of depression, anxiety, and PTSD illustrate the importance of psychosocial interventions that can help reestablish social networks and community engagement. These included spiritual and religious practices, the support of family and friends, and access to sources of income and material assistance (Lopes Cardozo et al., 2004).

Although physical dislocation is an obvious by-product of war, displacement itself may actually represent an essential step to adaptation and survival in conflict settings. Thompson and Eade (2002) found that women who were uprooted from local towns and villages throughout the 1980s civil war in El Salvador assumed leadership roles in forming new support systems and grassroots organizations. Such strategies were an essential step to help repair community networks and create civilian protection strategies to deal with pervasive state violence targeting rural populations. While these women suffered physical violence and psychological trauma, they were not simply victims. In this case, by engaging in collective action women took on the role of social actors contributing to their individual and collective empowerment, ultimately helping build support for an end to a brutal and long-running civil conflict (Thompson & Eade, 2002).

Research following the September 11, 2001 terrorist attacks reveals significant mental health impacts for those directly affected by the violence, as well as others who experienced heightened anxiety due to fear of future attacks on U.S. soil. This suggests that while it was unusual for such events to occur within the United States, the reaction to these traumatic incidents mirrored that experienced by people in other conflicts. For example, elevated levels of depression, anxiety and other psychological problems were found to be significant among residents of New York City following the attacks (Galea et al., 2002; Schlenger, 2005). A study of mental health seeking among parents of young children in Manhattan noted that all parents "reported some direct exposure to the attacks or the immediate aftermath" (DeVoe, Bannon, Klein, & Miranda, 2007, p. 312). Nearly two-thirds of parents sought at least one common form of mental health care following 9/11, while 37 percent received at least two types of treatment. Not only did most parents cite high amounts of psychological distress, but also significant levels of behavioral and sleeping problems were reported among their children, which contribute to greater parental distress and can undermine family functioning.

The long-term effects of exposure to the September 11 attacks differed among children in one study depending on their previous history of exposure to harmful events (Mullett-Hume, Anshel, Guevara, & Cloitre, 2008). Middle school youth with little (lifetime) exposure to traumatic events were found to have a "significant impact on PTSD symptomatology" from the World Trade Center attacks (Mullett-Hume et al., 2008, p. 106). Among nearly 200 youth in this study, more than 40 percent reported a range of symptoms that impaired their ability to function effectively and affected their level of happiness more than two years after the terrorist attacks – relationship problems, trouble completing schoolwork, and difficulties with family and friends. A survey of undergraduate college students at three public universities one year after September 11 noted that the attacks continued to produce a "residual level of symptoms and probable cases of PTSD" in significant numbers of students (Blanchard, Rowell, Kuhn, Rogers, & Wittrock, 2005, p. 149). Those living in greater proximity to New York City had a higher likelihood of such symptoms, a finding supported by other research (Galea et al., 2002).

While feelings of confusion, fear, and powerlessness were common following September 11, especially among those closest to the attacks (Beck & Buchele, 2005), they were pronounced among family members of dead or missing workers from the World Trade Center buildings. Boss, Beaulieu, Wieling, Turner, and LaCruz (2003) note that the trauma of the terrorist attacks was also aggravated for persons of color, as real or perceived incidents of discrimination, racism, and mistreatment increased in the immediate aftermath of 9/11. A study of resilience in Arab American couples also found a high level of personal experience (or knowledge of) discrimination against Arabs in the United States following the attacks (Beitin, Allen, & Allen, 2005). In addition, researchers found that Arab Americans faced a profound struggle over their identity – Arabs vs. Americans – "in the midst of pressure from the larger society to take sides" (p. 257).

Aside from the trauma directly linked to the attacks, different groups also experienced community disruption and a range of stressors following September 11. Krauss et al. (2003) describe how low-income residents of the Lower East Side of Manhattan, already dealing with an HIV epidemic and the impact of welfare reform, were suddenly faced with school closures, the fear of additional attacks, and rising levels of violence and ethnic conflict in their neighborhood. As familiar and "safe" spaces were restricted or closed off due to the attacks, many parents and their children were forced to navigate an environment increasingly seen as more unpredictable and dangerous. Among participants in focus groups and interviews, "nearly all parents mentioned that their child was now afraid to go to school . . . Now every school – elementary, junior high, high school – was a place were rumors about local dangers and threats were common" (Krauss et al., 2003, p. 525). Thus as feelings of safety were undermined, local residents and the larger community restricted or changed their behavior in public settings: "new dangers appeared to come from new places and new people under new rules" (p. 526).

Illustration and discussion

Social workers have a critical role to play as community agents helping to rebuild local communities disrupted from war and armed conflict. By emphasizing an empowerment-based, participatory approach to healing the wounds of war (both physical and psychological) they can address both the *psycho* and *social* aspects of conflict in order to strengthen social capital in local communities (Lee, 2001). The focus on integrating civilians and the victims of war into community life involves re-establishing key community functions: religious institutions, employment, and schools to name a few. This also suggests a need to prioritize community involvement to develop and hone community organizing skills – especially among those affected by armed conflict – which can be used in multiple phases of local reconciliation following war. In the following case illustration, a community social worker helps a family by focusing on different efforts that promote self-help and a community empowerment approach to deal with the varied disruptions caused by armed conflict. The use of interventions targeting the *social* is thus seen as key to psychological well-being and the promotion of health.

The family lives in a developing country that has experienced sustained ethnic and religious conflict for several years. Religious and ethnic minorities have been prominent victims of sustained violence. Significant numbers of this population have been forced to flee to safer parts of the country or abroad, resulting in the disintegration of many formerly thriving communities. Moreover, as a result of widespread armed conflict, the country's economic system has been severely disrupted, the health and educational systems have failed, and much of the population is reliant upon humanitarian assistance to meet basic needs. Throughout the country, key community leaders (religious figures, union members, and teachers) have been targeted for kidnapping and violence, and much of the country is marked by a lack of stability and community functioning.

Members of the family are among the hundreds of thousands of internally displaced persons (IDPs) uprooted from their local community in recent years due to pervasive armed conflict and targeted violence. Although the family has been displaced to a part of the country that is relatively stable, like most IDPs they are without access to adequate food, secure housing, regular work, and stable education for their children.

While the community they live in has experienced only a few acts of violence, the family remains fearful of retribution and/or violence based on their identity: they are members of a small religious minority in the country. During the ongoing conflict their sect has been targeted by members of the nation's dominant religious group in an effort to force it out of several local communities and promote "ethnic cleansing." During some of the most brutal fighting, the family's 19-year-old son was kidnapped from their home and tortured, while the father's brother was murdered by an extremist group operating in their former community.

After living in their new community for several weeks, the family approached a local community-based organization, which is supported by an international non-governmental organization (NGO), for a mattress and some basic material goods (food and cooking utensils). One of two social workers serving with the group did a full intake with the family to assess their overall situation (family status, their current work situation, education, health, and basic needs). The social worker identified a range of material needs for the family. Secure housing and access to adequate food were most pressing; but the family also lacked a stable income, while none of their three children were attending school.

During the course of the intake, the social worker determined that the father was suffering from severe depression, which manifested itself in his inability to sleep regularly, a noticeable withdrawal from interaction with his family, and sudden outbursts of anger. These conditions appeared to stem from his loss of job and displacement from the community where he lived his entire life. After some prodding, he also expressed unresolved trauma stemming from the death of his brother and the kidnapping of his son. He noted that his perceived inability to protect and provide for his family had eroded his self-confidence and, in his eyes, made him "less of a man." The family's two daughters initially attended school in their new community. But following an incident in which a schoolmate was harassed by several older boys, the father decided that it was unsafe for them to continue attending. Despite the protests of his older daughter, both girls stayed at home most of the day. The younger daughter, aged nine, reported having nightmares and was fearful of leaving the home. The son expressed a desire to contribute to the family; he had been working as a day laborer, but would have liked to secure a more stable form of employment and more regularly get out of the house. The mother, despite the disruption and multiple traumas affecting the family, took up *de facto* the role of head of household. She was bringing in a small income through domestic service which has afforded her a growing sense of accomplishment. She has also recently begun to participate in a women's cooperative making pickles and pastries for sale in the local market, an initiative supported by local and international NGOs.

A typical, western method of addressing some of the trauma and apparent mental health problems affecting this family would be to implement specific mental health interventions like individual therapy. However, given the conditions in the country, this was not the most realistic, feasible, or culturally acceptable means of serving this family. Due in part to a lack of local mental health capacity (training, services, education) there is no viable means to deal with the more severe mental health effects of war and displacement for most civilians. The country lacks an adequate workforce of trained social workers, psychiatrists, and mental health professionals. In this family situation, the social worker recognized the need to focus on helping with mental health issues via *community interventions*; in other words, promoting community rebuilding and reintegration of family members into the community.

The social worker recognized that dealing with more immediate material needs was a necessary precursor to working with this family on longer-term psychological problems. Direct mental health interventions are thus viewed as secondary to meeting the family's basic needs. Helping the family to overcome the social isolation produced by war was viewed as the most viable method to re-establish key social and community networks and their reintegration into mainstream society. Combating fear, the stress of poverty and family and community disruption by becoming functioning social actors were all seen by the social worker as part of promoting good mental health.

Efforts to provide education and training in marketable skills, especially for displaced youth, have been identified by humanitarian groups as a key method to promote youth participation and leadership in community rebuilding efforts. This is seen as essential given the large numbers of youth, especially young men, no longer attending school and who have irregular attachment to the labor force. Many of these youth are seen as prime candidates for joining the varied armed militias that continue to operate in the country and which offer young men money for carrying out violent attacks. The social worker, in conjunction with a local initiative between an international organization and the Ministry of Education, helped the son join a new vocational-technical program for young men that offers a stipend during training. This allowed the son to receive training that led to certification as a computer technician, to begin earning a small, but steady income, and to create a network of friends that helped facilitate his integration into the local community. While he continued to avoid discussion of his kidnapping, after several months in the program, the son was more engaged with his family and developed several close friends.

Based on information shared at meetings of community workers and NGO representatives, the social worker has recently developed a new appreciation of the urgency of addressing the needs of men. Given their growing social isolation, family disruption and the strains produced by a lack of work and income for many of these men, community workers now believe that integrating this population into the local community will help address a rise in domestic and gender-based violence; and it may likely confront the depression which seems common among displaced adult men in the community. As a result, the social worker has begun a project with an international humanitarian group to work with older men. After several unsuccessful attempts, the social worker has identified several (informal) community leaders who agreed to facilitate focus groups among male IDPs.

These discussion groups help highlight a number of previously ignored concerns that are critical to the identity of the male participants. These include a loss of a sense of self-efficacy which is linked to a lack of work and diminished leadership roles in the community. Indeed, the focus of a "livelihoods" approach that prioritizes economic empowerment of youth and women has made many of these men, who formerly worked in important positions in their community, feel isolated and ignored.

The focus groups have helped to articulate a number of ways that men can begin to be reintegrated into the local community. This includes using them to help plan economic development efforts and finding ways to work with/in local community institutions (educational, commercial, etc.), and to promote post-conflict reconciliation among disparate social groups. Aside from their own direct needs, the focus groups allow participants to identify other community functions that are currently deficient, such as the need for safe spaces for children to play. The effort is so successful that the social worker is able to gain the support and participation of religious and community leaders from several different ethnic and religious groups. This leads the father to volunteer to serve on a new community-based organization aimed at promoting dialogue between different religious and ethnic groups. Although he has been unable to secure full-time work, his newfound community leadership role and the increased stability of his family has positively affected his interactions with other family members. After initially fighting with his wife over her growing independence, the father now supports her employment and her effort to start her own small business. The family's two daughters eventually returned to school, although the youngest girl continues to struggle in her coursework. Despite repeated attempts to create an informal community counseling center, the social worker has been unsuccessful. Efforts to have the youngest daughter undergo formal therapy have also failed due to a lack of available (and affordable) local resources, as well as the resistance of her father. Ultimately, the social worker will need to maintain a long-term relationship with this family to ensure their continued social integration.

Some attention to the mental health needs of different family members has occurred in this situation, largely via their ability to adapt to their new community and the stabilization of key community functions. Yet larger, long-term issues remain unresolved. For example, there is still a need for formal methods to help rebuild trust among disparate community groups (ethnic, religious, etc.). Thus, mechanisms for promoting social reconciliation must be created or strengthened to adequately address the grievances that exist among different social groups. Experiences in other post-conflict settings suggest the efficacy of strengthening the capacity of displaced groups to participate in civil society and/or local government to ensure community involvement in such efforts. This could include promoting provisions related to transitional justice (such as local a "truth commission"); providing some training in mediation skills among displaced groups; or efforts to engage civilians in conflict resolution to ensure that the causes and consequences of conflict are adequately addressed. Much of this work may be beyond the scope of most social workers; however, those trained in community practice do possess the knowledge and basic skills to help facilitate some of these efforts.

Conclusion

Despite a need to provide both individual and community level interventions that address war trauma, there are critical obstacles to such efforts. Perhaps the most significant barrier to adequate mental health treatment and services is the differing capacity within states and communities to address the varied mental health needs of the victims of war. Capacity is often linked to geographic location, with rural settings lagging behind the development of mental health services for urban populations, especially in low-income countries. The growth of a nation's health and mental health sector is thus linked to its financial capacity, as well as the priority given to addressing mental health needs. While investments in public health have increased, in general the creation of a comprehensive mental health system has lagged in many developing countries – precisely where they are often needed most. The targeting of health sector and professional health care workers in war has also undermined local health and mental health capacity in many countries that have experienced conflict. The level and duration of armed conflict is another key influence on the prioritization of national assets, as resources devoted to the military often assume large portions of state budgets.

International organizations that provide humanitarian and development assistance in disaster and conflict settings have begun to address the need for mental health services. Given limited resources and competing demands, however, these groups face a tension between projects to address mental health-related issues (depression, child abuse, and gender-based violence) and broader economic concerns and civilian protection issues. Thus even among organizations with significant capacity and experience, treatment for trauma and mental health counseling are often a low priority given an overall hierarchy of needs to address.

To address these barriers and concerns, a task force established by the United Nations has established guidelines on mental health and psychosocial support in conflict and emergency settings (Inter-Agency Standing Committee, 2007). They recommend a range of measures, including developing among medical professionals the capacity to recognize the mental health needs of individuals, providing access to treatment for those with severe mental disorders, training aid workers in mental health and psychosocial support, and facilitating community mobilization and involvement in emergency response.

While important research has emerged on direct practice with refugees (Balgopal, 2000; Goodkind, 2007; Nash et al., 2006; Ovitt, Larrison, & Nackerud, 2003), attention to how social workers address the mental health needs of populations affected by war is limited. The emphasis on work with refugees in camps or clinical interventions represents a more traditional, individualized approach to war trauma. Increasingly, however, psychosocial interventions that attempt to recreate community ties and promote social (re-)integration are regarded as a more viable and culturally relevant approach with war-affected populations.

For example, the use of community development in post-conflict societies can help build social capital and reconstruct fractured communities (Ager, Strang, & Abebe, 2005). Social work is particularly suited to contribute to practice aimed at strengthening communities. Ideally, an empowerment-based model to community-building should recognize the strengths and potential contributions of those directly affected by war. What social work could bring to this concern with community-based psychosocial efforts is a focus on engaging local organizations and community leaders in designing and implementing programs addressing the trauma and disruption caused by war. This could occur in both post-conflict settings as well as in regions affected by significant refugee populations fleeing armed conflict. Such an approach follows the IASC recommendations for work in disaster and conflict settings which suggest

> mobilizing groups of disaster affected people to organize their own supports and participate fully in the relief effort. In this respect, local people are not passive beneficiaries but actors who have assets and resources, and support is provided from within the community as well as by outsiders.
>
> (IASC, van Ommeren, & van Wessells, 2007, p. 822)

Social work curriculum in the United States has addressed practice in conditions of disaster relief. However, the focus of such training has been on addressing natural disasters, a situation similar to social work literature on disaster (Harding, 2007). To address this limitation, more attention must be given to practice that directly confronts the effects of war on mental health and well-being of affected populations (Ramon, 2008). Considerable opportunity for social work contribution to this field exists.

Building on the insights of the United Nations Children's Education Fund and leading humanitarian organizations regarding principles for intervention with traumatized children, social workers could help emphasize "normalization" rather than specific therapeutic interventions. According to these principles, " 'trauma counselling' should *never* be the point of departure for psychological programming, because structured, normalizing, empowering activities within a safe environment will help the majority of the children recover over time" (as cited in Healy, 2008, p. 274). Thus, social workers trained to develop child-oriented programs focusing on establishing routines, structured play, and art-related activities would already be contributing to the "normalization" of daily life for children from war-affected areas.

Aside from opportunities working with those affected by war, social work should also play a central role challenging the assumptions that normalize war and armed conflict. Greater attention to peacemaking and global efforts for social justice is as necessary as developing ameliorative responses that fail to address the fundamental causes of war. In this sense, addressing war as a social problem intrinsically linked to community well-being and mental health would afford the profession the opportunity to contribute to structural change through advocacy and policy-making. Such an approach could help prevent armed conflict with its attendant destruction of community and significant mental health trauma.

Web resources

Center for Victims of Torture
www.cvt.org/

Coalition to Stop the Use of Child Soldiers
www.child-soldiers.org/

Courage to Care Campaign
www.usuhs.mil/psy/courage.html

Heartland Alliance
www.heartlandalliance.org/

Inter-Agency Standing Committee
www.humanitarianinfo.org/iasc/

International Campaign to Ban Landmines
www.icbl.org/

National Center for PTSD
www.ptsd.va.gov/

United Nations Development Fund for Women (UNIFEM)
www.unifem.org/

References

Abergavenny, R.D. (2000, December 16). Sanctions against Iraq "double" child mortality. *British Medical Journal, 321* (1490).

Ager, A., Strang, A., & Abebe, B. (2005). Conceptualizing community development in war affected populations: Illustrations from Tigray. *Community Development Journal, 40* (2), 158–168.

Angel, B., Hjern, A., & Ingleby, D. (2001). Effects of war and organized violence on children: A study of Bosnian refugees in Sweden. *American Journal of Orthopsychiatry, 73* (1), 4–15.

Attanayake, V., McKay, R., Joffres, M., Singh, S., Burkle Jr., F. & Mills, E. (2009). Prevalence of mental disorders among children exposed to war: A systematic review of 7,920 children. *Medicine, Conflict and Survival, 25* (1), 4–19.

Balgopal, P.R. (ed.). (2000). *Social work practice with immigrants and refugees.* New York: Columbia University Press.

Beck, R., & Buchele, B. (2005). In the belly of the beast: Traumatic countertransference. *International Journal of Group Psychotherapy, 55* (1), 31–44.

Beitin, B.K., Allen, K., & Allen, R. (2005). Resilience in Arab American couples after September 11, 2001: A systems perspective. *Journal of Marital and Family Therapy, 31* (3), 251–267.

Berthold, S.M. (2000). War trauma and community violence: Psychological, behavioral, and academic outcomes among Khmer refugee adolescents. *Journal of Multicultural Social Work, 8* (1–2), 15–46.

Blanchard, E.B., Rowell, D., Kuhn, E., Rogers, R., & Wittrock, D. (2005). Posttraumatic stress and depressive symptoms in a college population one year after the September 11 attacks: The effect of proximity. *Behaviour Research and Therapy, 43* (1), 143–150.

Boss, P., Beaulieu, L., Wieling, E., Turner, W., & LaCruz, S. (2003). Healing loss, ambiguity, and trauma: A community-based intervention with families of union workers missing after the 9/11 attack in New York City. *Journal of Marital and Family Therapy, 29* (4), 455–467.

Byers, M. (2005). *War law: Understanding international law and armed conflict.* New York: Grove Press.

Calhoun, C. (2004). A world of emergencies: Fear, intervention, and the limits of cosmopolitan order. *Canadian Review of Sociology and Anthropology, 41* (4), 373–395.

Carlton-Ford, S. (2004). Armed conflict and children's life chances. *Peace Review, 16* (2), 185–191.

Coalition to Stop the Use of Child Soldiers (2004). *Child soldiers global report 2004.* London: Coalition to Stop the Use of Child Soldiers.

Cortright, D., & Lopez, G.A. (1999). Are sanctions just? The problematic case of Iraq. *Journal of International Affairs, 52* (2), 735–755.

Declaration of Alma-Ata. (1978). International Conference on Primary Health Care, Alma-Ata, USSR (September 6–12). Retrieved May 17, 2009, from www.who.int/publications/almaata_declaration_en.pdf.

DeVoe, E.R., Bannon Jr., W.M., Klein, T.P., & Miranda, C. (2007). Post-September 11 mental health service help seeking among a group of highly exposed New York City parents. *Families in Society: Journal of Contemporary Social Services, 88* (2), 311–316.

Edelman, L., Kersner, D., Kordon, D., & Lagos, D. (2003). Psychosocial effects and treatment of mass trauma due to sociopolitical events: The Argentine experience. In S. Krippner & T.M. McIntyre (eds), *The psychological impact of war trauma on civilians: An international perspective* (pp. 143–154). Westport, CT: Praeger.

Eisenman, D.P., Gelberg, L., Liu, H., & Shapiro, M.F. (2003). Mental health and health-related quality of life among adult Latino primary care patients living in the United States with previous exposure to political violence. *Journal of the American Medical Association, 290* (5), 627–634.

Engelhard, I.M., Huijding, J., van den Hout, M.A., & de Jong, P.J. (2007). Vulnerability associations and symptoms of post-traumatic stress disorder in soldiers deployed to Iraq. *Behaviour Research and Therapy, 45* (10), 2317–2325.

Engstrom, D.W., & Okamura, A. (2004). A plague of our time: Torture, human rights, and social work. *Families in Society, 85* (3), 291–300.

Evidence-based prevention is goal of largest ever study of suicide in the military (2009, July 16). Washington, DC: National Institute of Mental Health. Retrieved July 27, 2009, from www.nimh.nih.gov/science-news/2009/evidence-based-prevention-is-goal-of-largest-ever-study-of-suicide-in-the-military.shtml.

Farwell, N. (2004). War rape: New conceptualizations and responses. *Affilia: Journal of Women and Social Work, 19* (4), 389–403.

Fiala, A. (2008). *The just war myth: The moral illusions of war.* Lanham, MD: Roman & Littlefield.

Galea, S., Ahern, J., Resnick, H., Kilpatric, D., Bucuvalias, M., Gold, J., & Vlahov, D. (2002). Psychological sequelae of the September 11 terrorist attacks in New York City. *New England Journal of Medicine, 346,* 982–987.

Garfield, R. (1999). *The impact of economic sanctions on health and well-being.* London: Relief and Rehabilitation Network, Overseas Development Institute.

Garfield, R. (2002). Economic sanctions, humanitarianism, and conflict after the cold war. *Social Justice, 29* (3), 94–107.

Garfield, R., & Leu, C.S. (2000). A multivariate method for estimating mortality rates among children under 5 years from health and social indicators in Iraq. *International Journal of Epidemiology, 29,* 510–515.

Ghobarah, H.A., Huth, P., & Russett, B. (2004). The post-war public health effects of civil conflict. *Social Science and Medicine, 59,* 869–884.

Ghosh, N., Mohit, A., & Murthy, R.S. (2004). Mental health promotion in post-conflict countries. *Journal of the Royal Society for the Promotion of Health, 124* (6), 268–270.

Gibbs, D.A., Martin, S.L., Kupper, L.L., & Johnson, R.E. (2007). Child maltreatment in enlisted soldiers' families during combat-related deployments. *Journal of the American Medical Association, 298* (3), 528–535.

Goodkind, J.R. (2007). Promoting Hmong refugees' well-being through mutual learning: Valuing knowledge, culture, and experience. *American Journal of Community Psychology, 37* (1–2), 77–93.

Gould, K.A. (2007). The ecological costs of militarization. *Peace Review, 19* (3), 331–334.

Gupta, S., Clements, B., Bhattacharya, R., & Chakravarti, S. (2002). The elusive peace dividend. *Finance and Development, 39* (4), 49–51.

Harding, S. (2007). Man-made disaster and development: The case of Iraq. *International Social Work, 50* (3), 295–306.

Healy, L.M. (2008). *International social work: Professional action in an interdependent world* (2nd ed.). New York: Oxford University Press.

Hicks, M.H.R., & Spagat, M. (2008). The dirty war index: A public health and human rights tool for examining and monitoring armed conflict outcomes. *PLoS Medicine, 5* (12), 1658–1664.

Hoge, C.W., Auchterlonie, J.L., & Milliken, C.S. (2006). Mental health problems, use of mental health services, and attrition from military service after returning from deployment to Iraq or Afghanistan. *Journal of the American Medical Association, 295* (9), 1023–1032.

Hossein-Zadeh, I. (2007). *The political economy of U.S. militarism.* New York: Palgrave Macmillan.

Human Rights Watch (HRW). (2008). www.hrw.org.

Inter-Agency Standing Committee (IASC) (2007). *IASC guidelines on mental health and psychosocial support in emergency settings.* Geneva: IASC.

Inter-Agency Standing Committee, van Ommeren, M., & van Wessells, M. (2007). Inter-agency agreement on mental health and psychosocial support in emergency settings. *Bulletin of the World Health Organization, 85* (11), 822–823.

International Catholic Migration Commission (ICMC). (2008). *Iraqi refugees in Syria.* Washington, DC: ICMC.

International Committee of the Red Cross (ICRC) (2009). *Annual report 2008.* Geneva: ICRC.

International Organization of Migration (IOM). (2008). *Assessment on psychosocial needs of Iraqis displaced in Jordan and Lebanon.* Amman and Beirut: IOM.

Jansen, G.G. (2006). Gender and war: The effects of armed conflict on women's health and mental health. *Affilia, 21* (2), 134–145.

Kaldor, M. (1999). *New and old wars: Organized violence in a global era.* Stanford, CA: Stanford University Press.

Karam, E.G., Mneimneh, Z.N., Dimassi, H., Fayyad, J.A., Karam, A.N., Nasser, S.C., Chatterji, S., & Kessler, R.C. (2008). Lifetime prevalence of mental disorders in Lebanon: First onset, treatment, and exposure to war. *PLoS Medicine, 5* (4), 579–586.

Keen, D. (2008). *Complex emergencies.* Malden, MA: Polity Press.

Kett, M.H. (2005). Internally displaced peoples in Bosnia-Herzegovina: Impacts of long-term displacement on health and well-being. *Medicine, Conflict and Survival, 21* (3), 199–215.

Kimmel, C.E., & Roby, J.L. (2007). Institutionalized child abuse: The use of child soldiers. *International Social Work, 50* (6), 740–754.

Kohert, B.A., Jordans, M.J.D., Tol, W.A., Speckman, R.A., Maharjan, S.M., Worthman, C.M., & Komproe, I.H. (2008). Comparison of mental health between former child soldiers and children never conscripted by armed groups in Nepal. *Journal of the American Medical Association, 300* (6), 691–702.

Kozaric-Kovacic, D., Folnegovic-Smalc, V., Skrinjaric, J., Szajnberg, N.M., & Marusic, A. (1995). Rape, torture, and traumatization of Bosnian and Croation women: Psychological sequelae. *American Journal of Orthopsychiatry, 65* (3), 428–433.

Krause, K., & Mutimer, D. (2005). Introduction. In *Small arms survey 2005*. Geneva: Graduate Institute of International Studies.

Krauss, B.J., Franchi, D., O'Day, J., Pride, J., Lozada, L., Aledort, N., & Bates, D. (2003). Two shadows of the twin towers: Missing safe spaces and foreclosed opportunities. *Families in Society: Journal of Contemporary Social Services, 84* (4), 523–528.

Krippner, S., & McIntyre, T.M. (2003). Overview: In the wake of war. In S. Krippner & T.M. McIntyre (eds), *The psychological impact of war trauma on civilians: An international perspective* (pp. 1–14). Westport, CT: Praeger.

Kroll, J. (2003). Posttraumatic symptoms and the complexity of responses to trauma. *Journal of the American Medical Association, 290* (5), 667–670.

Kuehn, B.M. (2009). Soldier suicide rates continue to rise. *Journal of the American Medical Association, 301* (11), 1111–1113.

Lacroix, M. (2006). Social work with asylum seekers in Canada: The case for social justice. *International Social Work, 49* (1), 19–28.

Lee, J.A. (2001). *The empowerment approach to social work practice* (2nd ed.). New York: Columbia University Press.

Levy, B.S., & Sidel, V.W. (2008). *War and public health* (2nd ed.). New York: Oxford University Press.

Lopes Cardozo, B., Kaiser, R., Gotway Crawford, C.A., & Againi, F. (2003). Mental health, social functioning, and feelings of hatred and revenge of Kosovar Albanians one year after the war in Kosovo. *Journal of Traumatic Stress, 16* (4), 351–360.

Lopes Cardozo, B., Bilukha, O.O., Gotway Crawford, C.A., Shaikh, I., Wolfe, M.I., Gerber, M.L., & Anderson, M. (2004). Mental health, social functioning, and disability in postwar Afghanistan. *Journal of the American Medical Association, 292* (5), 575–584.

Lutz, C. (2002). Making war at home in the United States: Militarization and the current crisis. *American Anthropologist, 104* (3), 723–735.

McCullough-Zander, K., & Larson, S. (2004). The fear is still in me: Caring for survivors of torture. *American Journal of Nursing, 104* (10), 54–64.

McIntyre, T.M., & Ventura, M. (2003). Children of war: Psychosocial sequelae of war trauma in Angolan adolescents. In S. Krippner & T.M. McIntyre (eds), *The psychological impact of war trauma on civilians: An international perspective* (pp. 39–53). Westport, CT: Praeger.

MedAct (2008). *Rehabilitation under fire: Health care in Iraq, 2003–2007*. London: MedAct.

Melman, S. (1974). *The permanent war economy. American capitalism in decline.* New York: Simon & Schuster.

Milillo, D. (2006). Rape as a tactic of war. Social and psychological perspectives. *Affilia, 21* (2), 196–205.

Mullett-Hume, E., Anshel, D., Guevara, V., & Cloitre, M. (2008). Cumulative trauma and posttraumatic stress disorder among children exposed to the 9/11 World Trade Center attack. *American Journal of Orthopsychiatry, 78* (1), 103–108.

Nash, M., Wong, J., & Trlin, A. (2006). Civic and social integration: A new field of social work practice with immigrants, refugees and asylum seekers. *International Social Work, 49* (3), 345–363.

Oakes, M.G., & Lucas, F. (2001). How war affects daily life: Adjustments in Salvadoran social networks. *Journal of Social Work Research and Evaluation, 2* (2), 143–155.

Ovitt, N., Larrison, C.R., & Nackerud, L. (2003). Refugees' responses to mental health screening. *International Social Work, 46* (2), 235–250.

Paulson, D.S. (2003). War and refugee suffering. In S. Krippner & T.M. McIntyre (eds), *The psychological impact of war trauma on civilians: An international perspective* (pp. 111–122). Westport, CT: Praeger.

Paulson, D.S., & Krippner, S. (2007). *Haunted by combat: Understanding PTSD in war veterans including women, reservists, and those coming back from Iraq.* Westport, CT: Praeger Security International.

Pedersen, J. (2007). Three wars later: Iraqi living conditions. In M.E. Bouillon, D.M. Malone, & B. Rowswell (eds), *Iraq: Preventing a new generation of conflict* (pp. 55–70). Boulder, CO: Lynne Rienner.

Pham, P.N., Weinstein, H.M., & Longman, T. (2004). Trauma and PTSD symptoms in Rwanda: Implications for attitudes toward justice and reconciliation. *Journal of the American Medical Association, 292* (5), 602–612.

Piachaud, J. (2008). Globalization, conflict and mental health. *Global Social Policy, 8* (3), 315–334.

Pilisuk, M. (2008). *Who benefits from global violence and war: Uncovering a destructive system.* Westport, CT: Praeger Security International.

Pittman, S., Drumm, R., & Perry, S. (2001). "IDDEAL" best practices as generated from the Albanian Kosovar refugees' personal reality. *Journal of Social Work Research and Evaluation, 2* (2), 227–236.

PLoS Medicine Editors (2009). Rape in war is common, devastating, and too often ignored. *PLoS Medicine, 6* (1), 1–3.

Ramon, S. (2008). *Social work in the context of political conflict.* London: Venture Press.

Ross-Sheriff, F. (2006). Afghan women in exile and repatriation: Passive victims or social actors? *Affilia, 21* (2), 206–219.

Santa Barbara, J. (2000). The psychological effects of war on children. In B.S. Levy & V.W. Sidel (eds), *War and public health* (2nd ed., pp. 168–185). New York: Oxford University Press.

Satcher, D., Friel, S., & Bell, R. (2007). Natural and manmade disasters and mental health. *Journal of the American Medical Association, 298* (21), 2540–2542.

Schlenger, W.E. (2005). Psychological impact of the September 11, 2001 terrorist attacks: Summary of empirical findings in adults. *Journal of Aggression, Maltreatment, and Trauma, 9,* 97–108.

Scholte, W.F., Olff, M., Ventevogel, P., de Vries, G.-J., Jansveld, E., Lopes Cardozo, B., & Gotway Crawford, C.A. (2004). Mental health symptoms following war and repression in eastern Afghanistan. *Journal of the American Medical Association, 292* (5), 585–593.

Sen, A.K. (1984). *Poverty and famines: An essay on entitlement and deprivation.* New York: Oxford University Press.

Snyder, C.S., Gabbard, W.J., Dean May, J., & Zulcic, N. (2006). On the battleground of women's bodies: Mass rape in Bosnia-Herzegovina. *Affilia, 21* (2), 184–195.

Sossou, M.A. (2006). Mental health services for refugee women and children in Africa: A call for activism and advocacy. *International Social Work, 49* (1), 9–17.

Tanielian, T.L., & Jaycock, L. (2008). *Invisible wounds of war: Psychological and cognitive injuries, their consequences, and services to assist recovery.* Santa Monica, CA: RAND.

Thompson, M., & Eade, D. (2002). Women and war: Protection through empowerment in El Salvador. *Social Development Issues, 24* (3), 50–58.

UNICEF. (1998). *Situation analysis of children and women in Iraq.* New York: UNICEF.

UNICEF. (2004). *The state of the world's children 2005: Childhood under threat.* New York: UNICEF.

United Nations Development Fund for Women (UNIFEM). (2008). *UNIFEM Annual Report 2008–2009.* New York: UNIFEM.

United Nations Development Program (UNDP). (2002). *Living conditions in Iraq.* New York: UNDP.

United Nations High Commissioner for Refugees (UNCHR) (2009). *2008 global trends: Refugees, asylum-seekers, returnees, internally displaced and stateless persons.* New York: UNCHR.

United Nations Security Council (2008, February 4). *Children and armed conflict.* Security Council Report No. 1. New York: UN Security Council.

U.S. Army Center for Health Promotion and Preventive Medicine (USACHPPM). (2009). *Epidemiologic consultation no. 14-HK-OB1U-09. Investigation of homicides at Fort Carson, Colorado: November 2008–May 2009.* Aberdeen, MD: Department of the Army.

Watts, S., Siddiqi, S., Shukrullah, A., Karim, K., & Serag, H. (2007). *Social determinants of health in countries in conflict: The Eastern Mediterranean perspective.* Cairo, Egypt: Commission on Social Determinants of Health, Health Policy and Planning Unit, Division of Health Systems and Service Development, World Health Organization.

Wheeler, D.P., & Bragin, M. (2007). Bringing it all back home: Social work and the challenge of returning veterans. *Health and Social Work, 32* (4), 297–300.

Witmer, T.A.P., & Culver, S.M. (2001). Trauma and resilience among Bosnian refugee families: A critical review of the literature. *Journal of Social Work Research and Evaluation, 2* (2), 173–187.

World Health Organization (WHO). (2002). *World report on violence and health.* Geneva: WHO.

6 Homelessness and its effects

Judith Bula Wise

Lyle and Mary stand on opposite street corners, lifting hand-lettered signs toward the averted, vacant, or rejecting eyes of most of the passing drivers. "Out of work. Stranded. Anything Helps. God Bless You." From mid-morning until sunset, they hope to gather enough for a meal before they return to the abandoned Ford station wagon in the vacant lot half mile away for a night's rest. Lyle sleeps in the back seat; his night terrors overwhelm him if he sleeps in the front seat.

Two miles away, Sharon tightens her grip on her five-year-old son's hand and joins a crowd gathering at the entrance to the Twelfth Street Shelter for the homeless. Her hope is to take away her son's hunger and his shivering from the February chill. She also hopes her violent, stalking husband won't find her for at least one more day. Her fear is a real one. She has the restraining order in her pocket, but many who say they want to help refuse to believe her. She has not been able to stop the shaking in her hands for three months. Before joining the lunch line, she met with a "social worker, in the best sense of that word" who handed Sharon the first child support payment from her husband, whose wages had been garnered. That afternoon the social worker was taking Sharon and her son to a "safe haven" residence that would allow her to have an address when she goes the next day for a job interview to work in an office supply store.

Near the center of town, Frank piles three plastic bags filled with his meager belongings under the bridge, on the south side out of the wind, then rolls his moth-eaten coat into a ball to serve as a pillow for his street friend, Mitch, who has had flu symptoms for three days. While Mitch sleeps, Frank finishes the next chapter in his ragged copy of Tolstoy's *War and peace* and then tries to get some rest. If only he could get the bugs to stop crawling around his feet. He's been told by one shelter worker that the bugs are hallucinations. He does know that every time he forgets to take his medicine, the bugs come back.

Rachel protects her corner cubicle in the public library during the day, leaving at four in the afternoon to claim the park bench closest to the steam grate to lessen the chance of freezing during the night. She reaches in her pocket for the yellow piece of paper and, for the sixth time in fifteen minutes, reads "Soup Kitchens: 1st Sunday of the month, Methodist Church, 2nd – Catholic, 3rd – Congregational, 4th – Presbyterian, 5th when there is one – Unitarian on the college campus." She lost her city map and, as hard as she tries to remember, she often confuses their locations and wanders the streets, disoriented and hungry. She hopes she is not losing her mind. The days when she felt comfortable asking for directions are over; she recalls the last time – when she was spit on by a young college student.

A "victim of circumstances" is the way Rachel answers the question of how she found herself suddenly homeless. A highly qualified researcher in pharmacology, she was among the second wave of her company's cutbacks. Only one year earlier, it had felt like an adventure to move across the country, away from family and friends, to accept a job that matched her training. Now, cut off from those supportive networks back in Chicago, her only acquaintances were those made at work. She lived on her savings for three months while looking for another job but was told repeatedly that she was either too specialized or overqualified. As her financial resources diminished, Rachel cut back on her anti-anxiety medications, no longer covered by her company's benefits plan. She tried to control her panic attacks through other methods, sometimes successfully but, more often, inadequate to address the continual increase of her fears. After one month's unpaid rent, Rachel was evicted from her two-bedroom apartment with no job, nowhere to live, 75 dollars in cash, and two tote bags filled with clothes, an extra pair of shoes, and several cans of food and boxes of cereal.

Lyle, Mary, Sharon, Frank, and Rachel are only a few of the hundreds who live without a permanent shelter, cope simultaneously with mental illness, and who seek help and support from human services workers in the communities in which they live. As devastating and continually stressful as it is to live without a roof over one's head, those who are faced with the added challenges of a mental illness find their lives filled on a daily, even hourly, basis with even more fearful uncertainties. Lyle, Mary, Sharon, Frank, and Rachel personify the persistence and resilience required to face the combined oppressions of job loss, health risk, poverty, and the shortage of affordable and accessible housing.

Yet, there is hope. "We know what works. Now we must put what we know to work" (Substance Abuse and Mental Health Services Administration (SAMHSA), 2003). This chapter describes steps toward doing exactly that, putting what we know to work. Lyle, Mary, Sharon, Frank, and Rachel are working with professionals and volunteers who know what works and who know how to gain access to resources that fit the needs of each person. To better understand these steps of moving from homeless to housed and mentally strong, definitions of homelessness plus social, economic, and political aspects of those definitions will be identified. Demographic information, including unique aspects of several multicultural variables, will be reported followed by a discussion on the association between "living on the street," in tent cities, or other temporary shelters and mental health/illness.

In recent years, advocates, policy makers, educators, and helping professionals seeking to end chronic homelessness for persons with serious mental illness have acknowledged that comprehensive understanding is needed regarding the multiple connections between *trauma response*, severe and chronic mental illness, and the lack of maintaining long-term housing. There has been a specific request for more advanced findings on trauma suffered, i.e. homelessness, and the coping responses to that trauma in relationship to perpetuating or diminishing the effects of homelessness (SAMHSA, 2003). The loss of one's home is often precipitated by a significant traumatic event such as a natural disaster, perhaps flood or hurricane, the onset of a major illness, the loss of employment, escape from a domestic violence situation, or a combination of several simultaneously occurring disasters. The consequences of these events spiral into other devastations and may include eviction, cutoffs from support networks, loss of health insurance, and onset of major depression. The greater the number and the longer these circumstances continue, the more likely it becomes to experience an escalation that can lead to even more severe challenges such as the onset of post-traumatic stress responses, daily risks of illness, hunger, malnutrition, and violence. If swift and thorough concrete responses, such as emergency funding, temporary shelter, medical attention for health needs, and access to employment are lacking, stressors escalate into heightened vulnerability, placing as many as 20 percent of persons who live without homes at risk for the onset or exacerbation of a mental illness, the roots of which are increasingly claimed to be in experiences of trauma (SAMHSA, 2003).

The cyclical nature of opportunity followed by disappointment followed by opportunity and so on, serves to trap homeless individuals and families in a situation of *ongoing and cumulative trauma*. Coordination efforts of the multiple systems involved are improving but are still often inadequate to meet the needs of the people served. Emergency room medical attention may be given but if shelter is unavailable after treatment, the person returns to the streets where they are immediately vulnerable to a reoccurrence of their illness. A job interview might be offered only to end prematurely because the person cannot provide a permanent address. And now, while facing what has been called the worst economic recession since the early 1900s, any chance to move toward becoming housed and mentally strong seems even more remote.

This chapter addresses the bidirectional relationships among complicated conditions such as trauma, trauma responses to homelessness and mental illness. The discussion of post-traumatic stress response is not exhaustive; here, the focus is upon the differentiation between a traumatic disorder and a response to a traumatic condition and is illustrated in a practice example. The stages of post-trauma recovery are identified, with suggested differential interventions appropriate to each stage.

Following the presentation of prevalence and multicultural variation, a practice illustration with assessment and intervention themes is presented. The life model of social work practice and the biopsychosocial model provide frameworks for discussion of the contributions of social work to our understanding of the problems of homelessness, particularly in relation to mental illness. Practice guidelines for work with those who live on the streets and who face co-occurring challenges to living mentally strong are also identified.

Separating the realities of homelessness from other social problems, including those identified in this volume, is imposible. Economic realities of homelessness, for example, are intimately connected with *poverty*. Difficulties finding housing are also extremely common for *immigrants*. Those anticipating release from the corrections system face initial decisions about where to live and how to afford that living arrangement. It is well documented that a significant number of homeless women and children are fleeing *violent domestic relationships*. When children and youth are *victimized physically and emotionally*, they flee their parental homes to escape the abuse, often without a plan for where they will live. And, finally, our *war veterans* are among those for whom the connection between post-traumatic stress response and living without permanent shelter is a tragic social reality.

Definitions of homelessness

One of six core values serving as the foundation for the *Blueprint for change: Ending chronic homelessness for persons with serious mental illness and co-occurring substance use disorders* is "supporting values that put people first" (SAMHSA, 2003).

(The other five core person-centered values are: choice, voice, empowerment, dignity and respect, and hope: SAMSHA, 2003.) This stance is consistent with a guiding rule from the empowerment approach: first, listen to the people. Here is what they, people who have been called "homeless," say:

I'm not homeless, ma'am. Don't you know? Home is where the heart is. I may not have a roof over my head at the moment, but I'm not homeless.

There are lots of people who care about us. You care about us. John cares about us. Mary cares about us. Street friends care about each other. This is where I feel at home, with the people who care about us.

For me, being hungry is the worst part. I can take everything else, the heat, the cold, the rain, even getting yelled at, but everything goes down hill when I don't get enough to eat. When I lived in Seattle, somebody started handing out food with poison in it to people begging on the street corners. I knew a couple of people who died from that. I stopped eating and got the hell out of there. It was a rough time.

I'm OK with the term "living on the streets" because that's *where* I am. But it's not *who* I am. I prefer that you see *me* first. I'm a person, I'm George. People don't say, "There goes Sheila; she's a two-bedroom apartment, or a one-story ranch style or a suburban tri-level." There's a lot more to me than the fact that I don't happen to have an address at the moment. When people see "homeless" as the first thing they know about me, we just don't get off to as good a start as when we find out what we have in common as people. And there's a lot we have in common, believe me, there's a lot.

These courageous statements challenge the stigma that comes with being called "homeless." The suffix "–less" immediately identifies deficit language (Wise, 2005), words that identify what is lacking rather than what is present. All who claim the validity of a strengths-based approach express caution about the use of deficit language. Each of the voices in these examples clearly speaks to what she or he does have, not to the homes they do not have at the moment. Not "homeless," they request, but at home within themselves, with the ones they love, or with the ones who care about them.

Other definitions are used among professionals in service, advocacy, research, and policy-making roles. These terms and definitions are used to identify patterns and to help establish a common language for cross-disciplinary and interdisciplinary understanding. Two of the most widely used definitions are best understood in a context-appropriate manner:

First, a homeless person is

one who lacks a fixed permanent nighttime residence, or whose nighttime residence is a temporary shelter, welfare hotel, or any other public or private place not designed as sleeping accommodations for human beings.

(National Coalition for the Homeless (NCH), 2009)

Second, a similar definition comes from the Stuart B. McKinney Act of 1994. A person is considered homeless who "lacks a fixed, regular, and adequate night-time residence" or who

has a primary night-time residency that is: (A) a supervised publicly or privately operated shelter designed to provide temporary living accommodations . . . (B) an institution that provides a temporary residence for individuals intended to be institutionalized, or (C) a public or private place not designed for, or ordinarily used as, a regular sleeping accommodation for human beings.

(U.S. Conference of Mayors (2004), 42 U.S.C. 11302(a))

This definition usually refers to the "literally homeless" who are sleeping in shelters or on the street. There are also many individuals and families who are known as the *hidden homeless*. In regions where there are fewer shelters available, such as in rural areas, people often double up with relatives and friends in substandard housing or sleep in cars or abandoned buildings (NCH, 2007). The term *episodically homeless* refers to those who cycle in and out of homelessness. They may be *situationally homeless*, without housing for a few nights, or *chronically homeless*, without housing for long periods of time (NCH, 2009).

The *episodically homeless* are those who have repeated brief periods of homelessness with each episode lasting a short time, several weeks to two to three months. Many of the episodically homeless are working hard to move forward, gathering resources, gradually working toward stabilizing a job situation, taking steps toward more permanent housing, building up the necessary protective resources to leave a violent domestic relationship, or managing health risks and expenses, all with enormous social and economic requirements and complications. The likelihood of setbacks is high and, when they do occur, these persons may be among those who cycle in and out of homeless shelters, utilizing the resources available to them for a few weeks or months until their own resources are strengthened to a point where they can again try independent living.

One example of the *situationally or temporarily homeless* are those who have been affected by the more than three million foreclosures which have occurred in the U.S. in 2007 and 2008. The working poor were the hardest hit and many in the middle class have also faced the shock of eviction from their homes: 76 percent of those foreclosed upon moved in with relatives or friends; 54 percent sought the services of emergency shelters. An estimated 40 percent turned to life on the streets or to tents, cars, trucks, or abandoned buses. Many individuals, couples, and families have used more than one form of temporary shelter. The time period between leaving a house in foreclosure and moving in with extended family, or into an affordable rental, ranged from a few hours or days to a few weeks, but rarely more than two months. Among *all* homeless in the United States, the estimate for the situationally or temporarily homeless is 80 percent (SAMHSA, 2003).

The *chronically homeless* usually have health and/or mental and behavioral health problems, additional conditions that contribute to becoming homeless and also add to the difficulty overcoming it. These additional conditions include substance use disorders (40 percent), physical disabilities or health-related disabling conditions (25 percent), and serious mental illness (20 percent) (SAMHSA, 2003). The association between homelessness and mental health/illness is the focus for the discussion in a later section. But first, there are social, economic, and political aspects of these definitions essential to understanding the complex nature of helping those who live on the streets or in temporary shelters and who also live with co-occurring mental illness.

Homelessness and mental health/illness

Social, economic, and political factors, which impact homelessness are overlapping rather than distinct influences. The association among social, economic, and political aspects is inseparable in the lives of those who live on the streets and yet, there are distinct patterns within each of these aspects that can help set the course for overcoming the oppression and hopelessness that too often come with living unhoused while, simultaneously, dealing with the challenges of a severe and chronic mentally illness.

Socially, the person who lives on the street, or who moves from one temporary shelter to another, is in continual contact with a variety of social networks. There are often ambivalent relationships with the person's family. Family members may lack understanding about the behaviors indicative of mental illness, may have rejected or abandoned the homeless person because of the inability to live up to the expectations of the family, or may lack helpful resources to assist their family member. Some family members wish to maintain contact with their homeless parent, sibling, or child but find that the person, instead, makes every effort to avoid them and may remain cut off from family contact for months or years at a time. Some youth have disconnected from their families because of the violence they have experienced in the home.

The communities in which the homeless live provide an additional social network which is sometimes supportive. The social connections that offer greater support may be the friendship network developed with others who live on the streets. A level of understanding grows from similar experiences, and through many examples of acceptance and concern, the homeless help each other. Never far away, however, is the reality that life on the streets increases environmental stresses and risk, such as victimization by violent crime, exposure to life-threatening temperatures, and vulnerability to illness. Those struck with physical and/or mental illness seldom have health insurance and its connections with a managed care network. They must turn to emergency room services for help, most often being released back onto the streets or to a temporary shelter after the crisis has passed.

As important as the social network and its supports are, homeless persons must simultaneously face the lack of access to the array of services necessary to move beyond subsistence levels. In their best efforts, the supports found at the community level integrate the social, economic, and political realities of homelessness, are responsive to immediate and concrete needs, and have the ability to follow through until the person, homeless and chronically mentally ill, can achieve greater stability. Unfortunately, this ideal scenario is often cut short due to lack of resources, funding, and personnel.

After the deinstitutionalization of mentally ill people from state hospitals in the mid 1950s, the introduction of psychotropic medications combined with Supplementary Security Income (SSI), Medicaid, and the Community Mental Health Services programs in the 1960s was an inadequate attempt to meet the complex needs of the mentally ill. When urban neighborhoods faced gentrification in the 1970s and 1980s, people with mental illness who had no assistance in meeting this transition were counted among those in the increasing numbers of homeless. A comprehensive and simultaneous array of services was needed.

The Community Support Program (CSP) was adopted as the answer to this need and was designed to enable "people with serious mental illness to live successfully outside of institutions" (SAMHSA, 2003). To this day, programs serving people who are homeless and who live with serious mental illness include elements from the initial program design: emergency shelters, outreach programs, drop-in centers, transitional housing, and health care.

> Outreach programs have been effective in reaching people with serious mental illnesses who are homeless, especially those who are unable or unwilling to accept help from more traditional office-based providers. In many cases, these efforts are literally saving people's lives.
>
> (SAMHSA, 2003)

Economically, every person standing on a street corner, lined up at a soup kitchen, or staring at a job listing on the computer at the local shelter is a clear and visible manifestation of severe poverty. Two trends historically contribute to increases in homelessness: a shortage of affordable rental housing and a rise in the numbers of those living at or below poverty levels of income ($12,740 for 1; $17,160 for 2; $21,580 for 3). "Persons living in poverty are most at risk of becoming homeless" (NCH, 2009). Poverty remains one of the major barriers to accessing adequate housing.

At the present time, we live in the ominous shadow of the worst recession and economic downturn since the Great Depression. One local program for homeless people has seen a 40 percent increase in the numbers served since the beginning of the recession (J. Eckstine, personal conversation, March 17, 2009). One disabled veteran with pelvic and back injuries was recently turned away by the Salvation Army because of a lack of funds. He turned to his county Community Action Group where he was told, "You make too much money." He found all of his local churches overwhelmed by the needs and requests of hundreds of people who had found themselves suddenly without a place to stay. Finally, he found a "local hero," a woman who was willing to rent to him. He needed $800 to move in which she would take in $50 per month increments. But he could find no one willing to loan him the money. He repeatedly called "211," a referral information line, but was passed from one recording to another. He exhausted his list of local charities, learning that they were all broke. Welfare was available only if he was so poor that there was no other way to live. "Tomorrow," he wrote, "I and everything I own will be on the street."

Public and private funding for all human services and charitable programs decreased significantly between 2007 and 2009, resulting in a lack of or inadequate income support systems through general relief such as the Temporary Assistance to Needy Families (TANF) program, Veterans Administration, unemployment benefits, SSI and Supplemental Security Disability Income (SSDI). In Chicago in the early 1990s, the difference between housed and unhoused mentally ill persons was found to be SSI (Eckstine, personal conversation, March 17, 2009). Since that time, many of these programs have seen changes in eligibility requirements and lifetime usage. Underfunded systems lead to long waiting periods during which the applicants are not allowed to work. Poorly funded congregate living situations add to the inadequacy of supports, as does a poorly funded mental health system.

The mental health system continues to struggle under the burden of historical deinstitutionalization. Prisons serve, in some instances, as de facto psychiatric institutions with mentally ill people disproportionately represented among those for whom solitary confinement and restraints are used. Prison staff as well as staff in other parts of the helping system, such as the fragmented and outdated substance abuse system, are lacking in sufficient training to be able to recognize the difference between mental illness and trauma response and/or responses to extreme stress. Many continue to hold biases against the mentally ill and the use of psychiatric medications and, lacking knowledge of more helpful ways to assist, may discriminate against those with mental illness.

Politicians identify a three-pronged structure that defines the interrelated causes for homelessness: a shortage of affordable housing, eroding work opportunities, and the cuts in public benefit programs (Cohen, 2001). President Barack Obama, riding on his campaign platform of hope and change included the following campaign messages regarding housing, job creation, health care, as well as supportive services and public assistance:

- Ensure public *housing* by a one-to-one replacement rule. Restore full funding to the Community Development Block Grant (CDBG) program. Provide housing counseling to tenants, homeowners, and other consumers. Create greater enforcement and stricter penalties for fraudulent mortgage lenders. Enact a 90-day moratorium on most home foreclosures. Create an Affordable Housing Trust Fund. [In August 2008, after the then Senator Obama began making this recommendation, a National Housing Trust Fund was enacted into law.]
- Invest $1 billion over five years in *job creation*, transitional jobs and career pathways programs. Create "green energy" jobs specifically for disconnected youth. Give employers a $3,000 tax credit for each new hire.

- Retain Medicaid, SCHIP [State Children's Health Insurance Program], and employer-provided *health care* insurance for those currently covered under those plans; create a public insurance program for those not currently covered. Mandate that all children are insured. Allow people who want private insurance to be able to seek it at a low cost by creating a watchdog organization for private insurance companies. Require employers to contribute to workers' health insurance. Provide a tax cut of up to 50 percent for businesses who pay employee premiums.
- Expand resources for *supportive services and public assistance,* and ex-offender job training and support services, including substance abuse programs Temporarily suspend tax on unemployment benefits through 2009. Improve existing services for veterans and expand homeless vouchers. Expand coverage of such programs to prevent at-risk veterans and veterans' families from falling into homelessness. Address the problems of violence against women and lack of affordable housing simultaneously.

(NCH, 2009)

Some of these proposed changes are beginning to take effect, such as the establishment of the National Housing Trust Fund and the Homes for Heroes Act that provides housing for low-income veterans. Others are facing resistance from Congress and strong lobbying bodies voicing opposition to such changes. Much remains to be seen in these efforts to meet the needs of our homeless populations.

Three kinds of federal policy affect people who live on the streets or in temporary shelters: first, homeless assistance programs that are part of the Stewart B. McKinney Homeless Assistance Act (known today as the McKinney-Vento Act); second, programs that include the homeless in their targeted populations; and third, federal programs not targeted specifically to people who are homeless or who live in temporary shelters, such as SSI, TANF, Veterans' Benefits, food stamps, and housing programs designed primarily for elderly people and/or those living in poverty. These programs provide the historical backbone to the programs serving the homeless today. Two programs receive further discussion here to provide a glimpse toward understanding, serving, and structuring policy for our homeless populations. They are the McKinney Homeless Assistance Act and the Bringing America Home Act (BAHA). Please note that a brief description of the Rural Homeless Assistance Act is also given in the later section on multicultural differentials.

The McKinney Homeless Assistance Act was first enacted into law in 1987 and included food and shelter programs that had been part of FEMA (Federal Emergency Management Agency), programs for transitional housing, for health and mental health needs to people with serious mental illnesses who were homeless, housing for disabled homeless people, and the prevention of homelessness. The fragmentation among these programs (twelve in the Department of Health and Human Services; six in the Department of Housing and Urban Development; four in the Department of Education; three each in the Departments of Agriculture, Defense, and Veterans Affairs; two in the Labor Department; and one each in FEMA, the General Services Administration, and the Department of Transportation) and the lack of coordination between and among them were major criticisms in the implementation phase of the initial version of this Act (NCH, 1999).

On the plus side, the McKinney Act required a Comprehensive Homeless Assistance Plan (CHAP), later replaced with the Comprehensive Housing Affordability Strategy (CHAS) by the National Affordable Housing Act. The CHAS required descriptions of the emergency and extended needs of homeless people in the given community plus the strategy to meet those needs. Amendments in 1988, 1990, 1992, and 1994 strengthened and expanded the original legislation.

In recent years, innovative programs and demonstration projects, built upon the experiences of implementing the earlier McKinney Act, are now funded by SAMHSA and Department of Housing and Urban Development (HUD) and offer findings on the most effective ways to serve people with serious mental illness who are homeless and who may also have co-occurring substance use disorders. One demonstration program, the "Homeless Adults with Serious Mental Illnesses" program, began in 1990. Each of the five project sites was "required to provide or arrange for outreach, intensive case management, mental health treatment, staff training, and service coordination. Results indicated that

> even people with the most serious mental illnesses who are homeless, once thought to be unreachable and difficult-to-serve, can be reached by the service system, can accept and benefit from mental health services, and, with appropriate supports, can remain in community-based housing.
>
> (SAMHSA, 2003)

The SAMHSA/CMHS Programs include Access to Community Care and Effective Services and Supports (ACCESS), the Supported Housing Initiative, and Projects for Assistance in Transition from Homelessness (PATH).

> PATH-funded providers nationwide have set a standard for the delivery of services to people with serious mental illnesses who are homeless. In 2001, with an allocation of nearly $36 million, 399 local PATH-funded organizations served more than 64,000 people with serious mental illnesses.
>
> (SAMHSA, 2003)

These findings can be found in the SAMHSA report, *Blueprint for change: Ending chronic homelessness for persons with serious mental illnesses and co-occurring substance use disorders* (2003). A list of its recommended practices and other essential services is presented in the Conclusion section of this chapter.

No discussion of the political aspects of our current definitions of homelessness would be complete without mentioning the Bringing America Home Campaign (BAHA), the national, broad-based initiative dedicated to the goal of ending homelessness. The proposed bill includes resolutions that require Congress to support housing as a basic human right as well as Universal Health Care and a Living Wage. Expansion of federal resources for affordable housing and programs for the homeless, for greater income and work supports for people experiencing homelessness, for temporary worker protections, and for civil rights protections for people experiencing homelessness are also part of the proposed bill. As mentioned above, the National Housing Trust Fund was enacted into law in August 2008 and represents a beginning to the requests made in this bill.

Perhaps the best summary of our societal, economic, and political obligations to our homeless populations is found in the statement of Core Principles upon which the National Coalition for the Homeless bases its actions. Those principles are:

1) Every member of society, including people experiencing homelessness, has a right to basic economic and social entitlements of which safe, decent, accessible, affordable, and permanent housing is a definitive component.
2) It is a societal responsibility to provide safe, decent, accessible, affordable, and permanent housing for all people, including people experiencing homelessness, who are unable to secure such housing through their own means.
3) All people, including people experiencing homelessness, who are able to secure safe,

decent, accessible, affordable, and permanent housing through their own means need economic and social supports to enable them to do so.

4) People experiencing homelessness deserve access to safe, decent, accessible, affordable, and permanent housing through the same systems and programs available to people with housing.

5) People experiencing homelessness have unique needs and life circumstances that may be addressed through housing programs designed specifically for them.

6) All people should have equal access to safe, decent, accessible, affordable, and permanent housing regardless of their unique needs or life circumstances.

7) Universal accesses to safe, decent, accessible, affordable, and permanent housing is a measure of a truly just society.

(NCH, 2009)

Demographically, an estimated 20–25 percent of all homeless face daily challenges of managing severe and persistent mental illness. "Recent estimates suggest that at least 40 percent have substance use disorders, 25 percent have some form of physical disability or disabling health condition, and 20 percent have serious mental illness" (Culhane, 2001). Approximately 25–50 percent of all who are homeless in the United States today suffer additionally from the stigma attached to labels of mental illness.

On any given night in the United States, an estimated 754,000 people, mostly minorities, were homeless on the streets, in cars, in abandoned buildings, or living in shelters in January 2005 (NCH, 2009). This translates into as many as 2.1 million in one year (Burt, Aron, Lee, & Valente, 2001). When children are included in the statistical count, that number rises to approximately 3 million (Burt et al., 2001).

Multicultural differentials reveal patterns of overrepresentation among our minority, marginalized, and vulnerable populations. Multicultural factors, as defined by the National Association for Multicultural Education, include ethnicity, age, gender, and sexual orientation, one's place in the life course, differing abilities, and geography. Each of these factors must be weighed as to its potential as a risk factor for those individuals and families who live on the streets or in temporary shelters and who are also living with a mental illness.

Homeless people are emphatically overrepresented among our various *ethnic and cultural* groups. In a 2004 survey, estimates for the homeless population nationwide were 49 percent African-American, 35 percent white, 13 percent Hispanic, 2 percent Native American, and 1 percent Asian (U.S. Conference of Mayors, 2004). The ethnic variation among the homeless is influenced by location. People experiencing homelessness in rural areas, for example, are more likely to be white, Native American or migrant workers (NCH, 2007).

Undocumented immigrants are allowed access to shelters [for the homeless] only if a child was born in the U.S. and is therefore a citizen. For legal immigrants to be eligible, at least one family member must be a citizen or a legally present immigrant.

(Mandell, 2009, p. 5)

Ethnicity and culture influence how individuals express mental health problems, how they seek help, and how their problems can best be resolved (U.S. Department of Health and Human Services (DHHS), 2001). Additionally, people of different ethnic and cultural backgrounds respond differently to psychiatric medications (SAMHSA, 2002). People of color may feel disconnected from the majority culture, making it difficult to connect with outreach workers and helping staff, especially if those individuals are not sensitive to cultural and linguistic needs.

Children under the age of 18 account for approximately 25 percent of the urban homeless population with unaccompanied minors numbering close to 3 percent of that urban homeless population. An estimated 51 percent of the homeless are aged 31 to 50 with a range of 2.5 percent to 19.4 percent identifying homeless persons in the 55 to 60 age range (U.S. Conference of Mayors, 2004).

The three most prominent groups by *gender* among homeless people are single men, single women, and mothers with children. Single homeless adults are more likely to be male than female. Single men were found to comprise 45 percent and single women were found to number 14 percent of the urban homeless population in the U.S. Conference of Mayors (2004) survey. Single women who were homeless without children were generally older, white women with higher levels of individual dysfunction, had been homeless longer than their counterparts with children, were more likely to have been in abusive relationships, have drinking problems and/or to admit to substance use, and were more likely to have received mental health services. A disproportionately high rate of sexual abuse and other trauma was found in the lives of women with serious mental illness who were also homeless. "People who have been abused are more vulnerable to ongoing stresses that may lead to mental illness, substance use, and homelessness" (SAMHSA, 2003).

One-third of the people who sought shelter from February through April 2005 were families with children (Brubaker, 2007). Homeless families are one of the fastest growing segments of the homeless population and have been found to constitute approximately 40 percent of people who become homeless (NCH, 2007). These families are most often headed by a single mother with one or two children. Single women homeless with children tend to be younger women with less than a high school education and a poor job history. African Americans are disproportionately represented among homeless single mothers. Homeless families describe a much greater incidence of spouse abuse, child abuse, greater use of illegal drugs, more mental health problems, higher rates of physical abuse as children, and weaker social support networks.

People who are homeless can be found in every segment of the life course. Children who are homeless with their parents average six years of age and constitute from 50–66 percent of the homeless family population (U.S. Conference of Mayors, 2004). Runaway youths escaping violent and abusive situations and "throwaways" (youth who have been thrown out of their homes) are two types of homeless youths, about half of whom have spent time in foster care. Many chronic runaways grow up to become homeless adults (NCH, 2009). The demographics and prevalence of the adult homeless populations have been documented above. Percentages of elders among the adult homeless populations range from 15 percent to 20 percent (SAMHSA, 2003).

Around 42 percent of homeless youth identify their *sexual orientation* as lesbian, gay, or bisexual (SAMHSA, 2003). Comparing GLBT (gay, lesbian, bisexual, transgender) homeless youth with their heterosexual counterparts, researchers have found that GLBT youth left home more frequently, were victimized more frequently, used highly addictive substances more frequently, and had more sexual partners than heterosexual homeless youth (Cochran, Stewart, Ginzler, & Cauce, 2002).

Gay homeless youth are more than twice as likely to have attempted suicide while living on the streets as heterosexual homeless youth (Van Leeuwen, 2007). Transgender individuals are especially stigmatized. They may become homeless as a direct result of job or housing discrimination. Researchers report that as many as 60 percent have been victims of harassment or violence, and 37 percent have experienced economic discrimination (Lombardi, 2001).

Geographically, homelessness in rural areas has been called "a silent epidemic afflicting thousands of individuals and families every year" (NCH, 2009). Higher rates of homelessness for women and young families in rural communities exist in the face of fewer resources available than in urban areas. Homeless assistance programs established by Congress and administered through HUD do not adequately serve rural communities. The Rural Assistance Homeless Act proposed by the National Coalition for the Homeless seeks to

> ensure that people in rural areas experiencing homelessness receive the same opportunities for homeless assistance as homeless persons in urban and suburban populations by establishing a rural homeless assistance program within the U.S. Department of Agriculture.
>
> (NCH, 2007)

The Department of Agriculture has been identified by NCH because of its greater expertise in rural development and its extensive outreach structure.

Geography also plays a role as a risk factor for homeless people when paired with climate concerns. In extreme cold or extreme heat, the homeless require additional protection. Such resources, though still inadequate to meet the needs of the increasing numbers of homeless, are more available in quantity and quality in urban areas than they are in rural areas.

Twenty-five percent of the people who sought shelter during the three-month period from February through April 2005 had *physical disabilities* (Brubaker, 2007). Disability, disease, and death are regular features of life on the streets and in shelters. For homeless women and men with chronic physical disabilities, homelessness can seem a way of life. Chronic health problems, the most lethal of which are HIV/AIDS and resurgent tuberculosis (National Health Care for the Homeless, 2001), compound the employment, housing, and problems of street-living. Not only do the homeless with disabilities require the economic assistance necessary for all who are homeless, but also they require ongoing physical rehabilitation, medical attention, and often the support of caregivers. *Learning disabilities* often interfere with a person's cognitive and information-processing abilities making it more difficult to find one's way logically through the morass of complications related to living on the streets or moving from one temporary shelter to another.

These risk factors associated with homelessness often occur simultaneously with the societal factors of poverty, lack of affordable housing, discrimination in housing, and lack of employment (SAMHSA, 2003). When combined with the struggles of living with a mental illness, homeless people also face risks associated with discrimination and housing barriers against people with mental illnesses, disability, and disadvantage. All of these risk factors can place the homeless person at an even greater risk of becoming a victim of criminal activity. "Homeless people, especially those with mental illnesses and/or co-occurring substance use disorders, come into frequent contact with the criminal justice system both as offenders and as victims" (SAMHSA, 2003).

Not all persons who live unhoused, without shelter, or who are temporarily sheltered suffer from mental illness. The homeless do tend to suffer with health and behavioral health problems that regularly interfere with their ability to manage tasks of daily living (SAMHSA, 2003) but only about 5 percent of people with *serious mental illness* are homeless at any given point in time. As many as 20 percent of all people with serious mental illnesses, however, have experienced homelessness at some point in their lifespan (Ahern & Fisher, 2001). Specific to those at the highest risk, 20 percent of the *chronic homeless* strive to manage a co-occurring *serious* mental illness. The association between these social, personal, political, biological, psychological, and emotional realities, long-embedded in historical and cultural influences, is vastly more complex than a simplistic, linear conclusion and is intertwined in a multiplicity of complicated factors. The questions remain: What risk and protective factors determine who among homeless people become mentally ill and who remain mentally resilient and strong? And who among mentally ill people become homeless and who remain housed?

People with serious mental illnesses can and do recover. Most mental illnesses, from a medical perspective, are considered treatable as general medical conditions (SAMHSA, 2003).

From a perspective of rehabilitation, people with serious mental illnesses move beyond the limitations of their illnesses and reclaim valued roles in society (Ahern & Fisher, 2001). People with serious mental illnesses become homeless because they are poor and because mainstream health, mental health, housing, vocational, and social services programs are unable or unwilling to serve them. They also are subject to ongoing discrimination, stigma, and even violence. Their ability to survive on the streets speaks volumes about their strength, resilience, and perseverance; all protective factors that can help them recover (SAMHSA, 2003).

Stressful situations can cause a reoccurrence or exacerbation of the symptoms of mental illness and these symptoms can, in turn, increase the person's vulnerability to becoming homeless. Their symptoms, for example, if untreated may include difficulty maintaining comfortable relationships with neighbors, neglecting housekeeping and cleanliness of their home and its surroundings, and confusion resulting potentially in job stress or in missed rent payments that may lead to eviction.

No other factor is as closely connected with homelessness as chronic alcohol dependence. Specific to the homeless population, substance use is both a precipitating factor and a consequence of being homeless (Zerger, 2002). As many as half of all people who are homeless have diagnosable substance use disorders. Increasingly, individuals who are homeless and have substance use disorders are younger and include women, minorities, poly-drug users, and individuals with co-occurring mental illnesses (McMurray-Avila, 2001). They have less education and fewer skills for daily living than their older counterparts. People with both disorders are at greater risk for homelessness because they tend to have more severe psychiatric symptoms, they tend to refuse treatment and medication, and they tend to abuse multiple substances. Untreated, they may be antisocial, aggressive, sometimes violent, and they have higher rates of suicidal behavior and ideation (SAMHSA, 2003).

Protective factors for persons who are homeless and who live with a mental illness include recovery from mental illness and subsequent stability with employment and housing and remaining sober if co-occurring substance abuse exists. Rates of recovery from serious mental illness have been found to occur with as many as 42 percent of formerly hospitalized patients who receive mental health services in their communities (SAMHSA, 2003). Recovery from homelessness has been defined as being sober, employed, and housed. Connection with others is viewed as the most significant protective factor in recovery from homelessness and it is often the outreach workers who make the first contact with the isolated homeless.

Illustration and discussion

Jane, a staff worker at a day program for the homeless in a midsized, central Colorado town, was first introduced to Jason, a distraught man in his early thirties, in the parking lot adjacent to the two-story brick building that housed that program. He was with two other staff members who were urging him to "talk with Jane." She recalls, with mild disbelief, that her first impression of Jason was how "sweet and helpful" he was trying to be, qualities that competed with, yet pushed through, his other, more distressing, symptoms: crying, shaking, depression, and suicidal thoughts.

Resources available in Jane's program could address many of the needs Jason described in this first meeting. They agreed to meet every two days. If participants come to the program without a referral from a mental health outreach worker or from the psychiatrist at the People's Clinic as Jason did, Jane assesses for mental illness, using a "low key" approach that she has found to be much more effective than a direct use of diagnostic labels. "Have you ever needed to use medication for sleep?" and, "Are there any medications you are allergic to?" are two questions that offer an opening for some people to admit their use of psychotropic medications. "Has anyone ever raised the question with you about an emotional or mental illness?" also frequently leads to the person's use of a label that they may have received at an earlier time.

During the first few weeks of their meetings, Jason was open with Jane about his psychiatric history, his addiction to methamphetamines, and the extreme domestic violence that resulted in permanent restraining orders against both Jason and his former wife, Chris. The couple had met during a time of sobriety for Jason but a time of alcohol addiction for her. Soon after they met, Chris discovered she was pregnant and they decided to get married. Incidents of domestic violence began after the birth of the first child and continued to escalate after the births of their second and third children. After a violent domestic dispute, Jason was taken to jail, Chris relapsed, and the children were taken into Child Protective Services after it had been reported that they were eating out of trash cans. Jason returned to using methamphetamines.

Jason blames his "severe meth addiction" as the reason his relationship with Chris ended. He also told Jane that he had been diagnosed with bipolar disorder during an earlier psychiatric hospitalization when he was depressed and suicidal. Following his time in jail after the violent domestic dispute, Jason could not return home because of the restraining order and, as a result, he had been episodically homeless since the end of that relationship, six months prior to his arrival at Jane's day program.

Jane believes it is never helpful to gloss over the horrendous aspects of a person's story. This only leads to a superficial connection, she says. The deeper connection required to help people cut through seemingly insurmountable odds to make changes from homelessness to housed and employed, is more likely to occur when they are honestly approached with, "Yes, all those things happened, you did all those things, *and* here are the strengths I see in what you are telling me now." When Jason began meeting with Jane, he was one month clean from meth but had also stopped taking the medication that helped regulate his swings between mania and depression. The depression, suicidal thoughts, and the sense of being overwhelmed that Jane observed the first time she met Jason were most likely the result, in part, of his lack of this medication.

During Jason's first few weeks of working with Jane, he agreed to use the services of several agencies. The first focus for their work was Jason's continued withdrawal from all substance abuse, his attendance at group support meetings, and monitoring what circumstances brought on his desire to use again. When these supports were solid for Jason after a few more weeks, Jane was better able to clearly discern the behaviors that had lead to a diagnosis of bipolar disorder. She reached for the NIMH checklist of symptoms for bipolar disorder and shared these with Jason "in a gentle way and at a time responsive to his need for such information." She continued with a low key and honest connection beginning her statements with such phrases as, "This is what I see . . ." or "I'm wondering if . . ." or "Have you ever known . . ." With Jason, she remarked on how he had used prescribed medications to help manage his symptoms and stabilize his moods earlier and wondered if he thought it "might be worth checking" to see if those medications would work now. Jason agreed to Jane's suggestion about meeting with the psychiatrist at the People's Clinic to assess this possibility.

Jane provided Jason with information about trauma and post-trauma response. She framed his observed behaviors – crying, shaking, depression, suicidal thoughts – and his reported behaviors – anger, numbness, difficulty processing information, heart palpitations, lack of energy, and startle responses – as his body's natural responses to terrifying events, the ways it tried to create distance from fearful circumstances for protection and survival. She also informed Jason of other post-trauma responses he might experience, such as intrusive memories of traumatic experiences, nightmares, confused thoughts and speech, exhaustion, irritability, sleep disturbances, and difficulty making decisions.

Other concrete services and resources provided by the day treatment program included food, how to access food stamps, clothing, transportation tokens, and rent money. Jane served as a broker for Jason to receive assistance from the Emergency Family Assistance Association (EFAA) and from several churches in the area for whom service to homeless people was part of their mission. When talking about his time in jail, Jason admitted he had to get his anger under control. Jane offered information about the differences between anger management and the kinds of help needed to redirect rage and violence behaviors. They discussed Colorado's AMEND (Angry Men Exploring New Directions) program as a possibility for Jason once his more immediate needs of housing and employment had been met.

Three weeks after his first meeting with Jane, Jason continued to live as a person who was episodically homeless. At the age of 32, he had cycled in and out of living on the streets or in temporary shelters, ten times. He had exhausted his list of family and friends who were willing to give him a place to stay. He had repeatedly tried and lost "eight or ten jobs, I can't remember exactly. I'd get enough to feed my addiction and would either quit the job or get fired." Jane asked about what was different now, how it happened that he had been off meth for the past month. "I got away from my suppliers and part of me wants to stay away from them. Realistically, though, I don't know. . . . I don't know if I can do it, but I'd like to give it a try."

Jane discussed job opportunities with Jason and discovered his interest in "food service positions." When she probed for more specifics, she learned that he was aiming for dishwashing at restaurants. Together they accessed Craig's List on one of the computers at the day treatment program, located several openings in local restaurants, and set up three interviews for Jason. He selected clothing from the program's interview clothing room and got a hair cut from one of the program volunteers. During these preparations, he appeared to be diligent, focused, and energized. When the time came for each of the interviews, Jason did not show up. A few weeks later, he came to see Jane "to say goodbye." He had found a "golden opportunity" in California and was leaving the next day to go find work there.

Two frameworks help conceptualize the assessment and intervention approaches for this discussion of Jane's practice with Jason: first, the life model of social work practice (Gitterman & Germaine, 2008), and second, the biopsychosocial framework. Biological, psychological, and social realities plus the interrelatedness of these three factors will be used for assessment and intervention observations from the second framework.

The impact of life transitions and traumatic life events, environmental pressures, and dysfunctional interpersonal processes, three focal points of *life-modeled practice*, frame the assessment of Jason's situation. Essential elements of life-modeled assessment include client participation, the level of fit between needs and resources, and viewing assessment as a moment-to-moment process (Gitterman & Germaine, 2008). Overlap and interrelatedness of these points is inevitable as they occur simultaneously in Jason's experiences.

Assessment of life transitions and traumatic life events   Developmentally, the "age 30 transition" typically raises a personal assessment about whether the major tasks of the twenties, of finding a primary relationship and becoming, or laying a foundation for becoming, financially independent from one's family of origin, have been successfully met or not. Jason had made attempts at both through his relationship with Chris (and probably earlier relationships unreported to Jane) and through cycles of brief employment, underemployment, and unemployment. Intertwined with behaviors indicative of a bipolar disorder, his highly energized, sometimes focused, sometimes violent behavior cycled with his depression, lack of energy, and sometimes suicidal behaviors. When unregulated without prescribed psychiatric medication, his mental illness interfered in profound ways with his making progress toward stable relationships and work experience. When stabilized on his medication, he was able to make steps toward mental health and secure a more steady income. Without his addiction to methamphetamines, Jason could have had a greater chance of managing his income in a way that could have led him out of homelessness, away from living on the streets and in temporary shelters, and into a more permanent residence. As long as he remains addicted, his chances of becoming housed and mentally strong will be a long reach for him. The simultaneous occurrence of behaviors related to his addiction, his mental illness, and his homelessness is a significant factor in the assessment of Jason's situation. Each of these realities feeds off of the other two. This assessment's connection to interventions, therefore, means that no separate treatment or form of help for only one will be as effective as the integrative treatment of all three at the same time.

Traumatic life events do not automatically lead to "post-traumatic stress disorders." Clarification of the difference between post-traumatic response and post-traumatic disorder is crucial for decisions made during assessment and intervention. Post-traumatic stress responses, such as those in Jason's situation, are appropriate to the events faced and are part of a natural healing process. Post-traumatic stress disorder (PTSD) and acute stress disorder (ASD), when used as specific diagnostic labels, require exposure to an extreme stressor, responded to by the presence of a specific constellation of behaviors, which occur over a designated period of time.

Examples of extreme stressors include

> natural disaster, rape or criminal assault, combat exposure, child sexual or physical abuse or severe neglect, hostage/imprisonment/torture/displacement as a refugee (or survivor of domestic violence), witness of a traumatic event, and the sudden unexpected death of a loved one.

> (Wise, 2007)

As reported to Jane, Jason did not reveal major traumas from his childhood or his adolescent years. One can only speculate about those years of his life. But, in the time they worked together, he did carry the memories of his own incidents of domestic violence, i.e. criminal assault, with Chris, and his subsequent arrest, incarceration, and homelessness.

The specific constellation of behaviors necessary for PTSD and ASD to be accurately used come from three main types of symptoms: the re-experiencing of the traumatic event through intrusive memories, flashbacks, nightmares, and/or triggers; avoidance and emotional numbing; and increased arousal indicated by sleep difficulties, irritability, anger, difficulty concentrating, hypervigilance, and exaggerated startle responses (Foa, Davidson, Frances, & Ross, 1999). Jason experienced a few of these symptoms but the majority were not part of his report to Jane at the time of their interactions making it premature to have used the label of "PTSD" for Jason.

The diagnostic term "acute PTSD" is used when symptoms last one to three months and, if longer than three months, "chronic PTSD." Neither of these terms fit Jason's situation making "post-trauma response" a more fitting description for him.

Assessment of environmental pressure   Loss of one's home represents one of the most devastating pressures in the relationship with one's environment. For Jason, environmental pressures occurred both before and after the loss of his home. Jason and Chris had very little time to know each other before the birth of their first child. They most likely lacked clarity about their roles as husband and wife together when they had to begin facing their obligations as parents at the same time. The family environment became an overwhelming environmental pressure for both of them, erupting in violence and resulting in forced restraints.

Environmental pressures related to Jason's work, and lack of work, would have been related to an inability to meet the financial needs of his family. He did not give information to Jane about whether or not Chris also had an income but, with their two addictions to substances, three children, and the employment ambitions he did mention to Jane, i.e. restaurant dishwashing, it is highly unlikely that the couple had the financial means to meet their needs and those of their children long before the children were taken into the custody of Child Protective Services.

The environmental pressures of living on the streets are enormous. Lack of cover during inclement weather, exposure to unsanitary conditions and disease, the risk of becoming a victim of violence, constant hunger and worry about whether there will be a next meal are only a few of the daily realities faced by those who are homeless. When also living with a mental illness, concerns about getting to appointments with psychiatrists for prescription medication refills as well as supportive work with other mental health professionals can increase the pressure felt by those who live on the streets.

Assessment of dysfunctional interpersonal processes Among the individuals, couples, and families who come to Jane's day program, it is not unusual to hear stories of how their friendship and family networks have been exhausted as places to turn for assistance and support. This was true for Jason. After being released from jail, he felt the friends and family who may have helped him earlier were "done" with him. The positive aspects of his relationship with Chris disintegrated into addiction and violence over time and placed their three children at extreme risk. Jason experienced his most emotionally healthy episodes when he was off methamphetamines and regulated through the use of psychiatric medication. However, once he felt he was doing better, he thought he could stop taking his medication. He quickly plummeted into depression or mania, became more vulnerable to substance abuse once again, and was less able to manage his violent behavior. Jason made a good first impression with Jane, seeming to be someone who "was trying to be helpful." This led Jane to believe that he might be someone who might try to help himself and, for a time, he did. In the end, however, Jason's dual cycles of manic depression and addiction carried the more compelling influence in the decisions he made.

Interventions in the work with Jane and Jason rested upon Jane's commitment to strengths-based and empowerment approaches to practice, both of which are reflected in the Life Model. Gender and age were the most noticeable differences between Jane and Jason. Jane was sensitive to Jason's concern about these differences and not only kept the work task-focused and responsive to his needs, but she also established a foundation for trust through acknowledging the horrific events that had brought him to the program and accepting him in spite of those events. This trust enabled Jason to be open about his past and his present needs so that the work could continue to move forward.

Empowerment practice interventions build on a person's strengths. Specific to the strengths revealed in the early stages of the work, helpful information is offered, the worker assists the person to make connections with others facing similar challenges, and skill enhancement necessary to moving forward becomes a primary focus for intervention.

After her straightforward acknowledgment of his addiction and violence, Jane went on to say, "Yes, you did all those things and here are the strengths I see in what you are telling me now." This statement built trust in two ways. First, Jason was truthful with Jane about his past as far as he was able at the time and she conveyed mutuality in also being truthful with him. Second, her readiness to leave that past in the past and move to the present also gave Jason permission to do the same. Jane provided information about addiction recovery support groups, about identification of behaviors that matched the bipolar diagnosis he had been given, and about natural responses to trauma that were separate from what was called an illness. She gave him information about where to find additional resources for food and shelter in the community. Connections with others in similar situations came for Jason as he participated in the various meetings offered in the day program. Skill enhancement came through the use of Craig's List to locate job opportunities and by helping Jason prepare for the job interviews.

Life modeled and empowering practice meant that Jane worked with Jason, addressing the most immediate and urgent needs as he described them, moving at a pace that provided relative comfort and safety for Jason. Without Jason's honest communication of his needs, Jane could not have provided services as closely connected with those needs; without Jane's help to use the relevant services in the program, Jason would have had a much more difficult time getting through those weeks. The services available through Jane's program were services Jason needed. Jason also had to agree to respect the rules of the program and, for example, never bring illegal substances on the premises nor act out in violent ways while there. Assessing which of Jason's behaviors could be attributed to his addiction and which behaviors were indicators of manic depression became a key factor in determining appropriate interventions and provided a good example of how assessment must be seen as ongoing. Jason's environmental pressures were assessed and included several life stories of what it had been like for him to live on the streets, stories that revealed not only the severe and dire circumstances he had faced, but also ones that showed just how resilient and resourceful he had been.

Jason's immediate needs for food and shelter were addressed the day of their first meeting. From there, additional concrete services were part of the plan for Jason: accepting his goals for employment then doing a job search together, setting up interviews, and taking steps for his preparation for those interviews. Supportive methods were also included through regular meetings with Jane and the recovery groups.

Jane's sensitivity to the three major steps in trauma recovery were evident in her timing of differential interventions with Jason at each of the respective stages: *safety* in finding protection away from threats, he had felt victimized by while living on the streets, and safety from environments that made it harder for him to stay away from abuse of substances; remembrance and mourning the loss of his home, his relationship with Chris and his children; and reconnection with others through the day program (Herman, 1997).

Jane's ongoing emphasis on Jason's personal and collective strengths was evidenced in the acknowledgement of Jason's response to the current crisis. With nowhere to go after his release from jail, he sought assistance with honesty and openness about what he had done to bring these circumstances upon himself. He agreed to renew his prescription to regulate his bipolar symptoms which, in turn, helped him stay drug free. He was focused and energized by his job search and participated in several groups; specifically in making the transition from homeless to housed and employed.

All did not always run smoothly between Jane and Jason. When Jane first observed Jason's level of distress, she was uncertain about his ability to make decisions that would help him move forward. She respected his initial discomfort at the possibility of seeing a psychiatrist at the People's Clinic for renewal of his bipolar medication and helped him understand the benefits and the risks involved if he chose to take that medication or not. Patience, perseverance, and understanding the impact of Jason's trauma responses helped Jane keep her professional perspective on the helping process during those times.

Biopsychosocial framework From a biological standpoint, Jane immediately observed Jason's responses that indicated physical reactions to earlier trauma: shaking and expressions of anger and fear. Commonly recognized physical reactions to trauma include nervous energy, jitters, muscle tension, upset stomach, rapid heart rate, dizziness, lack of energy, fatigue, and teeth grinding. Some behavioral reactions can also be seen as a subset of biological responses. These include being easily startled, exhibiting changes in eating and sleeping habits, losing or gaining weight, and experiencing restlessness (Rosenbloom & Williams, 1999). Once Jane knew Jason's history of taking methamphetamines, as well as psychiatric medications, she was aware that Jason's behaviors might also be biologically based in response to these drugs.

Psychologically, manifestations of Jason's mental and emotional states were changes in the way he thought of himself, his environment, and other people; intrusive memories of the trauma; fear related to the inability to feel safe; anger and irritability; loss of trust and emotional distance from others; and intense and extreme feelings. Other signs of psychological reactions to traumatic experiences include heightened awareness of surroundings (hypervigilance), difficulty concentrating, poor attention span or memory problems, difficulty making decisions, nightmares, sadness, grief, depression, guilt, numbness or lack of feelings, inability to enjoy anything, loss of self-esteem, feeling helpless, feeling chronically empty, and experiencing wide emotional swings such as having blunted, then extreme feelings (Rosenbloom & Williams, 1999).

Socially, this event in Jason's life included multiple losses. Because of the loss of his home and the restraining orders that prevented him from seeing his wife and children, Jason had to seek assistance from people previously unknown to him. He had to use social skills to build new social supports at a time when he was feeling overwhelmed, hopeless, and disoriented. Multiple losses in close succession are typically anxiety-producing and traumatic for even the strongest persons. For someone as vulnerable as Jason, multiple losses resulted in the onset of behaviors indicative of a trauma response. Other social indicators that a person is experiencing a trauma response are withdrawing from others, avoiding places or situations, becoming confrontational and aggressive, and experiencing an increase or decrease in sexual activity, all of which are also considered potential signs of depression and/or manic states.

Combined, the life model and the biopsychosocial frameworks for practice serve to provide an integrated approach to ongoing assessment and intervention. They complement, enhance, and strengthen each other, increasing the possibility that the client will be more thoroughly served because the assessments and intervention choices will have been shaped from a more holistic viewpoint.

Conclusion

There is hope. "We know what works. Now we must put what we know to work" (SAMHSA, 2003). Hopeful signs of change are on the horizon, signs of diminishing the impact of homelessness and its debilitating effects. Increased opportunities are arising from the crises that have been overwhelming in quantity and quality. Social work professionals stand in a pivotal position to be among those who are making these changes a reality.

SAMHSA's (2003) *Blueprint for change: Ending chronic homelessness for persons with serious mental illnesses and co-occurring substance use disorders* presents a clear set of practice principles and directions for ending chronic homelessness through "evidence-based and promising practices" as guidelines for practice and through other socially and environmentally essential services. Table 6.1 presents these essential service system components.

Table 6.1 Essential service system components

Evidence-based and promising practices

Outreach and engagement
- Meets immediate and basic needs for food, clothing, and shelter.
- Non-threatening, flexible approach to engage and connect people to needed services.

Housing with appropriate supports
- Includes a range of options from Safe Havens to transitional and permanent supportive housing.
- Combines affordable, independent housing with flexible, supportive services.

Multidisciplinary treatment teams/intensive case management
- Provides or arranges for an individual's clinical, housing, and other rehabilitation needs.
- Features low caseloads (10–15:1) and 24-hour service availability.

Integrated treatment for co-occurring disorders
- Features coordinated clinical treatment of both mental illnesses and substance use disorders.
- Reduces alcohol and drug use, homelessness, and the severity of mental health problems.

Table 6.1 Continued

Evidence-based and promising practices (continued)

Motivational interventions/stages of change
- Helps prepare individuals for active treatment; incorporates relapse prevention strategies.
- Must be matched to an individual's stage of recovery.

Modified therapeutic communities
- Views the community as the therapeutic method for recovery.
- Have been successfully adapted for people who are homeless and people with co-occurring disorders.

Self-help programs
- Often includes the twelve-step method, with a focus on personal responsibility.
- An important source of support for people who are homeless.

Involvement of consumers and recovering persons
- Can serve as positive role models, help reduce stigma, and make good team members.
- Should be actively involved in the planning and delivery of services.

Prevention services
- Reduces risk factors and enhances protective factors.
- Includes supportive services in housing, discharge planning, and additional support during transition periods.

Other essential services

Primary health care
- Includes outreach and case management to provide access to a range of comprehensive health services.

Mental health and substance abuse treatment
- Provides access to a full range of outpatient and inpatient services (e.g., counseling, detox, self-help/peer support).

Psychosocial rehabilitation
- Helps individuals recover functioning and integrate or reintegrate into their communities.

Income support and entitlement assistance
- Outreach and case management to help people obtain, maintain, and manage their benefits.

Employment, education, and training
- Requires assessment, case management, housing, supportive services, job training and placement, and follow-up.

Services for women
- Programs focus on women's specific needs, e.g., trauma, childcare, parenting, ongoing domestic violence, etc.

Low-demand services
- Helps engage individuals who initially are unwilling or unable to engage in more formal treatment.

Crisis care
- Responds quickly with services needed to avoid hospitalization and homelessness.

Family self-help/advocacy
- Helps families and domestic partnerships cope with family members' illnesses and addictions to prevent homelessness.

Cultural competence
- Accepts differences, recognizes strengths, and respects choices through culturally adapted services.

Criminal justice system initiatives
- Features diversion, treatment, and re-entry strategies to help people remain in or re-enter the community.

(Substance Abuse and Mental Health Services Administration, 2003)

Complex and multidimensional social challenges require focused, timely, and multifaceted responses. Homelessness, when experienced simultaneously with mental illness, is no exception. After decades of attempts, worthy though often inadequate, we have reached a level of knowledgeable response and coordination of services that is now providing evidence

> that people with serious mental illnesses and/or co-occurring substance use disorders who are homeless, once believed to be unreachable and difficult-to-serve, *can* be engaged into services, *can* accept and benefit from mental health services and substance abuse treatment, and *can* remain in stable housing with appropriate supports.
>
> (Lipton, Siegel, & Hannigan, 2000, p. 479)

U.S. Departments of HHS, HUD, and VA joined in 2003 to provide $35 million for the development of appropriate housing and supportive services for the Lyles and Marys, the Sharons and Franks, the Rachels and Jasons of our communities. Together these departments are also sponsoring policy academies for state and local policymakers to improve access to mainstream resources for those who live on the streets, in tent cities and other temporary shelters. The more we use our knowledge, the more we strengthen the hope that moving from homeless and mentally vulnerable to housed and mentally strong is not only a possibility but a visible and lasting reality.

Acknowledgement

The author wishes to express special thanks to Joy Eckstine, MSW, LCSW, Director of the Carriage House day program for those who live on the streets or in temporary shelters in Boulder, Colorado, for her hours of wise, compassionate, and energetic consultation so willingly given to contribute to this chapter.

Web resources

Corporation for Supportive Housing
www.csh.org

Covenant House
www.covenanthouse.org

Emergency Shelters International
www.esint.net

Foundation Center
www.foundationcenter.org

Health Care for the Homeless Information Resource Center
www.bphc.hrsa.gov/hchirc

Health Resources and Services Administration (Bureau of Primary Health Care)
www.bphc.hrsa.gov/

Locate Government Grant
www.LocateGovernmentGrant.com

National Alliance to End Homelessness
www.naeh.org

National Coalition for the Homeless
www.nationalhomeless.org

National Health Care for the Homeless Council
www.nhchc.org

National Institute of Mental Health
www.nimh.org

National Law Center on Homelessness and Poverty
www.nlchp.org

Salvation Army
www.salvationarmy.org

SAMHSA's National Mental Health Information Center
www.mentalhealth.samhsa.gov

SAMHSA's National Resource Center on Homelessness and Mental Illness
www.nrchmi.samhsa.gov

U.S. Department of Health and Human Services
www.hhs.org

U.S. Department of Housing and Urban Development
www.hud.org

U.S. Interagency Council on Homelessness
www.ich.gov

References

Ahern, L., & Fisher, D. (2001). Human services integration: Past and present challenges in public administration. *Public Administration Review, 51* (6): 533–542.

Brubaker, B. (2007). HUD study of homeless quantifies the problem. *Washington Post,* March 1.

Burt, M.R., Aron, L.Y., Lee, E., & Valente, J. (2001). *Helping America's homeless: Emergency shelter or affordable housing?* Washington, DC: Urban Institute Press.

Cochran, B.N., Stewart, A.J., Ginzler, J.A., & Cauce, A.M. (2002). Challenges faced by homeless sexual minorities: Comparison of gay, lesbian, bisexual, and transgender homeless adolescents with their heterosexual counterparts. *American Journal of Public Health, 92* (5): 773–777.

Cohen, M.B. (2001). Homeless people. In A. Gitterman (ed.), *Handbook of social work practice with vulnerable and resilient populations* (pp. 628–650). New York: Columbia University Press.

Culhane, C. (2001). Pre-conference institute presentation at *We Can Do This! Ending Homelessness for People with Mental Illnesses and Substance Use Disorders,* December 5, 2001.

Foa, E., Davidson, J., Frances, A., & Ross, R. (1999). Expert consensus treatment for posttraumatic stress disorder: A guide for patients and families. *Journal of Clinical Psychiatry, 60* (Suppl. 16), 69–76.

Gitterman, A., & Germaine, C. (2008). *The life model of social work practice: Advances in theory and practice* (3rd ed.). New York: Columbia University Press.

Herman, J.L. (1997). *Trauma and recovery* (2nd ed.). New York: Basic Books.

Lipton, F.R., Siegel, C., & Hannigan, A. (2000). Tenure in supportive housing for homeless persons with severe mental illness. *Psychiatric Services, 51* (4), 479–486.

Lombardi, E. (2001). Enhancing transgender health care. *American Journal of Public Health, 91,* 869–873.

Mandell, B.R. (2009). Homeless shelters: A feeble response to homelessness, *New Politics, 11* (3). Retrieved January 16, 2009, from www.wpunj.edu/newpol/issue43/BMandell43.htm

McMurray-Avila, M. (2001). *Organizing health services for homeless people: A practical guide* (2nd ed.) Nashville, TN: National Health Care for the Homeless Council.

National Coalition for the Homeless (NCH). (1999). *The McKinney Act: NCH fact sheet 18.* Washington, DC: NCH.

National Coalition for the Homeless (NCH). (2007). *NCH public policy recommendations: Rural Homeless Assistance Act.* Washington, DC: NCH.

National Coalition for the Homeless (NCH). (2009). *NCH public policy recommendations: Bring America Home Act.* Washington, DC: NCH.

National Health Care for the Homeless (2001). As cited in "Profile of Homelessness." *Priority home!: The federal plan to break the cycle of homelessness* (pp. 17–36). Washington, DC: Interagency Council on the Homeless.

Rosenbloom, D., & Williams, M.B. (1999). *Life after trauma.* New York: Guilford Press.

Substance Abuse and Mental Health Services Administration (SAMHSA). (2003). *Blueprint for change: Ending chronic homelessness for persons with serious mental illnesses and co-occurring substance use disorders.* DHHS Pub. No. SMA-04–3870. Rockville, MD: Center for Mental Health Services, Substance Abuse and Mental Health Services Administration.

U.S. Conference of Mayors (2004). *Hunger and homelessness 2004.* Washington, DC: U.S. Conference of Mayors.

U.S. Department of Health and Human Services (DHSS) (2001). *Mental health: Culture, race, and ethnicity. A report of the Surgeon General.* Washington, DC: U.S. Department of Health and Human Services.

Van Leeuwen, J. (2007). As cited in "Gay Youths Find Place to Call Home in Specialty Shelters" by Ian Urbina. Retrieved from www.nytimes.com/2007/17homeless.html

Wise, J.B. (2005). *Empowerment practice with families in distress.* New York: Columbia University Press.

Wise, J.B. (2007). Introduction: Empowerment as a response to trauma. In M. Bussey and J.B. Wise (eds), *Trauma transformed: An empowerment response* (pp. 1–12). New York: Columbia University Press.

Zerger, S. (2002). *Substance abuse treatment: What works for homeless people? A review of the literature.* Nashville, TN: National Health Care for the Homeless Council.

7 Corrections and its effects

Rudolph Alexander, Jr.

At the beginning of January, 2008, federal and state governments held 1,598,316 prisoners under their jurisdictions (West & Sabol, 2008). Six months earlier, Sabol and Minton (2008) reported that 780,581 detainees were held in local jails. The Bureau of Justice Statistics (2009) reported that as of June 30, 2008 federal and state correctional systems had custody of 1,610,584 prisoners. Within these prisons and jails, African American males were incarcerated at 6.6 times the rate for White males (Bureau of Justice Statistics, 2009). Put in another manner, 1 in 21 African American males were in prisons and jails compared to 1 in 138 White males (Bureau of Justice Statistics, 2009). More simply, on June 30, 2008, 846,000 African American males were in prisons and jails, 712,500 White males, and 427,000 Latino males (Bureau of Justice Statistics, 2009). Among females, the rates and numbers were lower, but racial differences exist. Among African American females, their rate of incarceration was 349 per 100,000 compared to 93 per 100,000 for White females and 147 per 100,000 for Latino females (Bureau of Justice Statistics, 2009). Combined, 207,700 women were incarcerated as of mid-year 2008 (Bureau of Justice Statistics, 2009).

James and Glaze (2006) estimated 56 percent of state prisoners, 45 percent of federal prisoners, and 64 percent of jail detainees had mental health problems. In 2007, 6,150,145 juveniles were arrested nationwide down from 6,550,864 juveniles arrested almost ten years earlier (Federal Bureau of Investigation, 2008). The Office of Juvenile Justice and Delinquency Prevention (OJJDP) administered the Juvenile Residential Facility Census (JRFC) every other year beginning in 2000. In 2004, OJJDP surveyed 3,257 public and private juvenile facilities and learned that they held 94,875 juveniles (Livsey, Sickmund, & Sladky, 2009). With these large numbers of adults and juveniles incarcerated, a high number of both groups are likely to include individuals with mental illness and have special needs (Borrill et al., 2003; Ferguson, Ogloff, & Thomson, 2009; Magaletta, Diamond, Faust, Daggett, & Camp, 2009; Way, Sawyer, Lilly, Moffitt, & Stapholz, 2008).

Advocates for incarcerated juveniles have charged that juveniles with mental disorders are denied adequate treatment (Lane, 2009). Assessing the population in juvenile correctional institutions, Fazel, Doll, and Langstrom (2008) reported gender differences in psychotic illness, major depression, attention deficit/hyperactivity disorder (ADHD), and conduct disorder. Among boys, 3.3 percent were diagnosed with psychotic illness, 10.6 percent with major depression, 11.7 percent with ADHD, and 52.8 percent with conduct disorder. Among girls, 2.7 percent were diagnosed with psychotic illness, 29.2 percent with major depression, 18.5 percent with ADHD, and 52.8 percent with conduct disorder (Fazell et al., 2008). Estrada and Marksamer (2006) reported that gay, bisexual, and transsexual youth were abused and mistreated in youth facilities, affecting their safety and mental health as a result. Hayes (2009) observed that while youth suicides within the communities have received public and professional attention, suicides by juvenile in confinement have very little attention. These statistics show high numbers of incarcerated juveniles with significant mental health issues. In 2008, a U.S. District Court in Ohio ordered massive changes in the provision of mental health treatment to all incarcerated juveniles in Ohio (*S. H. v. Tom Stickrath*, 2008).

For adults, the mental health issues within correction environments present a number of different problems and controversies (Alexander, 1991; Ashford, Wong, & Sternbach, 2008; Hartwell, 2001; Pollack, 2004; Swogger, Walsh, & Kosson, 2008; Vitacco, Neumann, & Wodushek, 2008). As mental health policy changed to reduced institutionalization of civilly committed persons, an increased mental health population occurred in both jails and prisons (Kinsler & Saxman, 2007; Reutter, 2008). In both correctional environments, prisoners and detainees have a right to mental health treatment. In the prison environment, this right is based on the Eighth Amendment to the U.S. Constitution because prisoners have been convicted, but in the jail environment, this right is based on the Fourteenth Amendment to the U.S. Constitution because most detainees have not been convicted and are being held for trial (Cohen & Gerbasi, 2005). While prisoners and detainees have the right to mental health treatment, often this right is violated. For example, a federal court concluded that prisoners with serious mental illnesses were not being given treatment and California had to spend about $8 billion to build hospitals to treat them, which California said it could not afford. Among some jail detainees who have been arrested for domestic violence suicide risk increased shortly after they have been arrested (Ludlow, 2009). Families have filed lawsuits when their relatives have committed suicides in jails or died due to the lack of proper mental health treatment ("Wrongful death suit against L. A. county jail settles for $750,000," 2008).

Further, a few prisoners and detainees have been diagnosed with Gender Identity Disorder, and they too have sued over the lack of mental health treatment (Chin, 2004; Dannenberg, 2008; *Estate of Miki Ann Dimarco v. Wyoming Department of Corrections*, 2007; *Long v. Nix et al.*, 1996; Tarzwell, 2006). This chapter covers these varied topics, including definition, issues, and controversies; developmental course and respective challenges; challenges for generational cohorts; cross-cultural issues; agency auspice and social work roles and methods; interventions and what works; case illustration; and conclusion.

Definitions of corrections

There are numerous definitions for treatment. In a hospital setting, psychiatric or mental health treatment includes not only contacts with a psychiatrist but also activities and contacts with the hospital staff designed to cure or improve the patient (Alexander, 1989). The American Psychological Association states that mental health treatment in a correctional setting is the use of a variety of mental health therapies, biological as well as psychological, in order to alleviate symptoms of mental disorders which significantly interferes with the inmate's ability to function in the particular criminal justice environment (Metzner, 2008). A California prison mental health professional testified an individual in state prison would have a serious mental disorder when he or she requires and is given access to the continuum of mental health care services if currently or within the past three years, he or she has had a significant disorder of thought or mood which substantially impairs or substantially impaired reality testing, judgment, or behavior. Also, a prisoner suffers from a serious mental disorder if she or he currently does not have the ability to meet the functional requirements of prison life without psychiatric intervention, including psychotropic medication (*Coleman v. Wilson et al.*, 1995).

The Washington Department of Corrections sought to create a program for seriously mentally ill prisoners but did not have a definition for serious mentally ill within the corrections population. So, it utilized a definition of serious mental illness employed by the Ohio Department of Corrections. There, serious mental illness was defined as:

A substantial disorder of thought or mood which significantly impairs judgment, behavior, and capacity to recognize reality or cope with the ordinary demands of life within the prison environment is manifested by substantial pain or disability. Serious mental illness requires a mental health diagnosis, prognosis and treatment, as appropriate, by mental health staff. It is expressly understood that this definition does not include inmates who are substance abusers, substance dependent, including alcoholics and narcotic addicts, or persons convicted of any sex offense, who are not otherwise diagnosed as seriously mentally ill.

(Lovell, 2008, p. 988)

Federal courts utilize an analytic framework for determining whether the mental health delivery system in prisons violates the Eighth Amendment prohibition against cruel and unusual punishment (Alexander, 1992). Indirectly, the courts have defined what a mental health delivery system is. The courts ask whether the challenged mental health delivery system operated by the prison system is so deficient that it deprives seriously mentally ill prisoners of access to adequate mental health care. To analyze that question, the courts have focused on the presence or absence of six basic, essentially common sense, components of a minimally adequate prison mental health care delivery system. These six components are: (1) a systematic program for screening and evaluating inmates to identify those in need of mental health care; (2) a treatment program that involves more than segregation and close supervision of mentally ill inmates; (3) employment of a sufficient number of trained mental health professionals; (4) maintenance of accurate, complete and confidential mental health treatment records; (5) administration of psychotropic medication only with appropriate supervision and periodic evaluation; and (6) a basic program to identify, treat, and supervise inmates at risk for suicide (*Coleman v. Wilson et al.*, 1995).

Ms. Elaine A. Lord, Retired Superintendent of Bedford Hills Correctional Facility in New York, discussed her over 20 years' experiences at this maximum security prison for woman with particular focus on women with serious mental illness (Lord, 2008). She discussed the failures of practices involving three mental health units that were governed by the Office of Mental Health, a New York state agency that operated within Bedford Hills. The three programs operated by the Office of Mental Health were a 13-bed inpatient unit that was shared with county jails, a Satellite Unit consisting of short-term cells and a small dormitory for women who were assessed as dangerous to themselves or others, and the Intermediate Care Program (ICP). The ICP was a therapeutic community for women who could not live in the general population due to their mental illness. A joint committee consisting of correctional staff and mental health staff decided admissions to the ICP, but a mental health professional decided admissions to the Satellite Unit. Despite these three programs, the number of women with mental illness exceeded these three programs and some women with mental illnesses were put in the general population. Apparently, Bedford Hill's Lord attempted to rotate some of the women who were in the three programs back into the general population but they learned that women who had been moved from the ICP to the general population were only able to stay for a few weeks before their behaviors became problematic. As a result, Lord reported the creation of a fourth program, the Set-up Program, and its success, although she did not systematically study this program.

One of the more controversial issues is the use or overuse of "super-maximum" prisons (Mears & Watson, 2006; O'Keefe, 2008) and the use of administrative segregation for inmates who are mentally ill (O'Keefe, 2007). Numerous professionals and courts have charged that supermax prisons cause mental illnesses in many prisoners or exacerbate existing mental illnesses that the prisoners have (*Dupuis v. Magnusson*, 2007; *Farmer v. Kavanagh*, 2007; O'Keefe, 2008; *Thomas et al. v. McNeil et al.*, 2009). While these prisons have been designed to house the alleged "worse of the worse" prisoners, critics note that these institutions where prisoners are isolated in cells for most of the day, facilitate mental illness (Cohen, 2008; Metzner, 2002). Rhodes (2005), an anthropology professor, received drawings from a prisoner in a super-maximum prison, and she concluded from analyzing these drawings that confinement in super-maximum prisons plays a role causing or exacerbating mental illness and affects the psychology and self-perceptions of prisoners. Lovell (2008) conducted a study of the prisoners in Washington's super-maximum and found that about 45 percent of them were seriously disturbed. Often, prisoners in super-maximum prisons do not receive mental health treatment, and when they have served their sentences, they are released into the community (Cohen, 2008). Some of these prisoners who have been in super-maximum prisons have serious problems adjusting to their communities, and some prisoners have committed very serious crimes upon their release (Kupers, 2008; Relly, 1999).

Another controversial mental health area is the use of the mental health system to deal with sex offenders. Although the U.S. Supreme Court has ruled that this policy is legal, it still remains controversial. In some states, convicted sexual offenders who have nearly served their sentences are given a civil hearing where they are committed to a mental health institution for treatment. Sometimes, these mental health units are within the prison grounds, and prisoners are simply moved from one part of the prison to another part. Many mental health professionals are opposed to the civil commitment of sex offenders because it is a guise to continue confinement using mental health laws (Alexander, 1995, 2000a). For instance, to civilly commit a person, the person must be both mentally ill and dangerous to self or others. When either dissipates, the person must be released from a mental health institution. Because prisoners must be released at the expiration of their sentences, one way to keep them confined is to declare in a civil forum that the offenders are seriously mentally ill.

Civil commitment for some sex offenders began in the United States during the 1930s. Minor sex offenders, such as individuals who engaged in voyeurism and genital exhibition, were civilly committed, whereas more serious offenders such as those who sexually assaulted individuals were incarcerated in the penal system. In the 1960s, most states repealed their civil commitment statutes based on civil rights violations and mental health professionals who questioned the etiology of sexual deviancy and who rejected the label of sexual psychopath as invalid and unreliable (Group for the Advancement of Psychiatry, 1977). In the 1980s, however, outraged citizens forced their legislators to retrieve civil commitment statutes after several highly publicized sexual assaults (Scheingold, Olson, & Pershing, 1992). A few states did not need to retrieve their civil commitment statutes because they never repealed them and only needed to amend their statutes in the 1980s. One such state was Minnesota.

In the late 1930s, Minnesota passed a statute permitting the civil commitment of a person who was assessed as having a "psychopathic personality" and who was sexually irresponsible. The Minnesota legislature defined a psychopathic personality as

> the existence in any person of such conditions of emotional instability, or impulsiveness of behavior, or lack of customary standards of good judgment, or failure to appreciate the consequences of personal acts, or a combination of any such conditions, as to render such person irresponsible for personal conduct with respect to sexual matters and thereby dangerous to other persons.
>
> (Hayes, 2009, *In re Blodgett*, 1994, p. 919)

Because of the broadness of the statute, the Minnesota Supreme Court narrowed the statute to

> those persons who, by habitual course of misconduct in sexual matters, have evidenced an utter lack of power to control their sexual impulses and who, as a result, are likely to attack

or otherwise inflict injury, loss, pain or other evil on the objects of their uncontrolled and uncontrollable desire.

(Hayes, 2009, *In re Blodgett*, 1994, p. 919)

Commitment under this statute could be indefinitely or until the treatment staff at the institution felt that the individual should be released. Initially, the law was used for persons who were caught peeping in windows, persons who exposed themselves publicly, and persons who engaged in consensual homosexual acts (Halvorsen, 1993). Later, it was applied to more serious offenders, but, unlike during its earlier use, it was being targeted at prisoners who were nearing the completion of serving their criminal sentences and being released back into the community. Alexander argued that social workers employed in civil commitment units for sex offenders faced a dilemma in that few states release committed sex offenders. Sex offenders must be assessed as being cured or not dangerous in order to be released; however, few clinicians are willing to make that assessment (Alexander, 1997).

Corrections and mental health/illness

The genesis for the right to mental health treatment for prisoners is a decision by the United States Supreme Court entitled *Estelle v. Gamble* (1976). In this case, a Texas prisoner named Gamble brought a lawsuit contending that he had been subjected to cruel and unusual punishment in violation of the Eighth Amendment because he was inadequately treated for a back injury. Although this prisoner lost his lawsuit, the U.S. Supreme Court established in this decision when a prisoner can make a valid claim of an Eighth Amendment violation based on medical issues. Justice Marshall, writing for the majority, stated that "in order to state a cognizable claim, a prisoner must allege acts or omissions sufficiently harmful to evidence deliberate indifference to serious medical needs" (*Estelle v. Gamble*, 1976, p. 106). Simply, a prisoner who has a serious medical problem that is being ignored by prison administrators is being inflicted with cruel and unusual punishment. The pain inflicted by a lack of medical treatment serves no legitimate penological interest. Echoing this sentiment with respect to juveniles, the Eleventh Circuit Court of Appeals held, first, that juveniles have the same right to medical treatment that was established in *Estelle v. Gamble* (1976), and a wait of three days to treat an injured juvenile constituted cruel and unusual punishment for which the superintendent was liable (*H.C. by Hewett v. Jarrard*, 1986).

With *Estelle v. Gamble* (1976) clearly establishing prisoners' right to medical treatment, it was quickly extrapolated to psychiatric care. Like Gamble, Bowring, the prisoner involved, did not prevail, but his lawsuit established the parameter for a right to mental health treatment. This prisoner was turned down for parole, in part, because a psychiatric report had indicated that his chance of success on parole was low because of a psychological problem. After getting his rejection for parole, he filed a lawsuit. He contended that because his freedom was being denied because of a psychological problem, the state had a duty to provide mental health treatment to him so that he could make parole. The U.S. District Court rejected the claim without a hearing, but the Fourth Circuit Court of Appeals reversed the District Court's decision and ordered a hearing on Bowring's claim (*Bowring v. Godwin*, 1977).

The Fourth Circuit Court of Appeals did not accept that Bowring had a psychological problem but that a hearing had to be held to determine the extent to which he had a serious medical problem. This hearing was necessary in light of *Estelle v. Gamble* (1976) because psychiatric treatment was considered to be medical treatment. Just as the U.S. Supreme Court had outlined how a prisoner could make a valid claim of an Eighth Amendment violation because of a medical issue, the Fourth Circuit Court of Appeals did the same with respect to a psychiatric problem. The Fourth Circuit Court of Appeals wrote that:

> A prison inmate is entitled to psychological or psychiatric treatment if a physician or mental health care provider, excising ordinary skill and care at the time of observation, concludes with reasonable medical certainty (1) that the prisoner's symptoms evidence a serious disease or injury, (2) that such disease or injury is curable or may be substantially alleviated; and (3) that the potential for harm to the prisoners by reason of delay or the denial of care would be substantial.
>
> (*Bowring v. Godwin*, 1977, p. 47)

Rationally extrapolated to *Estelle*, *Bowring* that prisoners with serious psychiatric problems have a right to be free from cruel and unusual punishment when they are allowed to suffer needlessly and painfully. *Bowring* does not mean that counseling must be provided for minor psychological distress. The psychological problem must be serious, such as a prisoner who is suffering from schizophrenia and is causing harm to himself or herself. A prisoner who is suffering from depression would not have a right to counseling for that depression, unless the depression is quite severe and is significantly affecting the prisoner's functioning in the institution. Numerous mental health professionals have lauded *Bowring* and federal courts throughout the country have adopted the *Bowring* principles (*Doty v. County of Lassen*, 1994; *Greason v. Kemp*, 1990; *Harris v. Thigpen*, 1991; *Lay v. Norris*, 1989; *Riddle v. Mondragon*, 1996; *Torraco v. Maloney*, 1991; *White v. Napoleon*, 1990). The widespread, national adoption of the principles in *Bowring* established the right to mental health treatment for prisoners suffering from major mental health difficulties. Among these circuits were the First, Sixth, Ninth, Tenth, and Eleventh. When a Court of Appeals Circuit rules on a case, it establishes the law for all states in that circuit.

When prisoners with mental illness acquired the right to mental health treatment, the courts ruled that only deliberate indifference to serious psychiatric problems would violate the Eighth Amendment prohibition against cruel and unusual punishment. As a result, courts did not consider prisoners suffering from *gender identity* disorder to meet the definition of serious psychiatric problems. However, one federal court ruled that a prisoner suffering from gender identity disorder was a serious mental disorder, triggering the protection of the Constitution and requiring that it be treated by correctional mental health professionals (*Jessica M. Lewis a/k/a Mark L. Brooks v. Berg et al.*, 2005; *Mariah Lopez a/k/a Brian Lopez v. The City of New York*, 2009). Issues occur over the placement of prisoners with gender identity disorder and their rights. For instance, the Tenth Circuit Court of Appeals reversed a decision in favor of Miki Ann Dimarco, a female with male genitalia. Dimarco was put on probation for check fraud and had her probation revoked for testing positive for drugs. While in the country jail, Dimarco was housed with women. When she was transferred to a prison for women, the prison officials discovered the male genitalia. Believing Dimarco posed a security problem, the officials put Dimarco in administrative segregation and kept her there for the duration of her sentence. Upon her release, Dimarco sued, arguing that she should have been given a right to challenge the conditions of her confinement. Although the trial judge ruled in her favor, the Court of Appeals reversed, holding that Dimarco had no liberty rights that Wyoming Department of Corrections violated (*Estate of Miki Ann Dimarco v. Wyoming Department of Corrections et al.*, 2007).

However, Orange County and the Sheriff settled a discrimination lawsuit based on the denial of treatment for a detainee who had a diagnosis of Gender Identity Disorder. The amount of the settlement was $49,000. Further, the Sheriff and the County agreed to provide all future detainees with similar diagnoses individualized treatment, provide staff training on gender identity disorder, and develop outreach to the Lesbian, Gay, Bi-Sexual and Transgender (LGBT) community. John Doe, as he was named in the lawsuit, was transgendering from female to male and was taking testosterone therapy every 14 days. He was given an injection of testosterone on August 6, 2004 but he was jailed on August 20, 2004. John Doe requested treatment, the injection, but the jail refused. When he was transferred eventually to a woman's prison in October 2005 where he did received treatment, John Doe had received no treatment in the county jail despite his primary physician advising the jail staff that the denial of treatment would have negative consequences for John Doe's health. In addition, Joe Doe was called by the jail staff a "freak," "sicko," and "that thing." After being released from the women's prison in September 2005, John Doe sued Orange County and the Sheriff for deliberate indifference to his medical problem, mental anguish, humiliation, and gender-based discrimination (Dannenberg, 2008).

The most controversial aspect of transsexuals in prisons is what treatment is due when a transsexual person is receiving treatment in the community before being arrested and convicted, and what treatment is required upon incarceration. One controversial aspect of this decision is that the mental health community recommends gender reassignment surgery ultimately as the last stage of treatment but the political system resists such treatment (Chin, 2004). Chin, who wrote that she was very sympathetic to the transgendered population, argued that prisoners with Gender Identity Disorder should not be given expensive reassignment surgery that is generally beyond the means of a poor person with Gender Identity Disorder in society. Chin agreed that prisoners with Gender Identity Disorder should not be subjected to cruel and unusual punishment, but they should not have a better life in prison. At the most, they are entitled to psychotherapy and diagnosis for their mental well-being (Chin, 2004).

Tarzwell (2006) provided a set of policy recommendations for the management of transgender prisoners. Tarzwell acknowledged that these recommendations would not provide an ideal environment but the recommendations would lead to an immediate improvement in the lives of transgender prisoners:

A: Transgender individuals (including prisoners both former and current), and transgender advocates must be included in the development and regular revision of written policies addressing the management of transgender prisoners.

B: A Management and Treatment Plan must be created for each transgender prisoner by a Transgender Committee.
   1: The Transgender Committee should include one prison medical official, one prison mental health official, one prison facilities or security official, a consultant specializing in transgender medical care, and a transgender legal advocate. The Committee must receive regular transgender-awareness training.
   2: The Management and Treatment Plan must be in writing, must justify placement and treatment choices, and must be reviewed regularly by the Transgender Committee.

C: Placement decisions must be based on the prisoner's subjective gender identity, placement preference, and safety.
   1: A prisoner's gender identity should be determined by asking with which gender the prisoner identifies. Additional information like photo identification, gender presentation, and medical records may be used to support a prisoner's gender identity narration, but are not required or sufficient.
   2: A prisoner's vulnerability should be assessed by asking questions such as: Have you been attacked before? Do people call you names, intimidate you, or harass you? Do

you think other people might harm you because of the way you look? If you have been in jail before, how were you treated by other inmates?

3: The Transgender Committee will determine whether the prisoner is properly placed in a men's or women's facility, and in the general population or in a vulnerable unit. Prisoners in vulnerable units must have access to the same services (including education, jobs, and drug treatment) as prisoners in the general population. Vulnerable units must not be so isolated from other facilities or prisoners that they effectively become administrative segregation.

4: Administrative segregation is an appropriate placement for a transgender prisoner only when the prisoner cannot safely be placed in any other housing. The Transgender Committee must immediately create a written plan for returning the segregated prisoner to less restrictive housing. Administrative segregation is a last resort, and must only be used for the period of time that the heightened risk exists, or until transfer to another facility can be arranged.

5: All correctional officers must participate in transgender awareness training.

D: The gender-affirming medical care available to a transgender prisoner should be determined by the Transgender Committee in consultation with the prisoner.

1: Established treatment regimens must be continued in the absence of compelling reasons for their suspension.

2: The inability to produce medical records of previous treatment shall not result in the conclusion that a prisoner has not received gender-affirming medical treatment, and must not be a bar to treatment.

3: The fact that a prisoner has not had previous gender-affirming medical treatment likewise must not be a bar to treatment. A prisoner confronting gender identity issues for the first time in prison must have the same access to counseling, hormones, and surgery as a prisoner who has already begun a sex-reassignment program.

4: Sex-reassignment surgeries must not be considered per se cosmetic or elective, and should be available to a transgender prisoner when the Transgender Committee determines that surgery is in the prisoner's best interests.

E: Prisoners must be screened for transgender identity and general vulnerability at intake; self-identification must be the primary mechanism for recognizing transgender prisoners.

1: All prisoners should be asked (in a professional and sensitive manner) their gender identity and whether they would like placement and/or treatment consideration by the Transgender Committee. All prisoners should be asked whether they fear victimization in the general population.

2: If intake staff believe that a prisoner is likely to be victimized because of gender expression, the intake staff may recommend the prisoner to the Transgender Committee.

3: Prisoner preferences should be respected unless compelling safety concerns demand alternative placement.

(Tarzwell, 2006)

In the *juvenile* environment noted proposed changes had been made and adopted by a U.S. District Court. In 2004, several juveniles filed a lawsuit against the Ohio Department of Youth Services, challenging the constitutionality of their confinement. The lawsuit evolved into a class action affecting future juveniles who might be incarcerated in Ohio. In 2007, the U.S. District Court approved a case management plan whereby a joint committee representing the plaintiffs and the defendants would undertake a fact-finding mission involving several juvenile facilities in the State of Ohio. Fred Cohen, a frequently used monitor of mental health care in court cases involving corrections, was selected as chair of this fact finding committee. Among the areas investigated by the committee were excessive use of force, arbitrary and excessive use of isolation and seclusion; arbitrary and excessive discipline; abusive violation of privacy; inadequate mental health care; inadequate health care; inadequate educational services; inadequate programming; failure to adequately train and supervise staff; failure to protect from harm; failure to provide an adequate grievance process; and failure to provide equal access to placement and services to females. In all these areas, the Cohen Report found serious deficiencies. As a result, the U.S. District Court entertained a stipulation for injunctive relief on April 9, 2008 and discussed the issues that the Ohio Department of Youth Services had to address (*S. H. et al. v. Tom Stickrath*, 2008).

Section VIII of the Court's decision addressed mental health care. An abbreviated list consisted of the following:

1. In general, the Department of Youth Services shall provide youth with a reasonably safe environment designed to effect proper development and prevent psychological deterioration.
2. The Department of Youth Services shall promote rehabilitation by developing, staffing, and implementing a comprehensive plan for a continuum-of-care mental health system that is attentive to the distinctive nature of adolescent cognitive, intellectual, emotional, social, and moral development.
3. The Department of Youth Services shall establish adequate policies and procedures that meet professional practice standards for every major area of mental health governance and service delivery.
4. The Department of Youth Services shall ensure that all youth have access to necessary inpatient psychiatric treatment at an appropriate facility.
5. The Department of Youth Services shall ensure that criteria for discharge from the mental health caseload are clearly articulated.
6. The Department of Youth Services shall provide adequate trained personnel, space, and time to accomplish these goals, including the addition of clinicians; independently licensed, or appropriately supervised Master's prepared social workers; psychiatric nurses, and clerical staff.
7. Clinical staffing goals shall be 1 clinician for each 15 girls diagnosed as mentally ill and in need of treatment; 1 clinician for each 20 boys diagnosed as mentally ill and in need of treatment; and 1 clinician for each 20 mentally ill youth in the general population.
8. The Department of Youth Services shall ensure that the mental health program will provide occupational therapy (OT) and general activity therapy in adequate number and quality.
9. The Department of Youth Services shall provide youth who are not on the mental health caseload with frequent, regular access to social work or other staff trained in the detection of depression and anxiety disorders, in order to prevent under-diagnosis due to masking or failure to report symptoms by youth who fear looking weak.
10. The Department of Youth Services shall ensure that treatment planning is based on professional standards, to include problem identification, solutions tied to the problem, identification of treatment response and current assets. The Department of Youth Services shall ensure that treatment programs are highly structured, consistent, intensive, and focused on changing specific behaviors and development of basic social skills.
11. The Department of Youth Services shall ensure that clinical staff, including psychology, expand and strengthen contact with the families, family surrogates, or other

significant adults in the lives of youth from reception through treatment and discharge planning.

12. The Department of Youth Services shall ensure that a mental health clinician meets regularly with girls on the mental health caseload for individualized non-crisis oriented treatment, and with the non-mental health caseload youth, in order to promote the early detection and treatment of depression. The Department of Youth Service shall strive to provide appropriate treatment for adolescent female depression.

13. Any youth who is currently on the mental health caseload or otherwise appears in need of assistance shall be provided with an advocate to assist such youth at any disciplinary hearing.

14. The Department of Youth Services shall establish, disseminate, and monitor clear, detailed protocols for quality assurance and peer review in the provision of mental health care.

15. The Department of Youth Services will ensure that mental health leadership at the Central Office level adequately recognizes and responds to the serious and complex needs of youth with mental illness in the correctional facilities.

16. The Department of Youth Services shall develop and implement its own core clinical training curriculum in order for all clinical staff to have requisite training and skills that are expected and supported by the agency.

17. The Department of Youth Services shall ensure that clinical staff develop specific individual treatment plans and goals for youth and assess progress toward these goals. Plans must include interventions that are strength-based, work toward specific individualized goals and include families whenever possible in treatment planning and delivery. Progress notes will be in standardized (SOAP) format.

18. The Department of Youth Services shall emphasize the need to distinguish a suicide gesture from an authentic attempt. Youth on suicide watch shall be seen daily by a psychologist during the week to provide appropriate intervention and support to assist the youth in developing the coping skills necessary to be removed from supervision and manage suicidal ideation.

(*S. H. et al. v. Tom Stickrath*, 2008, pp. 35–43)

McCorkle's (1995) study provided some knowledge of the *generational cohorts* for inmates with mental illness. McCorkle investigated gender, race, psychopathology, and institutional misbehavior. His variables were the history of medication or hospitalization, whether prisoners were on medication, marital status, education, whether the prisoner was employed prior to prison, whether the current offense was violent, whether the prisoner was confined in a medium security prison, and whether the prisoner was confined in a maximum security prison. The two other variables related to generational cohort were the age at first arrest and current age. Age at first arrest was not significant; however, current age was statistically significant at the 0.001 level for White males, Black males, White females, and Black females. Interpretatively, annual infraction rates increases for all four groups when these groups were younger (McCorkle, 1995). Put another way, older inmate groups with mental illness have fewer infractions than younger inmate groups with mental illness.

The mental health problems of juveniles differ from adult. According to findings detailed by Congress prior to the passage of the Mentally Ill Offender Treatment and Crime Reduction Act:

(1) According to the Bureau of Justice Statistics, over 16 percent of adults incarcerated in United States jails and prisons have a mental illness.

(2) According to the Office of Juvenile Justice and Delinquency Prevention, approximately 20 percent of youth in the juvenile justice system have serious mental health problems, and a significant number have co-occurring mental health and substance abuse disorders.

(3) According to the National Alliance for the Mentally Ill, up to 40 percent of adults who suffer from a serious mental illness will come into contact with the American criminal justice system at some point in their lives.

(4) According to the Office of Juvenile Justice and Delinquency Prevention, over 150,000 juveniles who come into contact with the juvenile justice system each year meet the diagnostic criteria for at least 1 mental or emotional disorder.

(5) A significant proportion of adults with a serious mental illness who are involved with the criminal justice system are homeless or at imminent risk of homelessness, and many of these individuals are arrested and jailed for minor, nonviolent offenses.

(The Mentally Ill Offender Treatment and Crime Reduction Act 108–414)

Hayes (2009) described the characteristics of juveniles who had committed suicides while in various facilities. From 1995 to 1999, 110 juveniles committed suicides, but Hayes had only 79 cases with completed data (Hayes, 2009). About 42 percent of the juveniles committed suicide in secure facilities, such as training schools; 37 percent of the juvenile suicides occurred in detention centers; 15 percent occurred in residential treatment centers, and 6 percent of the suicides occurred in a reception or diagnostic center. Racially, more than two-thirds of the suicides were White, 11 percent were African Americans and 6 percent were Latinos (Hayes, 2009).

Hayes (2005) also studied suicides in adult corrections and reported that over 400 suicide occur a year. Most of these suicides occur within the county jails and involve White males who take their life within 24 hours of being placed in the county jails. Researchers theorized that there are two causal factors in explaining jail suicides. One is that jails' physical structures are conducive to suicides and two the vulnerable persons jailed are in a crisis. From the jail detainees' viewpoint, the jail environment's characteristics and features promote suicides and suicidal behaviors. These are fear of the unknown, mistrust of the authoritarian environment, lack of control over the future, isolation from family and significant others, shame of incarceration, and the dehumanizing aspect of entering a jail. Moreover, certain characteristics are common among detainees in a crisis that could push them to suicides. Some of these are recent excessive drinking or drug use, recent loss of regular resources, severe shame or guilt over being arrested, current mental illness, previous suicidal behavior, and fear of going to court (Bonner, 1992).

Lewis (2005) reviewed the literature on lifetime prevalence of psychiatric diagnoses in female offenders in correctional institutions. She reviewed four studies. For major depressive disorders, the percentages were 16.9, 13, 38.8, and 21.3 for each of the four studies. Each study reported the percentages for post-traumatic stress disorder, and the percentages were 33.5, 30, 41.8, and 10.4. For dysthymia, the percentages were 9.6, 7.1, 4.1, and 8.0. Three studies reported the percentages for schizophrenia as 1.4, 1.6, and 0.8. The other study reported no information for schizophrenia (Lewis, 2005).

Numerous other mental health professionals have examined other social contexts of incarceration involving prisoners and detainees with serious mental illnesses. Grekin, Jemelka, and Trupin (1994) studied admissions to the Washington State Hospital and admissions to prisons for the individuals with mental illness. Their unit of analysis was counties. They found a significant three-way interaction among disposition, race, and counties. Particularly, they found that counties with a high proportion of a particular *minority* sent more of individuals with mental illness to prison than the State Mental Hospital. This practice was strongest for Latinos and African Americans were second. They concluded that race was a factor in how counties treated individuals with mental illness and determined which system, penal or non-penal, would handle them (Grekin et al., 1994).

Baillargeon et al. (2008) studied prisoners with psychiatric disorders involving bipolar schizophrenia, and depression diagnoses and their risks for HIV infection and HIV/hepatitis. Their sample consisted of 370,511 Texas prisoners from January 1, 2003 to July 1, 2006. They had categories of All HIV, HIV Only (Mono-infection), HIV/HCV (Hepatitis C Virus), and HIV/HBV (Hepatitis B Virus). For All HIV, 85 percent were male, 62 percent were African American, 12 percent for Latinos, and 26 percent were White. Age wise, 74 percent were between the ages of 30 to 49 and 19 percent were between the ages of 15 to 29. The percentages were somewhat similar for the other three groups of HIV categories. For All HIV, 18.1 percent had a psychiatric disorder, with 7.5 percent having a major depression and 3 percent having schizophrenia (Baillargeon et al., 2005).

Greenberg and Rosenheck (2008) studied the amount of homelessness among state and federal prisoners prior to their arrests with mental illness as one of the factors investigated too. These mental health factors were mania, depression, and psychoses. Among African Americans, 39 percent were homeless, for Whites, 53 percent were homeless, for Latinos 16.7 percent were homeless, and for other races 11 percent were homeless; 64 percent had symptoms of a mental health disorder, consisting of 53 percent for mania, 40 percent for depression, and 26 percent for psychoses. These researchers noted that practitioners need to better understand how some individuals become homeless and develop better interventions to prevent the cycling of inmates from homelessness to incarceration (Greenberg & Rosenheck, 2008).

A group of researchers investigated relationships involving male and female offenders in Iowa Department of Corrections who had borderline personality disorders. With respect to marital status and prisoners having a borderline personality disorder, 15.6 percent were divorced, 31.3 percent were married, 4.7 percent were single, and 48.4 percent were other. With respect to education, 58 percent had less than an high school education, 18.5 percent had a high school education or GED, and 23 percent had some college education. In terms of race and ethnicity, 67.7 percent were White, 15.4 percent were African American, and 16.9 percent were the Other category. For gender and those prisoners with borderline personality disorder, 81.5 percent were male and 18.5 percent were female (Black et al., 2007).

Wolff, Blitz, and Shi (2007) compared prisoners with and without mental disorders and their sexual victimization in prisons. Twelve of the prisons were for males and one was for females, with a sample size of 7,528; 93 percent of the sample were male. Within males, racially, 59 percent of the sample were African Americans, 16 percent were non-Hispanic Whites, 20 percent were Hispanic, and about 6 percent were of another race or ethnicity. Among female prisoners, 48 percent were African Americans, 31 percent were non-Hispanic White, 14 percent were Hispanic, and 7 percent were of another race or ethnicity. About 1 in 12 inmates with a mental disorder reported that they had been victimized sexually within the past six months, compared to 1 in 33 inmates without a mental disorder. Among males and females with mental disorders, females were three times more likely to be victimized sexually in prison (23.4 percent), compared to males (8.3 percent). Minority prisoners, African American and Hispanic, with mental disorders were more likely to be victimized than White prisoners with mental disorders. These researchers concluded that prisoners with mental disorders are more likely to meet with violence in prisons and these prisoners have further mental health issues. These prisoners should be screened for PTSD (Wolff et al., 2007).

Primm, Osher, and Gomez (2005) recounted the number of incarcerated persons, juveniles and adults, in the criminal justice system and the number of persons with mental illnesses as well as co-occurring substance abuse issues. They then discussed cultural competence in mental health treatment. Adopting a definition from the U.S. Department of Health and Human Services, they conveyed that cultural competence involved an array of behaviors, attitudes, and policies that coalesce by professionals in an agency or system to work effectively in cross-cultural interactions. Becoming skilled in cross-cultural interactions consists of a professional evolving over an extended period of time. This process requires institutionalization of principles and values as well as agencies or organizations having the ability to (1) value diversity; (2) conduct self-assessment; (3) manage the dynamics of difference; (4) acquire and institutionalize; (5) adapt to diversity and cultural contexts of the communities they serve (Primm et al., 2005). Based on previous work, Primm noted that African American and Latinos reported that at every stage of the criminal justice process, criminal justice professionals demonstrated inadequate cultural competence. Thus, recommendations by them to build cultural competence were systematic training, direction by leadership and advisory groups, guiding policies and principles that address treatment parity; linguistic assistance, accountability, advocacy and community outreach (Primm et al., 2005).

Severson and Duclos (2005) asked whether risk screening for suicide among American Indians was culturally sensitive and answered the question in the affirmative. They stressed that American Indian concept of mental illness might cause them to interpret screening questions differently than the general population of detainees. Instead of having a one size fits all approach, the suicide risk assessment protocol should be tailored to the cultural background of the detainee population. For example, if a mental health professional who is not culturally sensitive asks an American Indian about his or her mental health history, the question may be too confusing and the response may not be revealing. Many American Indians understand mental and emotional problems as being caused by external forces, not psychological conflict. Unwellness caused by external factors, such as consuming alcohol, is unnatural, whereas unwellness that is natural is caused by biological, social and/or cultural violations or taboos. Mental illness is a White person's disease that is shameful and unnatural, according to many American Indians and in many American Indians' communities, there is no word or conception for mental illness, per se. Wellness is viewed among American Indians as an undividable whole of the body, mind, and spirit (Severson & Duclos, 2005).

Utilizing a representative sample of prisoners that involved 14,500 of state prisoners, 3,700 federal prisoners, and 7,000 jail detainees, James and Glaze (2006) reported the percentages of incarcerated persons with mental health problems that had implications for cross-cultural considerations. They categorized race and ethnicity in four categories. In the Other category, consisting of American Indians, Alaska Natives, Asians, Native Hawaiians, other Pacific Islanders, and persons listing more than one race, James and Glaze (2006) indicated that 62 percent of those persons in state prisons had mental health problems compared to 62 percent of Whites, 55 percent of African Americans, and 46 percent of Hispanics. Within the federal prison system, 50 percent of the Other category had mental health problems compared to 50 percent of Whites, 46 percent of African Americans, and 37 percent of Hispanics. In local jails, 70 percent of the Others had mental health problems, 71 percent of Whites, 63 percent of African Americans, and 51 percent of Hispanics (James & Glaze, 2006).

Earle, Bradigan, and Morgenbesser (2001) provided insight into Native Americans in the New York prison system and their mental health needs. Renamed Iroquois by the French, the Haudenosaunee lived in upper New York for hundred of years. The Haudenosaunee consisted of five tribes: Mohawk, Oneida, Onodaga, Cayuga, and Seneca. Early mental health professionals at the close of the nineteenth century considered Native Americans to be mentally ill because they spoke with the dead, heard the dead, and saw the dead. They noted that many tribes adopted the Medicine Wheel consisting of four areas of functioning involving the social, mental, physical, and spiritual beings. All four must be in balance to determine what is healthy and what is unhealthy. Earle et al. (2001) examined records and interviewed some Haudenosaunees in a prison mental health unit to learn why the Haudenosaunees were in the mental health unit in higher proportion than the free world population. One Haudenosaunee revealed that "here you get referred if you act strange" with acting indicating that one was being quiet, keeping to one self, or acting aggressively (p. 127). Earle et al. (2001) concluded that

> counselors who work with American Indians in jail or in prison are encouraged to ascertain both the tribe to which a person belongs and the extent of affiliation, and learn whatever can be found regarding the cultural understandings and traditions of the Indian tribe or nation. Most importantly, the provider of service must ascertain the effect this will have on therapeutic interventions such as, for example the use of psychotropic medication.
>
> (Earle et al., 2001, p. 130)

Scott (2005) noted that despite the apparent need for mental health professionals who have been trained in providing care to the population of mentally ill prisoners, very few schools in psychiatry, psychology, and social work prepare students for this endeavor. The *correctional system* is an exclusive unique environment with specialized terminology, laws, rules, procedures, setting, and administrative management. In order for mental health professionals to provide effective care, they must understand the correctional world. Several professionals have discussed the impact of court decisions involving corrections and mental health (Perlin, 2001), and the roles of social workers in the area of mental health in corrections (Griffin, 2007).

Appelbaum (2005) described the psychiatrist role in the correctional culture, which is applicable to social work, although Appelbaum did not describe it as such. Among the areas that Appelbaum discussed were temperament, advocacy, medication use, consultation and liaison roles, forensic roles, and confidentiality. To be an effective correctional psychiatrist (Appelbaum, 2005, p. 38) or correctional social worker, he or she:

> 1. Understands the correctional culture; 2. Complies with institutional rules and regulations; 3. Maintains appropriate boundaries; 4. Uses correctional jargon appropriately; 5.Treats inmates, security staff, and other health care professionals with respect; 6. Collaborates with security staff; 7. Approaches patients in a professional, non-adversarial way; 8. Adapts with flexibility to the prison environment; 9. Advocates selectively; 10. Practices with sensitivity to fiscal and operational concerns; 11. Provides consultation and liaison service; and 12. Balances confidentiality with sharing of necessary information.

A social worker with a goal to attend law school, Griffin (2007) stated:

> With respect to professional obligations, the implications of social workers' concern for the dignity and worth of inmates with mental health problems spans all levels of practice. Perennial threats to funding for mental health treatment in jails and prisons, for example, provide opportunities for social workers to advocate for inmates at the macro-level. Since policy-makers regularly review and occasionally bolster extant treatment programs, social workers must intervene at the policy level to demand the proper treatment of mentally ill detainees. Organizations committed to human rights, such as Human Rights Watch, often act as media for the entrance of social workers into the world of policy-making. At the mezzo-level, social workers may address the problem of mental illness among inmates by becoming involved in programs that currently exist to meet the needs of detainees. Extant treatment programs in jails and prisons are chronically under-staffed, leaving an

unfortunate dearth of competent, caring mental health professionals. Given their comparatively broad training, social workers are well situated to "fill the gaps" that often plague treatment programs in correctional facilities.

(Griffin, 2007, p. 31)

Another social work professional discussed the essential elements of promising mental health services for jail detainees and the implications for social workers. A task force of the American Psychiatric Association identified four core elements of mental health services, and two criminal justice professional expanded them to six core elements. There expanded six elements are (a) screening, evaluation, and classification procedures; (b) crisis intervention and short-term treatment; (c) discharge planning mechanisms; (d) court liaison mechanisms; (e) diversion practices; (f) contracting procedures (Alexander, 1999). Alexander (1999) discussed these elements within the provision of privatization of mental health services for jails and the legal liability for social workers within the jail context. Alexander stressed that

> social workers should ensure that detainees are provided with professional services. At a minimum these services should include assessment of all prisoners for mental health problems. For suicidal detainees, crisis intervention should be provided. For seriously mentally ill detainees, service should include professional contacts designed to alleviate distress and improve functioning. While some detainees may need medication, individual and group counseling may be beneficial to them and others.
>
> (Alexander, 1999, p. 74)

Illustration and discussion

First, every correctional mental health program should establish a mission statement. In this mission statement should be (1) admission and discharge criteria; (2) treatment goals; (3) available interventions; (4) quality assurance and peer review; (5) contribution to safety and security of the institution and public safety; (6) methods of enhancing staff morale, including (a) respect for differences of opinion, (b) focus on conflict resolution, (c) regularly scheduled discussion and cross-training, (d) input and participation from all disciplines; (7) language that promotes a professional work environment (Chaiken, Thompson, & Shoemaker, 2005).

Judges have ruled that conducting assessments is essential to providing constitutionally accepted mental health treatment to prisoners. Ditton (1999) indicated that for a 1997 survey of inmates in federal and state prisons and detainees in jail involved the following questions that were answered yes or no in an effort to conduct initial screening:

(a) Do you have a mental or emotion condition?
(b) Have you ever been told by a mental health professional such as a psychiatrist, psychologist, social worker, or psychiatric nurse, that you had a mental or emotional disorder?
(c) Because of an emotional or mental problem, have you ever:
 (1) Taken a medication prescribed by a psychiatrist or other doctor?
 (2) Been admitted to a mental hospital, unit or treatment program?
 (3) Received counseling or therapy from a trained professional?
 (4) Received any other mental health services?

Adams and Ferrandino (2008) discussed the major issues that need to be addressed to improve inmate mental health care. Specifically, they cited (1) intake, screening, and assessment; (2) treatment and control; (3) risks and stakes; (4) risk management and treatment; (5) environments as therapy; (6) segregation and isolation; (7) medication; and (8) correctional officer involvement. In the intake, screening, and assessment areas, they note that professionals have debated the utility of clinical versus actuarial prediction models and the efficacy of them in assessing adults and juveniles with mental health problems. They noted too the assessment of psychopathy and dangerousness was important for the safety of the correctional staff and public. In the area of treatment and control, they stated that the relationship between them and determining an appropriate balance is a vital management issue. Regarding risks and stakes, Adams and Ferrandino (2008) said that

> a significant aspect of treatment strategies for mental disorders is trial and error. Clinicians use their experience to predict likely reactions to various treatments or interventions and then use their judgment to identify what would seem to be the best course of action. However, events do not always turn out as predicted, and so clinicians constantly modify their approaches with individual patients based on feedback as to what works best. In the context of correctional institutions, the trial-and-error aspect of mental health treatment has to be taken very seriously because some adverse outcomes, such as those involving violence, may be very harmful. Quite naturally, a conservative posture of risk avoidance and of adopting low-risk strategies is preferred.
>
> (Adams Ferrandino, 2008, p. 918)

Risk management and treatment consist of providing treatment to inmates with mental illness holistically and not an either or approach either changing the offender or controlling the offender. The environment as therapy means putting offenders with mental illness in the best environment possible. For instance, different prisons and different cell blocks or dormitories have different stressors which could lessen or aggravate prisoners' symptoms. Segregation and isolation are important factors for correctional administrators especially when they are used short term or long term for prisoners with mental illness. Providing medication is the primary method of administering treatment, but medications may be overused. Last, there is the continuing debate about the role of correctional officers in the treatment of prisoners with mental illness and providing them with training in mental illness besides the normal security training.

Treatment for prisoners with serious mental illnesses may be psychopharmacological or traditional therapies. Sometimes, correctional institutions have relied too heavily upon medications. Burns (2005) confessed that in the distant past, there was a tendency to use psychotropic drugs for their sedating effects "as a means of managing undesirable behaviors" (p. 89). Medications used in this manner, Burns noted, may violate prisoners' rights but she acknowledged that advances have been made and for many serious mental illnesses, medication is the preferred mode of treatment. Burn (2005) wrote, "I do not intend to imply that treatment with psychotropic medication is the sole requirement for appropriate mental health care of inmates; but rather, psychotropic medication is one component of a comprehensive treatment plan" (p. 90). Concurring, Chaiken et al. (2005) contend that the use of pharmacological treatment of mental illness is vital to the effectiveness of any correctional treatment program. The likelihood of medication compliance is increased by other therapeutic treatments. The most universal intervention used with mental health patients in correctional facilities are individual therapy, group therapy, recreational therapy, therapeutic community, substance abuse programs, assistance with daily living skills, and behavior incentive programs (Sacks, McKendrick, Hamilton, Cleland, Pearson, & Banks, 2008).

Elaborating upon Burn's acknowledgement that medication is not the only successful method for treating serious mental illnesses, Alexander (2000b) reported a group counseling program for seriously mentally ill persons who had been diagnosed with paranoid schizophrenia who were residing in Israel, contending that his approach could be successful in a correctional environment.

Particularly, Levine, Barak, and Granek (1998) conducted an experiment to learn if inducing cognitive dissonance would alter psychotic paranoid ideation in individuals who had been diagnosed with paranoid schizophrenia. Cognitive dissonance is the condition of having two dissonant beliefs at the same time. An individual feels tension and uneasiness when cognitive dissonance occurs. As a result, Levine et al. hypothesized that treatment that induced cognitive dissonance systematically would enable "patients who accepted the axiom to be gradually exposed to neutral, low and finally emotion-laden paranoid ideation in such a way that they eventually began to question the very existence of the paranoid system" (Levine et al., 1998, p. 11). In testing this hypothesis, the researchers randomly assigned 12 persons with diagnoses of paranoid schizophrenia to a treatment and control group. Before entering the cognitive-dissonance group individuals met with two therapists. One therapist posed a question to the other therapist, such as what may cause a traffic jam? The responding therapist answered perhaps a car out of gas and slowing traffic, engine trouble, a driver having a heart attack, construction work, traffic lights malfunctioning, or accidents. Then, the individual with mental illness is asked a similar question, which is neutrally selected by the therapists. After the individual has demonstrated some proficiency in providing several alternative explanations, one therapist declares that "it is axiomatic that any event has several alternative explanations perceived by the keen observer" (Levine et al., 1998, p. 6). This axiom is put on a piece of paper and the two therapists and the individual sign it. In effect, the higher functioning therapists influence the individual with mental illnesses and help to establish this norm for the group. When everyone has had this introduction, the group begins. Group counseling is structured and homework is given. When paranoid statements are made in group counseling, individual members remind all of the axiom and help to provide alternative explanations. The clinicians/researchers used the Positive and Negative Syndrome Scale (PANSS) to assess participants in both groups at baseline, two weeks, four weeks, six weeks, and ten weeks (i.e. follow-up). They found significant differences between the treatment and control group on thought disturbance scores and psychopathology (Levine et al., 1998).

Alexander (2000b) observed that cognitive-behavioral treatment was the most successful in treating adult and juvenile offenders. Three professionals have provided additional empirical support for the dominance of cognitive-behavioral treatment. They randomly assigned prisoners to three groups. One group received individual and group cognitive-behavioral intervention. Another group received just the individual cognitive-behavioral treatment, and the control group consisted of those prisoners on a waiting list for the individual group. The researchers measured all prisoners for level of mental disturbance at pre-test and post-test. Statistical analyses showed that both groups showed a decrease in the level of mental disturbance but the combination group had the greatest decrease (Khodayarifard, Pritz, & Khodayarifard, 2008).

Severson (1999) indicated that the jail environment is a system in which social workers can interact with multi-clients, and social workers have long understood that a system can include a prison or jail as a whole system or a subsystem. Two systems provide a review of prisoners and detainees with serious mental illness. First, *Frontline* broadcasted a presentation entitled the New Asylum. It noted that in most states, prisoners with serious mental illness receive little or no mental health treatment. However, Ohio was hailed as having developed a model of treatment for prisoners with serious mental illness and *Frontline* was given full access to Ohio prisons. Many prisoners with mental illness are placed at Ohio's maximum security prison at Lucasville, Ohio. These prisoners may begin serving their sentences at lower security prisons but are unable to follow rules within these institutions and thus spiraled into the maximum security prison. At the maximum security prison in Lucasville, Ohio, prisoners with mental illnesses are housed within a mental health unit. When these prisoners act out on the mental health unit, they may be placed in administrative segregation as punishment or they may go into the prison infirmary. From either place, a prisoner may be transferred to Oakwood Correctional Facility, which is a psychiatric hospital, located about 170 miles from Lucasville. Its goal is to provide short-term acute care for prisoners and once they are stabilized they are returned to Lucasville. One prisoner from the mental health unit at Lucasville had been placed in administrative segregation almost 100 times and frequently he had to be forcibly extracted from his cell by a special squad. This prisoner had been transferred to Oakwood and returned to Lucasville 18 times. He explained the differences between the two facilities, noting that the Oakwood mental health professionals are better and treat him better. He said he is not upset as much when he is at Oakwood. Fred Cohen, a mental health consultant, stressed that a maximum security prison is not suited to treat prisoners with mental illness and the environment in a maximum security prison is not conducive to psychiatric treatment (Navasky & O'Connor, 2005).

Debbie Nixon-Hughes, Chief of the Bureau of Mental Health Services within the Ohio Department of Rehabilitation, was interviewed by *Frontline* for the special on the New Asylum. She reported that a lawsuit had been filed to improve mental health services for prisoners with serious mental illness. As a result, the Department of Rehabilitation had evolved from a Department of Psychology to a Department of Mental Health, meaning that the Department created a continuum of services that were offered, from outpatient therapy, crisis services, and residential treatment services. It created its own inpatient psychiatric services and had increased staffing, including psychiatric nurses, social workers, psychologists, and psych assistants (PBS, 2005). Social workers were employed in various systems throughout the Ohio Department of Corrections but no social worker was specifically highlighted. In the New Asylum, a mental health professional was shown providing group therapy to five inmates. There were ten individual cells and each cell was a little larger than a telephone booth with one inmate in a cell. The cells curved in almost a half circle and the mental health professional set in a chair in the middle, counseling the inmates.

A second system, however, provides more specific social work involvement. A licensed Master's level social worker and two Master level social work students devised and implemented a psycho-educational group treatment program for woman jail detainees. The targeted areas for these women were stress, anxiety, depression, and trauma. Ultimately, the goal is to reduce the women's recidivism but the short-term goals were to address women's mental health issues. They drew from reality therapy, Lazarus' Model of behavior medication, cognitive theory, and empowerment theory to formulate their psychoeducational group intervention. The psychoeducational focus of the intervention was premised upon the assumption that these woman detainees had a number of emotional and mental health problems that made their stress worse and interfered with their ability to cope with being confined in a jail environment. Hence, the program was designed to intervene with these women's low self-esteem, victimization and depression, post-traumatic stress symptoms, high anxiety levels, and basic life issues, such as communication, problem solving and decision making, goal setting, and goal achievement. In that these social workers intended to conduct research on the effectiveness of their intervention, they used nonequivalent control group design (Pomeroy, Kiam, & Abel, 1998).

Considering the assessment and interventions skills displayed by these social workers, the intervention began with a social worker explaining to each individual member the program and intended research aspect of it. They were told that confidentiality was extremely important for all women to feel free to discuss and explore personal issues. Then, the women in both the experiment group and comparison group were administered various scales and instruments to measure their mental health issues to get their scores at pre-test. The intervention was to last five weeks, and the women were given resources and encouraged to contact these sources upon their discharge.

The introductory group session consisted of explaining the critical need for confidentiality, an explanation of group content and procedures, and the relationship between feelings and behaviors. Each woman was asked to examine their self-concept and their major life relationships. The social workers initiated trust-building exercises and related experiences. Then, these group leaders helped woman detainees acknowledge their feelings, thoughts, and actions. In this manner, the women would be able to transit from a failure identity to a success identity. As a consequence, the women experience less self-blame and shame. The women were provided with knowledge of the change process and asked to identify their strengths and assets. These detainees, consequently, developed positive affirmation statements based on their assessments and displayed these newer improved behaviors in the group. Once, a group member broke confidentiality and related comments made in the group to other women in the jail. Because of the seriousness of this breach and to reinforce the importance of confidentiality, the violator was removed from the group and recommended that she be placed in another part of the jail (Pomeroy et al., 1998). At the end of the five weeks, the treatment group had lower post-test scores than the comparison group. Further, the social workers relayed the success of one woman detainee who upon being criticized by jail staff for the cuts on her arms wrote down her feelings, as she was taught in group, instead of responding to the jail staff. Also, this woman detainee got out of jail, divorced her abusive husband, retrieved her children, and found a job (Pomeroy et al., 1998).

Conclusion

This chapter initially provided several definitions of mental health treatment and correctional mental health treatment. Then, it described a number of controversial topics involving mental health issues in corrections. Probably, the number one controversy is the use of super-max prisons which have been documented as causing mental illnesses and the release of prisoners negatively affected mentally from super-max prisons into the community. Another controversial area is the use of civil commitment to transfer essentially sex offenders from prison to a mental health unit to continue their confinement. Mental health clinicians are reluctant to say that a sex offender is cured or not dangerous, presenting an ethical dilemma.

This chapter reveals that pharmacological drugs, once used in an abusive manner, are the most appropriate for treating prisoners with serious mental illness. However, one experimental study revealed that individuals with serious mental illness in Israel who were paranoid could have their paranoia lessened by group treatment. A criminal justice professional stated that this could be used with prisoners with serious mental illness and who were paranoid. Further, criminal justice professionals contend that cognitive-behavioral approaches are very effective with prisoners with mental illness. The last section presents a case illustration of a system in Ohio, hailed as a model for the country, where prisoners with serious mental illness are housed in a maximum security prison, progressed through different areas of the prison, and then transferred to a mental hospital. When stabilized, they are returned to the maximum security prison and begin the cycle again. Some prisoners have traveled this circuit multiple times. If Ohio has a model system, then it says a lot about what is occurring in other states.

Web resources

Centers for Disease Control and Prevention: Correctional Health
www.cdc.gov/correctionalhealth/

Frontline, The New Asylum
www.pbs.org/wgbh/pages/frontline/shows/asylums/

Judge David L. Bazelon Center for Mental Health Law: Individuals with Mental Illnesses in Jail and Prison
www.bazelon.org/issues/criminalization/factsheets/criminal3.html.

SAMHSA: Substance Abuse Treatment in Adult and Juvenile Correctional Facilities
www.oas.samhsa.gov/ufds/correctionalfacilities97/5feda.htm

U.S. Department of Health and Human Services: Many in U.S. Prisons Lack Good Health Care
www.healthfinder.gov/news/newsstory.aspx?docID=623147

World Health Organization: Mental Health and Prisons
www.euro.who.int/Document/MNH/WHO_ICRC_InfoSht_MNH_Prisons.pdf

References

Adams, K., & Ferrandino, J. (2008). Managing mentally ill inmates in prisons. *Criminal Justice and Behavior, 35* (8), 913–927.

Alexander, R., Jr. (1989). The right to treatment in mental and correctional institution. *Social Work, 34,* 109–112.

Alexander, R., Jr. (1991). United States Supreme Court and an inmate's right to refuse mental health treatment. *Criminal Justice Policy Review, 5* (3), 225–240.

Alexander, R., Jr. (1992). Cruel and unusual punishment: A slowly metamorphosing concept. *Criminal Justice Policy Review, 6* (2), 123–135.

Alexander, R., Jr. (1995). Employing the mental health system to control sex offenders after penal incarceration. *Law and Policy, 17* (1), 111–130.

Alexander, R., Jr. (1997). The reconstruction of sex offenders as mentally ill: A labeling explanation. *Journal of Sociology and Social Welfare, 24* (2), 65–76.

Alexander, R., Jr. (1999). Social work and mental health services in jails. *Arete, 23,* 68–75.

Alexander, R., Jr. (2000a). Civil commitment of sex offenders to mental institutions: Should the standard be mental illness or mental disorder? *Journal of Health & Social Policy, 11* (3), 67–78.

Alexander, R., Jr. (2000b). *Counseling, treatment, and intervention methods with juvenile and adult offenders.* Pacific Grove, CA: Brooks/Cole.

Appelbaum, K.L. (2005). Practicing psychiatry in a correctional culture. In C.L. Scott and J.G. Gerbasi (eds), *Handbook of correctional mental health* (pp. 21–41). Washington, DC: American Psychiatric Publishing.

Ashford, J.B., Wong, K.W., & Sternbach, K.O. (2008). Generic correctional programming for mentally ill offenders: A pilot study. *Criminal Justice and Behavior, 35* (4), 457–473.

Baillargeon, J.G., Paar, D.P., Wu, H., Giordano, T.P., Murray, O., Raimer, B.G. et al. (2008). Psychiatric disorders, HIV infection and HIV/hepatitis co-infection in the correctional settings. *AIDS Care, 20* (1), 124–129.

Black, D.W., Gunter, T., Allen, J., Blum, N., Arndt, S., Wenman, G., & Sieleni, B. (2007). Borderline personality disorder in male and female offenders newly committed to prison. *Comprehensive Psychiatry, 48,* 400–405.

Bonner, R. (1992). Isolation, seclusion, and psychological vulnerability as risk factors for suicides behind bars. In M.R. Berman & J. Maltsberger (eds), *Assessment and prediction of suicide* (pp. 398–419). New York: Guilford Press.

Borrill, J., Burnett, R., Atkins, R., Miller, S., Briggs, D., Weaver, T., & Maden, A. (2003). Patterns of self-harm and attempted suicide among white and black/mixed race female prisoners. *Criminal Behavior and Mental Health, 13,* 229–240.

Bowring v. Goodwin, 551 F. 2d 44 (4th Cir. 1977).

Bureau of Justice Statistics (2009). Growth in prison and jail populations slowing:16 States report declines in the number of prisoners. Retrieved April 9, 2009, from www.ojp.usdoj.gov/bjs/pub/press/pimjim08stpr.htm.

Burns, K.A. (2005). Psychopharmacology in correctional settings. In C.L. Scott & J.G. Gerbasi (eds), *Handbook of correctional mental health* (pp. 89–108). Washington, DC: American Psychiatric Publishing.

Chaiken, S.B., Thompson, C.R., & Shoemaker, W.E. (2005). Mental health interventions in correctional settings. In C.L. Scott and J.G. Gerbasi (eds), *Handbook of correctional mental health* (pp. 109–131). Washington, DC: American Psychiatric Publishing.

Chin, L. (2004). A prisoner's right to transsexual therapies: A look at *Brooks v. Berg. Cardozo Women's Law Journal, 11*, 151.

Cohen, F. (2008). Penal isolation: Beyond the seriously mentally ill. *Criminal Justice and Behavior, 35* (8), 1017–1047.

Cohen, F., & Gerbasi, J.B. (2005). Legal issues regarding the provision of mental health care in correctional settings. In C.L. Scott and J.G. Gerbasi (eds), *Handbook of correctional mental health* (pp. 259–283). Washington, DC: American Psychiatric Publishing.

Coleman v. Wilson et al., 912 F. Supp. 1282 (USDC CA ED 1995).

Dannenberg, J.F. (2008, January). California jail settles gender-identify-disorder discrimination suit. *Prison Legal News, 19* (1), 31.

Ditton, P.M. (1999). *Mental health and treatment of inmates and probationers*. Washington, DC: Bureau of Justice Statistics.

Doty v. County of Lassen, 37 F.3d 540 (9th Cir. 1994).

Dupuis v. Magnusson, 2007 U.S. Dist. LEXIS 56143 (2007).

Earle, K.A., Bradigan, B., & Morgenbesser, L.I. (2001). Mental health care for American Indians in prison. *Journal of Ethnic and Cultural Diversity in Social Work, 9* (3–4), 111–132.

Estate of Miki Ann Dimarco v. Wyoming Department of Corrections et al., 473 F.3d 1334 (9th Cir. 2007).

Estelle v. Gamble, 429 U.S. 97 (1976).

Estrada, R., & Marksamer, J. (2006). Lesbian, gay, bisexual, and transgender young people in state custody: Making the child welfare and juvenile justice systems safe for all youth through litigation, advocacy, and education. *Temple Law Review, 79*, 415–438.

Farmer v. Kavanagh, 494 F. Supp. 2d. 345 (DC MD, 2007).

Fazel, S., Doll, H., & Langstrom, N. (2008). Mental disorders among adolescents in juvenile detention and correctional facilities: A systematic review and metaregression analysis of 25 surveys. *Journal of the American Academy of Child and Adolescent Psychiatry, 47* (9), 1010–1019.

Federal Bureau of Investigation (2008). *Uniform crime report, 2007*. Retrieved February 15, 2009, from www.fbi.gov/ucr/cius2007/data/table_33.html.

Ferguson, A.M., Ogloff, J.R.P., & Thomson, L. (2009). Predicting recidivism by mentally disordered offenders using the LSI-R:SV. *Criminal Justice and Behavior, 36* (1), 5–20.

Greason v. Kemp, 891 F. 2d 829 (11th Cir. 1990).

Greenberg, G.A., & Rosenheck, R.A. (2008). Homelessness in the state and federal prison population. *Criminal Behaviour and Mental Health, 18*, 88–103.

Grekin, P.M., Jemelka, R., & Trupin, E.W. (1994). Racial differences in the criminalization of the mentally ill. *Bulletin of the American Academy of Psychiatry and the Law, 22* (3), 411–420.

Griffin, R.C. (2007). The more things stay the same: A report on the mental health problems of inmates in America's jails and prisons. *Praxis, 7*, 26–33.

Group for the Advancement of Psychiatry (1977). *Psychiatry and sex psychopath legislation: The 30s to the 80s*. New York: Mental Health Materials Center.

Halvorsen, D. (1993, July 25). Sex criminal lockup law faces challenge. *Star Tribune*, pp. 1A, 10A, 11A.

Harris v. Thigpen, 941 F.2d 1495 (11th Cir. 1991).

Hartwell, S. (2001). Female mentally ill offenders and their community reintegration needs: An initial examination. *International Journal of Law and Psychiatry, 24*, 1–11.

Hayes, L.M. (2005). Suicide prevention in correctional facilities. In C.L. Scott and J.G. Gerbasi (eds), *Handbook of correctional mental health* (pp. 69–88). Washington, DC: American Psychiatric Publishing.

Hayes, L.M. (2009). *Characteristics of juvenile suicides in confinement*. Washington, DC: Office of Juvenile Justice and Delinquency Prevention. In *re Blodgett*, 510 N.W. 2d 910 (Minn. 1994).

H.C. by *Hewett v. Jarrard*, 786 F. 2d 1080 (11th Cir. 1986).

James, D.J., & Glaze, L.E. (2006). *Mental health problems of prison and jail inmates*. Washington, DC: Bureau of Justice Statistics.

Jessica M. Lewis a/k/a Mark L. Brooks v. Berg et al., 2005 U.S. Dist. LEXIS 39571 (2007).

Khodayarifard, M., Pritz, A., & Khodayarifard, S. (2008). The impact of group and individual cognitive-behavioral intervention on the mental health state of male prisoners. *International Journal of Psychotherapy, 12* (2), 50–66.

Kinsler, P.J., & Saxman, A. (2007). Traumatized offenders: Don't look now, but your jail's also your mental health center. *Journal of Trauma and Dissociation, 8* (2), 81–95.

Kupers, T.A. (2008). What to do with the survivors? Coping with the long-term effects of isolated confinement. *Criminal Justice and Behavior, 35* (8), 1005–1016.

Lane, M.B. (February 15, 2009). State devising competency standards for juveniles. *Columbus Dispatch*, pp. B1, B2.

Lay v. Norris, 876 F.2d 104 (6th Cir. 1989).

Levine, J., Barak, Y., & Granek, I. (1998). Cognitive group therapy for paranoid schizophrenics: Applying cognitive dissonance. *Journal of Cognitive Psychotherapy, 12*, 3–12.

Lewis, C.F. (2005). Female offenders in correctional settings. In C.L. Scott and J.G. Gerbasi (eds), *Handbook of correctional mental health* (pp. 155–185). Washington, DC: American Psychiatric Publishing.

Livsey, S., Sickmund, M., & Sladky, A. (2009). *Juvenile residential facility census, 2004: Selected findings*. Washington, DC: Office of Juvenile Justice and Delinquency Prevention.

Long v. Nix et al., 86 F. 3d 761 (8th Cir. 1996).

Lord, E.A. (2008). The challenges of mentally ill female offenders in prison. *Criminal Justice and Behavior, 35* (8), 928–942.

Lovell, D. (2008). Patterns of disturbed behavior in a supermax population. *Criminal Justice and Behavior, 35* (8), 985–1004.

Ludlow, R. (2009, March 5). Prisoner found hanged in cell. *Columbus Dispatch*, p. B3.

Magaletta, P.R., Diamond, P.M., Faust, E., Daggett, D.M., & Camp, S.D. (2009). Estimating the mental illness component of service need in corrections: Results from the mental health prevalence project. *Criminal Justice and Behavior, 36* (3), 229–244.

Mariah Lopez a/k/a Brian Lopez v. the City of New York, 2009 U.S. Dist. LEXIS 7645 (2009).

McCorkle, R.C. (1995). Gender, psychopathology, and institutional behavior: A comparison of male and female mentally ill prison inmates. *Journal of Criminal Justice, 23* (1), 53–61.

Mears, D.P., & Watson, J. (2006). Towards a fair and balanced assessment of supermax prisons. *Justice Quarterly, 23* (2), 232–270.

Metzner, J.L. (2002). Class action litigation in correctional psychiatry. *Journal of American Academy of Psychiatry & Law, 30*, 19–29.

Metzner, J.L. (2008). Correctional mental health. *American Medical Association Journal of Ethics, 10* (2), 92–95.

Navasky, M.R. (Writer, Producer, & Director), & O'Connor, K. (Writer, Producer, & Director). (2005, May 10). *The new asylums. Frontline* [Television broadcast].

O'Keefe, M.L. (2007). Administrative segregation for mentally ill inmates. *Journal of Offender Rehabilitation, 45* (1–2), 149–166.

O'Keefe, M.L. (2008). Administrative segregation from within: A corrections perspective. *Prison Journal, 88* (1), 123–143.

PBS (2005). Interview with Debbie Nixon-Hughes. Retrieved March 29, 2009, from www.pbs.org/wgbh/pages/frontline/shows/asylums/interviews/nixonhughes.html.

Perlin, M.L. (2001). Hidden agendas and ripple effects: Implications of four recent Supreme Court decisions for forensic mental health professionals. *Journal of Forensic Psychology, 1* (1), 33–64.

Pollack, S. (2004). Anti-oppressive social work practice with women in prison: Discursive reconstructions and alternative practices. *British Journal of Social Work, 34*, 693–707.

Pomeroy, E.C., Kiam, R., & Abel, E. (1998). Meeting the mental health needs of incarcerated women. *Health and Social Work, 23* (1), 71–75.

Primm, A.B., Osher, F.C., & Gomez, M.B. (2005). Race and ethnicity, mental health services and cultural competence in the criminal justice system: Are we ready to change? *Community Mental Health Journal, 41* (5), 557–569.

The Mentally Ill Offender Treatment and Crime Reduction Act 108–414.

Relly, J.E. (1999, May 3). Supermax: Inside, no one can hear you scream. *Tucson Weekly*, Retrieved March 13, 2009, from www.weeklywire.com/ww/05-03-99/tw_feat.html.

Reutter, D.M. (2008). Massachusetts's mental health treatment policies prove deadly for public, prisoners. *Prison Legal News, 19*, 1–6.

Rhodes, L.A. (2005). Pathological effects of the supermaximum prison. *American Journal of Public Health, 95* (10), 1692–1695.

Riddle v. Mondragon, 83 F.3d 1197 (10th Cir. 1996).

Sabol, W.J., & Minton, T.D. (2008). *Jail inmates at midyear 2007*. Washington, DC: Bureau of Justice Statistics.

Sacks, J.Y., McKendrick, K., Hamilton, Z., Cleland, C.M., Pearson, F.S., & Banks, S. (2008). Treatment outcomes for female offenders: Relationship to number of axis I diagnoses. *Behavioral Sciences and the Law, 26*, 413–434.

Scheingold, S., Olson, T., & Pershing, J. (1992). The politics of sexual psychopathy: Washington state's sexual predator legislation. *University of Puget Sound Law Review, 15*, 809–820.

Scott, C.L. (2005). Preface. In C.L. Scott and J.G. Gerbasi (eds), *Handbook of correctional mental health* (pp. xv–xvii). Washington, DC: American Psychiatric Publishing.

Severson, M.E. (1999). Social work education and practice in the jail setting. *Journal of Teaching in Social Work, 18* (1–2), 53–71.

Severson, M., & Duclos, C.W. (2005). *American Indian suicides in jail: Can risk screening be culturally sensitive*. Washington, DC: U.S. Department of Justice.

S.H. et al. v. Tom Stickrath, Stipulation for Injunctive relief. Case No. 2: 04-CV1206 (SD OH, 2008).

Swogger, M.T., Walsh, Z., & Kosson, D.S. (2008). Psychopathy subtypes among African American county jail inmates. *Criminal Justice and Behavior, 35* (12), 1484–1499.

Tarzwell, S. (2006). The gender lines are marked with razor wire: Addressing state prison policies and practices for the management of transgender prisoners. *Columbia Human Rights, Law Review, 38*, 167–202.

Thomas et al. v. McNeil et al., 2009 U.S. Dist. LEXIS 1208 (2009).

Torraco v. Maloney, 923 F.2d 231 (1st Cir. 1991).

Vitacco, M.J., Neumann, C.S., & Wodushek, T. (2008). Differential relationship between the dimensions of psychopathy and intelligence: Replication with adult jail inmates. *Criminal Justice and Behavior, 35* (1), 48–55.

Way, B.B., Sawyer, D.A., Lilly, S.N., Moffitt, C., & Stapholz, B.J. (2008). Characteristics of inmates who received a diagnosis of serious mental illness upon entry to New York state prison. *Psychiatric Services, 59* (11), 1335–1337.

West, H.C., & Sabol, W.J. (2008). *Prisoners in 2007*. Washington, DC: Bureau of Justice Statistics.

White v. Napoleon, 897 F.2d 103 (3rd Cir. 02/23/1990).

Wolff, N., Blitz, C.L., & Shi, J. (2007). Rates of sexual victimization in prison for inmates with and without mental disorders. *Psychiatric Services, 58* (8), 1087–1094.

Wrongful Death Suit Against L. A. County Jail Settles for $750,000. (2008, January). *Prison Legal News, 19* (1), 30.

8   Immigration and its effects

Gregory Acevedo and Manny J. González

In this chapter we present a discussion and analysis of one of the most vexing social problems –
immigration – and how its dynamics affect the array of vulnerabilities and risks for the
development of mental health problems among immigrant populations in the United States.
Immigration is a·multifaceted social phenomenon whose processes thread through most micro
and macro aspects of the fabric of human experience. Individuals, families, and communities
anchor the exchanges between sending and receiving nation-states. Social, political, and
economic forces that operate locally, nationally, regionally, and globally, channel immigration
flows. The profound dislocation of "place" that immigration involves reverberates throughout
the fabric of human experience in ways that powerfully affect mental health.

The emergence of social work itself can be seen as a response to the instabilities and social
problems that are concomitant with immigration (Acevedo & Menon, 2009). In the United
States, the birth of social work, under both the guise of the Charity Organization Society and the
Settlement House Movements, was in fact, the nation's efforts "on the ground" to contend with
immigration, urbanization, poverty, substandard housing, health and sanitation, and racial and
ethnic relations. Large numbers of immigrants came during the peak years of immigration in
U.S. history and inextricably linked to its political and economic development and the process
of "industrialization." In that era, immigration garnered much attention by the public, policy
makers, and social scientists. Today social workers provide direct services to immigrant
populations and influence the political dialogue about the status and human rights of all people.

We begin this chapter with an overview of the social, political, and economic process related
to the immigration phenomenon, provide a brief portrait of relevant demographics of the
immigrant population, and highlight how immigration affects mental health and mental illness.
The following section deploys the life model approach to delineate the matrix of risk and
resilience as it pertains to immigrant mental health and mental conditions. Next, we present a
practice illustration and discussion that underscores key issues with regard to assessment and
intervention. Last, we conclude with a focus on the important role that social work practice
plays in enhancing the mental health of immigrant populations in the United States.

With the ebb and flow of migration patterns, in recent decades the United States has again
been contending with large waves of immigration. During the Great Depression immigration to
the United States plummeted and it remained at low levels well into the post-World War II era.
In 1965, the amendments to the *Immigration and Nationality Act* abolished the national origins
system and established a visa category preference system. This shifted the exclusionary stance
that had dictated immigration policy since the Progressive Era, and in so doing, facilitated
immigration.

Since the 1980s, the United States has been receiving immigrants at a pace that rivals the
"golden door" era of immigration (see Table 8.1). Consequently, the topic of immigration
has reemerged as a matter of public concern and public policy, as well as gained renewed

Table 8.1 Immigration to the United States, 1861–2000

Decade	Number of immigrants
1861 to 1870	2,314,824
1871 to 1880	2,812,191
1881 to 1890	5,246,613
1891 to 1900	3,687,564
1901 to 1910	8,795,386
1911 to 1920	5,735,811
1921 to 1930	4,107,209
1931 to 1940	528,431
1941 to 1950	1,035,039
1951 to 1960	2,515,479
1961 to 1970	3,321,677
1971 to 1980	4,493,314
1981 to 1990	7,338,062
1991 to 2000	9,095,417

Source: U.S. Department of Homeland Security (2006).
Yearbook of immigration statistics: 2005. Table 25.

attention from the academy. However, unlike the waves of the past that were comprised primarily by Europeans, the new migration streams were flowing from nations and regions in the developing world, especially Latin America, the Caribbean, and Asia.

According to the most recent data in the U.S. Department of Homeland Security's (DHS) *Yearbook of Immigration Statistics: 2005*, the dominant source region in the nation's flow of immigrants is Latin America (53 percent), followed by Asia (25 percent) Europe, the principal source region in the golden era of U.S. immigration, yields a substantially smaller flow (13 percent) while the rest of the world accounts for 8 percent. The top ten immigrant-sending countries to the United States are all located in Latin America or Asia (in order: Mexico, China, India, Philippines, Cuba, Dominican Republic, Vietnam, Colombia, Korea and Haiti) (US DHS, 2006). This has been the trend since the late 1990s.

Africa remains a far less substantial source region to the United States than Latin America or Asia, but it does make up a good proportion of its refugee flows. In 2008, the top ten refugee-sending countries to the United States were Cuba, China, Somalia, Colombia, Haiti, Liberia, Ethiopia, Iran, India, and Uzbekistan (US DHS, 2008). This too has been a trend since the late 1990s. Under the "diversity" visa category (intended to diversify the immigrant in-flows to the country) the United States has made an attempt to encourage immigration from the African region. In 2008, the African region was number one in this category (18,060 of the total 44,538 diversity visas granted in 2008.) As we can see in Table 8.2, in 2008, most legal

Table 8.2 Persons obtaining legal permanent residence status by broad class of admission, 2008

Class of admission	Number (total=1,107,126)
Family-sponsored preferences	227,761
Employment-based preferences	166,511
Immediate relatives of U.S. citizens	488,483
Diversity visa	41,761
Refugees and asylees	166,392
Other	16,218

Source: U.S. Department of Homeland Security (2008). *Yearbook of immigration statistics: 2008.* Tables 3–5

permanent residents entered the United States under either the family-sponsored immigrants or as immediate relatives of citizens. The other major categories for class of admission, employment-based preferences and refugees and asylees, were fairly comparable (166,511 and 166,392 respectively.)

Immigration has also emerged as a *global concern*. The world's population is moving about the planet in unprecedented numbers: "Around 175 million persons currently reside in a country other than where they were born – about three per cent of the world's population. The number of migrants has more than doubled since 1975" (UN Department of Economic and Social Affairs (DESA), 2002, p. 2). This phenomenon is substantial for both developed and developing regions (see Table 8.3). The majority of the world's migrants (60 percent) currently reside in its more developed regions. Between 1990 and 2000, the number of migrants in the more developed regions increased by 23 million persons, or 28 per cent (UN DESA, 2002). While the greater proportion of the world's immigrant population are "economic" migrants, being pushed and pulled by economic conditions, since the 1970s, there has been an explosion in the world's refugee population (Zolberg, Suhrke, & Aguayo, 1989).

Definitions of immigration

Immigration is a phenomenon that has a long-standing association with social problems, such as poverty, racial and ethnic conflict, and disenfranchisement. Immigration is closely tied to two other powerful social processes: urbanization and economic development. The legacy of this nexus of social forces, immigration – urbanization – economic development, has included colonialism and slavery, the rise of tenements in the United States in the 1800s, and more recently, the shantytowns in the developing world; human trafficking; land consolidation and agro-business; and deforestation and pollution.

The legal and social designations of subgroups of immigrants: refugee, lawful permanent resident, undocumented persons and transnationals, are important in terms of the underlying ideological views associated with each and their eligibility for entitlement programs (Drachman & Ryan, 2001). For example a refugee as defined by the Refugee Act 1980 is a person who is outside his or her country because of fear of persecution on account of status in a persecuted

Table 8.3 Size and growth of migrant population by major area 1990–2000

Major area	1990	2000	Change: 1990–2000	
	Number (thousands)	*Number (thousands)*	*Number (thousands)*	*Number (thousands)*
World	153,956	174,781	20,825	13.5
More developed regions	81,424	104,119	22,695	27.9
Less developed regions	72,531	70,662	−1,869	−2.6
Least developed countries	10,992	10,458	−534	−4.9
Africa	16,221	16,277	56	0.3
Asia	49,956	49,781	−175	−0.4
Europe	48,437	56,100	7,663	15.8
Latin America and the Caribbean	6,994	5,944	−1,051	−15.0
Northern America	27,597	40,844	13,248	48.0
Oceania	4,751	5,835	1,084	22.8

Source: UN Department of Economic and Social Affairs (2002). *U.N. International Migration Report: 2002.*

group. These groups include race, religion, affiliation with a particular social group and political opinion (p. 653). Lawful permanent residents are granted permission to reside permanently in the United States and many require sponsorship to alleviate any potential economic "burden" upon the country's social welfare system. This economic concern influenced both the Personal Responsibility and Work Opportunity Reconciliation Act and the Illegal Immigration Reform and Immigrant Responsibility Act (IIRIRA), both enacted in 1996. These laws sharply curtailed the availability of federal services and benefits for immigrants and threaten those who choose to sponsor them. Social workers must be aware of the legal and ideological contexts in which each of these groups is subject; this will make a difference in terms of the immigrant's experience of acceptance/alienation and economic and social well-being. This is particularly so in the current climate of anti-immigration sentiment. Undocumented people are at particular legal, social and political risk. These are persons who must "fly under the radar;" they have no authorization to be in the United States and are at imminent risk of deportation. Because of this constant threat, they are unlikely to make themselves known to public or private agencies and truly live in the shadows. Another group of immigrants has been identified; transnationals are immigrant populations whose families, activities and support systems exist in both home and host countries. These individuals often maintain family connections in both countries, contribute economically to their home countries and migrate frequently.

Clearly, immigration is a "social fact" that affects the lives of people across the globe. Migration, the physical movement of large populations across territories, is a complex phenomenon. *Internal migration*, movements within the geopolitical boundary of the nation-state, can take the form of: rural to urban migration, characteristic of most countries experiencing large-scale economic and technological expansion; internally displaced populations (IDPs), such as those resulting from natural disasters or civil war; and forced migration, including slavery, human trafficking, and as part of "ethnic cleansing."

International migration, movements across geopolitical boundaries of nation-states, includes waves of both economic migrants and refugees. Globalization has been a driving force behind international migrations since the fifteenth century, and has had a displacing effect wherever it disrupts traditional social and economic relations. Globalization can be defined as the "long-term, large-scale processes of economic, historical and sociocultural change caused by the penetration of capitalist development into the non-capitalist zones of the world" (Acevedo, 2005, p. 138). The sharp increase in world migration in the post-World War II era, both economic migrants and refugee movements, has much to do with the escalating and intensified effects of the political, economic, and social dynamics of globalization.

Immigration is undeniably associated with labor and social welfare. Immigration today, as in previous eras, is connected to the political economic and sociocultural forces inherent in global integration (Menon & Acevedo, 2008). Immigrant labor is an integral part of U.S. economic productivity: "In 2006, foreign-born workers accounted for 15 percent of the U.S. labor force, and over the last decade they have accounted for about half of the growth in the labor force" (U.S. Council of Economic Advisers, 2007, p. 1). Immigration fuels U.S. macroeconomic growth and has significant labor market and fiscal effects. On average, the U.S. native-born population benefits from immigration and immigrants tend to complement (not substitute for) natives, raising their productivity and income. Immigration is an essential element in the U.S. economy and is a determinative component of its labor markets and wages and working conditions. Immigration is also a direct link between the United States and global economies. Immigration operates amidst both global and national-level dynamics.

There is also a link between *immigration and disenfranchisement, marginalization, and poverty*. For immigrants, poverty is often the principal push factor that instigates migration, whether from rural to urban areas within their country of origin, or from their nations of origin to nations with more expansive economic development. In search of higher wages and better working conditions, people living in the developing world often "choose" migration. Even refugee movements are linked to poverty; the civil wars and Cold War struggles that have destabilized regions are associated with the violent confrontation between the competing political-economic frameworks of "free-market" and "socialism," which at their core, were both models proposed as solutions to long-standing poverty in the non-developed world.

Among the foreign-born population in the United States, citizenship is highly correlated with increased economic and social mobility. For example, in 2007, 16.5 percent of immigrants fell below the U.S. poverty line (among the native-born the rate was 11.9 percent), but the poverty rate among naturalized citizens was only 9.5 percent compared to 21.3 percent for non-citizens (U.S. Census Bureau, 2008). Immigrants from Latin America are the largest immigrant cohorts in the country, but yet, the most economically disadvantaged in the United States. Compounding their economic disadvantage, Latin American immigrants also have the lowest rates of citizenship among regional source areas for the U.S. foreign-born population (Schmidley, 2001). However, even naturalization does not necessarily mean full-inclusion. After the immigration reforms of 1996, the rights of naturalized citizens to many public benefits were curtailed. This shift was part of the overall exclusionary bent of immigration policy that occurred with the passage of more punitive laws such as the Immigration Reform and Control Act 1986, and the Illegal Immigration Reform and Immigrant Responsibility Act 1996.

This move toward more restrictive immigration policies focused on curtailing both documented and undocumented immigration began in the 1980s, but it has escalated in the post-9/11 era and in the emphasis on border security. This has led to a rising concern related to the disenfranchisement and marginalization of immigrants in the marked rise in deportations (now called "removals") and detentions. There has been a substantial increase in the number of immigrants being held in detention centers, the conditions of which have been of grave concern to advocates (Bernstein, 2009). In general, worldwide, there has been an erosion of protections of immigrants' human rights: political, economic, social, and cultural.

The plight of the detained and deported is, but one of the myriad aspects of the traumas inherent to the migration experience (see Mitchulka, 2009). The migration experience involves profound "losses" of home, family and community. Informal and formal social connections are affected, from the most intimate of family and local community, through to the most abstract: "homeland." These losses are a necessary aspect of the migration process, but are quite often "ambiguous" (Falicov, 2003). All is not lost. For example, there remains in many migrants the longing and hope of returning to the homeland, therefore, the loss is neither necessarily complete nor final. Also too, there are visits, communications, remittances and other forms of connection that are, in fact, quite lively.

The journey of "before-during-and-after" presents numerous stressors and necessitates various accommodations and adaptations. Trauma in migration experience is "cumulative" and has the characteristic of "tension" trauma (Falicov, 2003). It is an extended process wherein tension is repeated and long-standing. This may or may not also include more specific and powerful traumatic events like being tortured, suffering acts of war or natural disaster and the like.

The central buffers to contending with migration are family and community. For all forms of social support, material to emotional, family is at the heart of the protective resources that buffer the stressors of migration. As noted previously, "immediate relatives of U.S. citizens" and "family-sponsored preferences" rank first and second as visa categories for legal permanent residents. Undocumented immigrants also rely on family ties in ways that mirror legal immigrant social networks. Managing migration stress draws heavily upon the "relational resilience" of immigrant family processes utilized to cope with stress (Falicov, 2003).

Immigrant communities often rest firmly on the foundation of co-ethnic families who live and often work in ethnically concentrated geographic areas: "ethnic enclaves." These communities are a powerful form of social connection. Many immigrants rely on ethnic enclaves and their economies as they transition into their new home. Enclaves represent a singular mode of integration into the host society for immigrants, and have done so since the 1800s. They create a form of social capital that encourages entrepreneurship and/or facilitates employment in particular sectors of an economy, often in the sector of community-based goods and services. Ethnic economies can serve as smaller-scale "protected" markets (or niches), or as "export-oriented" enterprises with extensive productive capacities that extend beyond a purely local market (Zhou, 1992). Both types of ethnic economies provide opportunities for employment and self-employment. They are important for the overall economic and cultural life of parti-cular ethnic groups and for the general economy (Light & Gold, 2000).

Family and community are essential aspects of the varied context of migration and reception that frames the migration experience. Falicov (2003, p. 281) delineates the factors that mediate the migration experience: degree of choice; proximity and accessibility to country of origin; gender; age; education; developmental stage of the family life cycle and its family form; community social supports; and the experience of racial or economic discrimination in their country of origin and adopted country. Segal and Mayadas (2005) underscore several factors that influence the immigrant and refugee experience that need to be appreciated:

1   The experience of the move from the home country to living in the United States;
2   Recognition of the phases of the immigrant and refugee experience;
3   The sociocultural heritage of the migrant;
4   Recognition of the problems and issues they encountered while relocating;
5   Being sensitive toward the migrant's psychosocial issues;
6   Familiarity with the policies, laws, and programs of U.S. Citizenship and Immigration Services;
7   Recognition of the differences and similarities between refugees and immigrants;
8   The impact of nativist and xenophobic reactions to immigrants and refugees.

Ultimately, the context of reception becomes the space within which the migrant adapts to their newfound circumstances, and also alters them as they weave their lives into the new country's social fabric. The reception they receive – welcome, unwelcome, or indifferent – has a powerful effect on what the outcomes will be for immigrants and refugees. One example, is the life courses of the children of immigrants (now comprising nearly one-fifth of the nation's children and youth) which vary from brilliant second-generation success stories to "oppositional cultures" rife with delinquency, such as gangs.

With the rise in the number of *children of immigrants*, social science has devoted much attention to their social and economic well-being (Fernandez-Kelly & Konczal, 2005; Kasinitz, Waters, Mollenkopf, & Holdaway, 2008). Much of the focus is on the various paths that children of immigrants take when *assimilating/acculturating* into mainstream society. "Segmented assimi-lation theory" (Portes & Rumbaut, 2001) proposes that children of immigrants have three potential outcomes: "assimilating" into a mainstream, "white," middle-class culture; "ethni-cization," which involves remaining within an ethnic or immigrant enclave culture; or "racialization," which entails embracing a native-born, urban, minority "oppositional" culture and identity. Only the first two outcomes lead to upward social mobility and generally positive outcomes, including educational success, for the second generation. Racialization, on the other hand, ultimately leads to downward social mobility, and antisocial behavior. Children of immigrants who are racialized become part of a diversifying "underclass."

Suárez-Orozco and Suárez-Orozco (2001) have developed a model of *"social mirroring"* to conceptualize how children of immigrants construct their ethnic identities. Their model is informed by W.E.B. Du Bois (1989) concept of "double-consciousness": the African-American experience of "looking at themselves through the eyes of others," i.e. dominant "white," middle-class culture. Suárez-Orozco and Suárez-Orozco (2001) also deploy Winnicott's concept of "reflected images," from the object relations theory, to build a conceptual framework for their model of social mirroring. The social mirror includes: public perceptions; racial distortions; day-to-day interactions; and the ascribed identity that children of immigrants "look into and see reflections," positive or negative. Media, the classroom, the "street," and the family, generate the most powerful reflected images. These images have their strongest effect among children of immigrants of color, such as African Caribbean and Latino children and youth.

Reactions to negative social mirroring are a principle determinant in the development of children of immigrants' ethnic identity style. "Hope" is the essential element in predicting the pathways to positive outcomes in response to negative social mirroring. Buffers that engender hope in children of immigrants are found in their: ethnic community, through supportive mechanisms like mentors and role models; family, through such protective buffering as reflecting positive mirroring and deflecting negative mirroring; and within themselves, through positive self-perceptions and resilient responses. In addition, material factors such as economic and educational opportunities play a crucial role in fostering a sense of hope and aspiration. Paths of hopelessness tend to lead to self-deprecation and self-doubt, which devolve into self-defeating behaviors and perhaps depression; or anger and acting-out behaviors. Material factors such as economic and educational opportunities are synergistically connected to place. The immigration experience lends itself quite well to analysis from an ecological perspective.

Migration does not root itself in ether. It is rooted in place (and time) and embedded in a distinct ecological niche. Housing stock, school districts, police-neighborhood relations, labor markets and transportation, faith-based organizations, and the social service network, are all grounded in place. Falicov (2003) presents a matrix of the influences that interact to form the ecological niche that a migrant inhabits: ethnicity and nation of origin; class and occupation; geography and climate; and religion. For all of these factors the characteristics of the immigrant or refugee may be well matched or mismatched to the host society. Matching, or fit, is most powerfully determined by the transactions between migrant and their ecological niche. While ethnicity/national origin, work, and religion are more obvious in their influence, geography and climate may not be; however, the transition from a tropical climate to a cold one, for example, is not an insignificant transition. Also too, there are issues related to geography that influence behaviors, such as speech, as demonstrated by the substantive differences between "mountain" and "lowland" people, and their linguistic dialect.

The ecological perspective with its emphasis on niche, adaptation, transactions, reciprocity and mutuality, and the goodness-of-fit between people and their environments is well suited to analyzing the migration experience. The life model (Germain & Gitterman, 1980; Gitterman & Germain, 2008), with its keen attention to social ecology, life course development, and vertical and horizontal stressors, offers a practice model that is able to account for the migration experience in its assessment and intervention strategies. This is clearly demonstrated when the life model is deployed to understand the mental health of immigrants and refugees.

Immigration and mental health/illness

Informed by the science of ecology, the *life model of social work practice* views the human organism as constantly adapting in an interchange with differential aspects of the social environment. Both the human organism and the social environment react to each other and change within a transactional matrix (see Gitterman & Germain, 2008). The person and the environment can be understood only in terms of their relationship, in which each continually influences the other within a particular context.

Gitterman (2009) has noted that throughout the life course people attempt to maintain a harmonious fit with their surrounding environments. This harmonious fit is usually achieved through a sense of self-efficacy – or when the human organism feels positive and hopeful about his or her capacity to survive and thrive within multiple social contexts – and the environment's responsiveness to human need via provision of life-sustaining resources. Conversely, this noted harmonious fit might be seriously compromised when the individual lacks adaptive coping capacities or when such capacities have been placed at risk by psychosocial stress and toxic environmental conditions. Within the life model (Germain & Gitterman, 1980), stress is conceptualized as a psychosocial state spawned by inconsistencies between the human organism's perceived needs and capacities and environmental qualities. As a psychosocial condition, stress is the by-product of complex person and environment transactions.

A central tenet of life modeled practice is that individuals will encounter stress or experience life stressors over the life course. From an ecological perspective, life stressors are caused by complex and precarious life issues that human organisms perceive as greater than their coping capacities and environmental resources (see Germain & Gitterman, 1995). According to the life model, life stressors and the associated stress will arise or become manifested in the following three interrelated areas of living: life transitions and traumatic life events, environmental pressures and dysfunctional interpersonal processes. Gitterman (1996, p. 398) has underscored the fact that while these three life stressors are interrelated, each takes on its own "force" and "magnitude" and provides direction for multi-method (e.g., individual, family, group and community practice) and integrative interventions with diverse client systems.

Intervention within the life model is informed by the historic purpose of the social work profession: to enhance the problem-solving and coping capacities of people; and to promote the effective and humane operation of systems that provide people with needed resources and services. While not prescriptive in nature, life modeled practice recognizes that social work practitioners require a broad repertoire of skills and techniques in addressing the needs of individuals and families who are overwhelmed by significant life stressors. These skills and techniques must be aimed at increasing a client's self-esteem, problem-solving and coping capacities; facilitating group functioning; and engaging and influencing organizational structures, social networks and social environmental forces (Gitterman & Germain, 2008). Payne (2005) has noted the type of therapeutic and socio-environmental skills or techniques that practitioners may employ when implementing a life model approach with identified clients. Some of these skills and techniques include: strengthening the client's motivation towards change, validation, support, management of emotionally laden content, modeling behavior, mobilization of environmental supports, case advocacy, mediation and teaching problem-solving skills.

Piedra and Engstrom (2009) have documented the relevancy of life modeled practice with immigrant families and their children. They note that the model's emphasis on factors that influence vulnerability and oppression, the impact of healthy and unhealthy environmental contexts, and the consideration of variations in the life course – the developmental path taken by the human organism – with attention to social and cultural determinants, provides a useful framework for social work intervention with immigrants. Echoing Piedra and Engstrom's (2009) assertion about the life model and provision of social services to immigrants, we also find that life modeled practice can be effective in meeting the needs of immigrants who suffer from an array of mental health conditions.

Life transitions, environmental problems and needs, the effects of acculturation stress and interpersonal conflict may often compel immigrants to seek out mental health services. Mental health practitioners (i.e., clinical social workers) then provide services to those recognized as conventional immigrants, refugees from a variety of cultural and regional origins, and an unspecified number of undocumented immigrants with a host of legal, economic, and health concerns. The varying needs of this diverse group constitute a challenge to social work practitioners as they attempt to ease the process of adjustment to a new society. The cultural norms about mental illness held by diverse immigrant groups complicate service delivery to this population. Mental illness, perhaps more than any other psychosocial condition, elicits powerful cultural responses. In many cultures, mental illness is a taboo subject, a cause for shame among families with a mentally ill member.

For example, Vietnamese have a cultural tendency to consider a mentally ill person to be born under an unlucky star and ill fated. For some, mental illness brings shame upon the family, affecting the fortunes and future of the whole family. As such, families are likely to try to care for the ill member within the confines of the family rather than seek outside help (Ganesan, Fine, & Lin Yi, 1989). From a life model point of view, this type of life stressor may readily produce dysfunctional interpersonal processes that may become evident in behaviors such as scapegoating, rigid alliances, social withdrawal and hostility (Gitterman & Germain, 2008).

Given that life modeled practice accounts for how specific social and cultural determinants may impact an individual's developmental trajectory, in working with immigrants social workers must understand how their culture views mental illness. Working within culturally sensitive frameworks can greatly enhance service delivery. For instance, one mental health center partnered with the local *curanderos* (faith healers) who, operating within a belief system that spirits inhabit the material world, utilize their healing arts with the Latin American immigrant community (see Rosenberg, 2000). The mental health center invited these local healers to help their clients. The clinical and administrative staff at the center found that the participation of the healers was symbolically important as an acknowledgement of their cultural place within the community, and as a result, they gained increased participation and credibility among the Latin American immigrant community. This organizational intervention is consistent with how the purpose of social work practice is conceptualized within the life model: "to help people mobilize and draw on personal and environmental resources for effective coping to alleviate life stressors and the associated stress; and to influence social and physical environmental forces to be responsive to people's needs" (Gitterman, 2009, p. 232).

For many immigrants entering a new country, establishing new relationships and leaving familiar ones and sources of social support represents a complex life transition that, to many, is traumatic in nature. Urrabazo (2000), for example, has noted the multiple traumas that undocumented Hispanic families have been exposed to in their attempt to cross the border into the United States: robbery, sexual assault and physical and psychological torture. The high rate of violent life events as well as high stress associated with the immigration experience can place immigrants and at increased risk of a number of the following clinical conditions, as detailed in the *Diagnostic and statistical manual of mental disorders* (DSM-IV-TR: American Psychiatric Association (APA), 2000): post-traumatic stress disorder, adjustment disorders and major mood disorders.

Post-traumatic stress disorder (PTSD) is a disabling psychiatric condition that develops subsequent to experience of a life threatening or traumatic event such as war combat, terrorism and violent attacks such as rape and assault (Herman, 1992). PTSD can severely interfere with daily functioning. Symptoms include: flashbacks, sleep problems and nightmares, feelings of isolation, guilt, paranoia and panic attacks. A person suffering from PTSD typically repeatedly relives the traumatic event through painful memories and is prone to intense feelings of fear, helplessness and horror. Often these feelings are accompanied by anxiety or panic attacks.

Studies of psychotherapy with South East Asian refugees provide numerous accounts of the severe hardship, including torture and other war-related horrific experiences (Ganesan et al., 1989). The vast majority of the Indochinese refugees who entered the United States following the 1975 collapse of the South Vietnam government were exposed to severe brutality and cruelty and debilitating living conditions. Such clients may struggle with depressed and irritable moods, pervasive feelings of being unsafe and feelings of intense guilt, especially if they survived when others did not.

Immigrant children are also vulnerable to traumatic stress disorders. When immigrant parents dream of bringing their children to the United States, they usually do so with the intention that their quality of life will improve. They flee political persecution, extreme economic desperation and look to the "land of opportunity," with the expectation that living in a democratic society will result in educational and employment opportunities. On arrival to the United States, however, the reality of sheer survival often becomes paramount. Finding housing and some type of employment become primary goals. Igoa (1995) has observed that, "In low-income immigrant families, it may be difficult for parents to nurture their children because the uprooting experience itself saps the parents' energy" (p. 40). The children in the family often are left to cope on their own, with the hope that they both (parent and child) learn English and acculturate as quickly as possible. The multiple losses the children and their families have gone through, the fears, confusion, sadness, and alienation they may feel often are left unattended. Yet it is these losses and "unspoken" traumas that immigrant children carry into their new schools, and teachers, educational administrators, and school mental health personnel (i.e., school social workers, school psychologists) must be prepared to respond to these noted traumatic concerns.

From an ecological perspective, the *adjustment and mood* conditions that are observed and diagnosed in immigrants and their children may be exacerbated by a minimally adequate or unfavorable person and environment fit. Germain and Gitterman (1995) have defined the person and environment fit as the actual fit between an individual's perceived needs, goal and capacities and the responsiveness and quality of the person's physical and social environment within a historical and cultural context. Immigrants are frequently diagnosed with adjustment disorders and depression (Yu, 1997). While such conditions are typically less severe in intensity and duration than traumatic stress disorders, they can be disabling and cause significant distress. According to the DSM-IV-TR (APA 2000), the central feature of adjustment disorder is distress that markedly exceeds what is normally expected by a stressor and impairment in job, academic or social functioning.

Major depression or dysthymic disorders are characterized by two or more of the following symptoms, appetite decrease or increase, sleep decrease or increase, fatigue or low energy, poor self-image, reduced concentration or indecisiveness and feelings of hopelessness. These symptoms cause clinically important distress or impair work, social or personal functioning (APA, 2000). These psychological disturbances are viewed as prevalent among immigrants and refugees because of the combination of past harrowing experiences in their country of origin and ongoing psychosocial stressors in the United States. In a study of 147 adult Vietnamese Americans, depression was correlated to acculturation problems (Tran, 1993).

In looking specifically at what is known about the incidence of mental health among Hispanic immigrant children and adolescents, studies consistently show that Hispanic youth seem to be particularly vulnerable. Psychiatric epidemiological studies of children and adolescents appear to suggest that Hispanic youth experience a significant number of mental health problems, and in most cases, more problems than non-Latino White youth (U.S. Department of Health and Human Services (DHHS), 2001). Glover, Pumariega, Holzer, Wise, and Rodriguez (1999), for example, found that Hispanic youth of Mexican descent in the southwest reported more anxiety-related problem behaviors than White students. Lequerica and Hermosa (1995) also found that 13 percent of Hispanic children screened for emotional-behavioral problems in pediatric outpatient settings scored in the clinical range on the Childhood Behavior Checklist (CBCL).

In addition to anxiety and behavioral problems, depression is a serious mental health predicament affecting the psychosocial functioning and adaptation of Hispanic youth. Studies of depressive symptoms and disorders have revealed more psychosocial distress among Hispanic youth than non-Latino White adolescents (U.S. DHHS, 2001). This finding may be related to the fact that about 40 percent of African American and Hispanic youth live in poverty, often in chaotic urban settings that disrupt family life and add considerable stress to their already fragile psychological condition (Allen-Meares & Fraser, 2004). Nationally, for example, Roberts, Chen, and Solovitz (1995) and Roberts and Sobhan (1992) have empirically noted that Hispanic children and adolescents of immigrant descent report more depressive symptomatology than do non-Latino White youth. In a later study that relied on a self-report measure of major depression, Roberts, Roberts, and Chen (1997) found that Hispanic youth of Mexican descent attending middle school were found to have a significantly higher rate of depression than non-Latino White youth at 12 percent versus 6 percent, respectively. These findings held constant even when level of psychosocial impairment and sociodemographic variables were taken into account. Life modeled practice underscores the importance of attachments, friendships, positive kin relationships and a sense of belonging to a supportive social network. The challenges of migration, however, may significantly compromise inter-personal connections with family members, friends and community. The impact of migration on children and families is profound. Family violence, marital problems and acting out among children and adolescents are some of the manifestations of family disruption Intergenerational tensions between parents who adhere to cultural traditions and their children who often acculturate at a faster pace are common. In the case of refugees, since 1997, a significant number of refugee applications have been granted for family reunification, typically when a spouse and children join a refugee already in the United States. Many of the recent refugees who arrived from Eastern Europe, Afghanistan and Ethiopia were for family reunification. The stressors impacting these families are severe, with such families likely to struggle with family dysfunction.

The mental health needs of immigrants vary considerably. The extent to which an individual is prepared for the transition to life in the United States, particularly with regard to educational and employment readiness, level of social support, and possession of adaptive coping capacities can impact on how well he or she adjusts to entrance into a new environment. Social work intervention with the immigrant population should be informed by a life model approach which draws attention to the normal life processes of growth, development and decline and conceptualizes dysfunctional processes of behavior and psychopathology as a by-product of person and environment transactional stress. Such a conceptualization does not deny the biopsychosocial dimensions of mental illness; rather, it highlights the importance of defining problems-in-living as a manifestation of person and environment exchanges.

Illustration and discussion

Roberto is a 37-year-old self-employed carpenter currently living in Miami with his wife. He came to the United States as a *balsero*. Balsero is the Spanish term that describes an individual who has left Cuba on a raft, or small boat. For many years he planned his exit out of Cuba. Roberto's training as a carpenter assisted his escape. Roberto built a 22-foot "lancha" (large wooden fishing boat) set a date, and in preparation held secret meetings with his family, and stole and stored food items for the trip. Finally one evening, he and twelve other family members set out for southern Florida. He reports that at the time he was thrilled, excited and very much afraid. Roberto, a fisherman for many years, felt competent about his knowledge of the sea and ability to navigate by the stars. While out at sea, the boat's motor failed and Roberto could not restart it. After drifting at sea for two days, he and his family were spotted by the U.S. Coast Guard and were brought to the Guantanamo Naval Base, where they remained for approximately three months. Roberto recalls that the conditions on the base were less than humane, with much illness, chaos and suffering. Thankfully, he and his family were admitted to the United States through the Catholic Charities Refugee Program. They were resettled in Syracuse, New York where they remained for approximately seven years, until the family jointly decided to relocate to Miami. Their decision was based on the family's need to live in a more tropical environment as well as a more culturally relevant community. Roberto moved to Miami first to establish enough of a firm footing to be able to be instrumental in assisting with relocating the rest of the family and facilitating their obtaining housing and employment. One year after settling in Miami, Roberto met his current wife and started his own carpentry business. He reports that his biggest issues are learning English and being poorly educated, but due to his work schedule there is little time left for him to go to school. Roberto states that he is feeling emotionally frustrated at times and he presents with symptoms consonant with a diagnosis of dysthymia. Nevertheless, he is resilient and optimistic about the future.

Roberto's cousin Ricardo was one of the twelve family members who had made the journey with him from Cuba. Ricardo is a 35-year-old unemployed SSI recipient who lives in a studio apartment. His father and paternal aunt had been living in Southern Florida for many years. Ricardo left Cuba with the expectation that he would be able to rely on their assistance as he made a new life for himself in the United States. Upon his arrival to Miami, however, he said that both his father and aunt rejected him. His father is now remarried and his new wife wasn't even aware that he existed. Ricardo reports that he has become extremely depressed as a result of his current family situation. Recently, his sister exited Cuba through the visa granting lottery system and joined him in Miami. Although the sibling reunion was a joyful occasion for Ricardo, the sister has been of minimal support to him since she too was facing the same family situation. Following the sister's arrival to Miami, his depressive symptoms exacerbated leading to his first suicide attempt and subsequently to his first psychiatric hospitalization. Following a few weeks of inpatient treatment, Ricardo was discharged from the hospital without a solidified outpatient treatment plan. Six months later a cousin – who had also entered the United States via the Mariel exodus – offered Ricardo a job in a small restaurant that he owned. He later discovered that the cousin had funded the venture with "fast money" that he had made through various illegal drug dealings. Unbeknown to Ricardo, this cousin began to use him as a "delivery man" in his drug business. Following a drug raid by the police, the restaurant closed, leaving Ricardo without a job. Once again he became extremely depressed, leading to a second suicide attempt and psychiatric hospitalization and ultimately discharged with a diagnosis of a schizoaffective condition. He reports feeling distraught at being shunned and rejected by his father and aunt, and only his sister is able to offer him some degree of emotional support. He states that he is sad that his father expects him "to make something out himself," to do something constructive with his life, but does not give him any emotional support or financial assistance. Ricardo tries to please his father by visiting him frequently and doing chores for him, but he says that he receives no parental recognition or validation in return.

The "journeys" of Roberto and Ricardo illustrate the central element of family in the immigrant and refugee experience. Their stories also punctuate many issues: surviving traumatic events and cumulative migration stress; the press of finding "good" work, and the value of education and language proficiency; the illicit economies that are sometimes a part of ethnic immigrant communities where economic opportunity is scarce. Even the issue of geography and climate is illustrated in the move back to the "tropics" from Upstate New York.

For Roberto and Ricardo, their mental health problems, as "private troubles" of milieu and as a public issue – the mental health of immigrants in the United States – were lived out in the world of family. González (2002) has noted that the ecological-systems perspective is a fruitful tool for the clinical practitioner working with Hispanic immigrants. The perspective facilitates an understanding of the various aspects of the migration experience and more effective assessment and interventions. González notes that as a result of a treatment approach premised on the ecological-systems perspective,

> The mental health problems of Hispanic immigrant patients will be significantly reduced if they are assisted in mediating complex social systems, in obtaining community resources, in attaining vocational/job skills, and in learning English as a second language. Likewise, the family reunification issues of Cuban Marielitos and balseros must be addressed via an ecologically based family treatment approach. Therefore, ecological structural family therapy, bicultural effectiveness training and the social/environmental change agent role model are recommended as viable treatment approaches that may ameliorate the family reunification dynamics and conflicts presented by Cuban immigrant/refugee patients.
>
> (González, Lopez, & Ko, 2005, p. 150)

Research evidence (Szapocznik et al., 1997) suggests that *ecological structural family therapy* is an effective treatment approach in addressing intergenerational conflict and acculturation differences in Cuban American families. The locus of mental illness is not only internal but also external in nature. This family approach highlights the stress of acculturation and its disruptive impact within the structure of the family. The intervention model pays careful attention to how normal family processes may interact with acculturation processes to create intergenerational differences and exacerbate intrafamilial conflict.

Based on structural family theory, *bicultural effectiveness training* is delivered as a twelve-session *psychoeducation* intervention approach, and has been empirically tested with Cuban American families experiencing conflict with their adolescent children. The training is specifically designed to decrease acculturation related stresses by two-generation immigrant families. For Cuban balsero patients who may be integrating into U.S.-based established family systems, this intervention model may be useful in treating family reunification dynamics.

Many Cuban American Marielitos and balseros did receive instrumental support from their U.S.-based extended families as they attempted to negotiate complex environmental conditions (e.g., employment, housing, health care, learning English as a second language). Atkinson, Thompson, and Grant (1993) developed the *social/environmental change agent role model* (a dimensional intervention approach) for ethnic-racial "minorities" with mental health problems. It recognizes the role of the social environment in promoting or handicapping psychological growth and development. This model encourages the social worker treating Cuban American patients to function as an agent for change or as a consultant or advisor to the "identified patient" acting to strengthen the patient's support systems. Based on the model, three factors should be assessed: (1) level of acculturation; (2) the perceived cause and development of the presenting problem (internally caused versus externally-environmentally caused); and (3) the specific goals to be attained in the helping process. Implementing this service model with Cuban Americans clients, however, challenges the mental health care providers to extend their professional role beyond that of psychotherapist to that of advocate, mediator, educator and broker (González, 2002).

The journeys of Roberto and Ricardo illustrate how the path to mental health for immigrants in the United States, involve many systems and institutions, via a complex ecology. Social work must field effective responses to the mental health needs of immigrants in multifaceted ways that utilize its full array of knowledge and skills for working with individuals, families, groups, and communities, and for policy and program development.

Segal and Mayadas (2005) note various social, economic, and cultural resources that migrants draw upon to integrate into their host country. They highlight the essential issues to consider when assessing immigrant and refugee families: discriminating between their realistic and unrealistic expectations; evaluating the families' problem-solving abilities and exploring their functioning within the context of their cultural heritage; identifying the transferability of their labor market experience; and gauging families' learning capabilities and motivation for adaptation.

In light of the vicissitudes of the migration experience and its stressors and traumas, the potential is high for mental health and social services needs to arise. Yet migrants, especially immigrants (because refugees tend to benefit from more available resources than economic migrants), face significant barriers to access and utilize health, mental health, and social services. Most notably there is poverty and its close association with benefits like insurance and public welfare. Citizenship status expands the array of benefits that immigrants are able to secure. Language and culture can become thick barriers to accessing and utilizing services.

Segal and Mayadas (2005) also provide a useful guide for structuring interventions with immigrants and refugees. They emphasize that work must focus on the following issues: economic self-sufficiency and asset building; equitable functioning in society; civic and political participation; empowerment; discussion and support groups; community organization; educational programs; individual counseling around tangible issues.

Obviously, the potential for the social work profession to aid immigrants and refugees in their myriad struggles in contending with the migration experience is vast. Mental heath is one crucial arena, but the profession needs to situate its clinical pursuits within a comprehensive view of the dynamics of immigration. The profession must enhance what it already does, but a great deal of the profession's knowledge and skills are still mired in nineteenth and twentieth century concepts. Social work needs to develop new ideas, and bold strategies and tactics that will effectively meet the challenges of the twenty-first century.

Conclusion

Professional organizations like the International Federation of Social Workers and National Association of Social Workers now have explicit policy statements on immigration (see the Web resources list). These are essential steps, but immigration as a social problem is so vexing that it poses a daunting challenge. They call upon the profession, as it did in the late 1800s and early 1900s, to marshal greater resources, and to deploy all it has to offer in its "tool kit;" via every tradition, method of practice, and by diffusing its knowledge and skills through all systems levels and varied settings.

Migration is perhaps the quintessential social problem to illustrate how social problems are always a matter of what C. W. Mills (1959) termed "the public issues of social structure," and their association with "the personal troubles of milieu." The mental health of immigrants and refugees are clearly connected to social forces, and are certainly a matter of milieu. The variegated nature of this social problem relates to the circumstances and needs of individuals, families, and communities. It is also inextricably related to issues of globalization, trans-nationalism, and economic development. The dynamics of social forces – like globalization and migration – influence and interact with social problems like inequality and institutional discrimination and have wide-sweeping implications for social justice and human rights. Indeed, immigration is a principle component in the determination of what we know as "human diversity."

Decades ago, Richard Titmuss (1968, 1987) argued that *disservices*, the costs of technological progress and economic development, were not distributed equally, or equitably. Titmuss emphasized that *diswelfares* costs leveled to the individual from social decisions and benefits, needed to be compensated. He made the case that society had a collective responsibility in ameliorating and eliminating diswelfares. Titmuss also made the case that society's account-ability lays in the responsibility of the state to meet the universal and selective needs of its population. Immigrants and refugees bear an unequal burden from the diswelfares which are the by-products of globalization and economic development.

Unfortunately, in the current era, many nations have been retrenching the welfare state, and immigrants and refugees have been a primary target for exclusion. These same nations have also shifted to restricting entrance, legal residence, and the path to citizenship. In concert with the retrenchment of the welfare state and exclusionary immigration policies, there has been a stunning rise in nativism, and its ugly nature has been exposed in increasing violent forms of repression like hate crimes against immigrants and refugees.

The risks inherent in the migration process are pronounced. In the current era they are exacerbated by social, political, and economic forces, which are now more globally inter-connected than ever. The resiliency among immigrant families and communities is remarkable for the ways it offsets the stressors of the migration experience. Immigrants and refugees now experience erosion of protections and rights that further strain their resilient capacities. The mental health of immigrants and refugees is a crucial aspect not only of their own socio-economic well-being, but also of the nations of which they are an essential element. Indeed, immigrants and refugees are key part of our global future. The social work profession should be at the forefront of addressing all aspects of immigration as a social problem; mental health is one of the most important.

Web resources

American Psychological Association, Public Policy Office, *The mental health needs of immigrants*
www.apa.org/about/gr/issues/minority/immigrant.aspx

Church World Service Immigration and Refugee Program
www.churchworldservice.org/site/PageServer?pagename=action_what_assist_main

International Organization for Migration
www.iom.int/

International Rescue Committee
www.theirc.org/

Lutheran Immigration and Refugee Services
www.lirs.org/

Migration Policy Institute
www.migrationpolicy.org/research/refugee.php

National Immigration Law Center (NILC)
www.nilc.org/immlawpolicy/index.htm
www.nilc.org/pubs/Guide_promo.htm
www.nilc.org/pubs/Guide_update.htm

Refugee Council USA
www.rcusa.org

United Nations Convention Relating to the Status of Refugees
www.unhcr.org/pages/49da0e466.html

United Nations High Commissioner for Refugees
www.unhcr.org

United Nations Refugee Agency
www.unhcr.org/cgi-bin/texis/vtx/home

U.S. Census Bureau on the Foreign-born Population
www.census.gov/population/www/socdemo/foreign/index.html

U.S. Citizenship and Immigration Services (USCIS), Residence and Citizenship
www.uscis.gov/portal/site/uscis

U.S. Committee for Refugees
www.refugees.org

U.S. Department of Homeland Security: Immigration-related services, benefits and activities
www.dhs.gov/files/immigration.shtm

U.S. Department of Homeland Security, Office of Immigration Statistics, *The yearbook of immigration statistics*
www.dhs.gov/files/statistics/publications/yearbook.shtm

U.S. Health and Human Services, Office of Refugee Resettlement
www.acf.hhs.gov/programs/orr/

U.S. State Department, Bureau of Population Refugees and Migration
www.state.gov/g/prm

References

Acevedo, G. (2005). Caribbean transnationalism and social policy formation. *Caribbean Journal of Social Work, 4*, 137–151.

Acevedo, G., & Menon, N. (2009). A breakwater in the waves: Social work and the history of immigration to the United States. *International Journal of Interdisciplinary Social Sciences, 4*, 123–137.

Allen-Meares, P., & Fraser, M.W. (2004). *Intervention with children and adolescents: An interdisciplinary perspective.* New York: Allyn & Bacon.

American Psychiatric Association (APA). (2000). *Diagnostic and statistical manual of mental disorders* (4th ed., text revision). Washington, DC: APA.

Atkinson, D.R., Thompson, C.E., & Grant, S.K. (1993). A three dimensional model for counseling racial/ethnic minorities. *Counseling Psychologist, 21*, 257–277.

Bernstein, N. (2009, December 3). Two groups find faults in immigrant detentions. *The New York Times.* Retrieved from www.query.nytimes.com/gst/fullpage.html?res=9E0DEEDE153DF930A35751C1A 96F9C8B63

Drachman, D., & Ryan, A.S. (2001). Immigrants and refugees. In A. Gitterman (ed.), *Handbook of social work practice with vulnerable and resilient populations* (2nd Ed., pp. 651–656). New York: Columbia University Press.

Du Bois, W.E.B. (1989) *The souls of Black folk.* New York: Bantam, 1903.

Falicov, C. (2003). Immigrant family processes. In F. Walsh (ed.), *Normal family processes: growing diversity and complexity* (pp. 280–300). New York: Guilford Press.

Fernandez-Kelly, P., & Konczal, L. (2005). "Murdering the alphabet": Identity and entrepreneurship among second generation Cubans, West Indians, and Central Americans. *Ethnic and Racial Studies, 28* (6), 1153–1181.

Ganesan, S., Fine, S., & Lin Yi, T. (1989). Psychiatric symptoms in refugees families from South East Asia: Therapeutic challenges. *American Journal of Psychotherapy, 43*, 218–228.

Gitterman, A. (1996). Life model theory and social work treatment. In F.J. Turner (ed.), *Social work treatment: Interlocking theoretical perspectives* (4th ed., pp. 389–408). New York: Free Press.

Gitterman, A. (2009). The life model. In A.R. Roberts (ed.-in-chief), *Social Workers' Desk Reference* (2nd ed., pp. 231–234). New York: Oxford University Press.

Germain, C.B., & Gitterman, A. (1980). *The life model of social work practice*. New York: Columbia University Press.

Germain, C.B., & Gitterman, A. (1995). Ecological perspective. *Encyclopedia of social work.* (19th ed., pp. 816–824). Silver Spring, MD: NASW Press.

Gitterman, A., & Germain, C.B. (2008). *The life model of social work practice: Advances in theory and practice* (3rd ed.). New York: Columbia University Press.

Glover, S.H., Pumariega, A.J., Holzer, C.E., Wise, B.K., & Rodriguez, M. (1999). Anxiety symptomatology in Mexican-American adolescents. *Journal of Family Studies, 8 (1)*, 47–57.

González, M.J. (2002). Mental health intervention with Hispanic immigrants: Understanding the influence of the client's worldview, language, and religion. *Journal of Immigrant and Refugee Services, 1* (1): 81–92.

González, M.J., Lopez, J.J., & Ko, E. (2005). The Mariel and Balsero Cuban immigrant experience: Family reunification issues and treatment recommendations. *Journal of Immigrant and Refugee Services* (The Haworth Social Work Practice), *3* (1–2), 141–153.

Herman, J. (1992). *Trauma and recovery*. New York: Basic Books.

Igoa, C. (1995). *The inner world of the immigrant child*. Mahwah, NJ: Lawrence Erlbaum Associates.

Kasinitz, P., Waters, M., Mollenkopf, J., & Holdaway, J. (2008). *Inheriting the city: The children of immigrants come of age*. New York and Cambridge, MA: Russell Sage and Harvard University Press.

Lequerica, M., & Hermosa, B. (1995). Maternal reports of behavior problems in preschool Hispanic children: An exploratory study in preventive pediatrics. *Journal of the National Medical Association, 87* (12), 861–868.

Light, I., & Gold, S.J. (2000). *Ethnic economies*. New York: Academic Press.

Menon, N., & Acevedo, G. (2008). "Hidden transcripts" of globalization: The role of social work in the development of social welfare in the United States. *Global Studies Journal, 1*, 39–48.

Mills, C.W. (1959). *The sociological imagination*. New York: Oxford University Press.

Mitchulka, D. (2009). Mental health issues in new immigrant communities. In F. Chang-Muy & E. Congress (eds), *Social work with immigrants and refugees: Legal issues, clinical skills, and advocacy* (pp. 135–172). New York: Springer.

Payne, M. (2005). *Modern social work theory* (3rd ed.). Chicago, IL: Lyceum.

Piedra, L.M., & Engstrom, D.W. (2009). Segmented assimilation theory and the life model: An integrated approach to understanding immigrants and their children. *Social Work, 54*, 270–277.

Portes, A., & Rumbaut, R. (2001). *Legacies: The story of the immigrant second generation*. Berkeley, CA: University of California Press.

Roberts, R.E., & Sobhan, M. (1992). Symptoms of depression in adolescence: A comparison of Anglo, African and Hispanic Americans. *Journal of Youth and Adolescence, 216* (6), 639–651.

Roberts, R.E., Chen, Y.W., & Solovitz, B.L. (1995). Symptoms of DSM-III-R major depression among Anglo, African and Mexican American adolescents. *Journal of Affective Disorders, 36* (1–2), 1–9.

Roberts, R.E., Roberts, C.R., & Chen, Y.W. (1997). Ethnic differences in levels of depression among adolescents. *American Journal of Community Psychology, 25* (1), 95–110.

Rosenberg, S. (2000). Providing mental health services in a culture other than one's own. *Reflections: Narratives of Professional Helping, 6*, 32–41.

Schmidley, A.D. (2001). U.S. Census Bureau, Current Population Reports, Series P23–206, *Profile of the foreign-born population in the United States: 2000*. Washington, DC: U.S. Government Printing Office.

Segal, U.A., & Mayadas, N.S. (2005). Assessment of issues facing immigrant and refugee families. *Child Welfare, 84*, 563–583.

Suárez-Orozco, C.S., & Suárez-Orozco, M.M. (2001). *Children of immigration*. Cambridge, MA: Harvard University Press.

Szapocznik, J., Kurtines, W., Santisteban, D. A., Pantin, H., Scopetta, M., Mancilla, Y. et al. (1997). The evolution of structural ecosystemic theory for working with Latino families. In J. Garcia & M.C. Zea (eds), *Psychological interventions and research with Latino populations* (pp. 156–180). Boston, MA: Allyn & Bacon.

Titmuss, R.M. (1968). *Commitment to welfare*. London: George Allen & Unwin.

Titmuss, R.M. (1987). *The philosophy of welfare*. B.A. Smith & K. Titmuss (eds). New York: Routledge.

Tran, T.V. (1993). Psychological traumas and depression in a sample of Vietnamese people in the United States. *Social Work, 18*, 184–194.

UN Department of Economic and Social Affairs (DESA) (Population Division) (2002). *International Migration Report: 2002*. New York: United Nations Publications.

Urrabazo, R. (2000). Therapeutic sensitivity to the Latino spiritual soul. In M.T. Flores & G. Carey (eds), *Family therapy with Hispanics: Toward appreciating diversity* (pp. 205–227). Boston, MA: Allyn & Bacon.

U.S. Council of Economic Advisers (2007). *Immigration's economic impact*. Washington, DC. Retrieved from www.whitehouse.gov/cea/cea_immigration_062007.html.

U.S. Census Bureau (2004) *The foreign-born population in the United States: 2003*. Washington, DC: Current Population Reports.

U.S. Census Bureau (2008). *Current population survey, 2007 and 2008: Annual social and economic supplements, Table 3. People and families in poverty by selected characteristics: 2006 and 2007*. Washington, DC: U.S. Government Printing Office.

U.S. Department of Health and Human Services (DHHS). (2001). *Mental health: Culture, race, and ethnicity – A supplement to mental health. A report of the Surgeon General*. Rockville, MD: DHHS.

U.S. Department of Homeland Security (2006). *Yearbook of immigration statistics: 2005*. Table 25. Washington, DC: U.S. Department of Homeland Security, Office of Immigration Statistics.

U.S. Department of Homeland Security (2008) *Yearbook of immigration statistics: 2008*. Washington, DC: Office of Immigration Statistics U.S. Department of Homeland Security.

Yu, M. (1997). Mental health services to immigrants and refugees. In T.D. Watkins & J.W. Callicutt (eds), *Mental health policy and practice today* (pp. 164–181). Thousand Oaks, CA: Sage.

Zhou, M. (1992). *Chinatown*. Philadelphia, PA: Temple University Press.

Zolberg, A.R., Suhrke, A., & Aguayo, S. (1989). *Escape from violence: Conflict and the refugee crisis in the developing world*. New York: Oxford University Press.

9 Child maltreatment and its effects

Carolyn Knight

Individuals with a history of childhood maltreatment are disproportionately represented among clinical populations who seek out or are required to seek social work services (Davies, 2003; Sachs-Ericsson, Blazer, Plant, & Arnow, 2005). In fact, in some settings like addictions, domestic violence and mental health, research suggests that the majority of clients will have experienced some sort of victimization in childhood (Dixon, Browne, & Hamilton-Giachritsis, 2005; Meeyoung, Farkas, Minnes, & Singer, 2007; Spatz-Widom, Marmorstein, & Raskin-White, 2006). In this chapter, the definition and nature of childhood maltreatment is examined, as are the long-term consequences. The relationship between adult problems in living and a history of childhood victimization also is discussed. Using a case illustration, principles of effective social work practice with clients with histories of childhood maltreatment are identified, and this includes ethical considerations.

Definitions of child maltreatment

Legally, child maltreatment generally is more narrowly defined as child abuse. Definitions vary by state and limit the age of victim (usually 16 or younger) and often require that the perpetrator serve in some sort of caretaking capacity in relationship to the child. Specific acts that constitute physical and sexual abuse, neglect, and in some cases, emotional abuse are identified in each state. Social workers should be familiar with relevant child abuse statutes, given mandatory reporting requirements. The National Association of Social Workers (NASW) Code of Ethics specifically addresses this issue in its section on commitment to clients:

> Social workers' primary responsibility is to promote the wellbeing of clients. In general, clients' interests are primary. However, social workers' responsibility to the larger society or specific legal obligations may on limited occasions supersede the loyalty owed clients, and clients should be so advised. (Examples include when a social worker is required by law to report that a client has abused a child or has threatened to harm self or others.)
>
> (NASW, 2008)

In this chapter, child maltreatment or victimization will be used to refer not only to what is legally defined as sexual or physical abuse, but also to acts of commission that could be defined legally as assault. Child maltreatment is defined as sexual and physical acts committed against children and youth 16 years of age or younger by someone in a position of power or authority. Child maltreatment includes but is not limited to fondling, masturbation, watching or participating in pornography, and anal and/or vaginal penetration in the case of sexual victimization, and hitting, punching, burning, and kicking in the case of physical victimization. Physical neglect is not included in this definition since research and theory both suggest that the associated long-term consequences are different and tend to be less severe.

Some states include emotional abuse in legal statues regarding child abuse, but this is much harder to specify and document (Rodriguez-Srednicki & Twaite, 2004). Sexual and physical maltreatment are, by nature, emotionally abusive. In fact, theorists and researchers focus more on the psychological, traumatic impact of physical and sexual victimization, rather than the specific acts of maltreatment, since this is what leads to the problems in living that adult survivors face.

Therefore, defining what is meant by "trauma" and "traumatizing" is also important. The earliest conceptualizations of trauma focused on the event that precipitated it. Bessel van der Kolk, one of the first theorists and researchers to study trauma, emphasized the dramatic, overwhelming nature of an event: "Trauma, by definition, is the result of exposure to an inescapably stressful event that overwhelms a person's coping mechanisms" (van der Kolk, 1987, p. 25). Increasingly, researchers and theorists have concentrated on an individual's subjective interpretation of an event. Williams and Sommer (2002, p. xix) note, "Trauma is in the eyes of a beholder."

McCann and Pearlman (1990) assert that an event is traumatic if it, "(1) is sudden, unexpected, or non-normative, (2) exceeds the individual's perceived ability to meet its demands, and (3) disrupts the individual's frame of reference and other central psychological needs and related schemas" (p. 10). An especially damaging aspect of child maltreatment is the power differential that exists between the child or youth and the perpetrator. Relative to the perpetrator, the victim is psychologically, physically, and emotionally powerless. The child's sense of powerlessness is often less about her or his physical stature relative to the perpetrator and more about psychological vulnerability. As Herman notes, "Captivity, which brings the victim into prolonged contact with the perpetrator, creates a special type of relationship – one of coercive control" (Herman, 1995, p. 87).

Another aspect of child maltreatment that contributes to its long-term traumatic impact is exploitation. The perpetrator takes advantage of the victim's trust, dependence, and her or his physical, emotional, social, and/or intellectual immaturity. Whether or not a caretaking relationship exists, it is the essential powerlessness of the victim, coupled with the betrayal inherent in the victimization, which is traumatizing to the youth or child.

Whether there is physical pain or not, child maltreatment leads to feelings of worthlessness and powerlessness. In the case of sexual abuse, especially, victims often feel like "damaged goods" (Browne & Finkelhor, 1986). Further, victims of child maltreatment tend to blame themselves and struggle with chronic feelings of guilt and responsibility for their victimization. Deep feelings of sadness, akin to grief, as well as feelings of anger and rage also are common (Green, 2000).

Psychological damage also occurs because the child's sense of self and self-worth are still evolving (Cloitre, Miranda, & Stovall-McClough, 2007). The victimization becomes intertwined with and begins to define the youth's or child's views of self and others. Many survivors of childhood maltreatment lack a sense of "intact self" or a coherent, stable sense of identity (Garfield & Leveroni, 2000; Janoff-Bulman, 1992). Victimization in childhood also interferes with the individual's ability to regulate emotions and often leads to a worldview characterized by mistrust, hostility, and suspicion as the results of numerous studies reveal (McCann & Pearlman, 1990; Resick, 2001).

The case of two sisters, both of whom were sexually abused in nearly identical ways, illustrates the concepts so far presented. Hannah and Rachel were sexually molested by their next door teenaged neighbor when each was between the ages of approximately 5 and 8. Neither sister was aware of the sexual abuse of the other. Hannah, the older of the two siblings, did not recall her sexual abuse until she was in her twenties (memory and child maltreatment is discussed in the section that follows). In contrast, Rachel, younger by four years, had always remembered the abuse. In both cases, the abuse occurred in the basement of the neighbor's home and involved oral sex, fondling, and mutual masturbation.

Hannah and Rachel, as well as their abuser, were members of the Orthodox Jewish community, and this presented some unique challenges to both of them. Within this community, sexual abuse is rarely discussed and was presumed to be non-existent. The siblings disclosed to their parents the sexual abuse on separate occasions and the disclosures were met with support and understanding; yet, the sisters struggled with intense feelings of isolation and being different, feelings that are common among survivors of sexual abuse, but were exacerbated by sexual abuse being so taboo in their community.

Despite the similarity of their victimization and their feelings of isolation resulting from their cultural background, Hannah and Rachel struggled in very different ways. As noted, Hannah did not even recall her victimization until she was an adult. Even before this, though, she struggled with feelings of low self-esteem, social isolation, and difficulties in interpersonal relationships. Her relationship with her parents was strained, she had few intimate relationships, and struggled to manage intense feelings of anger and resentment. Even after seeing a social worker for a significant length of time, she continued to struggle with the same issues. Rachel also struggled with feelings of low self-esteem and difficulties in social relationships. Unlike her sister, Rachel had an eating disorder. Further, and in contrast to her sister, her relationship with her parents was a positive one. Through her work with a social worker, she developed the ability to be sexually and emotionally intimate, managed her eating disorder, and began to enjoy her life and her relationships. In the section that follows, the relationship between childhood victimization and later problems in living is examined in more depth, as are reasons why the sisters' struggles were so different.

Child maltreatment and mental health/illness

Determining the *prevalence* of child maltreatment is complicated by several factors, most notably differing legal and operational definitions of what it is (Runyan et al., 2005; Shaffer, Huston, & Egeland, 2008). Research findings also are often based upon subjects' self-report of whether or not they were victimized, often years earlier. Survivors of child maltreatment often forget about their experiences or minimize the significance, so such self-report data can be very unreliable. In several studies between 40 and 60 percent of participants did not report childhood victimization for which there was independent, objective documentation (Fergusson, Horwood, & Woodward, 2000).

According to the U.S. Department of Health and Human Services, Administration for Children, Youth, and Families (DHHS, ACYF, 2009), there were almost 800,000 substantiated child protective service reports in the United States in 2007. Slightly more than 10 percent of cases involved physical abuse and 7 percent were sexual abuse cases. Emotional abuse accounted for less than 5 percent of the cases. The majority of confirmed cases involved neglect. The younger the child, with children under three being at greatest risk, the higher the rate of victimization. In the vase majority of cases (more than 85 percent), the perpetrator was a parent, relative, or unmarried partner of a parent (DHHS, ACYF, 2009).

When looking at child maltreatment more generally – that is, not just confirmed cases of child abuse – even a conservative estimate suggests that at least one-third of women and one-quarter of men experienced some form of sexual, physical, or emotional maltreatment prior to reaching age 18 (Breslau, 2002). In a national survey of children and youth aged 17 and under, almost 14 percent of the respondents reported experiencing some form of maltreatment, just within the previous year (Finkelhor, Ormrod, Turner, & Hamby, 2005). Three-quarters of those youth who reported maltreatment indicated they had been emotionally abused. Almost one-half indicated they had experienced physical abuse and 8 percent indicated they had experienced some sort of sexual victimization. Children and youth with histories of child maltreatment typically experience multiple exposures, often to more than one type of victimization (Finkelhor et al., 2005).

Research indicates that maltreatment in childhood or adolescence results in *serious and long-lasting consequences*, especially if it involves sexual victimization. Child and youth maltreatment have been found to be associated with: behavioral problems such as substance abuse, eating disorders, self-injury, aggression, and suicide and suicidal thoughts (Banyard, Williams, & Siegel, 2001; Weichelt, Lutz, Smyth, & Syms, 2005); psychiatric conditions such as borderline personality disorder, depression, PTSD, and dissociative identity disorder (Read & Ross, 2003; Spence et al., 2006); and physical and health problems (Brown, Schrag, & Trimble, 2005; Goodwin & Stein, 2004; Solomon & Heide, 2005).

A history of child maltreatment also has been found to be more likely among adults in treatment for issues associated with family and domestic violence and clients in forensic settings (Arata & Lindman, 2002; Spitzer, Chevalier, Gillner, Freyberger, & Barnow, 2006).

PTSD diagnosis is the one most commonly applied to individuals with traumatic histories, generally, and to those who have experienced maltreatment in childhood specifically. A stressful event is a necessary but not a sufficient condition for a diagnosis of PTSD, and the event must be one that involves actual or threatened death or serious injury, and/or a threat to the physical integrity of the person or others. The individual's response to the event must involve intense fear, helplessness, or horror (APA, 2000).

A diagnosis of PTSD also requires that the individual experience: one or more "re-experiencing symptoms" that trigger "intense psychological distress;" three or more "avoidance and numbing responses" in response to thoughts or memories of the event; and two or more "hyperarousal responses" like difficulty falling or staying asleep, problems with concentration, and irritability (APA, 2000). The symptoms must persist for at least one month and result in significant distress or impairment in functioning. "What distinguishes people who develop PTSD from people who are merely temporarily overwhelmed is that people who develop PTSD become 'stuck' on the trauma and keep reliving it in thoughts, feelings, or images" (van der Kolk, van der Hart, & Burbridge, 2002, p. 24).

Despite widespread use of the PTSD diagnosis, significant problems exist with its application, particularly in cases of child maltreatment. Most basically, the classification does not adequately take into account or explain individual differences (Bowman, 1999). Prior emotional functioning, temperament, developmental level, and cultural and social context all have been found to impact an individual's potential to develop PTSD In fact, in her review of available research, Bowman concludes, "Individual differences are significantly more powerful than event characteristics in predicting PTSD, with events contributing relatively little variance" (Bowman, 1999, p. 27). The role of culture is receiving increased attention, since it appears that:

the interactions between the individual and his or her environment/community play a significant role in determining whether the person is able to cope with the potentially traumatizing experiences that set the stage for the development of PTSD. Thus, PTSD reflects the sociocultural environment in which it occurs.

(DeVries, 1996, p. 400)

It also appears that the level, intensity, and length of the individual's exposure to an event are at least as, if not more, influential predictors of PTSD than the event itself.

Research consistently demonstrates that a diagnosis of PTSD typically co-occurs with at least one other major psychiatric classification like depression, substance abuse, and anxiety and panic disorders (Resick, 2001). What has yet to be determined is the direction of causality in this relationship, so the questions remain: Are psychiatrically fragile individuals more likely to develop PTSD in response to a traumatic event? Or, do individuals who develop PTSD face a greater risk of developing other psychiatric disorders?

It is increasingly accepted that traits and characteristics that predate an individual's exposure to trauma are especially predictive of subsequent psychiatric symptomology. For example, summarizing a broad range of epidemiological data, Breslau (2002) argues:

> only a small subset of trauma victims succumb to PTSD; most do not. Recent studies indicate that trauma victims who do not succumb to PTSD (that is most victims) are not at a markedly elevated risk for the subsequent first-onset of other psychiatric disorders, compared with unexposed persons. The excess incidence of the first onset of other disorders following trauma exposure is concentrated primarily in the small subset of trauma victims with PTSD. These observations suggest that PTSD identifies a subset of trauma victims at considerable risk for a range of disorders.

(Breslau, 2002, p. 928)

Research suggests that individuals who have been maltreated in childhood or adolescence, especially women who were sexually abused, often do exhibit many of the symptoms that are typically associated with PTSD. However, their childhood experiences may not conform to the requirements of the original diagnosis. For example, sexual abuse of a child often does not involve physical harm in the conventional sense or occur under circumstances that would be characterized as "cruel" or frightening (Herman, 1995). Further, among individuals who have experienced similar sorts of childhood maltreatment, the incidence rates of PTSD symptoms can vary widely.

The experiences of two clients illustrate the problems with the PTSD diagnosis.

When Ken was 12, his parents were killed in a car crash, and he and his seven siblings were each farmed out to live with relatives. Ken went to live with a maternal aunt and her husband. Within six months of moving in with his relatives, Ken's uncle began to fondle him. This progressed to oral and anal sex and ultimately included several other men who routinely gang-raped, sodomized, and tortured him. As an adult, Ken struggled with numerous problems in living, but he did *not* have any of the symptoms required for the PTSD diagnosis. In Ken's case, the precipitating events – the death of his parents and the increasingly violent, sadistic, and painful sexual abuse he experienced over a six-year period – conform to the traumatic event required for the diagnosis, but he evidenced none of the symptoms.

In contrast, Marianne's brother, older than her by 12 years, beginning when she was 7, sexually abused her. Marianne did not view this as rape or as sexual abuse, and her accounts suggest that her brother was never rough, threatening, or violent. He would "reward" her with toys, candy, flattery, and special attention. As an adult, Marianne experienced classic signs of PTSD. She had frequent nightmares about someone trying to hurt her and went to great lengths to avoid being a passenger in a car because of the anxiety it provoked in her (her brother often raped her in his car). Certain sights, smells, and sounds would trigger flashbacks to the abuse and panic attacks, and she reported she "froze" and "zoned out" whenever she was touched by a man.

A number of authors have argued that a new diagnostic classification, often referred to as complex PTSD, is required to adequately account for, describe, and understand the experiences of and symptoms associated with child maltreatment. Korn and Leeds (2002) note, for example, that trauma experienced in childhood is "not just an event" rather it is a "complex process, often embedded within a context of severe neglect, deprivation, and emotional invalidation" (p. 1465).

Child and youth maltreatment often is ongoing and long-standing, and in this way, it differs significantly from the original conceptualizations of the cause of PTSD. As discussed, exposure to maltreatment and the child's emotional and cognitive immaturity combine to produce particularly damaging consequences for later adult functioning. Ongoing research generally supports the need for a diagnosis of traumatic stress that takes into account these realities of child maltreatment, and the complex PTSD conceptualization continues to be refined and expanded upon. However, some authors argue that complex PTSD is actually a more severe variation on the original PTSD diagnosis. Whichever is the case, individuals who have been victimized in childhood face some particularly difficult challenges in adulthood. In summarizing these difficulties, Tinnin, Bills, and Gantt (2002) observe:

> A patient with complex PTSD . . . feels small, weak, and inadequate in a world that seems increasingly unmanageable and overwhelming. In time, the victim not only feels vulnerable, but unacceptable, secretly concluding that she or he is unworthy of love. This conclusion undermines even the hope of being loved and results in an image of a weak, inadequate, unlovable victim facing an indifferent, cold, and essentially hostile world which will easily crush him or her.
>
> (Tinnin et al., 2002, p. 105)

Individuals who have experienced child maltreatment have been found to be much more likely to be diagnosed with *borderline personality disorder* (BPD). Features of this condition include, among others, intense and ongoing feelings of abandonment, disruptions in relationships that alternate between extremes of attachment to and withdrawal from others, distorted and unstable views of self, recurrent suicidal threats and gestures, and impulsivity (Linehan, 1993). Korn and Leeds suggest that borderline personality disorder is best viewed as a "posttraumatic stress personality and relational adaptation to childhood abuse and neglect including disruptions of attachment and bonding" (2002, p. 1466).

Clients diagnosed with borderline personality are often viewed as particularly difficult to engage in a working relationship, and unlikely to benefit from intervention. Their deep mistrust of others leads to testing and other manipulative behaviors. However, their interpersonal difficulties reflect their attempts to manage their relationships as well as distortions in thinking about others, discussed in more detail below.

Adults with histories of child maltreatment also are likely to exhibit dissociative symptoms. Further, the majority of individuals diagnosed with dissociative identity disorder (DID) (formerly known as multiple personality disorder), which is the most extreme form of dissociation, have been found to have a history of maltreatment as a child. Dissociation is defined as, "a psychological process by which information – incoming, stored, or outgoing – is deflected from integration with its usual and expected associations" (Rodin, deGroot, & Spivak, 1997, p. 161). The DSM-IV-TR distinguishes dissociative disorders as those in which there is a "disruption in the usual integration of functions such as consciousness, memory, identity, and perception of the environment [that is associated with] impairment in social, occupational, or other areas of functioning" (Rodin et al., 1997, p. 161). In the case of DID, the individual lacks a coherent sense of self. Emotions, thoughts, feelings, and memories are split off into separate parts.

Dissociation, particularly DID, is typically viewed as extremely dysfunctional. But dissociation provides the individual with a valuable – and sometimes the only – way of coping with and surviving childhood maltreatment and is consistent with a child's capacity to fantasize and create an alternate, less painful reality. If the child can "pretend" that the awful things that are happening to her or him are not happening or are happening to someone else, it becomes easier to endure the psychic, physical, and/or emotional pain, as the following examples reveal.

Sam was sexually abused in the basement of his home by a family acquaintance, though his memories about this experience, which began when he was in elementary school and lasted through middle school, came back to him only in adulthood. He was sodomized and forced to perform oral sex on the perpetrator. When he began to recall his victimization, he described how "weird" it felt to him:

> I know that this was happening to me. Even now I can feel something in my mouth and I can feel pain in my rectum. But all I can see is the dryer. It's as if I wasn't there at all. I just see that white dryer.

Her father "for as long as she can remember" sexually and physically abused Serena. She has always had complete and vivid recall of her victimization, which included vaginal and anal rape and severe physical beatings that resulted in numerous hospitalizations. She has been permanently scarred by her father's assaults and sustained permanent internal injuries. She described her father's sexual assaults in the following way:

> I remember him coming into my bedroom at night. It would be very dark and I knew he was in the room. And then it all goes blank. The next thing I know it's morning and my sheets are stained, sometimes bloody, and I am sometimes very sore "down there," but I don't know exactly what happened.

Both of these clients were quite young at the time their victimization began, and they found ways to escape while they were being victimized, a phenomenon known as peritraumatic dissociation (Marmar, Weiss, & Metzler, 1997). Each of these clients relied upon one of the few adaptive skills they possessed – the ability to escape their victimization by retreating into a different reality. Research findings support the existence of peritraumatic dissociation, particularly among children who experience repeated, prolonged, frightening, and intrusive victimization (Banyard, Williams, & Siegel, 2001). Research also indicates that dissociation reflects neurobiological changes that occur as a result of being traumatized in childhood (Nemeroff, 2004).

Dissociation can become a more or less permanent way in which the individual copes in life. "Dissociation can develop into a conditioned response to any stressful situation. Thus, what served effectively as a problem-solving strategy in childhood can become a debilitating condition that may seriously impede healthy adult functioning" (Sutton, 2004, p. 24). The disconnect between feelings and actions is not limited to the maltreatment, but rather becomes the individual's habitual way of interacting and dealing with the world. A client, Sarah, summed it up well when she said:

> I know that I should feel things, but I don't feel anything. I know what I am supposed to feel, and I can fake it, but inside, I am empty. If you tell me to cry, I'll cry. If you tell me to laugh, I'll laugh. But it's all fake. None of it is real.

With dissociative identity disorder, the individual's thoughts, feelings, and experiences can become so compartmentalized that she or he experiences amnesia and can lose track of hours, even days, at a time. Some individuals with DID possess well-defined alters with distinctive personalities, conforming to the popular stereotypes of "multiple personality" found in books and movies. For many others, the fragmentation is less rigid, and there may be some awareness of the other parts of the self. Whichever is the case, the fragmentation serves an important protective function. The survivor's feelings and experiences can be split off and housed in different parts of the self, thus enhancing her or his ability to survive the maltreatment and manage its effects.

Many survivors of child and youth maltreatment have, at best, incomplete, and at worst, *little or no memory* of their victimization. "Motivated forgetting" (Reviere, 1996) can be viewed as a specific example of dissociation, serving a similar protective function:

> If a traumatic experience defies a child's ability to understand, categorize, and assimilate, and if accommodation poses a threat too great, memory for traumatic events may be impaired . . . In the absence of [psychic] structure (i.e., schematic understanding), which provides organization and meaning, traumatic experience cannot be represented or encoded in any mature meaningful way. Thus, while fragmented sensory impressions, stereotyped actions, physiological reactions, images, and affects may be loosely retained, these are all "prerepresentational." The integrated memory is lost to repression.
>
> (Reviere, 1996, p. 38)

A loss of memory about, or incomplete recall of, maltreatment experienced in childhood is viewed both as a psychological defense and as a consequence of the child's inability to cognitively process and understand the experience.

> The recollections of Betty, who was sexually abused beginning in toddlerhood, typify the role memory plays in childhood trauma. She did not have specific recall of the original abuse, in which she was forced to perform oral sex on an uncle who was caring for her while her mother was hospitalized. She did, however, experience physical symptoms, like

feeling as if her mouth was full, gagging, and soreness in her throat, that she neither understood nor could explain but which mirrored her earliest victimization.

Betty was sexually abused on subsequent occasions by this same uncle. Unlike this earliest abuse, she had memories, though somewhat fragmented, of these later experiences. Because of her cognitive and emotional immaturity and limited linguistic ability, Betty can be viewed as having a prerepresentational memory of her earliest sexual abuse. That is, the memory of what happened to her was stored physically, rather than cognitively, and therefore apparent through her physiological responses.

As van der Kolk (1996, p. 221) observes, in many instances, it's "the body that keeps the score," as opposed to the mind.

A number of theorists and researchers question the *validity of memory loss, recovered memories, and dissociation*, particularly dissociative identity disorder, in cases of child maltreatment (Goodman et al., 2003). Piper and Merskey (2004) observe that much of the research that supports the relationship between DID and child maltreatment relies solely upon the survivor's uncorroborated recollections. After reviewing all available evidence, in fact, they conclude, "as of this writing, no evidence supports the claim that DID patients as a group have actually experienced the traumas asserted by the disorder's proponents" (p. 595).

Summarizing the criticism leveled at the DID diagnosis specifically, Gleaves (1996) observes that in many instances, clinicians create the diagnosis: "Psychotherapists play the most critical role in the development of the condition by suggesting and legitimizing the concept of multiplicity, creating the symptomology through hypnosis, and then shaping the patient's behavior through differential reinforcement" (1996, p. 43). Critics argue that media coverage of individuals alleged to have "multiple personalities" as well as portrayals of these individuals in films and literature have served to further legitimize an already invalid diagnosis and, ironically, provide individuals with the knowledge necessary to develop the symptoms. Even when the symptoms of DID are not induced, it is argued that they reflect a client's need for attention rather than the existence of distinct alter personalities.

In the case of repressed memories, critics argue that these, too, may be the creation of clinicians who assume that the client must be a survivor of child maltreatment, given the symptoms and problems in living with which she or he presents. Critics note that uninformed use of hypnotic techniques and guided imagery can lead to false memories (Alison, Kebbell, & Lewis, 2006). Authors also question whether forgetting about childhood trauma is any different than forgetting about anything else that occurs in childhood (Loftus, Garry, & Feldman, 1994; McNally, 2003). Simply put, the older one gets, the more likely it is that events, persons, and experiences will be forgotten. Critics note that much of the research that supports the existence of traumatic forgetting is fundamentally flawed since it relies upon individuals' retrospective reports of experiences they allegedly had.

However, there remains abundant evidence that some survivors of child maltreatment *do* forget about their victimization and others *do* have experiences, memories, and feelings of which they have little or no awareness (Ghetti et al., 2006). Research also suggests that traumatic experiences are, more so than neutral or positive ones, likely to be fully or partially forgotten (Kluft, 1997). However, research also suggests that whether in response to traumatic events or more neutral ones, memories are not stored like videotapes and are always only more or less accurate versions of reality (Herman & Harvey, 1997). Therefore, memories may be psychologically true, even if they are not completely historically accurate (Barber, 1997).

Social workers must be mindful about the debate and controversy that surrounds dissociation and memory loss and recall. We must recognize that many of the clients who present themselves for treatment for problems characteristic of survivors of child maltreatment may not disclose this history because they simply do not remember it. They may have fragmented and disjointed memories of their victimization and a disjointed sense of self, and these may be disconcerting to both social worker and client.

Dissociation and memory loss can serve important adaptive functions for survivors of child maltreatment. We can normalize and validate these coping capacities and the experiences that necessitated them. We also can help clients with histories of child maltreatment become more affectively present and aware of the self. We can anticipate that as clients with histories of child maltreatment talk about the challenges and difficulties they face in the present and/or the past, memories of past victimization may surface. Memory recall is not an appropriate goal of social work intervention. Yet, when memories spontaneously surface, and they often do, they can signify the client's readiness to confront the trauma directly. Therefore, it is best to frame this work as "working with" client memories not "memory work," to which it is often referred. Finally, social workers also should assume that in some instances their clients will manifest signs of dissociation, which can range from subtle, such as exhibiting little or no affect and having no memory of what was discussed in a session to more overt, such as the client talking or acting differently, and having little or no awareness of this at the time or later.

We should strive for a position of neutrality (Alison et al., 2006; Courtois, 2001). This means we do not automatically assume that child maltreatment exists simply because the client presents with symptoms – including memory loss and dissociation – that are consistent with this history. This also means that we do not assume the client does not have complete recall of her or his maltreatment or that she or he engages in dissociative behavior. Finally, this means that the practitioner should work in partnership with the client, discussing with her or him possible treatment options, what presenting problems and symptoms might mean, and the like. Working in partnership with the client is consistent with the ethical principle of informed consent (Frischholz, 2001).

The problems in living and emotional and psychiatric problems described so far can be viewed as reflections of the adult survivor's attempts to make sense of what happened and the impact it has on her or his ability to engage in relationships with others. Both borderline personality disorder and dissociation reflect profound *disruptions in an individual's sense of self* and ability to manage affect (Diseth, 2005).

For reasons identified in the definition section, child maltreatment distorts individuals' core beliefs about themselves and the world in which they live:

> The individual's unique response to trauma is a complex process that includes the personal meanings and images of the event, extends to the deepest parts of a person's inner experience of self and world, and results in an individual adaptation.
>
> (McCann & Pearlman, 1990, p. 6)

Janoff-Bulman (1992) argues that child maltreatment shatters an individual's basic assumptions about her or his personal worth and invulnerability and the fairness of her or his world.

Survivors of child maltreatment will inevitably seek to understand and make sense of their experiences. Fundamentally, they will try to answer a question to which, ultimately, there will never be a satisfactory answer: "Why did this happen to me?" As a result of the child's cognitive and emotional immaturity, the likely response to this question is one that involves self-blame and a belief that the world, particularly the individual's social world, is unsafe and unknowable.

Relationships are avoided since they bring with them pain and open the individual up to further exploitation.

McCann and Pearlman (1990) have articulated a theory, based upon studies of survivors of child maltreatment that examines in depth how victimization affects the development of a sense of self. In their model, constructivist self-development theory (CSDT), the authors argue that child maltreatment interrupts or destroys the self-capacities that allow individuals to "maintain a consistent sense of identity and positive self-esteem" (1990, p. 21). These self-capacities include experiencing the full range of affective responses without disintegrating psychologically or being consumed by them; being able to be alone and comfortable with oneself; soothing and comforting oneself when distressed; and accepting criticism and negative feedback without it undermining one's sense of worth.

Ongoing research provides support for a number of the assumptions of constructivist self-development theory, beginning with how views of oneself shape views of others and the self-reinforcing nature of this relationship (Ali, Dunmore, Clark, & Ehlers, 2002). Survivors of child and youth maltreatment are particularly vulnerable to subsequent victimization as adults (Messman-Moore & Brown, 2004; Street, Gibson, & Holohan, 2005) and to experience difficulties in forming secure attachments (Waldinger, Schulz, Barsky, & Ahern, 2006). As McCann and Pearlman (1990) suggest, survivors of maltreatment in childhood and adolescence are more likely than individuals not exposed to such experiences to exhibit the distortions in thinking about self and others and to have difficulty regulating emotions (Cloitre et al., 2005).

Cultural factors influence an individual's experience of child maltreatment and help to explain the extent to which the victimization is traumatic (Elliott & Urquiza, 2006). For example, Bernard (2002) argues that when child maltreatment occurs within a context of racism, it not only intensifies the negative effects, but also compromises the individual's efforts at recovery. The example of Hannah and Rachel presented earlier clearly illustrates the role of culture. Given the secrecy that surrounded sexual abuse within the Orthodox Jewish community, both sisters had particularly intense struggles with feelings of isolation, despite the support of their family. In fact, their mother and father, and later two younger sisters (who were told about the abuse of their older sisters) sought out social work services to assist them with the feelings of isolation they themselves experienced.

Another client, Kay, was African American; she struggled not only with her history of sexual and physical abuse, but also with the silence she was forced to keep about what she endured. Kay grew up in the 1960s and described her parents as upwardly mobile and successful professionals. She reported that she always understood that there was no room in her family for "weakness" or flaws, that in order for them to make it in the white world, they all had to be perfect. Therefore, her feelings of worthless as a result of her victimization were especially acute.

Male clients may have an especially difficult time coming to terms with having been victimized, particularly when this involves sexual abuse, since it so violates culturally defined expectations about what it means to be a man (Hunter, 1990).

Rob, a client who was sexually abused by a priest when he was ten, commented, for example, "I'm not supposed to be the one who is weak and gets victimized. I'm supposed to be the 'knight in shining armor' who comes in and saves the damsel in distress."

Adversarial growth and resilience   Clearly, survivors of child and youth maltreatment face a number of struggles as a result of their victimization. However, it is important that the clinician also recognize that exposure to maltreatment actually can lead to what has been referred to as *adversarial or post-traumatic growth* (Linley & Joseph, 2004).

> Trauma is about devastation and resilience. The most damaged survivor may demonstrate strength that surpasses our expectations . . . It could be argued that such an individual is in some ways more resilient than others. If we measure posttraumatic growth by symptom checklists, or if we assume growth and impairment are polar opposites, we overlook the many individuals with severe symptoms who also have enormous strengths.
>
> (Saakvitne, Tenne, & Affleck, 1998, pp. 281–282)

Few clients with histories of maltreatment are likely to view themselves as either survivors or as having benefited in any way from what happened to them. When exploring with clients possible positive outcomes of their experiences, therefore, we must balance attending to and validating the many difficulties that have resulted with identifying and building upon the strengths and positive attributes that also may exist but go undetected.

A growing body of research demonstrates that, when asked, individuals exposed to trauma often identify positive gains they have made as a result of their victimization. However, findings also reveal that relative to other traumatic events like natural and human-made disasters, adversarial growth is more limited and more difficult to discern among survivors of child maltreatment (Bonanno, 2004; Linley & Joseph, 2004).

Evidence suggests that potential benefits can include stress inoculation whereby the individual's sense of self-efficacy and ability to cope with challenging events in the future are enhanced as a result of exposure to adversity. McMillen (1999) notes that what doesn't kill you makes you stronger. Surviving a traumatic event like maltreatment in childhood also may serve as a wake-up call, providing individuals with an opportunity to evaluate their priorities, enhance or create a sense of spirituality, and prompt them to live their lives in more fulfilling ways. Adversity also can create in individuals more empathy and sensitivity towards others.

Betty, a client described earlier, is a nurse who works with cancer patients, many of whom are terminally ill. Her compassion for her patients and her deep respect for their struggle and for the gift of life stem, at least in part, from her own experiences with abuse as a child.

Another client, Linda, was diagnosed with DID and also was dealing with a number of other problems, like her own physical health, the sexual abuse of her own young daughter, the risk of bankruptcy, and marital problems. Yet, she still found time to befriend a teenage neighbor, whom she "sensed" was a survivor of sexual abuse. Linda's instincts turned out to be correct, and as a result of her concern and with her guidance, the young woman got into treatment. Linda possessed not just a "sixth sense" about underlying sexual abuse, but also a great deal of insight.

Because it appears to be harder for victims of child maltreatment to identify positive gains, it likely that these will be realized only if the individual, with the assistance from the social worker, is deliberate in identifying them (Saakvitne et al., 1998). Social workers should appreciate the unique meaning clients with histories of maltreatment in childhood and adolescence have attached to the victimization as well as assist them in creating a frame of reference that is more empowering. For example, it is important to recognize and credit clients for having survived what happened to them. Regardless of the challenges they face in the present, clients with histories of maltreatment show resilience by simply surviving the victimization in the first place.

An ever-expanding body of theory and research has sought to identify factors that protect individuals and promote resilience. The literature available on *resilience* in the face of adversity was developed at least in part as a reaction to the fact that theories about the effects of trauma generally, and childhood maltreatment specifically, were based almost exclusively upon the study of individuals who developed problems as a result of their exposure and sought out or were required to seek treatment. The focus was squarely on pathology, and as Bonanno (2004) notes, this pathogenic emphasis resulted in viewing even the absence of problems in the wake of trauma as being yet another sign of pathology. Summarizing this research, Bonanno comments: "this evidence suggests that resilience is common, is distinct from the process of recovery, and can be reached by a variety of different pathways" (2004, p. 25).

A related body of research focuses on the factors that are associated with more positive outcomes in response to the traumatic effects of child maltreatment. Supportive relationships, at the individual and community level, both at the time of and long after the victimization, have been found to be especially helpful at mitigating the long-term effects of maltreatment (Feinauer, Hilton, & Callahan 2003; Twaite & Rodriguez-Srednicki, 2004). What is particularly important is the way that others respond to the victimization and to the child or youth. If a disclosure of maltreatment is met with belief and protection from future harm, this can lessen the long-term impact of the victimization. Similarly, if the adult discloses her or his childhood maltreatment and is responded to with understanding and validation, this accelerates the process of recovery. "Genuine positive, affirming relationships where positive coping skills are supported, identified, and modeled can create an environment in which hardiness can be generated" (Feinauer et al., 2003, p. 75).

Illustration and discussion

Both *individual and group modalities* have been found to be beneficial interventions for adult survivors of child maltreatment (Knight, 2009). Each offers survivors some unique advantages. In the case of individual treatment, clients can benefit simply from developing a relationship with someone that is non-exploitive, open, and honest. A working alliance between client and worker provides the client with a corrective emotional experience, exposing her or him to a relationship that is dramatically different from those she or he has experienced in the past. The social worker also can serve as a model of affective expression, demonstrating through her or his actions and reactions the self-capacities that the client needs to develop.

Because of their disappointments in past relationships and their victimization, clients with histories of child maltreatment are likely to approach the social worker with a mixture of suspicion and hostility. Transference issues can be powerful forces in the working relationship, providing the worker and client with valuable insights into and ways of challenging the assumptions about self and others that have resulted from the maltreatment (Pearlman & Saakvitne, 1995).

Participation in a group affords individuals with histories of child maltreatment the opportunity to be with others who have had similar experiences and feelings. Most basically, clients are able to experience the validation, affirmation, and acceptance that accompany being with others who are "all in the same boat" (Shulman, 2008). Group membership has the potential to decrease isolation and enhance esteem through fostering connections among members and providing them with the opportunity to assist one another (Knight, 2009). These benefits are in many ways unique to the group modality. In individual sessions with clients, social workers can normalize and reframe experiences and feelings, but this is simply not as persuasive or compelling as when it comes from others who know firsthand what it means to have been maltreated as a child or adolescent.

As with individual intervention, group membership provides survivors with a corrective emotional experience as others relate to them in non-exploitive ways. As in individual treatment, transference can be a powerful phenomenon in groups that include survivors of child maltreatment, given the number of relationships that exist (Klein & Schermer, 2000). Therefore, social workers facilitating groups for survivors of maltreatment must be prepared to pay close attention to group process issues that reflect members' distorted assumptions about one another and to identify and address these directly.

Five interrelated *practice considerations* have relevance for both individual and group work with clients with histories of child maltreatment (Knight, 2009). First, the social worker must remain mindful of her or his role and professional boundaries. Clients with histories of maltreatment tend to struggle with multiple problems in living and their (and our) sense of urgency may be so great as to lead us to offer more than our professional role allows. We also may be tempted to become too available to survivors, as well as too involved in their present-day lives.

Second, since child maltreatment so often leads to feelings of powerlessness and worthlessness and diminishes the client's self-capacities, the social worker should seek to enhance the client's feelings of mastery and competence, regardless of the specific purpose of the intervention. This empowerment orientation will also assist us in maintaining appropriate boundaries.

Third, we should strive to adopt a trauma-sensitive, not trauma-centered, focus. This means understanding the ways in which the individual's current problems in living and the way she or he relates to us reflect the childhood victimization. This also means adopting a neutral stance, as discussed previously.

Fourth, it is critical that we maintain an appropriate treatment focus, and determine whether the client should be encouraged to work in the present or to tackle the past. In some settings, the work will necessarily be concentrated in the present and on the problems in living that necessitated social work services. In many other settings, even when the individual client or group and the worker have the opportunity to explore in depth past history, the focus may still be on assisting the survivor in managing her or his life in the present more effectively. When we operate from a trauma-sensitive perspective, we quickly recognize that the past and present are inextricably linked. For example, as we talk with clients about their present challenges, we can reframe these in ways that point out the connection to the past. As we help clients focus on the past victimization, we can assist them in seeing the ways in which it intrudes in the present and help them to better manage these intrusions. And, as we help clients better manage their problems in the present and/or their reactions to the past, we are assisting them in altering the distortions in thinking about the self that lead to feelings of powerlessness and worthlessness.

Finally, social workers must recognize that working with survivors of child and youth maltreatment is personally and professionally challenging. As noted, survivors can be difficult to engage in a working relationship. The range and depth of problems in living they experience can be overwhelming, and their stories of exploitation can be painful to hear. Therefore, we must accept that we will be inevitably affected — indirectly traumatized — by our work with survivors child maltreatment (Knight, 2009). Manifestations of indirect trauma include intrusive symptoms analogous to those associated with PTSD, known as secondary traumatic stress (Figley & Kleber, 1995), and distortions in thinking about self and others, known as vicarious traumatization (McCann & Pearlman, 1990). Readers will note the parallels between these two phenomenon and those experienced by clients themselves. Indirect trauma also can be manifested in a diminished capacity to empathize with clients, known as compassion fatigue (Figley, 1995).

Indirect trauma is not the same as countertransference, which involves our reactions to particular clients, often in response to our own personal issues (Pearlman & Saakvitne, 1995). Indirect trauma is best viewed as an inevitable occupational hazard that accompanies our work with clients with histories of child maltreatment. Rather than seeking to avoid these reactions, we need to be proactive in taking care of ourselves and develop ways of minimizing the impact (Knight, 2009). This includes giving voice to our feelings and reactions, seeking out supervisory support, and maintaining and deepening our personal relationships.

The case that will be utilized to illustrate principles of effective practice as well as concepts previously presented is that of Kay, who was introduced earlier. Kay, an African American woman in her mid-fifties, sought out services after her daughter, age 14, disclosed to her that she had been molested by a relative. Initially, Kay went to a local rape crisis center, which limited client contacts to twelve sessions. During her time at the center, Kay disclosed her own history of abuse and assault, which consisted of being molested by two male teenaged neighbors when she was in elementary school and of being violently raped in college. Kay also reported that she was physically and emotionally abused by her mother, which consisted of frequent and severe beatings and being called a variety of demeaning names and told repeatedly that she was not wanted and that her mother wished she hadn't been born. Prior to this self-referral to the rape crisis center, Kay had not sought out any mental health services. She had been hospitalized once before for depression and suicidal thoughts. According to Kay, her history of maltreatment never came up in her inpatient treatment, and upon release, she did not pursue follow-up counseling as recommended.

Kay was referred to me as her sessions were winding down at the rape crisis center. Her daughter was referred for counseling elsewhere, and, as required by law, her daughter's molestation was reported to the proper authorities. Ultimately, the case was closed for lack of evidence. When Kay and I first met she was overwhelmed and described herself as being "depressed," "stressed out," and "stuck." She expressed a great deal of guilt about her daughter's molestation, as well as anger at her mother and the college football player who had raped her. Her memories of the fondling that occurred in childhood were fragmented and she questioned whether she had just made this up. She also hesitantly offered that she had a sense that her stepfather, who she considered her father, had "done something" to her, but she had no clear memory of this. She was unemployed, having left her job as a successful high school administrator in another state, when she left her husband of 25 years. Kay's husband remained at their home out of state, along with the couple's two older sons, ages 18 and 20.

Kay and her husband talked on a daily basis, and she acknowledged being financially and emotionally dependent upon him. He made it clear that he wanted to reconcile, but she maintained that she didn't think she loved him any more and she felt as if she was being "smothered" in their relationship. Kay's mother had passed away a number of years ago, as had her stepfather. She described her mother as being cold and uncaring throughout her life, but she viewed her stepfather and loving and supportive. She never knew who her biological father was. Kay had no brothers or sisters, nor any extended family with whom she kept in touch.

The beginning phase of work   Kay was eager to continue with the work she had begun, given her level of stress and feelings of desperation. Any mistrust or resentment of me as a possible helper resulting from the differences between us (I am white and am not a survivor of child maltreatment) and/or from any distortions in thinking that might have resulted from her maltreatment was mitigated by her sense of urgency.

Initially our sessions focused on several interdependent issues but concentrated largely on stabilization. First, we worked on helping Kay remain involved in and on top of the investigation into her daughter's molestation. This was not only necessary for her daughter's well-being, but it also promoted Kay's feelings of self-efficacy. This involved helping Kay to separate her guilt and feelings of powerlessness in response to her own experiences from her reactions to what happened to her daughter. This also involved helping her to acknowledge these feelings, as well as helping her identify the strengths she exhibited: Her daughter trusted her enough to tell her about the molestation; once Kay became aware of the abuse of her daughter she took appropriate action. She provided unconditional support, understanding, and nurturance to her daughter, even as she struggled with her own maltreatment as a child.

A second focus of our earliest sessions was assisting Kay in managing her feelings of stress and depression. As a result of these feelings, she was more or less paralyzed, unable to look for work or make any decisions about her separation. This resulted in a self-defeating cycle in which she had trouble getting out of bed or accomplishing anything during the day, which in turn reinforced feelings of powerlessness and worthlessness. Kay and I identified stress and relaxation techniques that could work for her, as well as talked directly about how out of control and hopeless about her situation she felt. We also began to identify small steps that she could take, such as developing a list of her expenses and a budget so she could work out a separation agreement.

I suggested that Kay consider consulting with a psychiatrist to see if she had a mood disorder that could be controlled through medication. Initially, she was reluctant to pursue this, claiming that she wasn't weak or crazy. Ultimately, Kay agreed and took an antidepressant for a period of time. She reported benefiting from this, as the medication helped her to keep her depression under control so she could "think clearly" and get things done.

In the excerpt that follows, Kay and I address her depression and the difficulties she had getting out of bed in the morning.

Kay (K): I can hardly drag myself out of bed in the morning, and then I lay around all day and do nothing and just think about how lousy things are. My daughter, my husband, I don't have a job. I'm just worthless! (*Starts to cry*)

Silence

Carolyn (C): So, it's tough just getting going in the morning. But, the problem is, the more you lay around, the worse you feel. You get stuck in this vicious cycle.

K: Yeah, I just can't get my self together.

C: It's hard, isn't it, when you are feeling so overwhelmed by so many things. But, let me ask you this. Even though you are feeling really lousy, you've still been getting Vanessa [her daughter] off to school each day. Right? And you are getting her to her appointments, following up with all the police stuff, helping her with her homework. Getting dinner, all that sort of stuff.

K: Right . . . I guess so.

C: Not you guess so, you know so! So you're still doing important things. So what I am wondering is this. How are you getting yourself to do these things, even though you feel so bad and depressed? Somehow you are getting these things done and staying on top of them. If we can figure this out, then we can help you to start to do some of the other things that you need to do.

K: Well, I don't know. Vanessa is everything to me. I would do anything for her.

C: I understand, but still, how did you take those feelings of love for her and use them to get you going to do the things you needed to do.

K: Well, I guess I just said, F— it! Vanessa needs you so get your sh— together and get moving.

C: Well, there you go. That's a strategy! So, you just sort of tell yourself that yeah, things are tough, but there's work to be done, and you've got to do it. I'm wondering if you could apply that same approach to something else that you need to take care of.

With many clients, especially those who have been victims of child maltreatment, it isn't enough to empathize with their feelings. We have to be prepared to help them start to do things differently, because as they *do* things differently, they start to *feel* differently about themselves and their situation (Shulman, 2008). In this example, what I helped Kay to do was identify things she was already doing to make her situation better. This is an application of solution-focused practice in which the worker asks about exceptions to problems and searches for differences that make a difference (DeShazer, 1991). My efforts concentrated on building upon the strength Kay demonstrated in caring for and protecting her daughter.

A third focus of our early work was on Kay's recollections of her abuse, and her feelings and reactions that resulted. Kay experienced some of the symptoms consistent with a diagnosis of PTSD, including nightmares of being chased and hunted down and panic attacks. She also reported flashbacks to her rape, which were fairly vivid, and to her molestation, which were vague and unclear. As noted, she also had begun to have a sense that her stepfather had "done something" to her, and experienced physical reactions in her legs and groin area that were disconcerting to her.

Our work in this area involved several interrelated strategies. First, as Kay reported the symptoms she experienced, I sought to normalize and validate them. Second, we spent time in our sessions processing in greater detail the nature of the flashbacks, what she saw, and the feelings that were evoked. Kay appeared to have full recall of her rape, but she was reluctant to talk about it. She also appeared to have full recall of her mother's physical and emotional abuse of her, but also was reluctant to discuss this in detail. Given the numerous other challenges Kay was dealing with, it was important to honor her desire not to explore in depth her mother's abuse of her or her rape as a way of helping her feel more in control of herself and her life.

Kay's recollections of her molestation by neighborhood youth were disconcerting to her, as were her questions about her stepfather's possible abuse. Kay expressed a desire to know, one way or the other, what happened in both situations. We decided to start with the neighborhood youths, since this was less overwhelming to her. We utilized guided imagery techniques, which have been found to help clients piece together their memories of child maltreatment, and which allow the social worker to remain neutral, as discussed previously. The most useful of these was the movie analogy in which Kay described what she was seeing in a "movie" that depicted the images she was seeing (Bisson, 2005: Leviton & Leviton, 2004). Rather than being *in* the movie, Kay acted as a *reporter* describing what she was seeing on the screen. This strategy enhances the client's ability to cope with what is remembered, since it deliberately encourages dissociation as a means of protecting clients from being flooded with feelings and memories.

Ultimately, Kay recalled being abused by two different teenagers. In one case, she recalled only one instance in which the youth forced her to masturbate him. In the second case, she believed that there were multiple instances that involved mutual masturbation and perhaps oral sex. She believed that she was in late elementary or junior high school. She could not recall who the boys were, nor how or why the abuse stopped. She was of the belief that she did not tell anyone, and she believed that both boys lived close to her but wasn't sure they knew one another. Kay's recollections are typical of those of clients with histories of child maltreatment. While she came to have a better understanding of what happened to her, there were still gaps in her memory. As noted previously, the goal of our work with survivors shouldn't be memory recall. In fact, in many instances, we will need to assist clients in tolerating gaps in memory, and assist them in making meaning of what they do remember (Knight, 2009).

The middle phase of work   It is not always clear when our work shifts from the engagement and beginning phase to the *middle phase*, but over time, the nature of our work does change, in response to the deepening relationship that exists and the greater willingness of the client to talk openly and honestly. In many social work settings, worker and client may not have the opportunity to pursue in greater depth the client's history of maltreatment. Their work together may be more short term and remain focused on stabilization, as was much of my work with Kay in the beginning phase. In fact, this focus was maintained in the middle phase, though there also was much greater attention devoted to Kay's past.

It was during the middle phase of our work that the opportunity for Kay to participate in a group arose. Kay had been attending a time-limited group for sexual assault survivors offered by the same rape crisis center from which she initially received counseling. When that group ended, the leader asked if I would take over the group, since members seemed eager to continue their work together. I agreed, but prior to doing so, Kay and I discussed the challenges associated with me becoming the group worker in addition to being her individual worker. Survivors' problems in relationships and their difficulties with boundaries can affect their ability to manage these sorts of dual relationships (Knight, 2009).

Initially Kay expressed some reservations about me becoming the group leader, claiming that she didn't want to "share" me. As we discussed this in greater detail, it became clear to both of us that Kay's reservations were a reflection of transference issues and were associated with her feelings about her mother's treatment of her and Kay's feelings of abandonment and rejection. These feelings became a focus of our work in individual sessions. Ultimately, Kay understood and accepted the different roles and responsibilities associated with my being her individual social worker and the social worker for the group.

In the first session of the group, I explored with members their thoughts, feelings, and reactions about transitioning from one worker to another, what they hoped to accomplish through their continued participation in the group, and their insights into what they had so far discussed and dealt with. I also clarified for them my role as Kay's individual worker, since, like the individual, members of a group that includes survivors of child maltreatment can struggle with what they perceive as the "special-ness" that one member has with the group worker (Knight, 2009).

Individual and group work provide clients with different, though complementary, benefits. In the group, the social worker is responsible for fostering mutual aid among all members, not conducting "casework in the group" (Kurland & Salmon, 2005). The worker can introduce topics that have surfaced in the group in the individual sessions with the client. The worker also can encourage the client to raise topics in group that have surfaced in the individual sessions.

Individual sessions with Kay   Kay's and my work in the middle phase was a continuation of what we had started earlier. We continued to focus on enhancing her ability to manage the challenges she faced on a daily basis, so that she could remain strong for her daughter and her feelings of self-efficacy could continue to develop. Kay and I also continued to examine her thoughts and feelings about her husband and her marriage with the goal of assisting her to make a decision about whether to formalize her separation or seek reconciliation. Ultimately, Kay decided to formalize the separation, without deciding whether it would be permanent or not. We also explored employment options and her thoughts about what she wanted to do to earn money. Kay wanted to become more financially and emotionally independent and believed that if she had employment of some sort she would feel better about herself.

We increasingly focused on helping Kay manage her feelings and reactions in response to her more complete memories of her molestation by the neighborhood youths. While still reluctant, Kay also began to talk in greater depth about what her mother had done to her, as well as her rape. In both instances, Kay worried that her feelings about these two experiences would overwhelm her. Therefore, as Kay talked in greater detail about what happened to her, we identified and worked on ways that she could manage the feelings that surfaced.

When our work with clients with histories of child maltreatment becomes more focused on the underlying trauma, it is important that we help clients both express and manage – or contain – feelings. Research reveals that if clients aren't helped to manage the feelings and reactions that surface as they explore their past, they are likely to be retraumatized and their feelings of power-lessness, rather than being diminished, are reinforced (Solomon & Johnson, 2002).

The following excerpt reveals the ways in which the social worker can help the client talk about the past – in this instance Kay's rape – at the same time that she or he assists the client in managing the feelings that result.

Carolyn (C): Okay, Kay, as we agreed, we're going to "go back there." We're going to help you talk about what happened to you in college, when you were raped. It's time to tell the story, get it out of you, and share the burden of it, so you don't carry it alone.

Kay (K): (*Begins to cry*)

C: So, liked we discussed, I want you to describe what you see when you close your eyes. You don't have to be there. You're here with me, and you're safe. Look around the room here. Make sure it looks safe and secure to you.

K: (*Looks around the room and nods her head*)

C: Okay, so you're safe in this room, and it's just you and me. Sonny [the football player] is nowhere around here. He's long gone, right?

K: (*Nods her head*)

C: Okay, so what do you see?

K: I am at this party. My girlfriend and I. We were freshman, thought we were cool and all. We didn't know anyone there . . . we felt so full of ourselves with all the football players and stuff. (*Continues to cry, starts rocking back and forth*)

C: Kay, are you okay? Remember you're not there; you're here. Would it help if you talked about it as a spectator, rather than using "I"?

K: No, I'm okay. I'm okay.

C: Okay, so what happened next?

K: So, then this really handsome guy comes up to me, and starts talking to me. He's like the star quarterback on the team, and he's talking to me. He starts kissing me and I'm like, "Cut that out, I don't even know you!" He laughed, and backed off. But then later, I went to find the bathroom, and before I knew it, I felt this big hand on my back, and I was pushed into a bedroom onto the bed. (*Crying*)

Silence

K: I was all confused. I didn't know what was happening, and I thought at first that someone was just playing around. Like my girlfriend or something. But then, I looked up and it was him. Sonny. I was on the bed, and he was holding me down by my neck. I started crying. I told him to let me up. He didn't say anything, he just started laughing, telling me that he was on the team, he could do what he wanted. That I'd thank him afterwards, because he was so good with the ladies.

Silence

C: You doing okay?

K: Yeah, I'm fine. So, then he pulls down my pants and pulls down his pants and he . . . he . . . rapes me. And it hurt really bad because he was so rough. I think someone came in to the room, and he told them to go away, he was busy with his "woman." I think I heard someone laughing and then the door closed. When he was done, he warned me not to say anything. Told me, again, that if I said anything, no one would believe me. I didn't say anything, ever. Not to my friend, not to my family. Not to anyone, until now.

Kay described an experience about which she had more or less complete recall. Though she had never talked about her rape in detail, for her, the memory was not new. Kay and I already had identified strategies that she could use that helped her feel less anxious and more in control. She found deep breathing and relaxation techniques helpful, consistent with the findings of research (Bisson, 2005; Leviton & Leviton, 2004). Cognitive-behavioral techniques that helped her distinguish the present from the past also were very useful, which also is consistent with research findings.

In contrast, in this next excerpt, Kay and I explore her "sense" that her stepfather had done something to her. This session occurred after the previous one and was in response to an increase in the number of physical sensations Kay was experiencing that were causing her great distress. As discussed earlier, it is often the "body that keeps the score," so that even when survivors of child maltreatment don't have an explicit memory of their victimization, they may experience physiological reactions and sensations that reveal what may have happened. Also as discussed previously, recalling memories of abuse should not be the goal of our work with clients with histories of child maltreatment. Yet, in a case such as Kay's, in which physical, emotional, and/or psychological reactions associated with the past become more intrusive, exploring the victimization – "working with" memories – can be an appropriate intervention.

Carolyn (C): So tell me more about these weird feelings you've been getting.

Kay (K): Well, it's like this burning feeling in my legs, on my skin. Like a cool, burning feeling at the same time. It goes up and down both of my legs. It kind of hurts, but it also kind of feels good.

C: I am wondering if you can feel those feelings now?

Silence

K: (*Closes her eyes*) Yeah, I can feel it sort of. It's like in my legs.

C: Are you seeing anything while you are feeling these feelings in your legs?

Silence

K: (*Eyes closed*) Well, yeah, I can see my . . . I can see my dad.

C: What is he doing?

K: He's . . . he's rubbing something on my legs. I don't know, like some kind of ointment. (*Crying harder*)

K: Yeah, that's it, he's rubbing this stuff up and down my legs. I took ballet lessons, I practiced all the time, and he would rub my legs when I would get home. They hurt soooo bad, and my mother, she would just tell me to stop whining and slap me if I complained about my legs.

C: I am wondering if you can see yourself, like see how old you were when your dad was doing this?

K: (*Closing her eyes*) Yes, I can see that. Wow, I can see that really well. I'm like – I look like I am about ten or so. I have this little outfit on, and I remember that outfit. Yes, I am in fourth or fifth grade I think.

C: Good, you're doing fine. So, what else are you seeing, or what else do you feel?

K: (*Crying harder*)

C: Kay, what is it? What are you seeing, feeling?

K: I have this feeling around my genitals, like inside myself. It burns!

C: So, you have this feeling inside of you? Is it that same feeling on your legs or different?

K: It's sort of the same, but it hurts more. It hurts inside of me really bad!

C: Can you see what is causing the hurt? What's making you hurt like that inside?

Silence

C: Kay, can you hear me? Remember where you are. You're here with me, okay. You're feeling these feelings in your legs and inside of you, but you are here with me. Not there, okay? Can you tell me more? What is causing the hurt?

| K: | (*Crying hard*) My dad. I see my dad's hands on my – on her – legs. He's going up and down, and then he stops. His hand is on my tummy. He's rubbing my tummy. Then he moves his hand . . . |

Silence

K:	His hand goes down to where I pee. I can feel him touching me there. It burns a lot! Why does it burn? OW! It hurts me so bad. Daddy, stop hurting me!
C:	Kay . . . Kay (*more loudly*). Kay, turn off the images now, okay? Let everything go black, now. Remember, you're here with me. Your dad isn't here, and your dad can't hurt you now. You're here. Take some deep breaths, okay? Take those deep breaths that help you feel more in control and more relaxed.
K:	Okay. Okay. The pain is going away now.

This excerpt typifies the ways in which the social worker can maintain a position of neutrality, but also help the client fill in the blanks of fragmented memories. Kay's disclosures and her descriptions of her physical reactions suggest that her father fondled her when he was massaging her legs. It is important to note that neither here, nor later, did I automatically conclude that this is what happened.

The excerpt also reveals the importance of continuing to assist the client in discussing her or his past in a way that is manageable. Unless clients are equipped with the necessary coping skills, remembering their past can be re-traumatizing and undermine feelings of self-efficacy. When we work with clients' memories of childhood maltreatment, ultimately what becomes most important is the psychological impact these memories have. Therefore, Kay and I concentrated our efforts on helping her identify and work through her feelings about what she had remembered, especially betrayal, anger, loss, and powerlessness.

Kay's involvement in group work   Generally, when discussing groups, the focus is on the group as a whole. This "two-client paradigm" recognizes that the social worker has two clients, the group as a whole and each individual member (Shulman, 2008). Attention is directed towards understanding what an individual member's behavior says about and how it relates to the group as a whole. However, given the focus of this chapter, I will concentrate on Kay's involvement in the group, and how she benefited from this.

In our individual sessions, Kay often expressed intense feelings of being different, crazy, and all alone. She remained extremely disconcerted by the range of symptoms she experienced and her fragmented memories. On the one hand, Kay expressed frustration that she couldn't recall more about what happened, and on the other, she worried that just when she thought she knew all that happened, something else would surface, and she'd be back to square one. Finally, even as she began to talk about what each of her parents had done to her, she struggled with accepting the reality of what she disclosed, since it was so painful. Her family was, in her words, the "perfect, Negro family of the 1960s," and it was hard for her to accept that her mother and father could have abused her.

Kay's reactions are common among clients with histories of child and adolescent maltreatment. I validated these feelings and reactions, assuring her that they were typical of others in her situation. I also conveyed acceptance and support. However, group members were in a much better position to do this. I consistently encouraged Kay to discuss in group what she was remembering and feeling. Initially, Kay was reluctant to do so, expressing embarrassment about what she remembered, even though others in the group had revealed equally sensitive and painful material. Ultimately, Kay opened up to members, and she was met with understanding and acceptance.

A particularly valuable aspect of Kay's participation was the reduced feelings of isolation that resulted. The following excerpt occurred approximately one-third of the way through the six-month group. In our individual sessions, Kay and I had been exploring her feelings associated with her father's possible molestation, as revealed through the memories she recalled. This coincided with the group's focus on new memories and betrayal by loved ones.

Jane disclosed that her father would insert objects in her and photograph this. She also revealed that her father would torture her younger sister (by 14 years – Jane felt like her mother) until Jane agreed to have sex with him. If she resisted his advances, at other times he would tie her, stomach down, to a barstool and rape her and insert objects like the handles of tools into her. As Jane talked about this, members reacted with disgust, sadness, and tears. Another member, Sue, then reported that when she was very young she had a leg problem that required her to use crutches. As a result, her father would often carry her around. She remembered being at a funeral and her father holding her and sticking his fingers inside of her. Sue recalled that she was crying and that the people her father was talking told her not to cry and that she was being childish. Kay then said that as Sue was talking, she was beginning to feel something physical in her vaginal area, and could see her father. Kay then exclaimed, "He [her father] stuck his fingers in me, he stuck his fingers or something in me!"

At this point, most members were crying. Kay and Sue were rocking back and forth, clenching their fists. I commented that members' revelations were very painful. I sensed their deep feelings of being violated in the most fundamental of ways. They had little control over their bodies, and those who were supposed to protect them were in fact exploiting them. I also noted that, in Kay's case, it appeared that her specific recollection that her father inserted his fingers in her was new and wondered what that was like for her to now have this information.

All six members jointed in this discussion, confirming their feelings of betrayal and anger. Kay stated that she felt some relief that she now "knew" what she had always known "in her gut" – that her father had violated her in this way, but she also questioned whether this was really true. She also said that part of her wished she hadn't had this memory, since it just made her angrier and feel more alone. Jane replied that she could really relate to this, since over the years, new memories had surfaced for her as well. She assured Kay that she *would* be okay and that she wasn't crazy. Another member, Linda, stated that she also could understand where Kay was coming from. Even though she had always known what happened to her, she still found it hard to accept, since it meant that her parents had hurt her and taken advantage of her; she wanted to hold on to the belief that her parents loved her.

Kay's memory of her father inserting his fingers inside of her occurred spontaneously in the group and no doubt was related to the discussion that members were having. This sort of spontaneous recall is even more likely to occur in group, since members' disclosures are likely to prompt recall of experiences in others. Over time, Kay came to accept that her father had, in fact, abused her and that it involved penetration with his fingers. Though Kay desired to know if anything else happened, her recollections never became any clearer. She did believe that her father engaged in this behavior on a regular basis, as she could see herself at different ages and in different situations. As noted earlier, an important aspect of our work with survivors of child maltreatment can be to help them accept that they may never have total recall of what happened to them. A complete recollection is not necessary for a client to come to terms with her or his past. What is necessary is for clients to confront and manage their affective reactions to what they have remembered and any feelings they may have about the incompleteness of their memories.

Members' responses to Kay's recollection were affirming to her in several ways. First, they could relate to and understand her sense of betrayal and violation at the hands of someone she loved and wanted to believe loved her. Second, members validated how disconcerting it was to have a memory come back so unexpectedly. Members also helped Kay accept the possibility that she would never remember everything. Finally, all members connected to her ambivalence about accepting what she remembered as being true. This affirmation, in turn, enhanced Kay's ability to manage her feelings and reactions and her feelings of self-efficacy.

I have noted on several occasions that racial issues compounded Kay's isolation and feelings of worthlessness. This included her mother's demeaning comments to her about the color of her skin and the pressure on her to be "perfect" so that her family could "make it" in the white world. This issue surfaced in a powerful way in the group. Of the six members of the group, Kay was the only African American; the other members were white. It is generally advisable to adhere to the "not the only one" principle (Gitterman, 2005) whereby no one member stands out in a way that is different from all others. In reality, this is not always possible, nor is it always easy to ascertain which characteristics are important considerations. In this particular group, Kay's race didn't seem to affect her participation or the members' responses to her, given their shared sense of urgency and purpose. However, in a later session of the group, race did surface as Kay continued to struggle with intense feelings of anger, betrayal, and abandonment.

> Members had been talking about how alone they felt, and how angry they were at those who didn't protect them, who knew something was wrong, and did nothing. Linda commented that she realized she was much angrier at her mother for not doing anything about the abuse than she was at her brother, who had abused her. Sue, agreed, observing that she tried to tell her uncle what her parents were doing to her, and her uncle simply told her to "stop making up stories." Kay remained silent for much of this discussion, and I asked her what was going on for her. Kay was initially reluctant to answer, but finally said, "Look, I don't want to sound mean or anything, but you all really don't know what it's like. Not really." When asked to explain what she meant, Kay hesitated and then said, "None of you ever had a mother tell you you were too black. You don't know what it's like to be black! To be spit at, stared at, told you had to be perfect to fit in! You just don't know what that's like!"

> Members were initially silent, and Kay quickly apologized for her outburst. I suggested there was no reason for her to apologize, that we all appreciated her ability to be so honest about such difficult feelings. Jane then said, "I'm really sorry, Kay. I never really thought about how it might be more difficult or different for you, because of having to deal with racism and all, in addition to the stuff we deal with." Marlene added, "Yeah, I can see where this is like doubly difficult for you." Linda then said, "I guess I see this, but I also think that we all feel isolated and alone, even if it's for different reasons. I mean, I could never understand why my mother singled me out to beat up on me. I had two brothers, and she didn't touch them. She just beat me. What was wrong with me? Why me? I'm sorry, I really am, that people treated you badly because you're black, because that's just ignorant. But I think that even if your mom hadn't said those things to you, you would have felt angry and bad, since she's your mom and she's supposed to protect you, not hurt you."

Members' comfort with one another is very evident in this exchange. Kay was able to be open about her resentment and bitterness, which initially is directed at others in the group. This is an example of the transference discussed previously. Their comfort also is evident in the support that Kay's comments elicited from others and in Linda's willingness to, in some ways, "take on" Kay. She didn't dismiss Kay's comments or become defensive; but she did astutely reframe Kay's feeling in a way that all could relate to. In fact, Linda's comments reflect how we can be responsive to our client's struggles in culturally sensitive ways. We can acknowledge the unique challenges the client may face, but also normalize her or his reactions.

The ending phase of work Kay ended her involvement in individual and group work abruptly and simultaneously. Her home out-of-state (in which her husband still lived with their two sons) burned down, and they lost all of their possessions. Kay's husband and sons were not hurt, but the whole family was, understandably, devastated. Kay decided to return to her home state to assist her husband with the clean-up and with dealing with the insurance company. While she intended to be gone for only a brief period of time, she ended up staying indefinitely, since problems developed with the insurance claim, and her husband developed some significant health issues.

Kay and I didn't really have a chance to terminate, nor did she have a chance to end with the group, or the members with her. She and I did meet one more time, and for much of that session, Kay discussed the stress and worry she was experiencing as a result of the fire. I suggested that we spend time talking about what she had accomplished so far, and what challenges might still lay ahead for her. While we did spend a bit of time on this, Kay's focus was clearly on her family. I provided her with some suggestions for resources that could be helpful to her and her daughter in the future.

Kay attended one more group meeting, and, as in our individual session, she spent a good bit of time talking about her feelings about what had happened. Members were supportive and understanding and expressed sadness at her leaving. Kay also expressed sadness, claiming that she would really miss the support that the group had provided to her.

This was not the sort of ending that readers learn about from textbooks. It was sudden and unexpected, and it left a lot of loose ends. Yet, this sort of thing happens a lot in social work practice, especially with clients who are survivors of maltreatment, given the number of challenges they face. Rather than focusing on what we could have accomplished had we had more time, in our brief discussion of ending, Kay and I concentrated on what she did accomplish. I attempted to solidify the gains that she had made. I also wanted to help Kay say goodbye to the group and to me, since it was important for her to acknowledge the connections to others she had developed. Even when we can't engage in the sort of termination activities that are recommended, we should do what we can to help survivors end their relationships with us in ways that are affirming, counter their distortions in thinking, and enhance their self-capacities and their willingness to seek out help in the future, should they need it.

Conclusion

Social workers are in an especially good position to be helpful to clients with histories of child and youth maltreatment. The ecological perspective and its emphasis on the biological, psychological, and social influences that shape individual behavior is well suited to understanding and responding appropriately to the many challenges that survivors experience. Further, our commitment to the client and our recognition of the importance of the working relationship also is consistent with survivors' need for corrective emotional experiences in which their beliefs about self and others are challenged.

The social work profession's problem-solving focus, coupled with its strengths orientation, also is well suited to the treatment needs of clients with histories of child maltreatment. Whether our work is more short term and concentrated on current problems in living or more long term, we are helping survivors deal with the long-term impact of their maltreatment when we assist them in better managing their present-day lives.

The value base of the profession also prepares us for work with survivors of childhood trauma and reinforces a number of the practice considerations discussed previously. The values of client's right to self-determination, acceptance, and non-judgmentalism reinforce the importance of helping survivors develop their self-capacities and enhance their feelings of self-worth. The ethics of cultural competence and uniqueness of the individual sensitize us to the influence that cultural factors play in explaining survivors' reactions to their maltreatment. Informed consent and professional competence serve as guides to the selection and use of intervention techniques and assist us in ascertaining when a referral to another resource, such as a psychiatrist for medication evaluation, is warranted.

The profession's commitment to lifelong learning and recognition of the important role that supervision plays in enhancing our practice effectiveness also prepares us for working with survivors of maltreatment. There have been dramatic changes in what are considered best practices in work with survivors of child maltreatment. Therefore, we must remain cognizant of current research and theory and refine our practice accordingly. Further, given the challenges that working with survivors of maltreatment presents to us as professionals, seeking out the support and guidance of others is critical to our effectiveness and to our own well-being. In my practice, I regularly consult with colleagues about the dilemmas I face. In Kay's case, this included my reactions to the brutal nature of her rape and to her mother's cruelty towards her and the abrupt, less-than-ideal ending that occurred between Kay and me, and the feelings of frustration I experienced as a result.

Finally, our understanding of mutual aid and the skills associated with creating and facilitating groups, also enhances our ability to be helpful to survivors of child and youth maltreatment. Group membership validates and affirms members' experiences and feelings and is empowering. Membership also provides them with yet another way to confront their distortions in thinking about themselves and others.

Web resources

Administration for Children and Families, U.S. Department of Health and Human Services: information on Child Maltreatment
www.acf.hhs.gov/programs/cb/stats_research/index.htm

Centers for Disease Control and Prevention: Child Maltreatment Prevention
www.cdc.gov/ncipc/dvp/CMP/default.htm

International Society for Traumatic Stress Studies
www.istss.org/

References

Ali, T., Dunmore, E., Clark, D., & Ehlers, A. (2002). The role of negative beliefs in posttraumatic stress disorder: A comparison of assault victims and non victims. *Behavioral and Cognitive Psychotherapy, 30*, 249–257.

Alison, L., Kebbell, M., & Lewis, P. (2006). Considerations for experts in assessing the credibility of recovered memories of child sexual abuse: The importance of maintaining a case-specific focus. *Psychology, Public Policy, and Law, 12*, 419–441.

American Psychiatric Association (APA). (2000). *Diagnostic and statistical manual of mental disorders* (4th ed., text revision). Washington, DC: APA.

Arata, C., & Lindman, L. (2002). Marriage, child abuse, and sexual revictimization. *Journal of Interpersonal Violence, 17*, 953–971.

Banyard, V., Williams, L., & Siegel, J. (2001). Understanding links among childhood trauma, dissociation, and women's mental health. *American Journal of Orthopsychiatry, 71*, 311–321.

Barber, J. (1997). Hypnosis and memory: A hazardous connection. *Journal of Mental Health Counseling, 19*, 305–317.

Bernard, C. (2002). Giving voices to experiences: Parental maltreatment of Black children in the context of societal racism. *Child and Family Social Work, 7*, 239–252.

Bisson, J. (2005). Adding hypnosis to cognitive-behavioral therapy may reduce some acute stress disorder symptoms. *Evidence-based Mental Health, 8* (4), 109.

Bonanno, G. (2004). Loss, trauma, and human resilience: Have we underestimated the human capacity to thrive after extremely aversive events? *American Psychology, 59*, 20–28.

Bowman, L. (1999). Individual differences in postraumatic distress: Problems with the DSM-IV model. *Canadian Journal of Psychiatry, 44*, 21–33.

Breslau, N. (2002). Epidemiological studies of trauma, posttraumatic stress disorder, and other psychiatric disorders. *Canadian Journal of Psychiatry, 47*, 923–929.

Brown, R., Schrag, A., & Trimble, M. (2005). Dissociation, childhood interpersonal trauma, and family functioning in patients with somatization disorder. *American Journal of Psychiatry, 162*, 899–905.

Browne, A., & Finkelhor, D. (1986). Impact of child sexual abuse: A review of the literature. *Psychological Bulletin, 99*, 66–77.

Cloitre, M., Miranda, R., & Stovall-McClough, K. (2005). Beyond PTSD: Emotion regulation and interpersonal problems as predictors of functional impairment in survivors of childhood abuse. *Behavior Therapy, 36*, 119–124.

Courtois, C. (2001). Commentary on "Guided imagery and memory": Additional considerations. *Journal of Counseling Psychology, 48*, 133–135.

Davies, S. (2003). The late-life psychological effects of childhood abuse: Current medical literature. *Pediatrics, 16*, 61–65.

Department of Health and Human Services, Administration for Children, Youth, and Families (DHHS, ACYF). (2009). *Child maltreatment 2007*. Washington, DC: Government Printing Office. Retrieved from www.acf.hhs.gov/programs/cb/pubs/cm07/cm07.pdf

DeShazer, S. (1991). *Putting differences to work*. New York: Norton.

DeVries, M. (1996). Trauma in cultural perspective. In B. van der Kolk, A. McFarlane, & L. Weisaeth (eds), *Traumatic stress: the effects of overwhelming experience on mind, body, and society* (pp. 398–413). New York: Guilford Press.

Diseth, T. (2005). Dissociation in children and adolescents as reaction to trauma: An overview of conceptual issues and neurobiological factors. *Nordic Journal of Psychiatry, 59*, 79–91.

Dixon, L., Browne, K., & Hamilton-Giachritsis, C. (2005). Risk factors of parents abused as children: A mediational analysis of the intergenerational continuity of child maltreatment (Part I). *Journal of Child Psychology and Psychiatry, 46*, 47–57

Elliott, K., & Urquiza, A. (2006). Ethnicity, culture, and child maltreatment. *Journal of Social Issues, 62*, 787–809.

Feinauer, L., Hilton, H., & Callahan, E. (2003). Hardiness as a moderator of shame associated with childhood sexual abuse. *American Journal of Family Therapy, 31*, 65–78.

Fergusson, D., Horwood, L., & Woodward, L. (2000). The stability of child abuse reports: A longitudinal study of the reporting behavior of young adults. *Psychological Medicine, 30*, 529–544.

Figley, C. (1995). Compassion fatigue: Toward a new understanding of the costs of caring. In B. Stamm (ed.), *Secondary traumatic stress: Self care issues for clinicians, researchers, and educators* (pp. 3–28). Lutherville, MD: Sidran Press.

Figley, C., & Kleber, R. (1995). Beyond "victim": Secondary traumatic stress. In R. Kleber, C. Figley, & B. Gersons (eds), *Beyond trauma: Cultural and societal dynamics* (pp. 75–98). New York: Plenum.

Finkelhor, D., Ormrod, R., Turner, H., & Hamby, S. (2005). The victimization of children and youth: A comprehensive national survey. *Child Maltreatment, 10*, 5–25.

Frischholz, E. (2001). Different perspectives on informed consent and clinical hypnosis. *American Journal of Clinical Hypnosis, 43*, 323–327.

Garfield, D., & Leveroni, C. (2000). The use of self-psychological concepts in a Veterans Affairs PTSD clinic. *Bulletin of the Menninger Clinic, 64*, 344–364.

Ghetti, S., Edelstein, R., Goodman, G., Cordon, I., Quas, J., Alexander, K. et al. (2006). What can subjective forgetting tell us about memory for childhood trauma? *Memory and Cognition, 34*, 1011–1025.

Gitterman, A. (2005). Group formation: Tasks, methods, and skills. In A. Gitterman & L. Shulman (eds), *Mutual aid groups, vulnerable and resilient populations, and the life cycle* (3rd ed., pp. 73–110). New York: Columbia University Press.

Gleaves, D. (1996). The sociocognitive model of dissociative identity disorder: A reexamination of the evidence. *Psychological Bulletin, 120*, 42–59.

Goodman, G., Ghetti, S., Quas, J., Edelstein, R., Alexander, K., Redlich, A. et al. (2003). A prospective study of memory for child sexual abuse: New findings relevant to the repressed memory controversy. *Psychological Science, 14*, 113–118.

Goodwin, R., & Stein, M. (2004). Association between childhood trauma and physical disorders among adults in the United States. *Psychological Medicine, 34*, 509–520.

Green, B. (2000). Traumatic loss: Conceptual and empirical links between trauma and bereavement. *Journal of Personal and Interpersonal Loss, 5*, 1–16.

Herman, J. (1995). Complex PTSD: A syndrome in survivors of prolonged and repeated trauma. In G. Everly & J. Lating (eds), *Psychotraumatology: Key papers and core concepts in post-traumatic stress* (pp. 87–100). New York: Plenum.

Herman, J., & Harvey, M. (1997). Adult memories of childhood trauma: A naturalistic clinical study. *Journal of Traumatic Stress, 10*, 557–571.

Hunter, M. (1990). *Abused boys: The neglected victims of sexual abuse.* Lexington, MA: Lexington Books.

Janoff-Bulman, R. (1992). *Shattered assumptions: Towards a new psychology of trauma.* New York: The Free Press.

Klein, R., & Schermer, V. (2000). Introduction and overview: Creating a healing matrix. In R. Klein & V. Schermer (eds), *Group psychotherapy for psychological trauma* (pp. 3–46). New York: Guilford Press.

Kluft, R. (1997). The argument for the reality of delayed recall of trauma. In P. Appelbaum, L. Uyehara, & M. Elin (eds), *Trauma and memory: Clinical and legal controversies* (pp. 25–60). New York: Oxford University Press.

Knight, C. (2009). *Introduction to working with adult survivors of childhood trauma: Strategies and skills.* Belmont, CA: Thomson Brooks/Cole.

Korn, D., & Leeds, A. (2002). Preliminary evidence of efficacy for EMDR resource development and installation in the stabilization phase of treatment of complex posttraumatic stress disorder. *Journal of Clinical Psychology, 58*, 1465–1487.

Kurland, R., & Salmon, R. (2005). Group work versus casework in a group: Principles and implications for teaching and practice. *Social Work with Groups, 28* (3–4), 121–132.

Leviton, C., & Leviton, P. (2004). What is guided imagery? The cutting edge process in mind/body medical procedures. *Annals of the American Psychotherapy Association, 7*, 22–29.

Linehan, M. (1993). *Cognitive-behavioral treatment of borderline personality disorder.* New York: Guilford Press.

Linley, P.A., & Joseph, S. (2004). Positive change following trauma and adversity: A review. *Journal of Traumatic Stress, 17*, 11–20.

Loftus, E., Garry, M., & Feldman, A. (1994). Forgetting sexual trauma: What does it mean when 38 percent forget? *Journal of Consulting and Clinical Psychology, 62*, 1177–1181.

Marmar, C., Weiss, D., & Metzler, T. (1997). Peritraumatic dissociation and posttraumatic stress disorder. In J. Bremner & C. Marmar (eds) *Trauma, memory, and dissociation* (pp. 229–247). Washington, DC: American Psychiatric Press.

McCann, I., & Pearlman, L. (1990). *Psychological trauma and the adult survivor.* New York: Brunner/Mazel.

McMillen, J.C. (1999). Better for it: How people benefit from adversity. *Social Work, 44*, 455–467.

McNally, R. (2003). Recovering memories of trauma: A view from the laboratory. *Current directions in psychological science, 12*, 32–35.

Meeyoung, M., Farkas, K., Minnes, S., & Singer, L. (2007). Impact of childhood abuse and neglect on substance abuse and psychological distress in adulthood. *Journal of Traumatic Stress, 20*, 833–844.

Messman-Moore, T., & Brown, A. (2004). Child maltreatment and perceived family environment as risk factors for adult rape: Is child sexual abuse the most salient. *Child Abuse and Neglect, 28*, 1019–1034.

National Association of Social Workers (2008). *Code of Ethics of the National Association of Social Workers.* Retrieved from www.socialworkers.org/pubs/code/code.asp

Nemeroff, C. (2004). Neurobiological consequences of childhood trauma. *Clinical Psychiatry, 65*, 18–28.

Pearlman, L., & Saakvitne, K. (1995). *Trauma and the therapist: Countertransference and vicarious traumatization in psychotherapy with incest survivors.* New York: W.W. Norton.

Piper, A., & Merskey, H. (2004). The persistence of folly: A critical examination of dissociative identity disorder. Part I. The excesses of an improbable concept. *Canadian Journal of Psychiatry, 49*, 592–600.

Read, J., & Ross, C. (2003). Psychological trauma and psychosis: Another reason why people diagnosed with schizophrenia must be offered psychological therapies. *Journal of the American Academy of Psychoanalysis and Dynamic Psychiatry, 31*, 247–268.

Resick, P. (2001). *Stress and trauma*. Philadelphia, PA: Taylor & Francis.

Reviere, S. (1996). *Memory of childhood trauma*. New York: Guilford Press.

Rodin, G., deGroot, J., & Spivak, H. (1997). Trauma, dissociation, and somatization. In J. Bremner & C. Marmar (eds), *Trauma, memory, and dissociation* (pp. 161–178). Washington, DC: American Psychiatric Press.

Rodriguez-Srednicki, O., & Twaite, J. (2004). Understanding and reporting child abuse: Legal and psychological perspectives. Part One: Physical abuse, sexual abuse and neglect. *Journal of Psychiatry & Law, 32*, 315–359.

Runyon, D., Cox, C., Dubowitz, H., Newton, R., Upadhyaya, M., Kotch, J. et al. (2005). Describing maltreatment: Do child protective service reports and research definitions agree? *Child Abuse and Neglect, 29*, 461–477.

Saakvitne, K., Tenne, H., & Affleck, G. (1998). Exploring thriving in the context of clinical trauma theory: Constructivist self development theory. *Journal of Social Issues, 54*, 279–299.

Sachs-Ericsson, N., Blazer, D., Plant, E., & Arnow, B. (2005). Childhood sexual and physical abuse and the 1 year prevalence of medical problems in the national comorbidity survey. *Health Psychology, 24*, 32–40.

Shaffer, E., Huston, L., & Egeland, B. (2008). Identification of child maltreatment using prospective and self-report methodologies: A comparison of maltreatment incidence and relation to later psychopathology. *Child Abuse and Neglect, 32*, 682–692.

Shulman, L. (2008). *The skills of helping individuals, families, groups, and communities*. Belmont, CA: Thomson Brooks/Cole.

Solomon, E., & Heide, K. (2005). The biology of trauma. *Journal of Interpersonal Violence, 20*, 51–60.

Solomon, S., & Johnson, D. (2002). Psychosocial treatment of posttraumatic stress disorder: A practice friendly review of outcome research. *In Session: Psychotherapy in Practice, 58*, 948–959.

Spatz-Widom, C., Marmorstein, N., & Raskin-White, H. (2006). Childhood victimization and illicit drug use in middle adulthood. *Psychology of Addictive Behaviors, 20*, 394–403.

Spence, W., Mulholland, C., Lynch, G., McHugh, S., Dempster, M., & Shannon, C. (2006). Rates of childhood trauma in a sample of patients with schizophrenia as compared with a sample of patients with non-psychotic psychiatric diagnoses. *Journal of Trauma and Dissociation, 7*, 7–22.

Spitzer, C., Chevalier, C., Gillner, M., Freyberger, H., & Barnow, S. (2006). Complex posttraumatic stress disorder and child maltreatment in forensic patients. *Journal of Forensic Psychiatry and Psychology, 17*, 204–216.

Street, A., Gibson, L., & Holohan, D. (2005). Impact of childhood traumatic events, trauma-related guilt, and avoidant coping strategies on PTSD symptoms in female survivors of domestic violence. *Journal of Traumatic Stress, 18*, 245–252.

Sutton, J. (2004). Understanding dissociation and its relationship to self-injury and childhood trauma. *Counseling and Psychotherapy Journal, 15*, 24–27.

Tinnin, L., Bills, L., & Gantt, L. (2002). Simple and complex post-traumatic stress disorder: Strategies for comprehensive treatment in clinical practice. In M.B. Williams & J. Sommer (eds), *Maltreatment and trauma* (pp. 99–118). Binghampton, NY: Haworth Press.

Twaite, J., & Rodriguez-Srednicki, O. (2004). Childhood sexual and physical abuse and adult vulnerability to PTSD: The mediating effects of attachment and dissociation. *Journal of Child Sexual Abuse, 13*, 17–38.

van der Kolk, B. (1987). *Psychological trauma*. Washington, DC: American Psychiatric Press.

van der Kolk, B. (1996). The body keeps the score: Approaches to the psychobiology of posttraumatic stress disorder. In B. van der Kolk, A. McFarlane, & L. Weisaeth (eds), *Traumatic stress: The effects of overwhelming experience on mind, body, and society* (pp. 214–241). New York: Guilford Press.

van der Kolk, B., van der Hart, O., & Burbridge, J. (2002). Approaches to the treatment of PTSD. In M. Williams & J. Sommers (eds), *Simple and complex PTSD: Strategies for comprehensive treatment in clinical practice* (pp. 23–46). New York: Haworth Press.

Waldinger, R., Schulz, M., Barsky, A., & Ahern, D. (2006). Mapping the road from childhood trauma to adult somatization: The role of attachment. *Psychosomatic Medicine, 68*, 129–135.

Weichelt, S., Lutz, W., Smyth, N., & Syms, C. (2005). Integrating research and practice: A collaborative model for addressing trauma and addiction. *Stress, Trauma, and Crisis, 8*, 179–193.

Williams, M.B., & Sommer, J. (2002). Trauma in the new millennium. In M. Williams & J. Sommer (eds), *Simple and complex PTSD: Strategies for comprehensive treatment in clinical practice* (pp. xix–xxii). New York: Haworth Press.

10 Intimate partner violence and its effects

Bonnie E. Carlson

Intimate partner violence (IPV), also known as domestic violence or abuse, spousal abuse, and wife abuse, was originally identified as a social problem in the 1970s by feminist activists. Early on, the focus was on physical violence of wives, with feminists and scholars assuming that domestic violence was a manifestation of the patriarchal rights of husbands to physically abuse their wives. But over time, it became clear that it was not only married women who were abused, and concern broadened to include unmarried women – dating, separated and divorced – as well as women and men in same-sex relationships. In addition, importantly, the focus broadened to include emotional or psychological abuse in addition to physical and sexual abuse. IPV is a very costly problem for American society, estimated by the Centers for Disease Control and Prevention to be $8.3 billion annually, approximately half of which goes for "direct medical and mental health care services" (National Center for Injury Prevention and Control, 2003, p. 2).

Definitions of intimate partner violence

IPV consists of physical violence, sexual abuse or assault, and emotional or psychological abuse that is perpetrated by partners or acquaintances, including current or former spouses, cohabiting partners, boyfriends or girlfriends, and dating partners. IPV includes abuse perpetrated in heterosexual as well as same-sex intimate relationships. The majority of victims of IPV are women, and the majority of perpetrators are men who are generally well known to the victims (Browne & Williams, 1993; Tjaden & Thoennes, 1998). *Physical violence* include acts of physical aggression that are intended to harm one's partner, for example pushing, grabbing, and shoving; punching; kicking, biting, or choking; beating up; and threatening to, or using a knife or gun.

Lesser consensus exists on a definition of *emotional or psychological abuse*, as noted in a recent review (Follingstad, 2009), but most definitions would include acts intended to denigrate, isolate or dominate an intimate partner. Examples of emotional abuse include extreme jealousy and possessiveness, monitoring of behavior, or unwarranted accusations of infidelity; threats to harm the victim's family, children, friends, or pets; verbal attacks such as insults, ridicule or name calling or harassment; isolating the victim from others or threats of abandonment or infidelity; denying access to resources such as family income; and or destroying the victim's personal property (Marshall, 1999). Understanding emotional abuse (EA) or maltreatment is important, because it typically precedes and/or accompanies physical abuse (Cascardi, O'Leary, Lawrence, & Schlee, 1995; O'Leary, Malone, & Tyree, 1994), although it also occurs in the absence of other types of abuse (Loring, 1994). Regardless of how it is defined, EA is much more prevalent and harmful than physical abuse and is considered by some to occur to some degree in virtually all intimate relationships (Marshall, 1994; O'Leary & Jouriles, 1994).

Legal definitions of *rape and sexual assault* vary by state, although virtually all stipulate the victim's lack of consent for sexual acts. The criminal codes of many states no longer use the term "rape," however rape is typically understood to mean forced or coerced penetration of the vagina, mouth or anus. In contrast, sexual abuse involves either threats of sexual behavior, coerced sexual behavior that does not involve penetration, or engaging in other sexual acts with a person who cannot give consent.

Women, too, are perpetrators of partner abuse in heterosexual relationships, during adolescence as well adulthood, most commonly emotional abuse. Abuse by women continues to be a controversial issue in the domestic violence arena (Holtzworth-Munroe, 2005). A telephone survey of 420 men reported that 5.5 percent were physically victimized in their lifetime by a female partner (Reid et al., 2008). Another 2008 study of 70,000 men and women using the CDC's Behavioral Risk Factor Surveillance System instrument found that fewer than 1 percent of men reported physical abuse or unwanted sex in the previous 12 months (Breidling, Black, & Ryan, 2008). A review of 62 studies concluded that although female violence toward partners is a "common occurrence," its prevalence varies considerably across studies as a function of type of study population, how IPV was defined and measured, and timeframe (Williams, Ghandour, & Kub (2008). The authors further concluded that we know relatively little about its prevalence over time, its developmental trajectory or impact. This abuse should not be minimized, however this chapter addresses victimization of women by intimate partners and its effects on their mental health. Readers interested in this topic may wish to consult the book by Buttell and Carney (2005) as well as a special issue of the journal *Violence and Victims* (2005, volume 20, number 2).

Intimate partner violence and mental health/illness

Since the late 1970s, much research has been conducted regarding the *incidence and prevalence of IPV*. Over this period of time, prevalence estimates based on national survey studies of IPV have varied widely, depending on when the surveys were conducted and the methodologies used, including the context of the survey (e.g., a study of crime victimization versus a study of family problems). For example, Straus and Gelles (1990) found that 12 percent of women reported victimization by an intimate partner during the previous year, whereas more recent studies have found much lower past year and lifetime prevalence. Tjaden and Thoennes (2000) found that only about 1 percent of women reported victimization in the previous year, as did R.S. Thompson et al. (2006). Whereas Tjaden and Thoennes (2000), in a study of crime victimization, reported the lifetime estimate of women's physical victimization by a male partner was to be about 20 percent, the Thompson et al. (2006) group reported a 30 percent lifetime prevalence of physical abuse. Two other large-scale studies found lifetime prevalence of physical violence to be 13.3 percent (Coker et al., 2002) and 20 percent (Breidling et al., 2008). The latter group reported a 12-month prevalence of physical abuse or unwanted sex to be 1.4 percent. Methodological differences, especially in how variables are operationally defined, are likely to account for the differences found.

Sexual victimization of women by intimate partners is a common experience. National studies have found that substantial numbers of women have been raped or otherwise sexually assaulted. The National Comorbidity study reported that 9.2 percent of women had been raped and 12.3 percent had been sexually molested (Kessler, Somnega, Bromet, Hughes, & Nelson, 1995). A report based on data from a nationally representative sample of 8,000 women and 8,000 men, interviewed as part of the National Violence Against Women Survey, stated that 17.6 percent women experienced rape in their lifetime, with younger women at higher risk (Tjaden & Thoennes, 2006). Furthermore, about 75 percent of all sexual assaults against women are perpetrated by an intimate partner or someone known to the victim, with 43 percent of rapes of women perpetrated by a current or former intimate partner (Tjaden & Thoennes, 1998, 2006). Finally, Coker et al. (2002) report 4.3 percent of women reported lifetime prevalence of sexual abuse, while Breidling et al. (2008) reported a lifetime prevalence of unwanted sex to be 10.2 percent.

A 2003 study of 3,370 court-involved battered women found that 80 percent reported previous psychological abuse (Henning & Klesges, 2003). In contrast, another study found much lower prevalence estimates: 12.1 percent of women reported psychological abuse by itself, with 90 percent of the almost 18 percent who reported physical or sexual abuse also reporting psychological abuse (Coker et al., 2002). Similarly, Thompson et al. (2006) found a lifetime prevalence of psychological abuse of 35 percent. These inconsistencies illustrate the effect of using different definitions of EA or psychological abuse. Surprisingly, little research on prevalence of various types of EA or psychological abuse is available. One study found that the most common types experienced were ridicule, restriction, and jealousy (Follingstad, Rutledge, Berg, Hause, & Polek, 1990). Sackett and Saunders (1999) found jealous control to be the most common form, followed by ridicule. Tolman (1989) reported the most frequently endorsed items from the Psychological Maltreatment of Women Inventory to be instances of verbal abuse such as yelling, showing insensitivity to feelings and not allowing the woman to talk about feelings, and bringing up the past with the intention of hurting. Henning and Klesges (2003) found the most common forms of EA were yelling, name-calling, and jealousy, all reported by more than half of those women reporting EA.

Essentially, over the course of their lifetimes, male partners victimize substantial numbers of women. This includes emotional or psychological abuse, physical abuse or assault, and sexual abuse or assault. IPV is not caused by a single factor. Three decades of research have found that there are *multiple and complex factors that elevate the risk* for IPV. The ecological framework is a useful conceptualization to organize these diverse factors that can be found to reside at the individual level, in perpetrators as well as victims, in relationships and family systems, at the community level, and in society as a whole (Gitterman, 2008).

We know a good deal about individual-level risk factors pertaining to abusers. Although women do use violence in intimate relationships, *male gender* is generally acknowledged to be an important risk factor for IPV. For example, Briedling et al. (2008) found that women were twice as likely as men to be victimized physically or sexually by an intimate partner over the course of their lifetimes. Men who perpetrate physical, sexual, and emotional abuse are disproportionately likely to be young, unemployed, and have low income (e.g., Bachman & Saltzman, 1995; Greenfeld et al., 1998; Straus & Gelles, 1986; Thompson et al., 2006; Tjaden & Thoennes, 1998). Another major risk factor is abuse of alcohol and drugs, which is related to physical violence (e.g., Aldarondo & Kantor, 1997; Caetano, McGrath, Ramisetty-Mikler, & Field, 2005; Leonard & Senchak, 1996; Testa, 2004) as well as sexual assault (Ullman, Karabatsos, & Koss, 1999). Some studies have found exposure to violence in one's family of origin, such as receiving violent discipline, being physically abused by caregivers, or witnessing violence between parents can serve as risk factors for perpetration of adult partner violence (e.g., Aldarondo & Kantor, 1997; Leonard & Senchak, 1996).

Although researchers have attempted to isolate personality characteristics or traits that increase the risk of perpetrating IPV, no single male personality type has been found to distinguish abusive men from men who do not sexually or physically abuse women. However, the following personality risk markers for male partner abuse were identified in a research review: emotional dependence and insecurity; low self-esteem, empathy and impulse control; poor communication and social skills; aggressive, narcissistic and antisocial personality types; and anxiety and depression (Kaufman Kantor & Jasinski, 1998). Other research has suggested that there may be at least two different subtypes of abusive men, one that is violent only toward a romantic partner and another that is violent toward people in general (Holtzworth-Munroe & Stuart, 1994). Because emotional or psychological abuse is so strongly associated with physical abuse (O'Leary, Malone, & Tyree, 1994), the use of EA can also be considered a risk factor for IPV.

Patterns have also been identified among *victims* of IPV. Low-income women are more likely to be victimized by intimate partners, and economic dependency on the abuser can also be a barrier to women being able to terminate an abusive relationship (e.g., Horton & Johnson, 1993; Sullivan, Campbell, Angelique, Eby, & Davidson, 1994; Thompson et al., 2006). Previous victimization is also a risk factor. Numerous studies have found that victimization as a child or adolescent, such as witnessing spousal abuse and being the direct recipient of physical and/or sexual abuse, greatly increases the risk for being sexually or physically assaulted by a partner (e.g., Gidycz & Koss, 1991; Maker, Kemmelmeier, & Peterson, 1998; Thompson et al., 2006; Weaver, Kilpatrick, Resnick, Best, & Saunders, 1997; Whitfield, Anda, Dube, & Felitti, 2003). Another risk factor for IPV victimization is alcohol or drug abuse and physical (Hien & Ruglass, 2009; Hilbert, Kolia, & VanLeeuwen, 1997; Plichta, 1996). Substance abuse may actually be both a cause and an effect of IPV, affecting young women and women of color in particular (Kilpatrick, Acierno, Resnick, Saunders, & Best, 1997).

Another factor whose effects may be bidirectional – both cause and effect – is social isolation which is related to victimization and has been found to occur both before and after partner violence (Nielsen, Endo, & Ellington, 1992). Abusive men are freer to initiate abuse and continue to abuse women who lack social networks. Much anecdotal evidence indicates that abusive men often control their partners by cutting them off from contact with significant others such as family members or friends. Thus, having a strong social network of supporters may be protective by reducing the risk of becoming abused, as well as buffering women from the adverse effects of being abused. As a consequence of abuse, social isolation may occur as abused women retreat from contact with others due to shame and stigma or others withdraw in frustration if a woman does not leave the abusive relationship or out of fear of the abuser.

At the level of the *couple*, two factors have been identified as increasing risk for IPV. First, relationship type is a risk factor: separated and cohabiting couples are at greatly increased risk for partner violence compared to married or dating couples (e.g., Bachman & Saltzman, 1995). Second, a review concluded that poor communication and social skills were risk factors for partner violence (Kaufman Kantor & Jasinski, 1998).

Factors at the *community level* have been found to increase risk for IPV. Urban areas have been found to have the highest rates of IPV (Greenfeld et al., 1998). In addition, the lack of services to address partner violence for either perpetrators or victims can be a risk factor. For example, rural areas, with smaller populations and fewer social services in general, may lack specialized services such as batterer intervention programs for abusive men or domestic violence shelters that allow women to terminative abusive relationships if they wish to (Sudderth, 2006).

Risk factors for IPV also exist at the *sociocultural level*. Such risk factors establish a broad context that has made many forms of IPV socially acceptable historically. Widespread agreement exists that sexism and gender-role stereotyping have operated as risk factors for women's victimization by intimate partners (Dobash & Dobash, 1979; Stark & Flitcraft, 1996). For example, rates of marital violence are highest in states where there is the most economic, educational, political, and legal inequality (Yllo & Straus, 1990). Another manifestation of sexism is the social stigma that victims of sexual assault and partner violence continue to feel, although the blame associated with being a victim of rape seems to be diminishing. For example, through the 1980s varying segments of the population held abused women at least partially if not completely responsible for the abuse they experienced (e.g., Ewing & Aubrey,

1987). Even in the twenty-first century, however, such attitudes and beliefs persist to some extent. For example, in a public opinion survey of New York state adults, almost one-quarter thought that some women who are abused secretly want to be treated that way, and almost half (46 percent) agreed with the statement that some violence is caused by the way women treat men (Carlson & Worden, 2005). Currently, many abused women feel criticized for not immediately terminating an abusive relationship, which is well supported in the public opinion research, where almost two-thirds believed that "most women could find a way to get out of an abusive relationship if they really wanted to" (Carlson & Worden, 2005, p. 1227). So the content of victim blaming appears to have shifted from "it's your fault you are being abused" to "it's your fault you are putting up with it," with little understanding of what is really involved in ending an abusive relationship.

The extent to which race and ethnicity serve as risk factors for IPV remains unclear. Some research indicates that Black and American Indian women experience higher rates of physical violence compared to white women (e.g., Tjaden & Thoennes, 1998; Zlotnick, Kohn, Peterson, & Pearlstein, 1998). In contrast, other studies have reported that white women have higher IPV rates as compared to Latinas (Sorenson, 1996). Yet other studies have failed to find racial/ethnic differences in IPV rates or have found higher rates for Latinos compared to other groups (Straus & Smith, 1990). Because there are important differences across ethnic/racial groups in previously discussed risk factors for partner violence such as income and place of residence (urban versus rural), research on the prevalence of IPV by racial/ethnic group must control for such factors so that any relationships found are not confounded by these other risk factors. Other aspects of culture are discussed below. Hispanics have become the largest U.S. ethnic minority group. Although there is much intergroup diversity within the Latino population, the majority (59 percent) come from Mexico (U.S. Census Bureau, 2004). Research on the prevalence of IPV in the *Latino population* is mixed regarding whether rates are higher, lower, or the similar to those of whites or other ethnic groups (Straus & Smith, 1990; Tjaden & Thoennes, 1998). It should be noted that Latinos as a group possess several factors that would elevate the risk of IPV, including a younger age structure than other groups, lower educational attainment, lower socioeconomic status, and high levels of exposure to violence in the home as children (Caetano, Shafer, Clark, Cunradi, & Raspberry, 2000; West, Kaufman Kantor, & Jasinski, 1998). In addition, the heavy drinking patterns of some Latino men place their female partners at higher risk for victimization (Caetano et al., 2000). Several core values are related to the risk for IPV as well as abused Latinas' options for extricating themselves from violent and abusive relationships. Latino culture is more collectivist than individualistic (Marin & Marin, 1991), and the value of *familismo* indicates that the family unit is tremendously important (Flores-Ortiz, 1993). Traditional Latino family structure is patriarchal, with gender roles rigidly prescribed. *Machismo* calls for men to be family protectors and breadwinners, but also honorable and courageous, whereas women should be the maintainers of family life and long-suffering, as prescribed by *marianismo* (Comas-Diaz, 1993). Their traditional Latino gender role expectations can be a risk factor for IPV. The values of *respeto* and *simpatia*, respectively, direct people to be deferent to authority and to maintain harmonious interpersonal relations (Comas-Diaz, 1993). Thus, family members, including wives, should defer to men, reinforcing the power differential between husbands and wives, and possibly contributing to IPV.

With such a substantial subgroup of Latinos born outside the United States, 38 percent, immigration and the acculturation issues create stress and may also increase the risk of partner violence, especially where gender roles are changing or if the female partner is able to obtain employment when the male partner cannot. Latinas have been said to encounter special challenges in coping with domestic violence such as immigration-related stress, acculturation issues, legal and language barriers, and financial strains (Mattson & Rodriguez, 1999). Both immigrants and refugees also often must deal with isolation from supportive family networks, which can be a risk factor for abuse or keep abused Latinas entrapped in abusive relationships (Ramos, Carlson, & Kulkarni, 2010). Undocumented status can increase the risk for domestic violence, with the abuser using threats of deportation to control the victims; fear of deportation can also serve as a major barrier to getting protection from law enforcement and assistance from some social agencies (Murdaugh, Hunt, Sowell, & Santana, 2004). Another challenge for abused Latinas is the cultural reluctance to seek help outside the family. Thus, agencies must demonstrate practice approaches that are sensitive to Latino culture in order for victims to utilize such services.

The literature is equivocal on whether *Black* women are at higher risk for violent victimization by male partners than women of other ethnicities (Heron, Twomey, Jacobs, & Kaslow, 1997). National studies have indicated lifetime prevalence estimates for IPV ranging from 11 percent (Greenfeld et al., 1998) to 26 percent (Tjaden & Thoennes, 1998). Regarding sexual victimization, the National Violence Against Women Survey found lifetime sexual assault rate of 19 percent for black women compared to 18 percent for white women (Tjaden & Thoennes, 1998). Thus, substantial numbers of African American women are physically and sexually victimized by romantic partners.

Regardless of prevalence estimates, it is clear that there are unique issues for black women in terms of IPV. For example, the negative societal stereotypes of black women as being oversexualized, as "sexual temptresses" (Asbury, 1987; Neville & Pugh, 1997), increase their risk for sexual victimization. On the other hand, more positive stereotypes of black women as strong and independent, able to handle things on their own, can nevertheless be barriers to seeking help for abuse if it occurs (Asbury, 1987; Moss, Pitula, Campbell, & Halstead, 1997). Growing up in poverty may exposure black children to violence of all kinds at an early age, leading them to see violence as normative (Asbury, 1987).

A history of oppression, racism, and discrimination strains the relationships of black couples, and the poor treatment of African American men by the American criminal justice system has resulted in reluctance by black female victims to access law enforcement when they are victimized by partners (Heron et al., 1997; Moss et al., 1997; Neville & Pugh, 1997). The limited opportunities for black men to be successful in the breadwinner role are viewed as particularly stressful for black couples and families (Barnes, 1999). The history of institutionalized racism and its impact on the self-image of black men is also seen by many as a major factor in why black men abuse their female partners (Brice-Baker, 1996). Black men's reduced access to important resources such as income and power is viewed as contributing to the use of violence against female partners by some as a compensatory resource (Barnes, 1999). The relative scarcity of black men, fueled by the large numbers in the custody of the criminal justice system, may make African American women especially reluctant to end abusive relationships because of the relatively poor prospects of finding another nonviolent relationship (Asbury, 1987; Barnes, 1999). Contacting the authorities may be perceived as being disloyal to the African American community (Neville & Pugh, 1997), effectively limiting black victims' ability to access help. The higher poverty rates of African Americans may be especially problematic for black women trying to extricate themselves from abusive relationships (Brice-Baker, 1996; Heron et al., 1997). African American women also have strengths that have facilitated their coping with violence and abuse, in particular seeking emotional support from other women and the black community and the use of spirituality (Few & Bell-Scott, 2002).

Limited research examines the consequences of abuse for black women in particular, but the few studies suggest that the mental health effects in particular are quite similar. A small qualitative study of black college students who had ended psychologically abusive relationships found that the survivors experienced depression, suicidal thoughts, and social isolation

(Few & Bell-Scott, 2002). Ramos, Carlson, and McNutt (2004), studying an HMO sample of 584 women, compared white and black experiencing seven types of abuse across the lifespan, including five types of adult abuse: recent (past year) emotional, recent physical, recent sexual, past physical, and past sexual. Black women were more likely than white to report recent emotional abuse (32 percent versus 19 percent), but equally likely to report the other types of abuse. For both black and white women, the more types of abuse reported over the lifespan, the greater the likelihood of reporting both depression and anxiety. Interestingly, at every abuse level, including no lifetime abuse at all, black women were more likely to report symptoms of depression and anxiety, compared to white women (Ramos et al., 2004).

IPV has been described as an epidemic in the *Asian* American immigrant community (Lee & Hadeed, 2009). Asian Americans are a diverse and heterogeneous community, composed of individuals and families who were born here or have resided here for many years as well as immigrants from numerous countries in East Asia (Japan, China (including Hong Kong), Korea, and Taiwan), South Asia (India, Pakistan, Bangladesh, Nepal, and Sri Lanka), as well as Southeast Asia (Vietnam, Malaysia, Singapore, Cambodia, Laos, Myanmar, Indonesia and the Philippines). The circumstances under which these groups have arrived in the United States are very different, and immigrants from these nations have come with different languages, customs, belief systems, food preferences, religions, and educational preparations. Although some have arrived at our shores as refugees (e.g., Cambodians), others have immigrated with higher education and excellent prospects for employment. However, there are some commonalities that are important to the victimization of women. Most Asian Americans come from cultures that are patriarchal and approve or accept aggression toward wives (Lee & Hadeed, 2009). Asian cultures also tend to espouse very traditional and rigid gender role norms that specify different roles for men and women and oftentimes view women as inferior to men. Women are often expected to be obedient and long suffering. Finally, maintenance of family harmony and family loyalty are said to be extremely important, making it very difficult for abused women to leave violent relationships (Lee & Hadeed, 2009). Several factors were identified in a recent review of research as being risk factors for abuse in Asian American immigrants in particular, beyond patriarchal norms: acculturation stress, status inconsistency, extremely high rates of physical punishment in childhood, conflict with in-laws, and alcohol abuse by males, especially in Korean and Chinese couples (Lee & Hadeed, 2009).

Native Americans comprise an extremely diverse community, spread all across the United States. Hundreds of federally recognized tribes exist, speaking many different tribal languages, and modern-day Indians live on reservations as well as in urban communities. Most prevalence research on IPV that has included Native Americans has found that American Indians report the highest levels of domestic violence. For example, the National Violence Against Women Survey found that 31 percent of American Indian women reported lifetime IPV victimization, compared to 21 percent of white women and Latinas, 26 percent of Black women, and 13 percent of Asian American women (Tjaden & Thoennes, 2000). Rates of sexual victimization were similarly higher for Native American women: 34 percent reported rape or attempted rape in their lifetime, double or triple the rate of other ethnic groups (Tjaden & Thoennes, 2000). Almost two-thirds of native women have experienced physical or sexual abuse in their lifetimes.

Several factors known to elevate risk for IPV are particularly problematic in American Indian communities, particularly unemployment, very low educational attainment, extreme poverty and alcohol abuse (Bohn, 1993; Robin, Chester, & Rasmussen, 1998). Robin et al. (1998) reported that heavy alcohol use by both parties was associated with the majority of IPV incidents they studied; 89 percent of the males and 57 percent of the females they studied reported lifetime rates of alcohol dependence or abuse. Both of these endemic problems are related to the institutional oppression perpetrated by Europeans and Americans, devastating native tribes. Two especially noteworthy aspects of this oppression were the seizure of lands rightfully owned by Native Americans and the forced removal from their families and placement of thousands of Indian children in boarding schools, wreaking havoc with family structure in affected Indian communities (Wahab & Olson, 2004). Abuse experienced as children is another potent risk factor for American Indian IPV (Bohn, 1993). Other issues include low reporting of IPV and rampant mistrust of white authorities, and jurisdictional issues in law enforcement between tribal communities and the states, complicating the problem of obtaining assistance when IPV occurs. Empowerment-based approaches to intervention with IPV have been recommended, as well as approaches that build and strengthen Native American communities, such as job creation (Wahab & Olson, 2004).

Although there is less research about abuse in *same-sex relationships*, it appears that lesbians (and gay men) are about as likely to be abused by a romantic partner as are heterosexual women. As is the case with women in heterosexual relationships, abuse can be physical, emotional, and/or sexual. There are many similarities in abuse of women in lesbian relation-ships, compared to women abused by male intimate partners, but there are also important differences. Similarities include stigma, self-blame, guilt and shame about being abused (Lie & Gentlewarrier, 1991; Renzetti, 1988); associated substance abuse (Farley, 1996; Renzetti, 1992); difficulty ending the abuse or extricating oneself from the relationship (Patzel, 2006); and dependency and power dynamics (Lockhart, White, Causby, & Isaac, 1994). But many differ-ences also exist. For example, people in same-sex relationships face a special form of abuse, namely being "outed" by a partner, that is, revealing his or her partner's sexual orientation without consent to family or employers (Elliott, 1996; West, 1998). Homophobia and internalized homophobia are other important differences. Abused lesbians of color have been said to be at "triple jeopardy" as they experience oppression from three sources: by being abused, by being lesbian, and by being a woman of color (Kanuha, 1990).

Gay men and lesbians face special challenges in disclosing abuse and obtaining help to address abuse due to homophobia and discrimination as well as a dearth of services sensitive to their special needs. Almost every published study on same-sex IPV discusses the special difficulties abused lesbians and gay men face in getting help. For example, lesbians in particular may be disbelieved due to the "myth of a lesbian utopia" or the abuse they report may be minimized (just a catfight between girls) (Hassouneh & Glass, 2008). Few agencies exist specifically dedicated to providing services to abused lesbians or gay men (Helfrich & Simpson, 2006). Although there are about 1,500 programs nationally providing shelter to abused women, none provides shelter exclusively to lesbians. Thus, seeking help from the formal service system may require disclosing one's sexual orientation, with potentially adverse consequences.

Based on the National Health Interview study, it is estimated that 15 percent of American women have one or more disabilities (LaPlant & Carlson, 1996). Research on IPV victimization among *women with disabilities*, physical and/or cognitive, is sparse, although it has been described as a "problem of crisis proportions" (Nosek, Howland, & Hughes, 2001a). A consensus has emerged that prevalence of physical, emotional, and sexual abuse are at least as common among women with disabilities as it is among able-bodied women (Chang et al., 2003; Curry, Hassouneh-Phillips, & Johnston-Silverberg, 2001; Hassouneh-Phillips & Curry, 2002; Milberger, Israel, LeRoy, Martin, Potter, & Patchak-Schuster, 2003). There are good reasons to think that women with disabilities are at even greater risk of abuse due to cultural devaluation of people with disabilities as well as long-term dependency on others, in particular family members, for care (Nosek et al., 2001a). Furthermore, there are disability-specific forms of abuse, such as withholding assistive devices, removing a wheelchair's battery, or refusing to assist with toileting or personal hygiene (Hassouneh-Phillips & Curry, 2002; Nosek, Foley, Hughes, & Howland, 2001b) that do not exist for women without disabilities.

Only one national survey of lifetime abuse comparing women with and without disabilities on abuse histories has been performed. The researchers found comparable levels of lifetime physical, emotional and sexual abuse: 62 percent. However, women with disabilities reported abuse of longer duration (Nosek et al., 2001b). It was found that "emotional, physical and sexual abuse are rooted in the need for perpetrators to exert power and control over victims" (Nosek et al., 2001b, p. 186), as is the case with non-disabled abused women. In an exploratory study using qualitative methods, Carlson (1998) interviewed 11 women with mental retardation and 19 key informants who were service providers in either the developmental disabilities or domestic violence field in regard to adult physical, emotional, and sexual abuse. All 11 women reported emotional abuse, 7 reported sexual abuse and 7 reported physical abuse. The key informants concurred that IPV was prevalent among women with mental retardation and that several factors made them especially vulnerable to being abused, including high levels of dependency on others for care and having low self-esteem, and not being familiar with resources to obtain help (Carlson, 1998).

Summarizing the very limited existing research, Hassouneh-Phillips and Curry (2002) concluded that abuse of women with disabilities tends to occur at home and is perpetrated by men, similar to the abuse of non-disabled women. The fact that women with disabilities are likely to have lower educational attainment as well as lower rates of labor force participation increases their isolation and decreases their involvement with people outside the home, increasing their vulnerability to abuse (Curry et al., 2001; Nosek et al., 2001b). In addition, certain disabilities involve cognitive impairments (e.g., traumatic brain injury) that may interfere with recognition of abuse and make seeking help or ending an abusive relationship especially challenging (Nosek et al., 2001b). Due to discrimination against women with disabilities and their marginalized status, some women feel so fortunate to have any relationship at all that they fail to label what is happening to them as abuse or are reluctant to challenge the abuse or end the relationship, fearing that they will never find another (Carlson, 1998; Curry et al., 2001). Such factors also dramatically increase the barriers to leaving an abusive relationship.

Help-seeking is especially challenging for abused women with disabilities. Some lack the physical ability to escape due to their disability (Milberger et al., 2003). Some are reluctant to report abuse due to their dependency on the abusers for their daily care; leaving may not represent a move toward greater independence as it does for non-disabled women but rather a move toward institutionalized care if the abuser has been their personal care provider (Curry et al., 2001). Few domestic violence programs are fully accessible, and even if they are, staff are seldom trained to assist women with physical or cognitive limitations. Staff who are lacking in expertise to assist clients with daily self-care may be uncomfortable serving women with special cognitive or physical needs.

Beginning in the 1980s, researchers began to realize that partner violence was not confined to married women or adult women but also occurred in college students. Shortly thereafter, *dating violence* in high school and middle school students was uncovered. Based on research conducted in the 1980s and 1990s, about one-third of college females were found to have experienced sexual violence in a dating relationship (Murray & Kardatzke, 2007). Research conducted in the 1990s revealed that dating violence occurs in the relationships of about one-third of high school students (Foshee et al., 1996; Jezl, Molidor & Wright, 1996; Molidor & Tolman, 1998). For example, O'Keefe (1997) reported that 43 percent of the female high school students she sampled from an ethnically diverse high school in southern California and 39 percent of the males reported perpetrating violence toward a dating partner. In a study of younger adolescents, predominantly white eighth graders in North Carolina, Foshee (1996) reported that over one-third of those who had dated reported being the victim of violence at the hands of a date, 37 percent of girls and 39 percent of boys. Substantially lower percentages admitted to inflicting violence on a dating partner, significantly more girls (28 percent) than boys (15 percent); girls, however, were more likely to say they had used violence in self-defense. Not surprisingly, boys were more likely to report perpetration of sexual violence (4.5 percent) compared to girls (1.2 percent) (Foshee et al., 1996). The most recent national data come from the 2003 Youth Risk Behavior Survey of more than 15,000 14–17-year-olds, ninth through twelfth graders. Researchers found that 9 percent of adolescents were victimized by an intimate partner during the prior year (Eaton, Davis, Barrios, Brenner, & Noonan, 2007). Most studies of dating violence find a very high level of bidirectional violence; that is, in most cases where there is violence, both partners are inflicting and sustaining it against each other (e.g., O'Keefe, 1997). Consistent with other large-scale studies, Eaton et al. (2007) found that girls' dating violence victimization was associated with smoking, drug and alcohol use, early sexual activity, and more sexual partners.

Emotional or psychological abuse has rarely been studied in adolescents, although White and Koss (1991) found it to be extremely prevalent in the dating relationships of college students: 81 percent of males admitted to perpetrating it and sustaining it, 87 percent of women had used it and been victimized by it. Foshee (1996) found emotional manipulation to be the most common type of psychological abuse reported by both boys and girls. Girls reported significantly more monitoring and emotional manipulation by their dating partners than boys, interestingly they also reported engaging in more emotional manipulation than did the boys (Foshee, 1996).

What motivates violence in young people who are not legally connected? In the O'Keefe (1997) study, male motivations for violence included anger, jealousy and control of the female partner whereas female motivations included anger, self-defense and jealousy. Clearly some dating violence is motivated by self-defense, perhaps half of girls' violence toward boys (Foshee et al., 1996) as well as retaliation for perceived wrongs such as infidelity. Other risk factors include seriousness of the relationship (Laner & Thompson, 1982; Stets & Pirog-Good, 1987). One review concluded that there was an association between substance use and dating violence (Lewis & Fremouw, 2001). A family history of exposure to family violence, child abuse or witnessing abuse between one's parents has also been identified as a risk factor (Foo & Margolin, 1995).

Initially, the perception was that injuries rarely occurred in cases of dating violence, largely because most of the aggression consisted of acts of minor violence such as pushing, slapping and shoving. However, Foshee (1996) found that 70 percent of the eighth grade girls who had sustained dating violence had been injured, significantly higher than the males who reported injuries (52 percent); almost 9 percent of the female victims had been seen in the emergency room for their injuries. It appears that very few adolescents involved in violent dating relationships seek help, informal or formal (Black, Tolman, Callahan, Saunders, & Weisz, 2008). Most adolescents who have experienced dating violence do not consult with adults about their experiences, typically because they expect criticism (e.g., Molidor & Tolman, 1998), but a small-scale study of high school students suggests that they may talk with a peer about it, especially girls (Black et al., 2008).

IPV can result in a wide range of adverse health and mental health consequences. Although not all female victims of IPV report adverse consequences, some do report that they experience several different types of mental health consequences. Self-blame, shame, and guilt are common in the aftermath of abuse. For many women, cessation of the abuse is sufficient for emotional distress to subside, but other victims may require professional intervention, even after an abusive relationship has ended, for well-being to resume (e. g., Zlotnick, Johnson, & Kohn, 2006).

One obvious *physical health consequence* is physical injury. IPV is one of the most common causes of injury to women in both population-based research (e.g., Coker et al., 2002) as well as research conducted in health settings such as emergency departments. For example, an early study based on a national sample found that 7.3 percent of severely physically abused women saw a doctor (Stets & Straus, 1990). One large, national study found that 42 percent of physical assault victims reported injuries, with minor injuries such as scratches and bruises being the most common (Tjaden & Thoennes, 2000). However, other adverse health consequences occur more often than do injuries. Abused women, compared to non-abused women, tend to experience poorer overall physical health and report more health problems and symptoms (e.g., McCauley et al., 1995). Some examples are gastrointestinal disorders, chronic pain, fatigue, dizziness, appetite problems, and gynecological problems such as sexually transmitted diseases (Carlson, 2007).

A broad range of *mental health* symptoms and problems have been identified in the aftermath of physical, emotional, and sexual abuse, including depression, PTSD, other forms of anxiety, and substance abuse (e.g., Campbell, Sullivan, & Davidson, 1995; Carlson, McNutt, & Choi, 2003; Gelles & Straus, 1990; Kilpatrick et al., 1997; Saunders, 1994). For example, a New Zealand study using the Diagnostic Interview Schedule to obtain DSM-III-R diagnoses of 15 mental disorders found that more than half of abused women met diagnostic criteria for at least one disorder in contrast to 38 percent of non-victims (Danielson, Moffitt, Caspi, & Silva, 1998). A study of 30 women staying in a domestic violence shelter found that although more than half the women studied manifested no mental disorders, the most common disorders in the remainder were PTSD (47 percent), major depressive disorder (37 percent), adjustment disorder (14 percent), personality disorders (10 percent), and substance abuse (6.7 percent) (West, Fernandez, Hillard, Schoof, & Parks, 1990). However, the most common adverse mental health consequence of IPV is probably generalized emotional distress not reaching the threshold of a diagnosable mental disorder.

Depression may well be the most commonly identified post-abuse mental health symptom, identified in a large number of small and large, clinical and population-based studies (Campbell, Kub, Belknap, & Templin, 1997; Cascardi & O'Leary, 1992; Danielson et al., 1998; Follingstad, Brennan, Hause, Polek, & Rutledge, 1991; Gelles & Harrop, 1988; Gerber, Leiter, Hermann, & Bor, 2005; McCauley, Kern, Kolodner, Derogatis, & Bass, 1998; Nicolaidis, Curry, McFarland, & Gerrity, 2004; Plichta, 1992; Saunders, Hamberger, & Hovey, 1993; Stets & Straus, 1990; Sutherland, Bybee, & Sullivan, 1998; Zink, Fisher, Regan, & Pabst, 2005; Zlotnick et al., 2006). A related concern is suicidal intent or behavior related to abuse history. One review concluded that whereas emotional abuse may be associated with depressive symptoms, research does not support emotional abuse leading to "clinically relevant levels of depression" (Follingstad, 2009, p. 283).

Alcohol and illegal drug abuse have been described as the second most common mental health problem observed in abused women (Abbott, Johnson, Koziol-McLain, & Lowenstein, 1995; Campbell, 2002; Danielson et al., 1998; Gerber et al., 2005; Kilpatrick et al., 1997; McCauley et al., 1998; Plichta, 1992). Some have questioned the causal order of IPV and substance use disorders. Substance abuse could precede the IPV, could be caused by the abuse, or could be both risk factor and effect, as was found by Kilpatrick et al. (1997). If substance use disorders follow partner violence, survivors could be self-medicating, abuse-related stress or other abused-related symptoms such as depression or PTSD. It is noteworthy that not all studies have found associations between substance abuse and IPA (e.g., Zlotnick et al. 2006).

Anxiety disorders are also associated with IPV, most commonly PTSD. Numerous studies have found a correlation between domestic violence and PTSD (e.g., Cascardi et al., 1995; McFarlane, Groff, O'Brien, & Watson, 2005; Silva, McFarlane, Soeken, Parker, & Reel, 1997) and Golding's (1999) meta-analysis of 11 studies has also documented an association. Golding (1999) concluded that the prevalence of PTSD in abused women was almost four times higher than in non-abused women, and another review of partner violence and PTSD concluded that 31 percent to 84 percent of women victimized by intimate partners develop PTSD (Jones, Hughes, & Unterstaller, 2001). A weakness of many studies of PTSD in abused women is that they have studied only help-seeking women, such as those receiving services from a domestic violence shelter, and such women represent a minority of all abused women. Women who seek help tend to be more severely abused; abuse severity, in particular how life threatening the experience is, has been shown to be predictive of PTSD intensity (Jones et al., 2001). However, it is not only seriously life threatening abuse that has been found to be associated with post-traumatic stress symptoms. Interestingly, even emotional abuse by itself has been associated with PTSD symptoms (Cascardi & O'Leary, 1992), and one study found psychological abuse rather than physical abuse predicted both PTSD and relationship termination (Arias & Pape, 1999). However, one review concluded that more research is needed on the extent to which psychological abuse leads to anxiety (Follingstad, 2009).

Several factors have been found to moderate the effects of partner abuse on mental health symptomatology. For example, abuse that is more long-lasting, severe, and frequent is associated with more symptoms (Follingstad et al., 1991; McCauley et al., 1998; Stets & Straus, 1990). We also know that multiple victimization experiences, especially adult victimization coupled with childhood physical or sexual abuse, significantly increase the risk for PTSD (e.g., Astin, Lawrence, & Foy, 1993; Astin, Ogland-Hand, Coleman, & Foy, 1995; Carlson, McNutt, & Choi, 2003; Cascardi et al., 1995; Follette, Polusny, Bechtel, & Naugle, 1996; Mullen, Martin, Anderson, Romans, & Herbison, 1996). This is important because childhood victimization by a family member increases the risk of partner violence victimization in adulthood, and many, maybe most, abused women also experienced interpersonal victimization as children (e.g., Astin et al., 1995; Briere, 1988; Chu, 1992; Gilbert, El-Bassel, Schilling, & Friedman, 1997; Weaver et al., 1997). For example, Carlson et al. (2003), studying 557 women from a health maintenance organization, found that recent abuse was associated with symptoms of both anxiety and depression, but past adult abuse and child abuse were also independently associated with anxiety, even when economic hardship was controlled.

Other anxiety diagnoses and symptoms have also been found to be associated with IPV in both population-based (e.g., Carlson et al., 2003; Follingstad et al., 1991; Plichta, 1992) and clinical samples (Gerber et al., 2005; McCauley et al., 1995; Sutherland et al., 1998). This is not surprising given numerous additional studies that have documented the stressfulness of partner abuse for women (e.g., Gelles & Harrop, 1988).

Consequences of sexual victimization by an intimate partner are quite similar to those of physical abuse. Short-term reactions commonly include shock and disbelief, emotional numbing, extreme fear, self-blame and a sense of being helpless (Goodman, Koss, & Russo, 1993). Self-blame and shame are not uncommon. Longer term reactions include PTSD and other anxiety disorders, depression and suicidality, substance abuse, sexual dysfunction and relationship difficulties (e.g., Goodman et al., 1993; Kilpatrick, Edmunds, and Seymour, 1992; Resick, 1993). One study found that 43 percent of sexual assault victims reported depression after the assault and 40 percent suffered from anxiety (Sorenson & Siegel, 1992). A national study found that 13 percent of rape victims had attempted suicide (Kilpatrick et al., 1992). Although symptoms for many victims begin to subside after about three months, for a subset of women painful symptoms can persist long term (Resick, 1993).

*Psychological or emotional abu*se, too, is associated with a variety of adverse mental health effects such as lowered self-esteem and depression (Follingstad et al., 1991; O'Leary, 1999; Sackett & Saunders, 1999). Interestingly, women who have experienced both physical and emotional abuse have reported that the emotional abuse is more harmful (Follingstad et al., 1990). As noted above, emotional abuse has also been associated with PTSD.

An issue that is of interest is how and why does IPV lead to these painful consequences and why do some abused women appear to be immune to adverse mental health consequences? Several factors may help to explain why some women appear to be relatively symptom-free, while others develop severe mental health problems. First, severity and duration of exposure to abuse matter. The more severe the abuse is, the greater the likelihood of experiencing symptoms (Carlson et al., 2003; Gelles & Harrop, 1988; Golding, 1999). Also, a history of previous adult or child victimization increases the risk for anxiety and depression, as discussed above. Carlson et al. (2003), using a stratified analysis, found that a higher cumulative lifetime abuse score that took into account childhood and adult abuse and their severity predicted the prevalence of both anxiety and depression.

Another potentially important factor that may influence whether abused women manifest mental health symptoms and their severity is the presence of protective factors. Although relatively little research has identified protective factors that make adults resilient in the face of multiple risks, the role of social support has been studied as a possible protective factor against the development of depression in abused women. Studies have found that abused women's perceptions of social support may directly affect their mental health, moderate their sense of well-being and mental health (Arias, Lyons, & Street, 1997; Tan, Basta, Sullivan, & Davidson, 1995), or mediate the relationship between abuse and mental health (Thompson, Kaslow, Lang, & Kingree, 2000). Studies of abused women's social support have yielded mixed findings. Some show that abused women have lower social support compared to non-abused women (e.g., Mitchell & Hodson, 1983; Nurius, Furrey, & Berliner, 1992; Thompson et al., 2000), whereas others have found similar levels of support (Carlson, McNutt, Choi, & Rose, 2002; Zlotnick et al., 1998). Social support may have a buffering effect by enhancing self-esteem and providing a confidant with whom to discuss concerns. One study found that abused women reporting symptoms of depression and anxiety were less likely to report all seven of the protective factors studied: partner support, non-partner support, good health, high self-esteem, advanced education, employment, and absence of economic hardship (Carlson et al., 2002). Furthermore, our analysis suggested that "at virtually every level of lifetime abuse, women with high levels of each protective factor were less likely to report depression and anxiety symptoms" (Carlson et al., 2002, pp. 733–734). This would suggest that these factors may buffer abused women from the adverse effects of depression and anxiety. The absence of financial hardship was found to be especially protective. Conversely, financial hardship may amplify the effects of abuse on mental health symptoms. In addition, there was evidence that the buffering effects of multiple factors accumulates such that at the highest level of lifetime abuse, more than half of the women with zero to three protective factors reported depression, in contrast to only 17 percent of women reporting four to seven protective factors (Carlson et al., 2002). Thus, strengthening protective factors may assist abused women still in abusive relationships as well as those who have left to enhance their functioning.

Protective factors in relation to development of PTSD in the aftermath of either childhood or adult interpersonal victimization are understudied. Resnick and Newton (1992) speculated that social support along with pre-trauma psychopathology (or the absence thereof) may influence whether survivors develop PTSD and if so its severity. One study compared two groups of abused women, a forensic sample of women who had attempted or committed homicide and a matched sample of help-seeking battered women, and found that social support had a main effect on one measure of PTSD but not another (Dutton, Hohnecker, Halle, & Burghardt, 1994). They concluded that social support may be less effective in buffering against PTSD than against depression or other forms of anxiety. Finally, PTSD was studied longitudinally in survivors of non-family assault in relation to coping strategies, including mobilization of social support. Social support was not related to PTSD scores two weeks following the assault, although a type of coping labeled "positive distancing" predicted lower PTSD three months post-assault (Valentiner, Foa, Riggs, & Gershuny, 1996). Future research should search for factors that may buffer women from the development of PTSD following exposure to IPV.

Professionals and the lay public alike often ask *why abused women remain in abusive relationships*, or at least why they do not leave sooner than they do. The reality is that many abused women do leave, almost half within two to five years in one community sample (Zlotnick et al., 2006). Service providers should understand the numerous practical and emotional barriers that interfere with victims being able to extricate themselves from abusive relationships. Most abused women are ambivalent about their relationships. Although they want the abuse to end, for a variety of reasons, not the least being an emotional attachment to the abuser, they are reluctant to leave (Barnett, 2000, 2001; Dutton & Painter, 1993; Patzel, 2006). A history of family victimization may also make it more difficult to leave because harmful treatment may seem more normal (Patzel, 2006). Self-blame may be another factor that prolongs abusive relationships, fueled by the perpetrator telling the victim that the abuse is her fault (Patzel, 2006). Another factor is the abuser's problems: his promises that he will change (Strube & Barbour, 1983) as well as the victim's belief that she can help to "fix" the offender (Patzel, 2006). When his change is not forthcoming, many such women will eventually leave (Strube & Barbour, 1983). Extreme fear of what the abuser will do if she tries to leave can also immobilize some women (Asbury, 1987; Barnett, 2000, 2001; Patzel, 2006; Strube & Barbour, 1983). Sadly, for some, leaving the relationship does not bring them safety from the abuser.

As a group, abused women are heterogeneous and have different needs and priorities. For example, although there is increasing acceptance that domestic violence is a crime (Worden & Carlson, 2005), and abused women are more likely than ever to seek redress from the criminal justice system, such as arrest or protective orders, many do not wish to avail themselves of these services, and seeking such services is still reported to be difficult and stigmatizing (Erez & Belknap, 1998). Some personnel in the justice system are frustrated and continue to be ambivalent toward victims (Toon & Hart, 2007).

Practical barriers to ending the relationship include being unable to find safe, affordable housing or to financially support oneself and one's children without a partner's contributions, a problem made worse when Temporary Assistance for Needy Families (TANF) legislation imposed limits on the length of time a woman can receive public assistance. Strube and Barbour (1983) found financial dependence on the abuser to be a barrier to leaving. Lack of social support is another practical barrier than many women face (Asbury, 1987; Barnett, 2000, 2001; Patzel, 2006).

Illustration and discussion

Emily is a 21-year-old white, part-time community college student who is also employed full-time as a clerk in a clothing store. She lives in an apartment by herself. For two years she has dated 26-year-old Jeremy, an intermittently employed man who sometimes deals drugs to support himself. She is currently four months pregnant by Jeremy. Although their relationship is far from perfect, Emily would desperately like to get married, but Jeremy has steadfastly refused. Even before she found herself pregnant, she wanted to get married, hopeful that marriage would help Jeremy to settle down and treat her better. It seems ironic to her that since she told Jeremy that she was pregnant, his behavior toward her has gotten worse rather than better. She really thought he would be as thrilled about being a father as she was about the prospects of being a mother.

Recently, her best friend Molly noticed some bruises on her arms caused by Jeremy grabbing and pushing her during yet another argument about the relationship. She really does not want her baby to be born out of wedlock and was trying to persuade Jeremy, again, to get married. When Molly confronted her about the bruises, Emily tearfully told her about the argument and with some prodding admitted that it wasn't the first time he had "gotten physical" with her. It was a relief to finally tell someone how difficult and disappointing the relationship had become after two years of dating. Molly expressed great concern and sympathy and conveyed to Emily that exposure to this kind of abusive behavior would be harmful to her child, trying to convince Emily that she should end the relationship rather than continuing to pressure Jeremy to get married. Molly had also noticed that Emily hadn't seemed like her old self in recent months. She was withdrawn, uninterested in getting together and doing things like she had been in the past, seemed exhausted all the time, and didn't seem to be eating either. So Molly was quite worried about Emily. Despite her concern, Molly told Emily that even though Jeremy was extremely possessive and jealous toward Emily, she had seen him in the recent past with other women in a local bar. Despite this, Emily clearly was not ready to break things off with Jeremy, but she agreed to have Molly accompany her on her next prenatal visit and discuss the situation with a medical professional. As it turned out, the nurse she saw at her health maintenance organization (HMO) screened Emily for intimate partner violence and Emily admitted that her partner was hurting her. The nurse followed up and referred Emily to see a social worker at the HMO. With Molly's encouragement, Emily agreed to see the social worker.

The social worker was skillful in engaging Emily, noticing immediately how ambivalent she was about the relationship, clearly not ready to terminate it. By encouraging Emily to tell her story about the relationship, she learned that extensive emotional/psychological abuse began at the beginning of the relationship, whereas the physical violence was more recent. The worker's dual objectives in the first session were to (1) form a supportive treatment alliance so that Emily would return and (2) to develop a safety plan (Rosen & Stith, 1993). She made sure that Emily had information about the local domestic violence program, including how to access its shelter, despite Emily saying that such services would not be necessary. The worker was able to convey a combination of concern for Emily's safety and well-being, as well as that of her unborn child, while clearly labeling what was happening to Emily as abuse. Labeling abusive treatment as "abuse" and validating a victim's thoughts and feelings can be powerful interventions that strengthen the relationship alliance, especially in the early stages of therapy (Walker, 1994). At the same time, the worker avoided a confrontational approach or pressuring Emily to commit to leaving the relationship that might make it difficult for her to return to future sessions. Examples of validations include: you are not alone, you do not deserve to be abused, you are not to blame for the abuse, you are not crazy, and what happened to you is a crime. The worker also noticed that Emily's mood seemed to be rather depressed, and upon questioning Emily admitted that she was feeling quite negative about herself and her future and rarely enjoyed the things she used to enjoy. She was sleeping a lot more than usual and not eating much, which she attributed to being pregnant, but might have been related to dysthymic disorder, or mild depression.

Future sessions would focus on confirming (or ruling out) a diagnosis of dysthymia, strengthening Emily's coping strategies, enhancing her social support, and helping her to evaluate, for herself and her child, the advantages and disadvantages of continuing the relationship with Jeremy versus the advantages and disadvantages of ending the relationship. Rosen and Stith (1993) also recommend three useful interventions: helping clients determine for themselves what would be the "last straw" for them (e.g., "If Jeremy hit you so that you fell down and miscarried, would you still be willing to stay in the relationship?"), using a timeline to assist clients in seeing the pattern of abuse in the relationship (to counteract the tendency to deny abuse and see each instance as singular or aberrant), and challenging clients' unrealistic fantasies about the future of the relationship. In Emily's case, her fantasies about Jeremy someday being a good husband and father are contradicted by his long-standing emotional abuse, poor employment history, drug dealing, seeing other women, and consistent refusal to really commit himself to the relationship or the baby.

Conclusion

Intimate partner abuse – physical, emotional, and sexual – is an all-too-common problem for women, a substantial minority of whom will experience such abuse, perpetrated by intimate partners, over the course of their lifetimes. IPV knows no bounds in terms of the types of women who are affected: white women, but also ethnic minorities; heterosexual women, but also lesbians; adult women, but also adolescents; and able-bodied women, but also women with mental or physical disabilities. Our understanding of why such abuse occurs has deepened since the late 1970s, and we have learned that it is a complex, persistent social problem with no single cause but rather numerous risk factors. Its effects can be short term or long term and are influenced by the type of abuse experienced, its duration and frequency, and its severity. IPV continues to be stigmatizing, causing its victims to experience shame and self-blame. In addition to causing physical injury and other non-specific health problems, IPV can lead to a range of mental health issues. These include depression, including suicidality; anxiety, including PTSD; and substance abuse. Sometimes these symptoms disappear when the abuse end, but for some victims they persist and require professional attention. Many abused women have difficulty acknowledging that they are being abused, and most are reluctant to terminate the abusive relationship, opting instead to try to get the abuse to stop. Typically, victims have tried to get the abuse to end using a variety of informal and formal help sources before they reluctantly leave the relationship.

Although addressing IPV as a social problem has been an interdisciplinary phenomenon, social workers have played an instrument role in establishing IPV as an important issue, preventing future abuse, and assisting victims and survivors. Social workers might encounter an abused woman in almost any setting, not merely those where IPV would be the presenting problem, such as a domestic violence program. Other settings where IPV is likely to be encountered include schools, child welfare settings such as Child Protective Services, and hospitals. Social workers are ideally suited to assist victims of IPV due to their focus on the importance of the social environment and use of the ecological perspective as a comprehensive framework for the understanding of human behavior. This viewpoint is an excellent fit for a complex, multiple-determined problem such as IPV. Other valuable social work principles in working with abused women include "starting where the client is" and self-determination. These can be challenging for practitioners, especially when a client is committed to a relationship that appears dangerous. Another useful social work approach is the identification of strengths. The willingness of social workers to address a client's needs comprehensively will also be valuable in working with abused women, who often need more than their mental health needs addressed, including concrete services such as finding housing, assistance with employment, services for children, and so forth.

Web resources

Family Violence Prevention Fund
www.endabuse.org

Minnesota Center Against Violence and Abuse
www.mincava.umn.edu/

National Coalition Against Domestic Violence
www.ncadv.org

National Resource Center on Violence Against Women
www.nrcdv.org

References

Abbott, J., Johnson, R., Koziol-McLain, J., & Lowenstein, R.R. (1995). Domestic violence against women: Incidence and prevalence in an emergency department population. *Journal of the American Medical Association, 273,* 1763–1767.

Aldarondo, E., & Kantor, G.K. (1997). Social predictors of wife assault cessation. In G.K. Kantor & J.L. Jasinki (eds), *Out of darkness: Contemporary perspectives on family violence* (pp. 183–193). Thousand Oaks, CA: Sage.

Arias, I., & Pape, K.T. (1999). Psychological abuse: Implications for adjustment and commitment to leave violent partners. *Violence and Victims, 14,* 55–67.

Arias, I., Lyons, C.M., & Street, A.E. (1997). Individual and marital consequences of victimization: Moderating effects of relationship efficacy and spouse support. *Journal of Family Violence, 12,* 193–210.

Asbury, J. (1987). African-American women in violent relationships: An exploration of cultural differences. In R. Hampton (ed.), *Violence in the black family: Correlates and consequences* (pp. 89–104). Lexington, MA: Lexington Books.

Astin, M.C., Lawrence, K.J., & Foy, D.W. (1993). Posttraumatic stress disorder among battered women: Risk and resiliency factors. *Violence and Victims, 8,* 17–28.

Astin, M.C., Ogland-Hand, S.M., Coleman, E.M., & Foy, D.W. (1995). Posttraumatic stress disorder and childhood abuse in battered women: Comparisons with maritally distressed women. *Journal of Consulting and Clinical Psychology, 63,* 308–312.

Bachman, R., & Saltzman, L.E. (1995). *Violence against women: Estimates from the redesigned survey.* Washington, DC: Bureau of Justice Statistics, U.S. Department of Justice.

Barnes, S.Y. (1999). Theories of spouse abuse: Relevance to African Americans. *Issues in Mental Health Nursing, 20,* 357–371.

Barnett, O.W. (2000). Why battered women do not leave, part 1: External inhibiting factors within society. *Trauma, Violence, and Abuse, 1,* 343–372.

Barnett, O.W. (2001). Why battered women do not leave, part 2: External inhibiting factors – social support and internal inhibiting factors. *Trauma, Violence, and Abuse, 2,* 3–35.

Black, B.M., Tolman, R.J.M., Callahan, M., Saunders, D.G., & Weisz, A.N. (2008). When will adolescents tell someone about dating violence victimization? *Violence Against Women, 14,* 741–758.

Bohn, D.K. (1993). Nursing care of Native American battered women. *AWHONN's Clinical Issues, 4,* 424–436.

Breidling, M.J., Black, M.C., & Ryan, G.W. (2008). Prevalence and risk factors of intimate partner violence in eighteen U.S. states/territories, 2005. *American Journal of Preventive Medicine, 34,* 111–118.

Brice-Baker, J.R. (1996). Domestic violence in African American and African Caribbean families. In R.A. Javier, W.G. Herron, & A.J. Bergman (eds), *Domestic violence: Assessment and treatment* (pp. 69–84). Norvale, NJ: Jason Aronson.

Briere, J. (1988). The long-term clinical correlates of childhood sexual victimization. *Annals of the New York Academy of Science, 528,* 327–335.

Browne, A., & Williams, K. (1993). Gender, intimacy, and lethal violence: Trends from 1976 through 1987. *Gender and Society, 7,* 78–98.

Buttell, F., & Carney, M.M. (2005). *Women who perpetrate relationship violence: Moving beyond political correctness.* Binghamton, New York: Haworth Press.

Caetano, R., Shafer, J., Clark, C.L., Cunradi, C.B., & Raspbery, K. (2000). Intimate partner violence, acculturation, and alcohol consumption among Hispanic couples in the United States. *Journal of Interpersonal Violence, 15,* 30–45.

Caetano, R., McGrath, C., Ramisetty-Mikler, S., & Field, C. (2005). Drinking, alcohol problems and the five-year recurrence and incidence of male to female and female to male partner violence. *Alcoholism, Clinical and Experimental Research, 29,* 98–106.

Campbell, J. (2002). Health consequences of intimate partner violence. *The Lancet, 359,* 1331–1336.

Campbell, J.C., Kub, J., Belknap, R.A., & Templin, T. (1997). Predictors of depression in battered women. *Violence Against Women, 3,* 271–294.

Campbell, R., Sullivan, C. M., & Davidson, W.S. (1995). Women who use domestic violence shelters: Changes in depression over time. *Psychology of Women Quarterly, 19,* 237–255.

Carlson, B.E., (1998). Domestic violence in adults with mental retardation: Reports from victims and key informants. *Mental Health Aspects of Developmental Disabilities, 1*, 102–112.

Carlson, B.E. (2007). Intimate partner abuse in health care settings. In K. Kendall-Tackett & S. Giacomoni (eds), *Intimate Partner Violence* (pp. 19.1–19.20). Kingston, NJ: Civic Research Institute.

Carlson, B.E., & Worden, A.P. (2005). Attitudes and beliefs about domestic violence: Results of a public opinion survey. II. Beliefs about causes. *Journal of Interpersonal Violence, 20*, 1219–1243.

Carlson, B.E., McNutt, L.A., Choi, D., & Rose, I.M. (2002). Intimate partner abuse and mental health: The role of social support and other protective factors. *Violence Against Women, 8*, 720–745.

Carlson, B.E., McNutt, L.A., & Choi, D.Y. (2003). Childhood and adult abuse among women in primary care: Effects on mental health. *Journal of Interpersonal Violence, 18*, 924–941.

Cascardi, M., & O'Leary, K.D. (1992). Depressive symptomatology, self-esteem, and self-blame in battered women. *Journal of Family Violence, 7*, 249–259.

Cascardi, M., O'Leary, K.D., Lawrence, E.E., & Schlee, K.A. (1995). Characteristics of women physically abused by their spouses who seek treatment regarding marital conflict. *Journal of Consulting and Clinical Psychology, 63* (4), 616–623.

Chang, J.C., Martin, S.L., Moracco, K.E., Dulli, L., Scandlin, D., Loucks-Sorrel, M.B. et al. (2003). Helping women with disabilities and domestic violence: Strategies, limitations, and challenges of domestic violence programs and services. *Journal of Women's Health, 12*, 699–708.

Chu, J.A. (1992). The revictimization of adult women with histories of childhood abuse. *Journal of Psychotherapy Practice and Research, 1*, 259–269.

Coker, A.L., Davis, K.E., Arias, I., Desi, S., Sanderson, M., Brandt, H.M., & Smith, P.H. (2002). Physical and mental health effects of intimate partner violence for men and women. *American Journal of Preventive Medicine, 23*, 260–268.

Comas-Diaz, L. (1993). Hispanic communities: Psychological implications. In D. Atkinson, J. Morton, & D. Sue (eds), *Counseling American Minorities* (pp. 241–296). Dubuque, IA: Brown & Benchmark.

Curry, M., Hassouneh-Phillips, D., & Johnston-Silverberg, A. (2001). Abuse of women with disabilities: An ecological model and review. *Violence Against Women, 7*, 60–79.

Danielson, K.K., Moffitt, T.E., Caspi, A., & Silva, P. (1998). Comorbidity between abuse of an adult and DSM-III-R mental disorders: Evidence from an epidemiological study. *American Journal of Psychiatry, 155*, 131–133.

Dobash, R.E., & Dobash, R. (1979). *Violence against wives: The case against patriarchy*. New York: The Free Press.

Dutton, D.G., & Painter, S. (1993). Emotional attachments in abusive relationships: A test of traumatic bonding theory. *Violence and Victims, 8*, 105–120.

Dutton, M.A., Hohnecker, L.C., Halle, P.M., & Burghardt, K.J. (1994). Traumatic responses among battered women who kill. *Journal of Traumatic Stress, 4*, 549–564.

Eaton, D.K., Davis, K.S., Barrios, L., Brenner, N.D., & Noonan, R.K. (2007). Associations of dating violence victimization with lifetime participation, co-occurrence, and early initiation of risk behaviors among U.S. high school students. *Journal of Interpersonal Violence, 22*, 585–602.

Elliott, P. (1996). Shattering illusions: Same-sex domestic violence. *Journal of Gay and Lesbian Social Services, 4*, 1–8.

Erez, K., & Belknap, J. (1998). In their own words: Battered women's assessment of the criminal processing system's responses. *Violence and Victims, 13*, 252–268.

Ewing, C.P., & Aubrey, M. (1987). Battered women and public opinion: Some realities about the myths. *Journal of Family Violence, 2*, 257–264.

Farley, N. (1996). A survey of factors contributing to gay and lesbian domestic violence. *Journal of Gay and Lesbian Social Services, 4*, 35–44.

Few, A.L., & Bell-Scott, P. (2002). Grounding our feet and hearts: Black women's coping strategies in psychologically abusive dating relationships. *Women and Therapy, 25*, 59–77.

Flores-Ortiz, Y. (1993). La mujer y la violencia: A culturally based model for the understanding and treatment of domestic violence in Chicana/Latina communities. In N. Alarcon (ed.), *Chicano Critical Issues* (pp. 169–182). Berkeley, CA: Third Woman Press.

Follette, V.M., Polusny, M.A., Bechtel, A.E., & Naugle, A.E. (1996). Cumulative trauma: The impact of child sexual abuse, adult sexual assault, and spouse abuse. *Journal of Traumatic Stress, 9*, 25–35.

Follingstad, D.R. (2009). The impact of psychological aggression on women's mental health and behavior. *Trauma, Violence, and Abuse, 10,* 271–289.

Follingstad, D.R., Rutledge, L.L., Berg, B.J., Hause, E.S., & Polek, D.S. (1990). The role of emotional abuse in physically abusive relationships. *Journal of Family Violence, 5,* 107–120.

Follingstad, D.R., Brennan, A.F., Hause, E.S., Polek, D.S., & Rutledge, L.L. (1991). Factors moderating physical and psychological symptoms of battered women. *Journal of Family Violence, 6,* 81–95.

Foo, L., & Margolin, G. (1995). A multivariate investigation of dating violence. *Journal of Family Violence, 10,* 351–377.

Foshee, V.A. (1996). Gender differences in adolescent dating abuse prevalence, types and injuries. *Health Education Research, 11,* 275–286.

Foshee, V.A., Linder, G.F., Bauman, K.E., Langwick, S.A., Arriaga, X.B., Heath, J.L. et al. (1996). The Safe Dates project: Theoretical basis, evaluation, design, and selected baseline findings. *American Journal of Preventive Medicine, 12,* 39–47.

Gelles, R.J., & Harrop, J.W. (1988). Violence, battering, and psychological distress among women. *Journal of Interpersonal Violence, 4,* 400–420.

Gelles, R.J., & Straus, M.A. (1990). The medical and psychological costs of family violence. In R.J. Gelles & M.A. Straus (eds), *Physical violence in American families: Risk factors and adaptations to violence in 8,145 families* (pp. 425–430). New Brunswick, NJ: Transaction.

Gerber, M.R., Leiter, K.S., Hermann, R.C., & Bor, D.H. (2005). How and why community hospital clinicians document a positive screen for intimate partner violence: A cross-sectional study. *BMC Family Practice, 19,* 48–56.

Gidycz, C.A., & Koss, M.P. (1991). Predictors of long-term sexual assault trauma among a national sample of victimized college women. *Violence and Victims, 6* (3), 176–190.

Gilbert, L., El-Bassel, N., Schilling, R., & Friedman, E. (1997). Childhood abuse as a risk for partner abuse among women in methadone maintenance. *American Journal of Drug and Alcohol Abuse, 23,* 581–595.

Gitterman, A. (2008). Ecological framework. In Y. Mizrahi & L. Davis (eds), *Encyclopedia of social work* (20th ed., pp. 97–102). New York: Oxford University Press.

Golding, J.M. (1999). Intimate partner violence as a risk factor for mental disorders: A meta-analysis. *Journal of Family Violence, 14,* 99–132.

Goodman, L.A., Koss, M., & Russo, N.F. (1993). Violence against women: Physical and mental health effects. Part I: Research findings. *Applied and Preventive Psychology, 2,* 79–89.

Greenfeld, L.A., Rand, M.R., Craven, D., Klaus, P.A., Perkins, C.A., Ringel, C. et al. (1998). *Violence by intimates: Analysis of data on crimes by current or former spouses, boyfriends, and girlfriends.* Washington, DC: Bureau of Justice Statistics, U.S. Department of Justice.

Hassouneh, D., & Glass, N. (2008). The influence of gender-role stereotyping on women's experience of female same-sex intimate partner violence. *Violence Against Women, 14,* 310–325.

Hassouneh-Phillips, D., & Curry, M. (2002). Abuse of women with disabilities: State of the science. *Rehabilitation Counseling Bulletin, 42,* 96–104.

Helfrich, C.A., & Simpson, E.K. (2006). Improving services for lesbian clients: What do domestic violence agencies need to know? *Health Care for Women International, 27,* 344–361.

Henning, K., & Klesges, L.M. (2003). Prevalence and characteristics of psychological abuse reported by court-involved battered women. *Journal of Interpersonal Violence, 18,* 857–871.

Heron, R.J., Twomey, H.B., Jacobs, D.P., & Kaslow, N.J. (1997). Culturally competent interventions for abused and African American suicidal women. *Psychotherapy, 34,* 410–424.

Hien, D., & Ruglass, L. (2009). Interpersonal partner violence and women in the United States: An overview of prevalence rates, psychiatric correlates and consequents and barriers to help seeking. *International Journal of Law and Psychiatry, 32,* 48–55.

Hilbert, J.C., Kolia, R., & VanLeeuwen, D.M. (1997). Abused women in New Mexico shelters: Factors that influence independence on discharge. *Affilia, 12* (4), 391–407.

Holtzworth-Munroe, A. (2005). Female perpetration of physical aggression against an intimate partner: A controversial new topic of study. *Violence and Victims, 20,* 251–259.

Holtzworth-Munroe, A., & Stuart, G.L. (1994). Typologies of male batterers: Three subtypes and the differences among them. *Psychological Bulletin, 116* (3), 476–497.

Horton, A.L., & Johnson, B.L. (1993). Profile and strategies of women who have ended abuse. *Families in Society, 74*, 481–492.

Jezl, D.R., Molidor, C.E., & Wright, T.L. (1996). Physical, sexual and psychological abuse in high school dating relationships: Prevalence rates and self-esteem issues. *Child and Adolescent Social Work Journal, 13*, 69–87.

Jones, L., Hughes, M., & Unterstaller, U. (2001). Post-traumatic stress disorder (PTSD) in victims of domestic violence. *Trauma, Violence, and Abuse, 2*, 99–119.

Kanuha, V. (1990). Compounding the triple jeopardy: Battering in lesbian of color relationships. *Women and Therapy, 9*, 169–184.

Kaufman Kantor, G. & Jasinski, J.L. (1998). Dynamics and risk factors in partner violence. In J.L. Jasinski & L.M. Williams (eds), *Partner violence: A comprehensive review of 20 years of research* (pp. 1–43). Thousand Oaks, CA: Sage.

Kessler, R.C., Somnega, A., Bromet, E., Hughes, M., & Nelson, C.B. (1995). Posttraumatic stress disorder in the National Comorbidity Survey. *Archives of General Psychiatry, 52*, 1048–1060.

Kilpatrick, D.G., Edmunds, C.N., & Seymour, A.K. (1992). *Rape in America: A report to the nation*. Arlington, VA: National Victim Center.

Kilpatrick, D.G., Acierno, R., Resnick, H.S., Saunders, B.E., & Best, C.L. (1997). A 2-year longitudinal analysis of relationships between violent assault and substance abuse in women. *Journal of Consulting and Clinical Psychology, 65*, 834–847.

Laner, M., & Thompson, J. (1982). Abuse and aggression in the context of dating and sex. *Deviant Behavior, 3*, 229–244.

LaPlant, M., & Carlson, D. (1996). *Disability in the United States: Prevalence and causes, 1992*. Retrieved from www.disc.ucsf.edu/repl/index.html

Lee, Y., & Hadeed, L. (2009). Intimate partner violence among Asian American immigrant communities. *Trauma, Violence, and Abuse, 10*, 143–170.

Leonard, K.E., & Senchak, M. (1996). Prospective prediction of husband marital aggression within newlywed couples. *Journal of Abnormal Psychology, 105*, 369–380.

Lewis, S.F., & Fremouw, W. (2001). Dating violence: A critical review of the literature. *Clinical Psychology Review, 21*, 105–127.

Lie, G.Y., & Gentlewarrier, S. (1991). Intimate violence in lesbian relationships: Discussion of survey findings and practice implications. *Journal of Social Service Research, 15*, 41–59.

Lockhart, L.L., White, B.W., Causby, V., & Issac, A. (1994). Letting out the secret: Violence in lesbian relationships. *Journal of Interpersonal Violence, 9*, 469–492.

Loring, M.T. (1994). *Emotional abuse*. New York: Lexington Books.

Maker, A.H., Kemmelmeier, M., & Peterson, C. (1998). Long-term psychological consequences in women of witnessing parental physical conflict and experiencing abuse in childhood. *Journal of Interpersonal Violence, 13*, 574–589.

Marin, G., & Marin, B.V.O. (1991). *Research with Hispanic populations*. Newbury Park, CA: Sage.

Marshall, L.L. (1994). Physical and psychological abuse. In W.R. Cupach & B.H. Spitzberg (eds), *The dark side of communication* (pp. 281–311). Hillsdale, NJ: Lawrence Erlbaum Associates.

Marshall, L.L. (1999). Effects of men's subtle and overt psychological abuse on low-income women. *Violence and Victims, 14* (1), 69–88.

Mattson, S., & Rodriguez, E. (1999). Battering in pregnant Latinas. *Issues in Mental Health Nursing, 20* (4), 405–422.

McCauley, J., Kern, D.E., Kolodner, K., Dill, L., Schroeder, A.F., De Chant, H.K. et al. (1995). The "battering syndrome": Prevalence and clinical characteristics of domestic violence in primary care internal medicine practices. *Annals of Internal Medicine, 123*, 737–746.

McCauley, J., Kern, D.E., Kolodner, K., Derogatis, L.R., & Bass, E.B., (1998). Relation of low-severity violence to women's health. *Journal of General Internal Medicine, 13*, 687–691.

McFarlane, J.M., Groff, J.Y., O'Brien, J.A., & Watson, K. (2005). Prevalence of partner violence against 7,443 African American, white and Hispanic women receiving care at urban public primary care clinics. *Public Health Nursing, 22*, 98–107.

Milberger, S., Israel, N., LeRoy, B., Martin, A., Potter, L., & Patchak-Schuster, P. (2003). Violence against women with disabilities. *Violence and Victims, 18*, 581–590.

Mitchell, R.E., & Hodson, C.A. (1983). Coping with domestic violence: Social support and psychological health among battered women. *American Journal of Community Psychology, 11*, 629–654.

Molidor, C., & Tolman, R.M. (1998). Gender and contextual factors in adolescent dating violence. *Violence Against Women, 4*, 180–194.

Moss, V., Pitula, C.R., Campbell, J.C., & Halstead, L. (1997). The experience of terminating an abusive relationship from an Anglo and African American perspective: A qualitative descriptive study. *Issues in Mental Health Nursing, 18* (5), 433–454.

Mullen, P.E., Martin, J.L., Anderson, J.C., Romans, S.E., & Herbison, G.P. (1996). The long-term impact of the physical, emotional, and sexual abuse of children: A community study. *Child Abuse and Neglect, 20*, 7–21.

Murdaugh, C., Hunt, S., Sowell, R., & Santana, I. (2004). Domestic violence in Hispanics in the Southeastern United States: A survey and needs analysis. *Journal of Family Violence, 19* (2), 107–115.

Murray, C.E., & Kardatzke, K.N. (2007). Dating violence among college students: Key issues for college counselors. *Journal of College Counseling, 10*, 79–89.

National Center for Injury Prevention and Control. (2003). *Costs of intimate partner violence against women in the United States.* Atlanta, GA: Centers for Disease Control and Prevention.

Neville, H.A., & Pugh, A.O. (1997). General and cultural-specific factors influencing African American women's reporting patterns and perceived social support following sexual assault. *Violence Against Women, 3*, 361–381.

Nicolaidis, C., Curry, M., McFarland, B., & Gerrity, M. (2004). Violence, mental health, and physical symptoms in an academic internal medicine practice. *Journal of General Internal Medicine, 19*, 893–895.

Nielsen, J.M., Endo, R.K., & Ellington, B.L. (1992). Social isolation and wife abuse: A research report. In E.C. Viano (ed.), *Intimate Violence Interdisciplinary Perspectives* (pp. 49–59). Washington, DC: Hemisphere.

Nosek, M.A., Howland, C.A., & Hughes, R.B. (2001a). The investigation of abuse and women with disabilities. *Violence against Women, 7*, 477–499.

Nosek, M.A., Foley, C.C., Hughes, R.B., & Howland, C.A. (2001b). Vulnerabilities for abuse among women with disabilities. *Sexuality and Disability, 19*, 177–189.

Nurius, P.S., Furrey, J., & Berliner, L. (1992). Coping capacity among women with abusive partners. *Violence and Victims, 7*, 229–243.

O'Keefe, M. (1997). Predictors of dating violence among high school students. *Journal of Interpersonal Violence, 12*, 546–568.

O'Leary, K.D. (1999). Psychological abuse: A variable deserving critical attention in domestic violence. *Violence and Victims, 14*, 3–32.

O'Leary, K.D., & Jouriles, E.N. (1994). Psychological abuse between adult partners. In L. L'Abate (ed.), *Handbook of developmental family psychology and psychopathology* (pp. 330–349). New York: John Wiley & Sons.

O'Leary, K.D., Malone, J., & Tyree, A. (1994). Physical aggression in early marriage: Prerelationship and relationship effects. *Journal of Consulting and Clinical Psychology, 62*, 594–602.

Patzel, B. (2006). What blocked heterosexual women and lesbians in leaving their abusive relationships. *Journal of the American Psychiatric Nurses Association, 12*, 208–215.

Plichta, S.B. (1992). The effects of women abuse on health care utilization and health status: A literature review. *Women's Health Issues, 2*, 154–163.

Plichta, S.B. (1996). Violence and abuse: Implications for women's health. In M.M. Falik & K.S. Collins (eds), *Women's health: The Commonwealth fund study* (pp. 237–232). Baltimore, MD: Johns Hopkins University Press.

Ramos, B.M., Carlson, B.E., & McNutt, L. (2004). Lifetime abuse, mental health, and African American women. *Journal of Family Violence, 19*, 153–164.

Ramos, B., Carlson, B., & Kulkarni, S. (2010). Culturally competent practice with Latinas. In L.L. Lockhart and F.S. Danis (eds), *Domestic violence mosaic: Culturally competent practice with diverse populations.* New York: Columbia University Press.

Reid, R.J., Bonomi, A.E., Rivara, F.P., Anderson, M.L., Fishman, P.A., Carrell, D.S., & Thompson, R.S. (2008). Intimate partner violence among men: Prevalence, chronicity, and health effects. *American Journal of Preventive Medicine, 34*, 478–485.

Renzetti, C.M. (1988). Violence in lesbian relationships: A preliminary causal analysis. *Journal of Interpersonal Violence, 3*, 381–399.

Renzetti, C.M. (1992). *Violent betrayal: Partner abuse in lesbian relationships.* Newbury Park, CA: Sage.

Resick, P.A. (1993). The psychological impact of rape. *Journal of Interpersonal Violence, 8,* 223–255.

Resnick, H.S. & Newton, T. (1992). Assessment and treatment of post-traumatic stress disorder in adult survivors of sexual assault. In D.W. Foy (ed.), *Treating PTSD: Cognitive-behavioral strategies* (pp. 99–126). New York: Guilford Press.

Robin, R.W., Chester, B., & Rasmussen, J.K. (1998). Intimate violence in Southwestern Indian tribal community. *Cultural Diversity and Mental Health, 4,* 335–344.

Rosen, K., & Stith, S. (1993). Intervention strategies for treating women in violent dating relationships. *Family Relations, 42,* 427–433.

Sackett, L.A., & Saunders, D.G. (1999). The impact of different forms of psychological abuse on battered women. *Violence and Victims, 14,* 105–117.

Saunders, D.G. (1994). Posttraumatic stress symptom profiles of battered women: A comparison of survivors in two settings. *Violence and Victims, 9,* 31–44

Saunders, D.G., Hamberger, L.K., & Hovey, M. (1993). Indicators of woman abuse based on a chart review in a family practice center. *Archives of Family Medicine, 2,* 537–543.

Silva, C., McFarlane, J., Soeken, K., Parker, B., & Reel, S. (1997). Symptoms of post-traumatic stress disorder in abused women in a primary care setting. *Journal of Women's Health, 6,* 543–552.

Sorenson, S.B. (1996). Violence against women: Examining ethnic differences and commonalities. *Evaluation Review, 20,* 123–145.

Sorenson, S.B., & Siegel, J.M. (1992). Gender, ethnicity and sexual assault: Findings from a Los Angeles study. *Journal of Social Issues, 48,* 93–104.

Stark, E., & Flitcraft, A. (1996). *Woman at risk: Domestic violence and women's health.* Thousand Oaks, CA: Sage.

Stets, J.E., & Pirog-Good, M.A. (1987). Violence in dating relationships. *Social Psychology Quarterly, 50,* 237–246.

Stets, J.E., & Straus, M.A. (1990). Gender differences in reporting marital violence and its medical and psychological consequences. In M.A. Straus & R.J. Gelles (eds), *Physical violence in American families: Risk factors and adaptations to violence in 8,145 families* (pp. 151–165). New Brunswick, NJ: Transaction.

Straus, M.A., & Gelles, R.J. (1986). Societal change and change in family violence from 1975 to 1985 as revealed by two national surveys. *Journal of Marriage and the Family, 48,* 465–478.

Straus, M.A., & Gelles, R.J. (1990). How violent are American families? Estimates from the national Family Violence Resurvey and other studies. In M.A. Straus & R.J. Gelles (eds), *Physical violence in American families: Risk factors and adaptations to violence in 8,145 families* (pp. 95–112). New Brunswick, NJ: Transaction.

Straus, M.A., & Smith, C. (1990). Violence in Hispanic families in the United States: Incidence rates and structural interpretations. In M.A. Straus & R.J. Gelles (eds), *Physical violence in American families: Risk factors and adaptations to violence in 8,145 families* (pp. 341–368). New Brunswick, NJ: Transaction.

Strube, M.J., & Barbour, L.S. (1983). The decision to leave an abusive relationship: Economic dependence and psychological commitment. *Journal of Marriage and the Family, 45,* 785–793.

Sudderth, L.K. (2006). An uneasy alliance: Law enforcement and domestic violence victim advocates in a rural area. *Feminist Criminology, 1,* 329–353.

Sullivan, C.M., Campbell, R., Angelique, H., Eby, K.K., & Davidson, W.S. (1994). An advocacy intervention program for women with abusive partners: Six-month follow-up. *American Journal of Community Psychology, 22,* 101–122.

Sutherland, C., Bybee, D., & Sullivan, C. (1998). Long-term effects of battering on women' health. *Women's Health: Research on Gender, Behavior, and Policy, 4,* 41–70.

Tan, C., Basta, J., Sullivan, C.M., & Davidson, W.S. (1995). The role of social support in the lives of women exiting domestic violence shelters. *Journal of Interpersonal Violence, 10,* 437–451.

Testa, M. (2004). The role of substance use in male-to-female physical violence: A brief review and recommendations for future research. *Journal of Interpersonal Violence, 19,* 1494–1505.

Thompson, M.P., Kaslow, N.J., Lang, D.B., & Kingree, J.B. (2000). Childhood maltreatment, PTSD, and suicidal behavior among African American females. *Journal of Interpersonal Violence, 15,* 3–15.

Thompson, R.S., Bonomi, A.E., Anderson, M., Reid, R.J., Dimer, J.A., Carrell, D., & Rivara, F.P. (2006). Intimate partner violence: Prevalence, types, and chronicity in adult women. *American Journal of Preventive Medicine, 30,* 447–457.

Tjaden, P., & Thoennes, N. (1998). *Prevalence, incidence and consequences of violence against women: Findings from the National Violence Against Women Survey. Research in Brief* (NCJ 172837). Washington, DC: U.S. Department of Justice, National Institute of Justice, and U.S. Department of Health and Human Services, Centers for Disease Control and Prevention.

Tjaden, P., & Thoennes, N. (2000). *Extent, nature, and consequences of intimate partner violence* (NCJ 181867). Washington, DC: Office of Justice Programs, U.S. Department of Justice.

Tjaden, P., & Thoennes, N. (2006). *Extent, nature, and consequences of rape victimization: Findings from the National Violence against Women Survey.* Washington, DC: Office of Justice Programs, U.S. Department of Justice.

Tolman, R.M. (1989). The development of a measure of psychological maltreatment of women by their male partners. *Violence and Victims, 14,* 159–176.

Toon, R., & Hart, B. (2007). *System alert: Arizona's criminal justice's response to domestic violence.* Phoenix, AZ: Morrison Institute for Public Policy, Arizona State University.

Ullman, S.E., Karabatsos, G., & Koss, M.P. (1999). Alcohol and sexual assault in a national sample of college women. *Journal of Interpersonal Violence, 14* (6), 603–625.

U.S. Census Bureau (2004). *Hispanic population in the United States: Census 2000 brief.* Washington, DC: U.S. Government Printing Office.

Valentiner, D.P., Foa, E.B., Riggs, D.S., & Gershuny, B.S. (1996). Coping strategies and posttraumatic stress disorder in female victims of sexual and nonsexual assault. *Journal of Abnormal Psychology, 105,* 455–458.

Wahab, S., & Olson, L. (2004). Intimate partner violence and sexual assault in Native American communities. *Trauma, Violence, and Abuse, 5,* 353–366.

Walker, L.E.A. (1994). *Abused women and survivor therapy.* Washington, DC: American Psychological Association.

Weaver, T.L., Kilpatrick, D.G., Resnick, H.S., Best, C.L., & Saunders, B.E. (1997). An examination of physical assault and childhood victimization histories within a national probability sample of women. In G.K. Kantor & J.L. Jasinski (eds), *Out of darkness: Contemporary perspectives on family violence* (pp. 35–46). Thousand Oaks, CA: Sage.

West, C.G., Fernandez, A., Hillard, J.R., Schoof, M., & Parks, J. (1990). Psychiatric disorders of abused women at a shelter. *Psychiatric Quarterly, 61,* 295–301.

West, C.M. (1998). Leaving a second closet: Outing partner violence in same-sex couples. In J.L. Jasinski and L.M. Williams (eds), *Partner violence: A comprehensive review of 20 years of research* (pp. 163–183). Thousand Oaks, CA: Sage.

West, C.M., Kaufman Kantor, G., & Jasinski, J.L. (1998). Sociodemographic predictors and cultural barriers to help-seeking behavior by Latina and Anglo American battered women. *Violence and Victims, 13,* 361–375.

White, J.W., & Koss, M.P. (1991). Courtship violence: Incidence in a national sample of higher education students. *Violence and Victims, 6,* 247–256.

Whitfield, C.L., Anda, R.F., Dube, S.R., & Felitti, V.J. (2003). Violent childhood experiences and the risk of intimate partner violence in adults: Assessment in a large health maintenance organization. *Journal of Interpersonal Violence, 18,* 166–186.

Williams, J.R., Ghandour, R.M., & Kub, J.E. (2008). Female perpetration of violence in heterosexual intimate relationships. *Trauma, Violence and Abuse, 9,* 227–249.

Worden, A.P., & Carlson, B.E. (2005). Attitudes and beliefs about domestic violence: Results of a public opinion survey. I. Definitions of domestic violence, criminal domestic violence, prevalence. *Journal of Interpersonal Violence, 20,* 1197–1218.

Yllo, K.A., & Straus, M.A. (1990). Patriarchy and violence against wives: The impact of structural and normative factors. In M.A. Straus & R.J. Gelles (eds), *Physical violence in American families: Risk factors and adaptations in 8,145 American families* (pp. 383–399). New Brunswick, NJ: Transaction.

Zink, T., Fisher, B.S., Regan, S., & Pabst, S. (2005). The prevalence and incidence of intimate partner violence in older women in primary care practices. *Journal of General Internal Medicine, 20,* 884–888.

Zlotnick, C., Kohn, R., Peterson, J., & Pearlstein, T. (1998). Partner physical victimization in a national sample of American families. *Journal of Interpersonal Violence, 13,* 156–166.

Zlotnick, C., Johnson, D.M., & Kohn, R. (2006). Intimate partner violence and long-term psychosocial functioning in a national sample of American women. *Journal of Interpersonal Violence, 21,* 262–275.

11 Community violence exposure and its effects

*Vanessa Vorhies, Neil B. Guterman, and
Muhammad M. Haj-Yahia*

Youth community violence exposure (CVE) is a problem of widespread proportions, although it continues to go frequently unrecognized, under-assessed, and under-addressed by professional social workers. Despite this, the startling prevalence rates of youth CVE across ethnic groups and the subsequent psychosocial outcomes for individuals, families, schools, and communities has resulted in the recognition of CVE as a significant public health problem (Carmona 2007; Koop & Lundberg, 1992; Krug, Dahlberg, Mercy, Zwi, & Lozano, 2002). For youth, the mental health outcomes can be as severe as those associated with child maltreatment, disasters, and witnessing domestic violence (Rosenthal & Wilson, 2008). In addition to CVE disproportionately affecting ethnic minorities (Attar, Guerra, & Tolan, 1994; Christofel, 1990; Jenkins & Bell, 1994), a number of risk factors on multiple levels (e.g. individual, family, school, and community) are associated with CVE and subsequent psychosocial outcomes. Although CVE is commonly believed to be a problem of poor urban neighborhoods, significant prevalence rates of CVE have been reported in rural and suburban communities as well (Jenkins & Bell, 1997). Despite the broad prevalence of the problem, social workers rarely assess CVE (Guterman & Cameron, 2003) and few have evaluated the effectiveness of clinical treatment and prevention methods.

Understanding the risks and protective factors associated with CVE and subsequent psychosocial outcomes, as well as, assessment strategies, treatment modalities, and prevention approaches will help to ameliorate a problem and the associated personal and communal outcomes. This chapter first defines CVE, discusses research limitations, and political implications of CVE; second, it describes youth CVE prevalence rates and risk/protective factors; third, it describes associated mental health outcomes and risk/protective factors; fourth, it provides a few examples of youth descriptions of CVE; finally, it provides guidelines for CVE assessment, intervention, and prevention.

Definitions of community violence exposure

At its most basic, the term *community violence* denotes acts of interpersonal violence that occur in community settings. However, "community violence exposure" is a complex term as the types of settings, violence, and exposure vary. Community violence can occur in various settings, such as neighborhoods, streets, schools, shops, playgrounds, or other community locales. The type of community violence can include, but is not limited to, gang violence, homicides, rapes, shootings, knifings, beatings, muggings, bullying, or threats (Krug et al., 2002). CVE can occur on both micro and macro levels, such as exposure through family member violence in the home or exposure to social unrest or riots in community settings (Guterman, Cameron, & Staller, 2000). Finkelhor, Ormrod and Turner (2007), in their development of a CVE model, identify multiple levels of community violence for youth, including the macrosystem (economic patterns, cultural beliefs, stigma of violence, policies and laws and social exlusion; exosystem (including school and afterschool programs, mental health systems, child welfare and the community at large); and mesosystems and microsystems, including the family, childcare organizations, community physical space, gangs, peers, and church (Finkelhor et al., 2007). Youth can also be directly or indirectly involved in violence either as victims, perpetrators, witnesses (Brady, Gorman-Smith, Henry, & Tolan, 2008; Margolin & Gordis, 2000), or some combination of these roles. Important to note is that witnessing community violence or simply hearing about community violence occurring has been linked to just as serious negative mental health outcomes as direct exposure through victimization or perpetration (Duckworth, Hale, Clair, & Adams, 2000; Scarpa, Hurley, Shumate, & Haden, 2006). Only assessing those directly involved in a violent incident overlooks youth who either witness or simply hear about community violence through their relationships with others.

Although the location and persons involved in the violence often shape whether an act of violence is considered community violence, no clear consensus yet exists as to what boundaries demarcate community violence from other forms of violence. One can see how it is debatable if bullying at school or in the home of a classmate should be considered youth community violence exposure. Or if witnessing familial physical fighting should be considered "child maltreatment" or community violence exposure. In fact, different forms of violence may overlap with or even "spill over" into community violence and vice versa as community violence may be alternately labeled as "domestic violence," "crime," "gang violence" or "school violence" depending on the victim, perpetrator, setting, and situation. For youth, the victimization and perpetration of violence in the community are often intimately intertwined (American Psychological Association (APA), 1993). The ecological perspective provides a framework for understanding CVE as a child's social context includes a number of subsystems of family, peers, school, church, and neighborhood that are embedded within larger systems with certain policies, institutions, and belief systems (Bronfenbrenner, 1999; Gitterman, 2008).

The lack of clear and precise demarcation of the term "community violence" makes it difficult to accurately track the magnitude of the problem, monitor changing trends over time, to identify risk and protective factors, or to know where, when, or how to intervene in order to prevent or best address youth exposed to community violence (Guterman et al., 2000). Addressing the many factors associated with CVE are necessary, including contextual elements such as schools, community organizations, the physical neighborhood, family life, in addition to influential social policies and individual characteristics, which all impact the risk that a youth will be exposed to CVE or develop psychosocial problems after exposure. Social workers are in a unique position to alter the rates of community violence and address the associated psychosocial outcomes because social work emphasizes the person and environment perspective and social workers are positioned in many key contexts (i.e. schools, hospitals, agencies that serve families and youth, government and advocacy groups) that can directly and indirectly impact CVE (Gitterman & Germain, 2008).

Community violence exposure and mental health/illness

Youth aged 18 and younger represent 26 percent of the U.S. population, yet they account for approximately 50 percent of the witnesses and victims of violent acts (U.S. Census Bureau, 2003). Compared to adults, youth are twice as likely to be victims or witnesses of severe victimization outside of the home (i.e. being mugged or physically assaulted) and have three times the risk of lower level victimization (i.e. threats) (Snyder & Sickmund, 1999). Although there has been a decline in community violence reports since the 1990s, these rates may be highly underestimated as it has been conservatively estimated that at least half of community violence events fail to be reported (Snyder & Sickmund, 1999).

Nationally representative surveys have found that in a given year between 50 and 75 percent of youth are the direct victims of severe violence (e.g. physical and sexual assault, attempted kidnapping) and/or less severe violence (e.g. theft or bullying) (Boney-McCoy & Finkelhor, 1995; Finkelhor, Ormrod, Turner, & Hamby, 2005). Additionally, youth who experience one direct victimization have a 69 percent chance of an additional victimization in the same year and, on average, youth with any exposure to community violence experienced three victimizations per year (Finkelhor et al., 2005).

In addition to prior history of violence exposure, a number of risk factors are associated with CVE, including, but not limited to: being poor, male, gang affiliated, living in a high-crime neighborhood, having a mental illness, being a child of a single parent (particularly an adolescent mother), and being Latino or African American (i.e., Bell, Taylor-Crawford, Jenkins, & Chalmers, 1988; Breslau, Davis, & Andreski, 1995; DuRant, Pendergrast, & Cadenhead, 1994; Resnick, Kilpatrick, Best, & Kramer, 1992). However, the complexity of CVE, poor research design, and discrepancies in research findings or interpretations of findings, make it difficult to determine which risk factors are independent predictors of CVE and which are merely co-occurring with CVE. For example, although race/ethnicity has been found to be associated with increased risk for CVE, Lauritsen (2003) found that the differences in youth CVE between white and black adolescents disappears once family and community factors are taken into account, suggesting the importance of considering how CVE risk factors interact with or mediate each other. Often, disentangling individual level factors from family and community level factors is difficult as they are often associated with one another (e.g. being a minority living in poverty in an urban neighborhood). The following discussion highlights the many factors that have been found associated with CVE, which are broad trends and by no means one-to-one predictors of violence exposure risk.

Race and ethnicity Although all ethnic groups are exposed to community violence in the United States, similar to rates of poverty, the rates of exposure among ethnic minorities are disproportionately high (Attar et al., 1994; Jenkins & Bell, 1994; O'Carroll, 1988). Homicide is the leading cause of death for African Americans, the second leading cause of death for Latinos, and the third leading cause of death for American Indians, Alaska Natives, and Asian/Pacific Islanders between the ages of 10 and 24 (Centers for Disease Control and Prevention (CDC), 2006). Compared to other racial and ethnic groups, African Americans tend to experience the highest levels of exposure to violent crimes (Attar et al., 1994; U.S. Bureau of Justice Statistics, 2008) and, compared to Caucasian youth, are ten times more likely to be victims of homicide (Anderson & Smith, 2005; Uniform Crime Reports, 2002), often committed by other African American youth who the victims know (CDC, 2000). The relationship to the victim or perpetrator has significant implications for psychosocial functioning and may disproportionately affect African American youth because they are more likely to be personally connected to the perpetrator of violence.

In 2009, prevalence rates of school and community violence exposure in Latino youth were reported to be similar to African American urban populations (Kataoka et al., 2009), with approximately 75 percent exposed to school violence and 50 percent exposed to community violence annually. Compared to Caucasian students in urban public schools, Latino and African American students were over two times more likely to witness at least one act of shooting or stabbing in a single year (Schwab-Stone et al., 1995). Asian American youth also report significant levels of CVE with reported victimization occurring both within and across racial groups (Le & Chan, 2001; Rennison, 2001). Additionally, one study reported American Indians experienced rates of violence between 1992 and 2002 at least twice as high as African Americans, Caucasians, and Asian Americans (Rennison & Rand, 2003).

Age Older youth are at greater risk for CVE than younger youth (Richters & Martinez, 1993; Weist, Acosta, & Youngstrom, 2001). This relationship between age and rates of CVE appears to be strong although there is some inconsistency in the findings. Official homicide reports show that the risk for violent death from a non-family perpetrator remains low until adolescence, then rises dramatically, and peaks at approximately 20 years, with a gradual decline through the rest of the lifespan (Snyder & Sickmund, 2006). Several self-report studies on non-fatal violence exposure corroborate this pattern; however, the findings of this relationship are not uniform, and may, in part, depend upon the subgroups studied. For example, urban samples of ethnic minorities reveal high rates of CVE among all age groups (Linares, Heeren, Bronfman, Zuckerman, Augustyn, & Tronick, 2001; Miller, Wasserman, Neugebauer, Gorman-Smith, & Kamboukos, 1999; Taylor, Zuckerman, Harik, & Groves, 1994). The rates of violence exposure (i.e. victimization or witnessing shooting, stabbing, or beating) for urban African American elementary school students is approximated at over 30 percent (Bell & Jenkins, 1993; Schiff & McKay, 2003), while the rate for African American high school students is approximated at between 61 and 71 percent (Jenkins & Bell, 1994; Pastore, Fisher, & Friedman, 1996; Uehara, Chalmers, Jenkins, & Shakoor, 1996; Voisin, 2003). Also, high rates of CVE exist even for extremely young African American children in urban settings: 47 percent of parents of children aged one to five years report their children have heard gun shots and 10 percent reported their children having witnessing a shooting or stabbing (Taylor et al., 1994). Other studies estimate that 78 percent of children aged three to four were exposed to at least one act of community violence (Shahinfar, Fox, & Leavitt, 2000) and that in a one-year period, 42 percent of children had witnessed at least one violent act and 21 percent had witnessed three or more violent acts (Linares et al., 2001).

Gender   Male children and adolescents are overall more likely than females to experience and witness violent incidents in the community, across socioeconomic gradients and ethnic groups (Boney-McCoy & Finkelhor, 1995; Fitzpatrick & Boldizar, 1993; Gladstein, Rusonis, & Heald, 1992; Schwab-Stone et al., 1995; Selnor-O'Hagan, Kindlon, Buka, Raudenbush, & Earls, 1998; Singer, Anglin, Song, & Lunghofer, 1995). Some evidence suggests that while males are at greater risk of personally experiencing and witnessing physical violence, females are at greater risk of exposure to sexual assaults (Rudoph & Hammen, 1999), though the findings on gender are not uniform. Some evidence suggests that gender differences in CVE may vary according to age. For example, studies have reported no gender differences in preschool children's exposure to community violence (Shahinfar et al., 2000), and one study found that girls in elementary school reported greater CVE than did boys of the same age, although those differences disappeared in a follow-up study conducted two years later (Attar et al., 1994).

Psychosocial-behavioral factors   Little empirical evidence to date sheds light on the individual-level psychosocial or behavioral factors that increase or decrease risk to CVE. Some preliminary evidence has indicated that the use of illicit psychoactive substances is associated with greater community violence exposure. For example, a multi-country study including over 3,000 adolescents in urban communities (Antwerp, Belgium; Arkangelsk, Russia; and New Haven, Connecticut) found that higher rates of smoking, alcohol use, marijuana use, and hard drug use were associated with higher levels of CVE (Vermeiren, Schwab-Stone, Deboutte, Leckman, & Ruchkin, 2003). Not surprisingly, adolescents with aggressive behavior problems are at a higher risk for violence exposure, particularly so for males who also show depressive symptoms (Lambert et al., 2005).

Peer influence   Peers are important to youth development, especially for adolescents. Witnessing community violence appears to be associated with affiliation with delinquent peers (Halliday-Boykins & Graham, 2001), and a number of studies have found that youth victims of community violence are more likely to have peers who are perpetrators and victims of violence (Felson, 1997; Lauritsen & Davis-Quinet, 1995; Lauritsen, Sampson, & Laub, 1991; Sampson & Lauritsen, 1990). In addition, some evidence suggests that negative and harsh parenting might place children at a higher risk of community violence exposure by shaping the children's own aggressive behavior, and by affecting their socializing patterns with more delinquent peers (Centers & Weist, 1998; Lauritsen, Laub, & Sampson, 1992).

Family level factors Household composition and structure, as well as parental attitudes, have been implicated in risk for CVE. Living in a single-female-headed household was associated with increased risk of youth CVE (Lauritsen, 2003). In fact, risk of violent victimization and CVE is 50 percent higher in single-parent families than among youth who live in two-parent families despite community location, socioeconomic factors, and race-ethnicity of family (Lauritsen, 2003). Parental interactions with youth also appear to influence CVE as poor parental monitoring and ineffective, inconsistent discipline are related to delinquency and violent behavior (Capaldi & Patterson, 1996; Dishion, Patterson, Stoolmiller, & Skinner, 1991; Gorman-Smith, Tolan, Zelli, & Huesmann, 1996; Patterson, Reid, & Dishion, 1992). Consequently, delinquency and violent behavior are associated with increased risk for CVE (Centers & Weist, 1998; Lauritsen et al., 1992).

Community level factors Schools are often thought of as safe havens from CVE, yet violence is often reported on school grounds, often in "un-owned places" or public spaces that no one has personal responsibility over (e.g. hallways, playgrounds) (Astor, Meyer, & Behre, 1999). Youth in urban neighborhoods are also exposed to high rates of CVE on their routes to and from school (Meyer & Astor, 2002). Although relatively infrequent compared to other types of school violence, school-related shootings continue to occur, are highly publicized by the media, and have major implications for student distrust, fears, and engagement in violence. Significant decreases in single-victim school-related homicides were observed from 1992 to 2006, yet, although fewer in number (8 of last 109 incidents), multiple-victim homicide rates remained stable (CDC, 2008).

Poverty In general, CVE is associated with community settings characterized by high concentrations of poverty, as indicated by low incomes, poor housing conditions, and high rates of residential instability (Cooley-Quille, Turner, & Beidel, 1995; Fitzpatrick, 1997; Horowitz, Weine, & Jekel, 1995; Moses, 1999; Overstreet, Dempsey, Graham, & Moely, 1999). For youth living in urban communities, direct victimization ranges from approximately 18 to 60 percent depending on the study (Margolin & Gordis, 2000; Richters & Martinez, 1993), whereas witnessing community violence is much more prevalent with rates of youth exposure estimated between 50 and 100 percent (Buka, Stchick, Birthistle, & Earles, 2001; Margolin and Gordis, 2000; Richters & Martinez, 1993; Stein, Jaycox, Kataoka, Rhodes, & Vestal 2003). Severe violence is common for youth in poor, urban communities as 67 percent of urban youth in one study reported having witnessed a shooting, 50 percent witnessed a stabbing, and 25 percent were personally victimized through a form of severe violence (Jenkins & Bell, 1997).

Urban settings Urban youth, when compared to suburban youth, report higher rates of exposure to severe violence and knew of more people who had been personally injured, but a significant number of youth in suburban communities reported exposure to violence (Gladstein et al., 1992). Yet, youth living in middle-class suburban and rural settings also face significant risk for violence exposure outside the home (O'Keefe & Sela-Amit, 1997; Singer et al., 1995; Slovak & Singer, 2002; Sullivan, Kung, & Farrell, 2004). High rates of exposure to gun violence were found in rural settings with 25 percent of youth, who were not defined as poor, reported exposure to gun violence at least once (Slovak & Singer, 2002).

Violent milieu The combination of poverty and location seems to play an important role in CVE. Public housing is associated with increased rates of community violence: 83 percent of African American middle-school students living in public housing knew someone who was violently killed in the community; 55 percent had witnessed a shooting; 43 percent had seen a dead body in the neighborhood; and 37 percent had been direct victims of physical violence

(Overstreet et al., 1999). Youth who witness murder are more likely to witness other incidents of severe violence indicating that high rates of homicide are tied to other incidents, which create a "violent milieu" for youth to develop in (Bell & Jenkins, 1993). Parents are often either unaware or in denial of community violence exposure as more than 50 percent of the parents in both low and high violence neighborhoods stated that their children had not been exposed to violence in the community (Hill & Jones, 1997).

Collective efficacy   Conditions in poor urban neighborhoods are thought to intensify levels of personal and social stress, and are also viewed as more prone to illicit behaviors such as drug trafficking and gang activities from which violent behavior may often originate (Attar et al., 1994; Gabarino, Dubrow, Kostelny, & Pardo, 1992; Neugebauer, Wasserman, Fisher, Kline, Geller, & Miller, 1999). However, concentrated poverty and community disorganization are not the only community-level factors that appear to be linked with heightened risk for violence exposure. "Collective efficacy" has been found to be a potent mediator between the low economic status of a neighborhood and violence, directly explaining how poverty shapes violent behavior. Collective efficacy of a neighborhood is characterized by the degree to which residents perceive positive social cohesion among one another, and the degree to which they exercise informal social control to maintain positive social norms (Sampson, Raudenbusch, & Earls, 1997). Levels of violence directly vary according to levels of collective efficacy, and poverty is a direct predictor of neighborhood collective efficacy.

The term "community violence" risks politicization, or worse, lends itself to be used in a biased or pejorative way, such as to purvey racist, classist, or ageist stereotypes about "violent communities" or demographically defined groups. In reality, youth CVE is prevalent across varying socioeconomic classes and cultures in urban, suburban, and rural settings. However, our culture's individualistic tendencies to ignore the role of institutional structures and policies and focus on the internal interpersonal relationships as the primary factors in "collective pathology" (Smith, 2007, p. 50), in addition to, our culture's tendency to label problems to create awareness, such as "community violence" and "urban war zone," "normalizes" the problem, suggesting that there is something about the interpersonal relationships in poor urban communities which "normalizes" results in high rates of CVE. Pathologizing communities as violent not only increases the incorrect assumption that CVE is a phenomenon specific to poor urban minority communities, it has a profound effect on how those who live within these communities view themselves and how outsiders view these communities and the people who live in them. Individuals exposed to multiple risks and stressors who witness media portrayals of their communities as violent and unsafe experience "an internalized sense of marginalization, powerlessness, and sense of despair among the most vulnerable" (Aisenberg & Herrenkohl, 2008).

Social workers must be aware of color-blind racism in which "minimization" of the problem or "blaming the victim" (Bonilla-Silva, 2003) are used to conceptualize youth CVE and its associated mental health outcomes. Blaming minorities for choosing to reside in poor or high crime neighborhood pathologizes populations by placing the root of the problem within poor minority families' as possessing a "lack of effort" or "inappropriate values" (Bonilla-Silva, 2003, p. 40). This is an incorrect assumption as many factors are associated with CVE, such as "residential instability, concentration of poor female-headed families with children, multiunit housing projects, and disrupted social networks, appear to stem directly from planned governmental policies at local, state, and federal levels" (Sampson & Lauritsen, 1990), not simply from individual choices or characteristics.

"Normalization" of CVE   Research of racism and the justification for racist beliefs reveal that those in power or the majority group tend to "normalize" events that could otherwise be interpreted as "racially motivated" or "racist" by interpreting events as *"natural"* or claiming *"that's the way it is"* (Bonilla-Silva, 2003, p. 37). According to sociologist Bonilla-Silva (2003,

p. 37), few things that occur in the social world are "natural," particularly things pertaining to race matters. Isolated urban communities where poor African Americans reside in were no accident as they "constructed through a series of well-defined institutional practices, private behaviors, and public policies by which whites sought to contain growing urban black populations" (Massey & Denton, 1993, p. 10). By viewing the problem of "community violence" as "natural" and the "way it is" for urban minority communities, society is at risk of further neglecting the problem of CVE and its deleterious effects. For example, decreased police responsiveness in poor urban communities is linked to beliefs about urban communities. "Officers come to believe that certain crimes are normative" in poor urban communities and thus not worth their effort, and they often view victims in such settings as deserving (Klinger, 1997). By accepting community violence as a "normal" experience for youth in urban neighborhoods and not directly addressing it, we are reinforcing stereotypes, preventing community integration, aiding in the increase of distrust of urban dwellers, which then break down the community cohesion that may have served or does serve as a protective factor to community violence exposure (Massey & Denton, 1993, p. 92).

Outcomes to youth CVE   The most devastating outcome of community violence exposure is death. Tragically, murder is one of the leading causes of death in children and adolescents (CDC, 2006) and therefore we believe prevention of violent victimization should be first on both the research and political agendas. First, CVE was thought to primarily influence aggression, delinquency, and criminal behavior (e.g., Herrara & McCloskey, 2003), however CVE has been associated with many other psychosocial outcomes including internalizing symptoms, such as depression, anxiety, and post-traumatic stress as well as poor educational outcomes, problems with social relations, and poor health status (Bair-Merritt, Blackstone, & Feudtner, 2006; Delaney-Black et al., 2002; Kitzmann, Gaylord, Holt, & Kenny, 2003; Lynch, 2003; Margolin & Gordis, 2000; Wolfe, Crooks, Lee, McIntyre-Smith, & Jaffe, 2003; Wright et al., 2004).

Violence exposure affects youth development. Victimization through family violence has been associated with developmental delays in social, cognitive, affective, and language development in youth (Bower & Stivers, 1998; Osofsky & Scheeringa, 1997). Similarly, CVE interferes with many of the primary developmental tasks in childhood and early adulthood (the period of greatest exposure risk), such as the development of trust, emotional regulation, and the ability to form and establish social relationships (Garbarino, Kostelny, & Dubrow, 1991; Margolin, 1998; Margolin & Gordis, 2000). Witnessing CVE in childhood has also been associated with increased risk for psychological problems later on in adolescence and adulthood, such as substance use issues and anxiety, depression, and PTSD (Aisenberg, 2001; Buka et al., 2001; Gorman-Smith, Henry, & Tolan, 2004; Hammack, Richards, Luo, Edlynn & Roy, 2004; Saltzman, Pynoos, Layne, Steinberg, & Aisenberg, 2001).

Externalizing symptoms   Clear links between CVE and externalizing symptoms such as increased aggression, delinquency, and weapons-carrying have been well established in the research literature. Increased fighting after witnessing a shooting or stabbing has been observed in African American grade school students in urban high-crime neighborhoods (Bell & Jenkins, 1993). Witnessing community violence has been highly associated with aggression in youth in both cross-sectional (Schwartz & Proctor, 2000) and longitudinal studies, the latter of which point out CVE independently predicts future aggression (Farrell & Bruce, 1997; Gorman-Smith & Tolman, 1998; Guerra, Huesmann, & Spindler, 2003; Miller et al. 1999). Antisocial behavior and willingness to use aggression have been shown to be more closely associated with witnessing violence than internalizing symptoms such as anxiety, depression, and somatization (Schwab-Stone et al., 1999). Studies of the sequelae of CVE have reported that aggressive acting out behaviors are a more prevalent consequence in boys than in girls (O'Keefe & Sela-Amit, 1997).

Minority youth and criminal behavior African American youth are overrepresented in the juvenile justice system compared to other racial or ethnic groups (Snyder & Sickmund, 2006), which may be associated with the higher rates of CVE that African Americans are at increased risk for. Longitudinal studies of youth who experienced CVE reveal these youth have increased involvement with the juvenile justice system and serious criminal behaviors (Margolin & Gordis, 2000; Widom, 1989). Cross-sectional studies support these findings. Juvenile offences has been positively associated with community violence victimization in a sample of 12 to 18-year-old African Americans (McGee & Baker, 2002) and of detained youth, those who engaged in serious criminal behaviors were four times as likely to experience CVE (Preski & Shelton, 2001). Increased witnessing of violence in the neighborhood was associated with increased self-report assaultive behavior and weapon carrying (Patchin, Hueber, McCluskey, Varano, & Bynum, 2006). Longitudinal studies have been able to document that increases in aggression *follow* violence exposure, providing evidence that CVE may evoke violence perpetration from victims more than the reverse, suggesting a rippling "contagion" effect of community violence (Farrell & Bruce, 1997; Gorman-Smith & Tolan, 1998) and the need for a discussion of the blurred lines between victim and perpetrator of community violence. Utilizing aggressive behaviors may be viewed as one attempt at coping with victimization experiences.

CVE and other externalizing symptoms Youth exposed to community violence report engagement in high levels of risky behaviors, including greater HIV-related risk behaviors (e.g., engaging in sex without condoms, sex with multiple partners, and using drugs during sex) (Berenson, Wiemann, & McCombs, 2001; Voisin, 2003) and greater use of alcohol and illicit psychoactive substances (Kilpatrick, Acierno, Saunders, Resnick, Best, & Schnurr, 2000; Margolin & Gordis, 2000; Schwab-Stone et al., 1995). Mediating factors emerging after CVE, such as increased psychological distress, academic issues, and risk for belonging to peer groups endorsing risk norms, have been proposed as factors influencing engagement in high risk taking behaviors (Voisin & Guilamo-Ramos, 2008). Also, risk taking behaviors, such as substance use, have been cited as possible coping mechanisms that youth utilize to cope with the stress associated with exposure to community violence (Kilpatrick et al., 2000).

Identification with the aggressor or aggressive individuals in the community may result from feelings of anxiety and fear and influence the carrying of weapons and engagement in violence (DuRant et al., 1994; Schwab-Stone et al., 1995). Most importantly, speculation as to why engagement in remorseless acts of aggression and retribution occur has lead to the consideration of CVE affecting youths' moral development. Not only has CVE been speculated to "truncate" youth moral development (Fields, 1987, cited in Garbarino et al., 1992), which is intensified by the lack of opportunities to discuss moral dilemmas with trusted adults (Garbarino et al., 1992), youth exposed to community violence may develop "nonchalant" attitudes, view "violence as a way of life" (Wilson, 1991, p. xii), and experience literal desensitization or hypersensitization to violence (Krenichyn, Saegert, & Evans, 2001; Wilson, Kliewer, Teasley, Plybon, & Sica, 2002). It is also posited that the fatalistic beliefs and behaviors, as well as, a sense of futurelessness often associated with youth CVE, especially adolescents (DuRant et al., 1994; Schwab-Stone et al., 1995; van der Kolk, 1987) may partially explain the high rates of suicide in adolescents (Rathus, Asnis, & Wetzler, 1995).

Internalizing and physical symptoms Youth cognitively process the experience of violence exposure differently than adults (Kliewer, Lepore, Oskin, & Johnson, 1998; Schwartz & Proctor, 2000) and may have more adverse reactions and less effective skills to cope with trauma. In children of all ages, witnessing community violence has been associated with stress reactions such as worries about safety, fearing for one's life, and recurrence of upsetting thoughts and feelings of loneliness (Bell & Jenkins, 1993; Osofsky, Wewers, Hann, & Fick, 1993; Voison, 2003). Cognitive theories of trauma posit that traumatic events remain "active" in our memories as "intrusive recollections" until they can assimilated into our existing schemas of our environment and ourselves, or until existing schemas adapt to integrate the traumatic event (Creamer, Burgess, & Pattison, 1992). CVE may have an indirect, rather than direct, effect on anxiety, as intrusive thoughts appear to influence the subsequent levels of anxiety (Kliewer & Sullivan, 2008). Also, youth exposed to community violence exhibit increased states of either physiological hypoarousal and hyperarousal (Krenichyn et al., 2001; Wilson et al., 2002), which result in desensitization to violence for some youth while others experience high levels of anxiety, both which may impact psychosocial functioning. Disrupted production patterns of cortisol, a hormone that is released when people experience stress or anxiety, have been linked to stress resulting from CVE exposure, with overall higher levels of cortisol present over the course of the day, especially in afternoons and evenings (Suglia, Staudenmayer, Cohen, & Wright, 2009). This research is important as these symptoms often go undetected by physicians (Suglia et al., 2009) as well as by social workers.

Not surprisingly, with the psychobiological research of CVE, post-traumatic stress disorder, an anxiety disorder commonly manifested after exposure to a traumatic event, has been linked to CVE exposure in numerous studies with children of different ages and race/ethnicities including African American, Latino, Asian, and Caucasian youth (Berthold, 1999; Cooley-Quille, Boyd, Frantz, & Walsh, 2001; Duckworth et al., 2000; Fitzpatrick & Boldizar, 1993; Ozer & Weinstein, 2004; Ozer & McDonald, 2006). CVE is also associated with heightened anxiety (Aisenberg, Trickett, Mennen, Saltzman, & Zayas, 2007) and depression (Gorman-Smith & Tolan, 1998; Ozer & McDonald, 2006), as well as somatic complaints that may be related to anxiety such as sleep disturbances, headaches, stomach aches, and increased symptoms of asthma (Campbell & Schwarz, 1996; Cooley-Quille et al., 2001; Dodge, Pettit, & Bates, 1997; Fitzpatrick, Piko, Wright, & LaGory, 2005; Foster, Kuperminc, & Price, 2004; Graham-Berman & Levendosky, 1998; Margolin & John, 1997; Mazza & Reynolds, 1999; Osofsky et al., 1993; Ozer & Weinstein 2004; Schwab-Stone et al., 1999; Singer et al., 1995). CVE has been linked to subsequent disturbances in self-esteem, trust, and emotion regulation, as well as, difficulties in interpersonal relationships and isolation from positive peer groups (Dell, Siegel, & Gaensbauer, 1993).

Factors influencing internalizing symptoms Internalizing symptoms appear to be moderated by age and timing of violence exposure. Younger students (sixth grade versus seventh and eighth graders) in a large urban sample were more likely to have symptoms of internalizing stress compared to older students and it has been theorized that this may be due to pubertal changes, the stress of the transition to junior high, or lower cognitive coping abilities (Schwab-Stone et al., 1999). Although girls tend to report more anxiety than boys in studies (Edlynn, Gaylord-Harden, & Richards, 2008), there is inconsistency in the findings that anxiety responses differ by gender (Kliewer & Sullivan, 2008; Schwab-Stone et al., 1999). Internalizing symptoms appear to be more prevalent soon after CVE, whereas externalizing behaviors are more prevalent as time passes and the child grows older. For example, after witnessing community violence, more internalizing symptoms were present at baseline and compared to two years later where more externalizing behaviors were present in a sample of 1,100 urban middle school students (Schwab-Stone et al., 1999). The relationship between the victim and perpetrator appears to affect psychological distress levels, as family victimization, witnessed or not, was associated with similar levels of psychological distress as victimized adolescents (Jenkins & Bell, 1994).

Academic achievement Traumatic stress and internalizing symptoms may impact youth academic achievement (Delaney-Black et al., 2002; Saltzman et al., 2001). Exposure to community violence has been associated with increased school and academic problems in youth (Delaney-Black et al., 2002; Kelly, Murphy, Sikkema, & Kalichman, 1993; Ozer, 2005; Schwab-Stone et al., 1995), although some studies report that community violence exposure is unrelated to academic achievement (Attar et al., 2004; Hill & Madhere, 1996). Longitudinal studies show that youth exposed to such violence are more likely than peers not exposed to violence to have poor educational outcomes (Allen & Tarnowski, 1989; Leiter & Johnsen, 1994). Stress affects sleep, concentration, memory, and intrusive thoughts which may impact academic performance. Among adolescents exposed to violence, severe PTSD has been associated with impaired school functioning (Saltzman et al., 2001), and interventions that focused on the reduction of PTSD symptoms were associated with improved academic performance (Lynch, 2003). CVE may also increase the level of fear associated with traveling to school or attending school as higher level of CVE predicted declines in school attendance and increases in school behavior problems in sixth through twelfth graders (Bowen & Bowen, 1999).

Mix of symptomology and cumulative exposure to stressors   More often than not, it is a complex mix of externalizing and internalizing behaviors that are observed or reported by youth who were exposed to community violence including low school achievement and high levels of anger, anxiety, aggression, antisocial behaviors, and alcohol use (Boney-McCoy & Finkelhor, 1995; DuRant, Getts, Cadenhead, Emans, & Woods, 1995; Schwab-Stone et al., 1995; Singer et al., 1995). Kliewer & Sullivan (2008) theorize that modeling may drive externalizing symptoms and identification with those observed (more of a social learning model) and internalizing symptoms may be a function of reflecting on how exposure threatens things that are important to you. Both externalizing and internalizing symptoms have strong implications for the building of meaningful and supportive relationships for youth as both symptom types effect how a youth trusts and engages in the community.

Community violence does not occur in a vacuum. Youth are often exposed to a number of life stressors in addition to often chronic violence in the home, at school, and/or in the community, which together negatively impact youth development psychological functioning (Margolin & Gordis, 2000). Poor community infrastructure, lack of social and economic opportunities, parents' problems with substance abuse and psychopathology, and chaotic living environments further intensify levels of stress and increase tolerance for violence (Elliot, Wilson, Huizinga, Sampson, Elliot, & Rankin, 1996; Gabarino et al., 1992; Leventhal & Brooks-Gunn, 2000; Moore, 2005; Repetti, Taylor, & Seeman, 2002). The most powerful predictor of symptom levels in youth with exposure to community violence was the inclusion of daily hassles in life (Ozer & Weinstein, 2004). Contextual factors including parent distress level and parent-child relations, family conflict also influence CVE outcomes. Margolin et al. (2009) found that youth are exposed to multiple kinds of violence, including parent-to-youth aggression and community violence, and exposure is related to youth behavior problems, which increased in families where fathers reported high levels of global distress symptoms. Similarly, Buka et al. (2001) found family conflict and domestic violence to moderate (and exacerbate) the relationship between community violence and youth psychosocial outcomes. Youth living within disadvantaged neighborhoods have higher CVE levels, but they typically experience fewer opportunities for positive relationships and adult role models than do other youth (Lynch & Cicchetti, 2002).

In addition to the combinations of risk factors associated with CVE and negative outcomes, the interrelationships among different kinds of community violence exposure are often neglected, as more often than not, exposure involves experience of multiple kinds of violence (Finkelhor et al., 2005). For example, bullying frequently entails physical assaults, property crimes, and sexual harassment (Nansel, Overpeck, Haynie, Ruan, & Scheidt, 2003). To take this one step further, other victimizations are often "precursors" or "catalysts" for exposure to violence (Finkelhor et al., 2005). For example, children abused by parents, for example, appear more likely to be bullied at school (Perry, Hodges, & Egan, 2001). Social learning theory posits that what behaviors children are exposed to will be modeled by the child and children, especially boys, learn to be violent by modeling aggression and violent behaviors as observed in their home, school, and community families (O'Keefe & Sela-Amit, 1997).

Type and Severity of CVE Method of violence exposure, type of violence, and frequency of exposure are important and understudied factors affecting youth psychosocial outcomes associated with CVE. Direct exposure to community violence is not necessary for youth to experience adverse outcomes. Witnessing violence has been associated with increased PTSD symptoms in urban youth after adjusting for direct victimization experiences (Duckworth et al., 2000). Also, simply hearing about community violence is associated with increased levels of anxiety, depression, and aggression among 18–21-year-olds (Scarpa et al., 2006). Different types of violence are likely to affect youth in different ways (Trickett, Durán, & Horn, 2003). For example, being robbed at gunpoint or witnessing a fistfight or hearing a drive-by shooting are clearly unique incidents, which affect youth differently (Horn & Trickett, 1998; Trickett et al., 2003).

Protective factors associated with CVE outcomes Despite the high prevalence of CVE within poor urban communities, the majority of youth do not have serious behavioral, social, or emotional problems (Tolan & Henry, 1996), indicating the existence of protective factors or resiliency characteristics in youth, their families, schools, and communities. Yet, little research examines community or family level factors that buffer risk among youth exposed to community violence (e.g. Gorman-Smith & Tolan, 2003; Ozer & Weinstein, 2004) or individual differences in coping with CVE that may serve as buffers to exposure or negative outcomes (Finkelor et al., 2005). Of the few studies that explore factors that appear to mediate or moderate the relationship between CVE and mental health outcomes, the youths' environment, level of social support, and number of combined risk factors appear to be important protective factors.

School environment Schools are commonly believed to protect youth from violence exposure, but they have rarely been studied as such. For urban adolescents, it's been theorized that schools may function as a zone of relative safety for youth, but are also settings in which youth are victimized or engage in violence (Kann et al., 1996). Similar levels of violence are present in schools and communities. In the United States and Europe, approximately 80 percent of youth have witnessed verbal aggression and 75 percent physical aggression in schools (Flannery, Wester, & Singer, 2004; Galand, Philippot, Buidin, & Lecocq, 2004; Singer et al., 1999), which are as high or higher than CVE rates. However, perceptions of safety associated with the school environment have been associated with educational and psychological outcomes (e.g. self-concept and control) (U.S. Department of Education, 1997). Thus, for some youth, school may be a protective factor and for others it may not. Interestingly, perceived support from school (teachers and peers) appears to promote resilience to a number of stressors and be more important for older youth (high school aged), whereas parent support and coping strongly promotes resilience in younger youth (middle-school aged) (O'Donnell, Schwab-Stone, & Muyeed, 2002).

Home environment and family The home environment, family structure, and relationships with parents also serve as protective factors to CVE. Safer home environments in high-crime neighborhoods are associated with better functioning among youth (Richters & Martinez, 1993). Family cohesion, closeness with parents, and time spent with family are identified protective factors for youth exposed to community violence (Gorman-Smith & Tolan, 1998; Hammack et al., 2004; Plybon & Kliewer, 2001), while being raised without a stable male figure in the home has been associated with increased levels of anxiety and aggression in youth exposed to community violence (Fitzpatrick & Boldizar, 1993) and less helpful mothers have been associated with higher depressive symptoms in youth as their overall CVE increased (Ozer & Weinstein, 2004), while positive coping on the part of parents and family cohesion serve as buffers to negative outcomes associated with CVE (Buka et al., 2001; Plybon & Kliewer, 2001).

Secure attachments in early family relationships has been speculated to be an important moderator of CVE for youth (Luthar, 2006) and having a secure attachment with at least one parent or other adult appears to buffer effects of CVE (Engle, Castle, & Menon, 1996; Katz & Gottman, 1997; Werner, 1995). Working with parents to assist them in building meaningful relationships with their children, learning ways to effectively cope with environmental stressors to create a sense of security and confidence in their children may lead children to have higher-self-esteems and improved ability to cope with CVE (Garbarino et al., 1992).

Social support   Social support from the youth's parents, school, and peer group has been found to be important in mitigating the negative impact repeated CVE (Hill & Madhere, 1996; O'Donnell, Schwab-Stone, & Muyeed, 2002). However, mixed findings exist as to the role of social support acting as having a direct impact on resiliency when exposed to community violence (Masten & Coatsworth, 1998). Higher perceived social support from peers and adults has been associated with less PTSD symptoms in youth (Berman, Kurtines, Silverman, & Serafini, 1996; Ozer & Weinsten, 2004), yet in another study, low family support was associated with increased anxiety symptoms over time, but family support did not moderate the relationship between exposure to violence and anxiety symptoms in youth with community violence exposure (White, Bruce, Farrell, & Kliewer, 1998). Improved coping has been related to having the opportunity to talk about exposure to community violence. For example, lower perceived constraints to discuss violence has been associated with less PTSD symptoms in youth (Ozer & Weinsten, 2004).

Coping skills and appraisal of violence   Youth's exposure to community violence may alter how they cognitively appraise violence. Coping behaviors have been theorized to play an important role in linkages between violence exposure and externalizing behavior problems (Rosario, Salzinger, Feldman, & Ng-Mak, 2003), but coping behaviors may differ depending on if the youth is a victim, witness, or perpetrator of violence, availability of people to talk to, and the youths' individual characteristics. After witnessing violence, avoidant coping was associated with increased stability, whereas approach coping was associated with increased anxiety over time for African American sixth and seventh graders in an urban setting (Edlynn et al., 2008). Witnessing violence is less likely to result in adjustment problems compared to personal victimization (Kliewer & Sullivan, 2008). This has been attributed to the theory that victimization threatens a youth's core needs for competence, relatedness, and autonomy to a greater extent than does witnessing violence (Kliewer & Sullivan, 2008; Skinner & Wellborn, 1994), which may explain why exposure to community violence negatively affects relationships and school performance. Coping behaviors also appear to be moderated by gender, but research findings have been inconsistent in this area (Edlynn et al., 2008). Also, coping behaviors were found to have a direct effect on youth physical and mental health, but did not mediate physical and mental health outcomes after exposure to violence (Fredland, Campbell, & Haera, 2008), suggesting that coping behaviors do not impact psychosocial functioning after exposure to violence, but do play a role in overall health.

Level of acculturation   Acculturation may be related to coping as it appears to impact the outcomes of youth CVE. Ho (2008) found that higher rates of bicultural orientation (i.e. when ethnic minorities adopt or identify with the values and lifestyle of both the dominant culture and one's own ethnic culture) were associated with lower externalizing and traumatic-stress symptoms when exposed to stress and community violence, but bicultural orientation did not moderate psychological symptomatology in Vietnamese and Cambodian adolescents. Increased acculturation in Latino youth is associated with increased health behavior risks when exposed to community violence (Balcazar, Peterson, & Cobas, 1996; Harris, 1999; Katoaka et al., 2003). Increased English language fluency was associated with higher levels of CVE and PSTD symptoms than those with lower fluency (Katoaka et al., 2003). This highlights the theories of tight-knit recently immigrated communities as being a protective factor for youth, yet as youth and their families become more Americanized, they are more likely to be exposed to violence in the community and experience increased risk for negative psychological outcomes.

Community factors Community involvement through adult mentoring and engagement in activities with community organizations (e.g., health, educational, religious, cultural, recreational, and social service organizations) appear to impact youths' resiliency to CVE (Fergus & Zimmerman, 2005; Luthar & Zelazo, 2003). The neighborhood context is important as it directly impacts crime levels (Agnew, 1999); influences the collective efficacy of residents in community child supervision (Sampson, Morenoff, & Gannon-Rowley, 2002); and appears to mitigate the buffering effects of social support for youth exposed to community violence if the community is particularly violent (Hammack et al., 2004). CVE affects how youth perceive their communities. As "danger replaces safety as the organizing principle" (Garbarino et al., 1992), youth may exhibit an underdeveloped or damaged sense of basic security in the world. This experience has implications for the youths' psychological health, as well as, engagement in community activities or violence.

Importance of assessment and role of social work Despite the prevalence of CVE and associated negative psychosocial outcomes and the opportunity for assessment by professionals, CVE is not routinely assessed in the fields of mental health (Guterman & Cameron, 1998), special education (U.S. Department of Education, 1997), child welfare, and juvenile justice systems (U.S. Department of Health and Human Services, 2001; Widom, 1999). Moreover, since many adult psychosocial problems may have their beginnings in childhood, early detection of violence exposure and its negative effects is important to prevent problems from becoming more ingrained during adulthood (Margolin & Gordis, 2000; Margolin & John, 1997). Although the child protective services system is an entire service system dedicated to specifically protecting, preventing, intervening, and educating society when children are exposed to violence inside the home, parallel mandated protocols and services have not been created for mental health, medical, or education professionals when children are exposed to violence outside the home.

Given that CVE is as prevalent as child maltreatment, if not more so, and often leads to similar detriment in youths' mental health and other psychosocial functioning, it is unclear as to why social workers have not paid more attention to the deleterious effects of CVE. Possibly, community violence is viewed as a normal experience by many social workers who work with poor minority youth in high crime neighborhoods or it is assumed that youth are not affected by community violence. Whatever the reason, social workers face a unique opportunity to effectively address youth exposure to community violence given that social workers engage youth at high risk of CVE exposure in numerous community settings, including hospitals, schools, child welfare agencies, community centers, and clinics (Guterman & Cameron, 1998).

Social work as a profession also uniquely emphasizes understanding contextual factors in relation to a client's presenting problems (i.e. person-in-environment model), which places social workers as important agents in assessing problematic behaviors or deteriorating mental health and considering not only individual and family level factors as impacting the youth, but also the influence of community-based experiences on the youth's functioning. Evidence-based approaches within social work are sorely needed to address the multilevel challenges for youth and their families at risk for CVE.

Illustration and discussion

Assessment Without assessing for CVE, it is impossible to influence future exposure or outcomes to exposure. The safety and protection of the youth is the first and foremost goal of assessment of

CVE. Inclusion of CVE questions must occur in every assessment a social worker conducts with a child or adolescent. It is common practice to assess the youth's problematic behaviors and psychological functioning; the context of the child's life, such as familial structure and relationship; and any child maltreatment. As we have learned, the psychological outcomes associated with CVE are as serious as those associated with child maltreatment. CVE is associated with a number of psychological sequelae, such as anxiety, depression, and aggression, which may be incorrectly attributed to other factors if CVE is not included in the assessment.

Social workers must not only work with youth or address specifically mental health issues associated with CVE. Social workers must also assess and work with youths' families, school system, and communities in order to decrease future CVE risk and mitigate psychosocial outcomes. Beyond assessment and treatment of CVE, social workers must engage in "community building, mediation, and advocacy" (Guterman & Cameron, 1998) in order to prevent community violence and build resiliency in individuals and communities with chronic violence exposure. Often the worst outcomes of CVE are for youth with the greatest number of individual and environmental stressors (Garbarino et al., 1992). Guterman & Cameron (1998) provide a framework for assessing CVE in youth that involves a four-step process using the acronym "I.S.L.E." (see Table 11.1).

The I.S.L.E. process is not intended to be a linear process, but rather one that is cyclical and complimentary. The four domains are "domains" of assessment, not "steps" to assessment, thus they can be approached in whichever order best fits the uniqueness of the individual's characteristics and the nature of CVE. The following are illustrations of youth exposed to community violence and key elements that social workers must be aware of while engaging in the I.S.L.E. process.

> Jenna an outgoing 15-year-old female residing in an urban neighborhood, disclosed that when she was 9 years old, she was pushed into the street with oncoming traffic by an older male classmate. Jenna reported that the assistant principal "got mad" at her and suspended her. Jenna became depressed, quiet, and felt nobody liked her because she got into fights all the time. She talked to teachers, the principal, and her mother about the fighting, but felt that none of them helped or "really listened" to her. Her mother told her to "stop fighting," but eventually suggested she talk to someone and she began talking to the school counselor, which she reported was helpful. More recently, Jenna reported that she and her boyfriend witnessed a young male fall to the ground, incoherent and bloodied after being beaten by a group of older kids near school. Jenna's boyfriend called the police, but she stated she did not tell her mother or discuss the incident with the school counselor. In response to how often violence occurs, Jenna stated, "You don't count the days, even month, every week. You just see it [violence]. It's there. It comes right out of the blue. It could happen anytime . . . you never know when."

Urban female youth are typically unassessed for CVE although they are often subject to physical and sexual violence in the community (Miller, 2008). Due to training or personal life experiences, social workers may not naturally consider community violence as a factor contributing to mental health symptoms in youth. In fact, adults are not always receptive to youth who come to them to discuss violence occurring in schools or communities. Adults may be in denial that violence is occurring, feel helpless to address a problem that seems literally "out of their hands" as it is occurring outside of their homes, or simply do not know what to say. Social workers have the unique position of being available and willing to talk with youth about violence exposure. More importantly, social workers can be trained in trauma-informed approaches in order to minimize undue stress as discussions about violence can often be "emotionally charged" (Guterman & Cameron, 1998).

Social workers, teachers, parents, and other community members may be exposed to community violence as well, which presents a unique challenge in addressing the issue. Although it is

Table 11.1 I.S.L.E. process

---

1 Identify: the youth's involvement in CVE and nature of the involvement
Individuals involved (victims, witnesses, perpetrators, accomplices)
Youth's relationship to those involved
Chain of events leading up to exposure – determine if events are malleable or entrenched
Location of incident
Youth's behavioral, affective, and cognitive coping responses to the events
Youth's sense of responsibility and control with regard to the incident

2 Sequelae assessment: Determine the impact of CVE PTSD

Anxiety	Inability to concentrate	Reckless behavior
Depression	Isolation	Somatic complaints
Aggression	Withdrawal from activities	Post-traumatic stress symptoms
Violence	Academic failure	

3 Lethality assessment: Determine to degree to which youth is in imminent or ongoing danger
Youth's proximity to the violence exposure
Relation to those involved in the violence
Motivation or inclination to be involved in violence
Suicidal ideation, especially for adolescents
Access to weapons
Identification with the aggressor

4 Ecological assessment: Determine risk and protective factors for youth
Religious & political beliefs
Social network & support – quality of relationships with these individuals
Willingness of social network to engage in intervention
Other stressors & protective factors:
– past exposure to violence
– family violence
– other traumatic experiences
– personal or family substance use
Poverty
Neighborhood
Access to supportive adults
Parental attitudes and psychological functioning
Problematic relationships
Gang involvement
Physical condition of neighborhood
The extent to which violence is used as a common way to have needs met

---

important to gain an understanding of the youth's developmental stage and "perceptual set," or the perceptive lens by which events are filtered, in order to understand how particular youth make sense of the violence and cope with it (Guterman & Cameron, 1998), it is equally important for the social worker to understand how he or she, as well as the community typically copes with violence exposure. It may be difficult to empathize with youth exposed to violence if social workers may not have personal experiences with violence or may be personally experiencing the effects of traumatization due to CVE. Taking stock of one's personal experiences, fears, and coping mechanisms around violence is important in order to be effective in working with youth exhibiting mental health symptoms post-CVE.

The process of youth sharing information about community violence with a trusted adult is as important as assessment. Youth often have difficulty approaching adults to discuss the subject of community violence, as adults (e.g. parents and teachers) tend to minimize the experience; attempt to problem solve rather than process; or focus on cheering up the victim or witness and/or punishing and shaming the perpetrator. Adults must be available and willing to discuss violence and respond in such a way that does not shut down communication, punish, or raise fear of being placed at even great risk by open discussion with the youth for witnessing or being involved in violence. This may be a delicate task as school rules and community laws in place to maintain safety emphasize punishment as a response, and traditionally, youth with aggressive or violence behaviors are often labeled as "trouble-makers" and held responsible for their actions, despite the numerous social and environmental factors that influence youth behavior. Adult responses to youths' disclosure of witnessing or involvement of violence may have a strong impact on mental health symptoms. In the previous case example, it is difficult to determine whether Jenna appears to have become isolated, stigmatized, and depressed due to violence exposure or due to the way in which the adults in her life responded to her attempts to talk about it. Most likely, it is combination of both, which is why there are number of interventions developed to assist schools and communities with effectively responded to CVE.

> Robby, a 17-year-old male living in the projects with his mother and sister, discusses his history of dealing drugs, the ease with which he can get a gun, and how friends of his were recently locked up for killing someone. Robby describes how when he was in second grade, he was beaten up on the playground, but didn't tell his mother because her response is "if you see a fight, keep to yourself, and go home." He also believes that "everybody sees things they don't want to see, so why tell someone?" Robby reports that knives don't scare him, but he has been threatened with a gun twice and uses verbal threats to protect himself and his sister, such as: "If you kill me, somebody's going to kill half your family." He states that "sometimes it is just talk," but "you just know . . . you can tell if people are serious. You have to be careful." Robby reports feeling normal when he plays basketball, but when especially "tired," he reports getting mad instantly when people look at him because he thinks they want to fight him. Robby grew up "fighting" with his cousin, but feels that fighting with friends is a waste of time, his advice, "only fight when you really have to."

Youth use many different ways to cope with violence exposure and much of it may be adaptive, such as increasing in toughness or exhibiting aggressive behaviors, but are misinterpreted by adults as maladaptive coping (Freeman, Schaffer, & Smith, 1996). Youth may develop a "braggadocio" attitude and blunt or inappropriate affect due to the psychological numbing associated with violence exposure (Guterman & Cameron, 1998). Thus, youth may seem unaffected by CVE, or on the other hand, exhibit severe aggression or irritability, which may be misattributed to personal characteristics or situations and not CVE. If violence is a respected method of getting one's needs met and idealized by youth in a particular community due to the use of violence by family members or other powerful or wealthy individuals (Gabarino et al., 1992), care must be taken by social workers to understand the intricate relationships between the youth, the violence, and the community in order to choose an appropriate method of intervention.

Safety planning and harm reduction strategies are contingent on social workers being familiar with state, school, or agency policies and confidentiality limits so that the appropriate parties are notified and solicited to participate in a plan to protect the youth, their family, and potentially the school and/or community. When assessing CVE, social workers must be prepared to enter into a crisis intervention mode if necessary. Any sharing of information must be done so with extreme care, as the youth may experience increased isolation, harassment, or retribution from family, peers, or others in the community for their disclosure. An inherent dialectic in these complex situations that the social workers must be aware of is that youth want to talk to you, but they don't want to talk to you at the same time. Working with males may be particularly difficult as they are often threatened to acknowledge their feelings and the fear of disclosing too much information about oneself or a family member or a friend has a strong bearing over what details a social worker will be clued in on. However, as evidenced by the example above, Robby was willing to discuss many of his experiences and beliefs about community violence with an interviewer, albeit someone he was not familiar with, when given the opportunity to do so. Talking with youth about their experiences and intervening after an incidence of violence in the community is a starting point for preventing violence and a number of intervention and prevention methods have been developed to address CVE on individual, family, school, and community levels.

Intervention More often than not, social workers must be creative in determining the best approaches for intervening with youth, as both internalizing and externalizing symptoms may be present, as well as, a myriad of influential environmental factors. A number of psychosocial interventions have been developed to treat youth exposed to trauma or abuse, including grief-based, expressive arts and play, and cognitive-behavioral therapies, yet little empirical evidence exists for their effectiveness with youth exposed to community violence. However, social workers can draw from the literature of effective treatments for youth PTSD (e.g. American Academy of Child and Adolescent Psychiatry (AACAP), 1998; Cohen, Berliner, & March, 2000) and harm reduction interventions to address youth mental health symptomatology resulting from CVE.

Grief-based approaches For youth exposed to a specific traumatic event, such as a school shooting, individual or group *"psychological first aid"* has been suggested as helpful and allows for the screening of significant mental health symptoms in the aftermath of trauma. Psychological First Aid can be administered in school or mental health settings in two or three sessions and includes discussions clarifying the facts of the incident, normalization of the youths' responses, and the teaching of problem-solving techniques to deal with difficult thoughts and feelings (Pynoos & Nader, 1988). Traumatic bereavement therapy, an adaptation of adult grief therapeutic techniques specifically for youth who witness or who are co-victims of homicide, includes counseling in acceptance, expression of emotion, retaining a positive view of the deceased, and adjustment to life without the individual (Pennels & Smith, 1994). Cognitive behavioral interventions have also been combined with traumatic grief interventions for children exposed to war crimes (Layne et al., 2001) and crimes related to interpersonal violence or terrorism (Cohen, Mannarino, Greenberg, Padlo, & Shipley, 2002).

Expressive arts and play therapy and cognitive behavior therapy Expressive arts and play therapy are commonly used with youth exposed to trauma or abuse. Incorporation of toys, games, and dolls in treatment and assessment assists children with feeling comfortable with a social worker while simultaneously serving as a vehicle for communication and an opportunity for further assessment and discussion of safety and harm prevention strategies (Gil, 1991). Empirically supported psychosocial interventions for traumatized youth informally incorporate play, such as structured parental counseling-child therapy (Cohen & Mannarino, 1993). Play therapy has also been formally integrated with cognitive behavior therapy (CBT) (e.g. Knell, 1998; Ruma, 1993). For older children and adolescents who are able to better articulate their experiences with single-event traumas, natural disaster, or ongoing trauma that has ended, cognitive behavior therapy has been found to be effective in mitigating mental health symptoms (e.g. Deblinger, Steer, & Lippmann, 1999). Posttraumatic stress in youth is often treated with CBT (e.g. Aisenberg & Mennen, 2000), which assists the youth with discovering new ways of thinking, challenging false beliefs, expressing feelings, and anxiety management through relaxation techniques (e.g. Finch, Nelson, & Moss, 1993).

Cognitive behavioral play therapy (CBPT) is directive and incorporates modeling and systematic desensitization techniques, yet CBPT allows youth to develop a sense of control within the structure created by the social worker in order to increase behavioral competence, correct maladaptive beliefs and/or instill adaptive thoughts and emotions (Knell, 1998; Ruma, 1993). Play and expressive arts that incorporate CBT must be done so in a developmentally appropriate way and skills must be provided to identify, process, and regulate emotions and behaviors (Deblinger &

Heflin, 1996), while also addressing misattributions of guilt, blame, and responsibility during the recalling of the incident (Banyard & Williams, 2007; Ross & O'Carroll, 2004).

Family interventions   For youth exposed to community violence, families are significant sources of resilience (Aisenberg & Mennen, 2000). Not only is it important for families to have an ability to provide a developmentally appropriate response to their children in the wake of CVE (Osofsky, 1997), but also to provide guidance and maintain communication with youth (Sweatt, Harding, Knight-Lynn, Rasheed, & Carter, 2002) and re-establish a sense of order and routine for their children (Groves, 2002). Often children and their families are exposed to the same acts of community violence and intervention with families is important for treating mental health symptoms (Vostanis, Tischler, & Cumella, 2001). For these families, it may be particularly important for parents to receive psychoeducation around increasing parental competencies, children development, the effects of violence exposure on child's functioning, and safety (Holland, Koblinskey, & Anderson, 1995; Osofsky & Fenichel, 1996) as well as therapeutic services that may positively impact personal well-being, coping strategies for daily living and trauma exposure, and parenting capacities (Osofsky & Fenichel, 1996).

Therapeutic approaches that work simultaneously with both the parent(s) and child(ren) may also be effective in addressing the mental health sequelae of CVE. Using attachment as the foundation, play therapy techniques allow the child to express emotion and work through the CVE while also allowing the parent to gain an increased understanding of the child's behavior as a way of coping with of his/her violence exposure (Davies, 1991; Osofsky & Fenichel, 1996). Also, comprehensive family support programs that blend parent education, mentoring, and mental health services that focus on parental self-sufficiency and being emotionally available to young children exposed to violence are linked to reduced conduct difficulties in children (Yoshikawa, 1994). Although not empirically supported, additional family support may be achieved through involvement with other traumatized families in community organizations, such as the Save Our Sons And Daughters (SOSAD) group, which provides support and crisis intervention for parents whose children have been killed, victimized, or witnesses of community violence (Osofsky & Fenichel, 1996).

School interventions and multimodal approaches   School interventions can provide psychoeducation, improve coping mechanisms, and increase social support. Brief CBT groups for immigrant Latino children exposed to community violence have been implemented in schools and has been found to significantly decrease symptoms of PTSD and depression in third to eighth graders (Kataoka et al., 2003). A manualized trauma-and-grief-focused treatment program, focused on increasing coping skills, adaptive grieving, psychoeducation, and normalization of CVE, has been found effective in significantly reducing grief and PTSD symptoms as well as improving academic performance (Saltzman et al., 2001). Programs that have been developed for communities with high rates of youth violence exposure include year-long intervention with youth in school-based groups, parental CBT and psychoeducation, community-based mentoring, and inclusion of key community players, such as teachers and police (e.g. Murphy, Pynoos, & James, 1997).

Prevention   Preventing CVE is accomplished through three different routes: primary prevention (interventions implemented universally to prevent the onset of CVE), secondary prevention (interventions implemented selectively a particular populations who are at high risk for CVE), and tertiary (interventions focusing on youth with previous CVE). Much information is available for intervening with youth who are violent, but little empirical evidence exists for effective prevention or treatment of CVE as the nature of CVE is complex and the research of CVE is plagued with inadequate study design and a lack of consistent data between studies preventing intervention comparisons (Limbos et al., 2007). However, scientific standards or "blueprints" of prevention strategies that significantly decrease violent behavior, crime, antisocial behavior, and substance use have been identified (Center for the Study and Prevention of Violence, 2004), as well as intervention methods that effectively mitigate negative psychosocial outcomes post-CVE.

More often than not, the social worker must be creative in determining the best approach for intervening with youth, as many youth will exhibit both internalizing and externalizing symptoms, and be exposed to a number of environmental factors that play some role in the CVE. The following are effective methods of intervention and harm reduction for youth with internalizing and externalizing mental health symptoms.

Kellerman, Fuqua-Whitley, Rivara, & Mercy (1998) assessed individual and community level violence prevention methods and although finding that most methods had "disappointing" or "mixed" results, they did find that interventions introduced in later childhood and adolescence do not appear as effective in preventing youth violence compared to those introduced between the prenatal period and six years of age (Kellerman et al., 1998), thus age appears to influence program effectiveness. CVE prevention occurs at four levels: individual, family, school, and community. Determining which prevention method is most appropriate for a subpopulation (i.e. age, race/ ethnicity, rural or urban) has been clinically recognized as important to address CVE. A number of internet websites have compiled youth violence prevention and treatment methods by specific population, situation, or location (see Web resources section below).

Strategies to reduce violence among youth often include improving *social skills and problem solving* (Tolan & Guerra, 1994). Programs such as Interpersonal Cognitive Problem Solving (ICPS) and Providing Alternative Thinking Strategies (PATHS) have been evaluated in school settings with youth, but need longitudinal study to see if reduced behavior problems and improved problem-solving skills are maintained over time (Kellerman et al., 1998). These programs tend to focus on: anger management, behavior modification, social perspectives, moral development, social skill building and problem solving, and conflict (Guerra & Williams, 1996). Methods that build social skills and increase problem-solving capacity are linked to reduced youth violence (Hawkins, Catalano, Kosterman, Abbott, & Hill, 1999; Howell & Bilchick, 1995; Thornton, Craft, Dahlberg, Lynch, & Baer, 2000). The learned social skills, emotion management, and increased moral aware-ness may influence how youth respond when harassed, provoked, or passively involved and/or witnessing a violent incident in the community.

Although most family prevention research has been focused on solely preventing youth from becoming violent or aggressive, working with youths' primary caregivers, in order to improve *family* relations through improving parenting skills and communication with their children, as well as educating them about the factors associated with violence, may be beneficial in preventing CVE and associated negative outcomes. An intervention method for families with aggressive children is the coercion model, which changes parental tactics and teaches different responses. It is composed of eight weekly family groups and four individual family sessions and has been found to reduce aggressive behaviors in youth and increase family cohesion (Patterson et al., 1992). Not only are family interventions important for children with behavior problems or aggressive tendencies, but also family involvement with the community establishes social ties and support that are important for strong families as increased social isolation has been associated with community and family violence (Carter, 2003). The Family Strengthening Policy Center (FSPC) maintains that families are strongest when supported by "safe and thriving" neighborhoods, which suggests that community functioning is associated with family functioning (FSPC, 2005). Thus, altering community level factors may have an impact on family factors and vice versa. More programs that specifically target families for CVE prevention must be explored as family issues, such as abuse and unemployment, increase the risk for youth CVE.

Although *schools* are often believed to be "safe" zones for exposure to CVE, violence occurs in schools. Strategies for addressing school violence vary greatly from school to school, depending upon student population and the community. Certain environmental risk factors, such as laws and cultural norms that support violence and punishment, access to guns, racial discrimination, increase the probability of youth violence (Hawkins et al., 2000). For youth who exhibit violent tendencies, early assessment and comprehensive and developmentally appropriate prevention methods including individual and family counseling, inpatient mental health programs, and alternative education programs have been suggested (Cunningham & Sandhu, 2000). Peer mediation and school violence curricula are two CVE prevention methods that have been evaluated. School violence prevention curricula have been found to increase knowledge of violence and conflict while decreasing physical aggression in school-aged children (Grossman et al., 1997) and self-reported rates of aggressive and violent behavior in adolescents, but were found to not alter adolescent attitudes towards violence or violence rates (Hammond & Yung, 1991; Webster, 1993). Peer mediation programs include a number of different treatment modalities, such as programs that focus on either or some combination of social, cognitive, or behavioral skills and incorporate counseling or group work (Wilson & Lipsey, 2005). Despite the type of treatment approach, aggressive behaviors commonly observed in schools, such as fighting, name-calling, intimidation, and other problematic interpersonal behaviors, generally decrease with adoption of peer mediation programs in school, especially for those students at increased risk for violence or exposure to violence (Wilson & Lipsey, 2005). However, peer mediation programs, as well as other violence prevention programs have not been evaluated for more serious school violence, such as shootings (Wilson & Lipsey, 2005).

Collaborations between parents, schools, and communities are common and are often the foundation for violence prevention planning (McDonald & Frey, 1999) and *communities* are now recognized as important stake-holders with expertise and resources to contribute to the systematic process of developing, implementing, and evaluating comprehensive plans for violence prevention (Cunningham & Sandhu, 2000). Community engagement in preservation of social ties and community cohesion has an impact on family and community violence (Carter, 2003). Ceasefire is an example of an evidence-based community violence prevention program targeting entire communities through street level outreach, public education, community mobilization, and involvement of faith leaders and law enforcement (Skogan, Hartnett, Bump, & Dubois, 2008). Ceasefire in Chicago has been found to decrease the number of shootings and the concentration and density of shootings, as well as, significantly decrease gang homicide patterns (Skogan et al., 2008).

CVE reduction cannot occur without an engaged and mobilized community with resources and partnerships with institutions that support consistent community involvement, ownership, and commitment to meet the actual needs of people in the community (Carter, 2003). Although a multitude of CVE risk factors exist, primary prevention may be the most powerful approach to ameliorate youth CVE, that is, preventing violence from occurring in the first place. In general, primary prevention methods that attempt to address the root causes of CVE have been given little attention. Additionally, strengths and needs-based approaches must be explored as opposed to "deficit"-based approaches when addressing CVE (National Human Services Assembly, 2005). According to sociological theory, little occurs naturally. Individual behaviors and community violence are a reflection of community and cultural norms, biases, and lack of opportunities (National Human Services Assembly, 2005). Thus, it is imperative that primary prevention strategies involve many different stakeholder and focus not on individual outcomes, but on community outcomes in order to prevent community violence.

The strategies suggested for addressing violence at state and local levels by the National Human Services Assembly (2005) include increasing awareness of "underlying contributors to violence," increasing community accountability through the establishment of formal organizations within communities that work with schools, law enforcement, hospitals, and organizations to create a "set of shared violence prevention principles" in order to address violence. These principles must be informed by key stakeholders (e.g. youths, families, schools, and communities) and can guide the development and process of strategic planning for intervention implementation and evaluation.

Conclusion

> Violence is a complex phenomenon arising from individual, systematic and societal factors; therefore, responses that combat it should be comprehensive and arise from local community contexts, and solutions must engage a broad array of disciplines and sectors.
>
> (Bowen, Gwiasda, & Brown, 2004, p. 357).

Social workers have a unique opportunity to impact youth CVE rates. If community stakeholders are to organize and work together to address CVE, then there is a need for connections and communication between these different groups. Social workers can be these connections because they are employed in the settings that should be involved in addressing CVE: various community organizations (e.g. YMCA, afterschool programs), law enforcement, hospitals, schools, and the government. Social workers are also trained to look beyond individual symptoms or situations and are aware of the influence that institutions, cultural beliefs, and society has on individuals. Social workers also tend to work with poor, disenfranchised, and marginalized populations, which are at higher risk for CVE. The field of social work must challenge accepted beliefs that poor, minority, urban neighborhoods are violent and expected to be so, because this is not the case. Also, typical western school and community beliefs regarding youth violence must be challenged in order to move away from punishment, isolation, and blaming/shaming of the youth to understanding the many factors involved in youth violence and to increase information sharing among youth, schools, and community organizations. However, first, social work's mission is to increase awareness of the high rates of CVE and the myriad of associated negative psychosocial outcomes. Then, social work's mission is to move beyond individual youth as primary targets for assessment and intervention in order for contextual factors, such as school policies or the physical condition of the neighborhood, to be assessed and addressed as well. Finally, social work's goal is to develop effective prevention approaches that are empirically supported.

Web resources

Center for Disease Control Violence Prevention
www.cdc.gov/ViolencePrevention/index.html

Center for the Study and Prevention of Violence
www.ibs.colorado.edu/cspv/blueprintsquery/

Community Youth Development Journal
www.cydjournal.org/contents.html

Guide to Community Preventive Services
www.thecommunityguide.org/violence/index.html

Institute for Community Peace
www.instituteforcommunitypeace.org/icp/

Prevention Institute
www.preventioninstitute.org/violenceprev.html

Promising Programs
Ceasefire: The Campaign to Stop the Shooting
www.ceasefire.com

National Youth Violence Prevention Center
www.safeyouth.org/scripts/topics/community.asp

Partners for Violence Prevention
www.partnersforviolenceprevention.org/cvp.html

References

Agnew, R. (1999). A general strain theory of community differences in crime rates. *Journal of Research in Crime and Delinquency, 36* (2), 123–155.
Aisenberg, E. (2001). The effects of exposure to community violence upon Latina mothers and preschool children. *Hispanic Journal of Behavioral Sciences, 23* (4), 378–398.
Aisenberg, E., & Herrenkohl, T. (2008). Community violence in context: Risk and resilience in children and families. *Journal of Interpersonal Violence, 22* (3), 296–315.
Aisenberg, E., & Mennen, F.E. (2000). Children exposed to community violence: Issues for assessment and treatment. *Child and Adolescent Social Work Journal, 17*, 341–360.
Aisenberg, E., Trickett, P.K., Mennen, F.E., Saltzman, W., & Zayas, L.H. (2007). Maternal depression and adolescent behavior problems: An examination of mediation among immigrant Latina mothers and their adolescent children exposed to community violence. *Journal of Interpersonal Violence, 22* (10), 1227–1249.
Allen, D.M., & Tarnowski, K.G. (1989). Depressive characteristics of physically abused children. *Journal of Abnormal Child Psychology, 17*, 1–11.
American Academy of Child and Adolescent Psychiatry (AACAP). (1998). Summary of practice parameters for the diagnosis and treatment of posttraumatic stress disorder in children and adolescents. *Journal of the American Academy of Child and Adolescent Psychiatry, 37* (9), 997–1001.
American Psychological Association (APA). (1993). *Violence and youth: Psychology response. Volume I: Summary report of the American Psychological Association Commission on violence and youth.* Washington, DC: APA.
Anderson, R.N., & Smith, B.L. (2005). Deaths: Leading causes for 2002. *National Vital Statistics Reports, 53* (17), 1–90.
Astor, R.A., Meyer, H.A., & Behre, W.J. (1999). Unowned places and times: Maps and interviews about violence in high schools. *American Educational Research Journal, 36* (1), 3–42.
Attar, B.K., Guerra, N.G., & Tolan, P.H. (1994). Neighborhood disadvantage, stressful life events, and adjustment in urban elementary school children. *Journal of Clinical Child Psychology, 23*, 391–400.
Bair-Merritt, M., Blackstone, M., & Feudtner, C. (2006). Physical health outcomes of childhood exposure to intimate partner violence: A systematic review. *Pediatrics, 117*, 278–290.
Balcazar, H., Peterson, G., & Cobas, J.A. (1996). Acculturation and health related risk-behaviors among Mexican-American pregnant youth. *American Journal of Health Behavior, 20*, 425–433.
Banyard, V.L., & Williams, L.M. (2007). Adolescent survivors of sexual abuse: Developmental outcomes. *Prevention Researcher, 14* (2), 6–10
Bell, C.C., & Jenkins, E.J. (1993). Community violence and children on Chicago's southside. *Psychiatry, 56*, 46–54.
Bell, C.C., Taylor-Crawford, K., Jenkins, E.J., & Chalmers, D. (1988). Need for victimization screening in a Black psychiatric population. *Journal of the National Medical Association, 80*, 41–48.
Berenson, A.B., Wiemann, C.M., & McCombs, S. (2001). Exposure to violence and associated health-risk behaviors among adolescent girls. *Archives of Pediatric and Adolescent Medication, 155*, 1238–1242.
Berman, S., Kurtines, W., Silverman, W., & Serafini, L. (1996). The impact of exposure to crime and violence on urban youth. *American Journal of Orthopsychiatry, 66*, 329–336.
Berthold, S.M. (1999). The effects of exposure to community violence on Khmer refugee adolescents. *Journal of Traumatic Distress, 12* (3), 455–471.
Boney-McCoy, S., & Finkelhor, D. (1995). Psychosocial sequelae of violent victimization in a national youth sample. *Journal of Consulting and Clinical Psychology, 63*, 726–736.
Bonilla-Silva, E. (2003). *Racism without racists.* Lanham, MD: Rowman & Littlefield.
Bowen, L.K., Gwiasda, V., & Brown, M.M. (2004). Engaging community residents to prevent violence. *Journal of Interpersonal Violence, 19* (3), 356–367.
Bowen, L.K., & Bowen, G.L. (1999). Effects of crime and violence in neighborhoods and schools on the school behavior and performance of adolescents. *Journal of Adolescent Research, 14*, 319–342.

Bower, G.H., & Stivers, S. (1998). Cognitive impact of traumatic stress. *Developmental Psychology, 10*, 625–653.

Brady, S.S., Gorman-Smith, D., Henry, D.B., & Tolan, P.H. (2008). Adaptive coping reduces the impact of community violence exposure on violent behavior among African American and Latino male adolescents. *Journal of Abnormal Child Psychology, 36*, 105–115.

Breslau, N., Davis, G.C., & Andreski, P. (1995). Risk factors for PTSD-related traumatic events: A prospective analysis. *American Journal of Psychiatry, 152*, 529–535.

Bronfenbrenner, U. (1999). Environments in developmental perspective: Theoretical and operational models. In S.L. Friedman & T.D. Wachs (eds), *Measuring environment across the life span* (pp. 1–28). Washington, DC: American Psychological Association.

Buka, S.L., Stchick, T.L., Birdthistle, I., & Earles, F.J. (2001). Youth exposure to violence: Prevalence, risks, and consequences. *American Journal of Orthopsychiatry, 71* (3), 298–310.

Campbell, C., & Schwarz, D. (1996). Prevalence and impact of exposure to interpersonal violence among suburban and urban middle school students. *Pediatrics, 98*, 396–402.

Capaldi, D.M., & Patterson, G.R. (1996). Can violent offenders be distinguished from frequent offenders: Prediction from childhood to adolescence. *Journal of Research in Crime and Delinquency, 33*, 206–231.

Carmona, R.H. (2007). *Family violence as a public health issue.* Retrieved July 20, 2009, from www.surgeon general.gov/news/speeches/violence08062003.htm.

Carter, J. (2003). *Domestic violence, child abuse, and youth violence: Strategies for prevention and early intervention.* Family Violence Prevention Fund. Retrieved July 1, 2009, from www.mincava.umn.edu/link/documents/fvpf2/fvpf2.shtml.

Center for the Study and Prevention of Violence (CSPV). (2004). *Blueprints for violence prevention: Overview and model programs.* Boulder, CO: CSPV. Retrieved July 20, 2009, at www.colorado.edu/cspv/blueprinst/index.html.

Centers, N.L., & Weist, M.D. (1998). Inner-city youth and drug dealing: A review of the problem. *Journal of Youth and Adolescence, 27*, 395–411.

Centers for Disease Control and Prevention (CDC). (2000). Firearms injury surveillance study, 1993–1998. Unpublished data.

Centers for Disease Control and Prevention (CDC) (2006). *Leading causes of death reports, 1999–2006.* National Center for Injury Prevention and Control. Retrieved July 1, 2009, from www.webappa.cdc.gov/sasweb/ncipc/leadcaus10.html.

Centers for Disease Control and Prevention (CDC). (2008). School-associated student homicides – United States, 1992–2006. *Morbidity and Mortality Weekly Report, 57* (2), 33–36.

Christofel, K.K. (1990). Violent death and injury in U.S. children and adolescents. *American Journal of Disease Control, 144*, 697–706.

Cohen, J.A., & Mannarino, A.P. (1993). A treatment model for sexually abused preschool children. *Journal of Interpersonal Violence, 8*, 115–131.

Cohen, J.A., Berliner, L., & March, J.E. (2000). Guidelines for treatment of PTSD: Treatment of children and adolescents. *Journal of Traumatic Stress, 13* (4), 566–568.

Cohen, J.A., Mannarino, A.P., Greenberg, T.A., Padlo, S., & Shipley, C. (2002). Childhood traumatic grief: Concepts and controversies. *Trauma, Violence and Abuse, 3* (4), 307–327.

Cooley-Quille, M.R., Turner, S.M., & Beidel, D.C. (1995). Emotional impact of children's exposure to community violence: A preliminary study. *Journal of the American Academy of Child and Adolescent Psychiatry, 34* (10), 1362–1368.

Cooley-Quille, M., Boyd, R.C., Frantz, E., & Walsh J. (2001). Emotional and behavioral impact of exposure to community violence in inner-city adolescents. *Journal of Clinical Child Psychology, 30* (2), 199–206.

Creamer, M., Burgess, P., & Pattison, P. (1992). Reaction to trauma: A cognitive processing model. *Journal of Abnormal Psychology, 101*, 452–459.

Cunningham, N.J., & Sandhu, D.S. (2000). A comprehensive approach to school–community violence prevention. *Professional School Counseling, 4* (2), 126–133.

Davies, D. (1991). Intervention with male toddlers who have witnessed parental violence. *Families in Society, 72*, 515–524.

Deblinger, E., & Heflin, A.H. (1996). *Treating sexually abused children and their nonoffending parents: A cognitive behavioral approach*. Thousand Oaks, CA: Sage.

Deblinger, E., Steer, R., & Lippmann, J. (1999). Two-year follow-up study of cognitive behavioral therapy for sexually abused children suffering posttraumatic stress symptoms. *Child Abuse and Neglect, 23*, 1371–1378.

Delaney-Black, V., Covington, C., Ondersma, S.J., Nordstrom- Klee, B., Templin, T., Ager, J. et al. (2002). Violence exposure, trauma, and IQ and/or reading deficits among urban children. *Archives of Pediatrics and Adolescent Medicine, 156*, 280–285.

Dell, M., Siegel, C., & Gaensbauer, T. (1993). Post-traumatic stress disorder. In C. Zeanah (ed.), *Handbook of infant mental health* (pp. 291–304). New York: Guilford.

Dishion, T.J., Patterson, G.R., Stoolmiller, M., & Skinner, M.L. (1991). Family, school, and behavioral antecedents to early adolescent involvement with antisocial peers. *Developmental Psychology, 27*, 172–180.

Dodge, K., Pettit, G., & Bates, J. (1997). How the experience of early physical abuse leads children to become chronically aggressive. *Rochester Symposium on Developmental Psychology, 8*, 263–288.

Duckworth, M.P., Hale, D.D., Clair, S.D., & Adams, H.E. (2000). Influence of interpersonal violence and community chaos on stress reactions in children. *Journal of Interpersonal Violence, 15*, 806–826.

DuRant, R.H., Pendergrast, R.A., & Cadenhead, C. (1994). Exposure to violence and victimization and fighting behavior by urban black adolescents. *Journal of Adolescent Health, 15* (4), 311–318.

DuRant, R.H., Getts, A., Cadenhead, C., Emans, S.J., & Woods, E.R. (1995). Exposure to violence and victimization and depression, hopefulness, and purpose in life among adolescent living in and around public housing. *Journal of Developmental and Behavioral Pediatrics, 16*, 233–237.

Edlynn, E., Gaylord-Harden, N., & Richards, M. (2008) African American inner-city youth exposed to violence: Coping as a moderator for anxiety. *Journal of Orthopsychiatry, 78* (2), 249–258.

Elliot, D.S., Wilson, W.J., Huizinga, D., Sampson, R.J., Elliot, A., & Rankin, B. (1996). The effects of neighborhood disadvantage on adolescent development. *Journal of Research in Crime and Delinquency, 33* (4), 389–426.

Engle, P.L., Castle, S., & Menon, P. (1996). Child development: Vulnerability and resilience. *Social Science and Medicine, 43*, 621–635.

Family Strengthening Policy Center (FSPC). (2005). Community violence prevention as a family strengthening strategy: A program of the National Human Services Assembly, Policy Brief No. 5. Retrieved July 6, 2009, from www.nassembly.org/fspc/practice/documents/vpdraft_2_.pdf.

Farrell, A.D., & Bruce, S.E. (1997). Impact of exposure to community violence on violent behavior and emotional distress among urban adolescents. *Journal of Clinical Child Psychology, 26*, 2–14.

Felson, R.B. (1997). Routine activities and involvement in violence as actor, witness, or target. *Violence and Victims, 12*, 209–221.

Fergus, S., & Zimmerman, M.A. (2005). Adolescent resilience: A framework for understanding healthy development in the face of risk. *Annual Review of Public Health, 26*, 399–419.

Finch, A.J., Nelson, W.M., & Moss, J.H. (1993). Childhood aggression: Cognitive-behavioral therapy strategies and interventions. In A.J. Finch, W.M. Nelson, & E.S. Ott (eds), *Cognitive-behavioral procedures with children and adolescents: A practical guide* (pp. 148–205). Boston, MA: Allyn & Bacon.

Finkelhor, D., Ormrod, R., Turner, H., & Hamby, S.L. (2005). The victimization of children and youth: A comprehensive, national survey. *Child Maltreatment, 10*, 5–25.

Finkelhor, D., Ormrod, R.K., & Turner, H.A. (2007). Polyvictimization and trauma in a national longitudinal cohort. *Development and Psychopathology, 19*, 149–166.

Fitzpatrick, K.M. (1997). Aggression and environmental risk among low-income African-American youth. *Journal of Adolescent Health, 21*, 172–178.

Fitzpatrick, K.M., & Boldizar, J.P. (1993). The prevalence and consequences of exposure to violence among African-American youth. *Journal of the American Academy of Child and Adolescent Psychiatry, 32*, 424–430.

Fitzpatrick, K.M., Piko, B., Wright, D., & LaGory, M. (2005). Depressive symptomatology, exposure to violence, and the role of social capital among African-American adolescents. *American Journal of Orthopsychiatry, 75*, 125–137.

Flannery, D.J., Wester, K.L., & Singer, M.I. (2004). The impact of exposure to violence in school on child and adolescent mental health and behavior. *Journal of Community Psychology, 32*, 559–573.

Foster, J.D., Kuperminc, G.P., & Price, A.W. (2004) Gender differences in posttraumatic stress and related symptoms among inner-city minority youth exposed to community violence. *Journal of Youth and Adolescence, 33*, 59–69.

Fredland, N.M., Campbell, J.C., & Haera, H. (2008). Effect of violence exposure on health outcomes among young urban adolescents. *Nursing Research, 57* (3), 157–165.

Freeman, L.N., Schaffer, D., & Smith, H. (1996). Neglected victims of homicide: The needs of young siblings of murder victims. *American Journal of Orthopsychiatry, 56*, 337–345.

Galand, B., Philippot, P., Buidin, G., & Lecocq, C. (2004). Violences à l'école en Belgique francophone: Différences entre établissement et evolution temporelle [School violence in Belgium: Differences between institutions and temporal evolution]. *Revue Française de Pédagogie, 149*, 83–96.

Garbarino, J., Kostelny, K., & Dubrow, N. (1991). What children can tell us about living in violence. *American Psychologist, 46*, 376–383.

Garbarino, J., Dubrow, N., Kostelny, K., & Pardo, C. (1992). *Children in danger: Coping with the consequences of community violence*. San Francisco, CA: Jossey-Bass Social and Behavioral Science Series.

Gil, E. (1991). *The healing power of play*. New York: Guilford Press.

Gitterman, A. (2008). Ecological framework. In Y. Mizrahi and L. Davis (eds), *Encyclopedia of social work* (20th ed.). New York: Oxford University Press.

Gitterman, A. & Germain, C.B. (2008). *The life model of social work practice: Advances in knowledge and practice* (3rd ed.). New York: Columbia University Press.

Gladstein, J., Rusonis, E.S., & Heald, F.P. (1992). A comparison of inner-city and upper-middle class youth's exposure to violence. *Journal of Adolescent Mental Health, 13*, 275–280.

Gorman-Smith, D., & Tolan, P. (1998). The role of exposure to community violence and developmental problems among inner-city youth. *Development and Psychopathology, 10* (1), 101–116.

Gorman-Smith, D., & Tolan, P.H. (2003). Positive adaptation among youth exposed to community violence. In S.S. Luthar (ed.), *Resilience and vulnerability: Adaptation in the context of childhood adversities* (pp. 392–413). New York: Cambridge University Press.

Gorman-Smith, D., Tolan, P.H., Zelli, A., & Huesmann, L.R. (1996). The relation of family functioning to violence among inner-city minority youth. *Journal of Family Psychology, 10*, 115–129.

Gorman-Smith, D., Henry, D.B., & Tolan, P.H. (2004). Exposure to community violence and violence perpetration: The protective effects of family functioning. *Journal of Child Clinical and Adolescent Psychology, 33*, 439–449.

Graham-Berman, S., & Levendosky, A. (1998). Traumatic stress symptoms in children of battered women. *Journal of Interpersonal Violence, 13*, 111–128.

Grossman, D.C., Neckerman, H.J., Koepsell, T.D., Liu, P.Y., Asher, K.N., Beland, K. et al. (1997). The effectiveness of a violence prevention curriculum among children in elementary school. *Journal of the American Medical Association, 277* (20), 1605–1611.

Groves, B.A. (2002). *Children who see too much: Lessons from the child witness to violence project*. Boston, MA: Beacon.

Guerra, N.G., & Williams, K.R. (1996). *A program planning guide for youth violence prevention: A risk-focused approach*. Boulder, CO: Center for the Study and Prevention of Violence, University of Colorado.

Guerra, N.G., Huesmann, L.R., & Spindler, A. (2003). Community violence exposure, social cognition, and aggression among urban elementary school children. *Child Development, 74* (5), 1561–1576.

Guterman, N., & Cameron, M. (1998). Assessing the impact of community violence on children and youths. In P.L. Ewalt, E.M. Freeman, & D.L. Poole (eds), *Community building: Renewal, well-being, and shared responsibility* (pp. 117–129). Washington, DC: NASW Press.

Guterman, N.B., & Cameron, M. (2003). Assessing the impact of community violence on children and youths. *Social Work, 42* (5), 495–505.

Guterman, N., Cameron, M., & Staller, K. (2000). Definitional and measurement issues in the study of community violence among children and youths. *Journal of Community Psychology, 28* (6), 571–587.

Halliday-Boykins, C.A., & Graham, S. (2001). At both ends of the gun: Testing the relationship between community violence exposure and youth violent behavior. *Journal of Abnormal Child Psychology, 29*, 383–402.

Hammack, P.L., Richards, M.H., Luo, Z., Edlynn, E.S., & Roy, K. (2004). Social support factors as moderators of community violence exposure among inner-city African-American young adolescents. *Journal of Clinical Child and Adolescent Psychology, 33*, 450–462.

Hammond, W.R., & Yung, B.R. (1991). Preventing violence in at risk African American youth. *Journal of Health Care for the Poor and Underserved, 2*, 359–373.

Harris, K.M. (1999). Health status and risk behaviors of adolescents in immigrant families. In D.J. Hernandez (ed.), *Children of immigrants: Health adjustment and public assistance* (pp. 286–347). Washington, DC: National Academy Press.

Hawkins, J.D., Catalano, R.F., Kosterman, R., Abbott, R., & Hill, K.G. (1999). Preventing adolescent health-risk behaviors by strengthening protection during childhood. *Archives of Pediatrics and Adolescent Medicine, 153*, 226–234.

Hawkins, J.D., Herrenkohl, T.I., Farrington, D.P., Brewer, D., Catalano, R.F., Harachi, T.W., & Cothern, L. (2000). *Predictors of youth violence.* Juvenile Justice Bulletin. Rockville, MD: Office of Juvenile Justice and Delinquency Prevention.

Herrara, V.M., & McCloskey, L.A. (2003). Sexual abuse, family violence, and female delinquency: Findings from a longitudinal study. *Violence and Victims, 18*, 319–334.

Hill, H.M., & Jones, L.P. (1997). Children's and parents' perceptions of children's exposure to violence in urban neighborhoods. *Journal of the National Medical Association, 89*, 270–276.

Hill, H.M., & Madhere, S. (1996). Exposure to community violence and African-American children: A multidimensional model of risks and resources. *Journal of Community Psychology, 24*, 26–43.

Ho, J. (2008). Community violence exposure of southeast Asian American adolescents. *Journal of Interpersonal Violence, 23*, 136–146.

Holland, C., Koblinskey, S., & Anderson, E. (1995). Maternal strategies for protecting Head Start children from community violence: Implications for family-focused education programs. Paper presented at the Head Start Association Annual Meeting, Washington, DC.

Horn, J.L., & Trickett, P.K. (1998). Community violence and child development: A review of research. In P.K. Trickett & C. Schellenbach (eds), *Violence against children in the family and community* (pp. 103–138). Washington, DC: APA Books.

Horowitz, K., Weine, S., & Jekel, J. (1995). PTSD symptoms in urban adolescent girls: Compounded community trauma. *Journal of the American Academy of Child and Adolescent Psychiatry, 34*, 1353–1361.

Howell, J.C., & Bilchick, S. (eds). (1995). *Guide for implementing the comprehensive strategy for serious violent and chronic juvenile offenders.* Washington, DC: Office of Juvenile Justice and Delinquency Prevention, U.S. Department of Justice.

Jenkins, E.J., & Bell, C.C. (1994). Violence among inner-city high school students and post-traumatic stress disorder. In S. Friedman (ed.), *Anxiety disorders in African Americans* (pp. 76–88). New York: Springer.

Jenkins, E.J., & Bell, C.C. (1997). Exposure and response to community violence among children and adolescents. In J.D. Osofsky (ed.), *Children in a violent society* (pp. 9–31). New York: Guilford Press.

Kann, L., Waren, C.W., Harris, W.A., Collins, J.L., Douglas, K.A., Collins, M.E. et al. (1996). *Youth risk behavior surveillance, 1995.* Atlanta, GA: Centers for Disease Control and Prevention.

Kataoka, S., Stein, B.D., Jaycox, L.H., Wong, M., Escudero, P., Tu, W. et al. (2003). A school-based mental health program for traumatized Latino immigrant children. *Journal of the American Academy of Child and Adolescent Psychiatry, 42* (3), 311–318.

Kataoka, S., Langley, A., Stein, B., Jaycox, L., Zhang, L., Sanchez, N., & Wong, N. (2009). Violence exposure and PTSD: The role of English language fluency in Latino youth. *Journal of Child and Family Studies, 18*, 334–341.

Katz, L.F., & Gottman, J.M. (1997). Buffering children from marital conflict and dissolution. *Journal of Clinical Child Psychology, 26*, 157–71.

Kellerman, A.L., Fuqua-Whitley, D.S., Rivara, F.P., & Mercy, J. (1998). Preventing youth violence: What works? *Annual Review of Public Health, 19*, 271–292.

Kelly, J., Murphy, D., Sikkema, K., & Kalichman, S. (1993). Psychological interventions to prevent HIV infection are urgently needed: New priorities for behavioral research in the second decade of AIDS. *American Psychologist, 48* (10), 1023–1034.

Kilpatrick, D.G., Acierno, R., Saunders, B.E., Resnick, H.S., Best, C., & Schnurr, P.P. (2000). Risk factors for adolescent substance abuse and dependence: Data from a national sample. *Journal of Consulting and Clinical Psychology, 68,* 19–30.

Kitzmann, K.M., Gaylord, N.K., Holt, A.R., & Kenny, E.D. (2003). Child witnesses to domestic violence: A meta-analytic review. *Journal of Counsulting and Clinical Psychology, 71* (2), 339–352.

Kliewer, W., & Sullivan, T.N. (2008). Community violence exposure, threat appraisal, and adjustment in adolescents. *Journal of Clinical Child and Adolescent Psychology, 37* (4), 860–873.

Kliewer, W., Lepore, S., Oskin, D., & Johnson, P. (1998). The role of social and cognitive processes in children's adjustment to community violence. *Journal of Consulting and Clinical Psychology, 66,* 199–209.

Klinger, D.A. (1997). Negotiating order in patrol work: An ecological theory of police response to deviance. *Criminology, 35,* 277–306.

Knell, S.M. (1998). Cognitive behavioral play therapy. *Journal of Clinical Child Psychology, 27* (1), 28–33.

Koop, C.E., & Lundberg, G.B. (1992). Violence in America: a public health emergency. Time to bite the bullet back. *Journal of the American Medical Association, 267* (22), 3075–3076.

Krenichyn, K., Saegert, S., & Evans, G.W. (2001). Parents as moderators of psychological and physiological correlates of inner city children's exposure to violence. *Applied Developmental Psychology, 22,* 581–602.

Krug, E.G., Dahlberg, L.L., Mercy, J.A., Zwi, A.B., & Lozano, R. (eds). (2002). *World report on violence and health.* Geneva: World Health Organization.

Lambert, S.F., Ialongo, N.S., Boyd, R.C., & Cooley, M.R. (2005). Risk factors for community violence exposure in adolescence. *American Journal of Community Psychology, 36,* 29–38.

Lauritsen, J.L. (2003). *How families and communities influence youth victimization.* OJJDP Juvenile Justice Bulletin. Washington, DC: Office of Juvenile Justice and Delinquency Prevention, U.S. Department of Justice.

Lauritsen, J.L., & Davis-Quinet, K.F. (1995). Repeat victimization among adolescents and young adults. *Journal of Quantitative Criminology, 11,* 143–166.

Lauritsen, J.L., Sampson, R.J., & Laub, J.H. (1991). The link between offending and victimization among adolescents. *Criminology, 29,* 265–292.

Lauritsen, J.L., Laub, J., & Sampson, R.J. (1992). Conventional and delinquent activities: Implications for the prevention of violent victimization among adolescents. *Violence and Victims, 7* (2), 91–108.

Layne, C.M., Pynoos, R.S., Saltzman, W.R., Arslanagic, B., Black, M., Savjak, N. et al. (2001). Trauma/grief focused group psychotherapy: School based postwar intervention with traumatized Bosnian adolescents. *Group Dynamics, 5,* 277–290.

Le, T., & Chan, J. (2001). *Invisible victims: Asian/Pacific Islander youth.* Oakland, CA: National Council on Crime and Delinquency.

Leiter, J., & Johnsen, M.C. (1994). Child maltreatment and school performance. *American Journal of Education, 102,* 154–89.

Leventhal, T., & Brookes-Gunn, J. (2000). The neighborhoods they live in: The effects of neighborhood residence on child and adolescent outcomes. *Psychological Bulletin, 126,* 309–337.

Limbos, A.M., Chan, L.S., Warf, C., Schneir, A., Iverson, E., Shekelle, P., & Kipke, M.D. (2007). Effectiveness of interventions to prevent youth violence: A systematic review. *American Journal of Prevention Medicine, 33* (1), 65–74.

Linares, L.O., Heeren, T., Bronfman, E., Zuckerman, B., Augustyn, M., & Tronick, E. (2001). A meditational model for the impact of exposure to community violence on early child behavior problems. *Child Development, 72,* 639–652.

Luthar, S.S. (2006). Resilience in development: A synthesis of research across five decades. In D. Cicchetti & D.J. Cohen (eds), *Developmental psychopathology: Risk, disorder, and adaptation* (2nd ed., pp. 739–795). New York: John Wiley & Sons.

Luthar, S.S., & Zelazo, L.B. (2003). Research on resilience: An integrative review. In S.S. Luthar (ed.), *Resilience and vulnerability: Adaptation in the context of childhood adversities* (pp. 510–549). New York: Cambridge University Press.

Lynch, M. (2003). Consequences of children's exposure to community violence. *Clinical Child and Family Psychology Review, 6* (4), 265–274.

Lynch, M., & Cicchetti, D. (2002). Links between community violence and the family system: Evidence from children's feelings of relatedness and perceptions of parent behavior. *Family Process, 41,* 519–532.

Margolin, G. (1998). Effects of domestic violence on children. In P.K. Trickett & C.J. Schellenbach (eds),

Violence against children in the family and the community (pp. 57–102). Washington, DC: American Psychological Association.

Margolin, G., & Gordis, B. (2000). The effects of family and community violence on children. *Annual Review of Psychology, 51,* 445–479.

Margolin, G., & John, R.S. (1997). Effects of domestic violence on children. In G.K. Kantor & J.L. Jasinski (eds), *Contemporary perspectives on family violence* (pp. 57–102). Washington, DC: American Psychiatric Association.

Margolin, G., Vickerman, K.A., Ramos, M.C., Serrano, S.D., Gordis, E.B., Iturralde, E. et al. (2009). Youth exposed to violence: Stability, co-occurrence, and context. *Clinical Child Family and Psychological Review, 12,* 39–54.

Massey, D.S., & Denton, N.A. (1993). *American apartheid: Segregation and the making of the underclass.* Cambridge, MA: Harvard University Press.

Masten, A.S., & Coatsworth, D.J. (1998). The development of competence in favorable and unfavorable environments. *American Psychologist, 53*(2), 205–220.

Mazza, J.J., & Reynolds, W.M. (1999). Exposure to violence in young inner-city adolescents: Relationships with suicidal ideation, depression, and PTSD symptomatology. *Journal of Abnormal Child Psychology, 27,* 203–213.

McDonald, L., & Frey, H.E. (1999). *Families and schools together: Building relationships.* Juvenile Justice Bulletin. Washington, DC: Office of Juvenile Justice and Delinquency Prevention, U.S. Department of Justice.

McGee, Z., & Baker, S. (2002). Impact of violence on problem behavior among adolescents: Risk factors among an urban sample. *Journal of Contemporary Criminal Justice, 18,* 74–93.

Meyer, H.A., & Astor, R.A. (2002). Child and parent perspectives on routes to and from school in high crime neighborhoods. *Journal of School Violence, 1* (4), 101–128.

Miller, J. (2008). *Getting played.* New York: New York University Press.

Miller, L.S., Wasserman, G.A., Neugebauer, R., Gorman-Smith, D., & Kamboukos, D. (1999). Witnessed community violence and antisocial behavior in high-risk urban boys. *Journal of Clinical Child Psychology, 28,* 2–11.

Moore, C.F. (2005). An unhealthy start in life: What matters most? *Psychological Science in the Public Interest, 6* (3), i–ii.

Moses, A. (1999) Exposure to violence, depression, and hostility in a sample of inner city high school youth. *Journal of Adolescence, 22,* 21–32.

Murphy, L., Pynoos, R.S., & James, C.B. (1997). The trauma/grief-focused group psychotherapy module of an elementary school-based violence prevention/intervention program. In J.D. Osofsky (ed.), *Children in a violent society* (pp. 223–255). New York: Guilford Press.

Nansel, T.R., Overpeck, M.D., Haynie, D.L., Ruan, W.J., & Scheidt, P.C. (2003). Relationships between bullying and violence among U.S. youth. *Archives of Pediatric Adolescent Medicine, 157,* 348–353.

National Human Services Assembly (2005). *Community violence prevention as a family strengthening strategy.* Family Strengthening Policy Center Policy Brief No. 5. Retrieved August 8, 2009, from www.nassembly.org/fspc/practice/documents/vpdraft_2_.pdf

Neugebauer, R., Wasserman, G.A., Fisher, P.W., Kline, J., Geller, P.A., & Miller, L.S. (1999). Darryl: A cartoon based measure of cardinal posttraumatic stress symptoms in school-aged children. *American Journal of Public Health, 89,* 758–761.

O'Carroll, C.W. (1988). Homicides among black males 15–24 years of age, 1970–1980. *Morbidity and Mortality Weekly Report, 37,* 543–545.

O'Donnell, D.A., Schwab-Stone, M.E., & Muyeed, A.Z. (2002). Multidimensional resilience in urban children exposed to community violence. *Child Development, 73,* 1265–1282.

O'Keefe, M., & Sela-Amit, M. (1997). An examination of the effects of race/ethnicity and social class on adolescents' exposure to violence. *Journal of Social Service Research, 22* (3), 53–71.

Osofsky, J.D. (ed.). (1997). *Children in a violent society.* New York: Guilford Press.

Osofsky, J.D., & Fenichel, E. (eds). (1996). *Islands of safety: Assessing and treating young victims of violence.* Arlington, VA: Zero to Three/National Center for Clinical Infant Programs.

Osofsky, J.D., & Scheeringa, M.S. (1997). Community and domestic violence exposure: Effects of development and psychopathology. In D. Cichetti & S. Toth (eds), *Rochester symposium on developmental psychopathology, 8: Developmental perspectives on trauma* (pp. 155–180). Rochester, NY: University of Rochester Press.

Osofsky, J.D., Wewers, S., Hann, D.M., & Fick, A.C. (1993). Chronic community violence: What is happening to our children? *Psychiatry, 56*, 36–45.

Overstreet, S., Dempsey, M., Graham, D., & Moely, B. (1999). Availability of family support as a moderator of exposure to community violence. *Journal of Clinical Child Psychology, 28*, 151–159.

Ozer, E.J. (2005). The impact of violence on urban adolescents: Longitudinal effects of perceived school connection and family support. *Journal of Adolescent Research, 20* (2), 167–192.

Ozer, E.J., & McDonald, K. (2006). Exposure to violence and mental health among Chinese American urban adolescents. *Journal of Adolescent Health, 39* (1), 73–79.

Ozer, E.J., & Weinstein, R.S. (2004). Urban adolescents' exposure to community violence: The role of support, school safety, and social constraints in a school-based sample of boys and girls. *Journal of Clinical Child and Adolescent Psychology, 33* (3), 463–476.

Pastore, D.E., Fisher, M., & Friedman, S.B. (1996). Violence and mental health problems among urban high school students. *Journal of Adolescent Health, 18*, 320–324.

Patchin, J.W., Hueber, B.M., McCluskey, J.D., Varano, S.P., & Bynum, T.S. (2006). Exposure to community violence and childhood delinquency. *Crime and Delinquency, 52* (2), 307–332.

Patterson, G.R., Reid, J.B., & Dishion, T.J. (1992). *Antisocial boys: A social interactional approach*. Eugene, OR: Castalia.

Pennels, S.M., & Smith, S.C. (1994). *The forgotten mourners: Guidelines for working with bereaved children*. Bristol, PA: Jessica Kingsley Publishers.

Perry, D.G., Hodges, E.V.E., & Egan, S.K. (2001). Determinants of chronic victimization by peers: A review and new model of family influence. In J. Juvonen & S. Graham (eds), *Peer harassment in school: The plight of the vulnerable and victimized* (pp. 73–104). New York: Guilford Press.

Plybon, L.E., & Kliewer, W. (2001). Neighborhood types and externalizing behavior in urban school-age children: Tests of direct, mediated, and moderated effects. *Journal of Child and Family Studies, 10*, 419–437.

Preski, S., & Shelton, D. (2001). The role of contextual, child and parent factors in predicting criminal outcomes in adolescence. *Issues in Mental Health Nursing, 22*, 197–205.

Pynoos, R.S. & Nader, K. (1988). Psychological first aid and treatment approach to children exposed to community violence: Research implications. *Journal of Traumatic Stress, 1* (4), 445–473.

Rathus, J.H., Asnis, G.M., & Wetzler, S. (1995, May). Exposure to violence and posttraumatic stress disorder in urban adolescents. Paper presented at the annual meeting of the American Association of Suicidology, Phoenix, Arizona.

Rennison, C.M. (2001). *Violent victimization and race, 1993–1998. Bureau of Justice Statistics, Special Report.* Washington, DC: U.S. Department of Justice.

Rennison, C.M., & Rand, M.R. (2003). *Criminal victimization 2002* (NCJ 187007). Washington, DC: U.S. Department of Justice.

Repetti, R.L., Taylor, S.E., & Seeman, T.E. (2002). Risky families: Family social environments and the mental and physical health of offspring. *Psychological Bulletin, 128*, 330–366.

Resnick, H.S., Kilpatrick, D.G., Best, C.L., & Kramer, T.L. (1992). Vulnerability-stress factors in development of posttraumatic stress disorder. *Journal of Nervous and Mental Disease, 180* (7), 424–430.

Richters, J.E., & Martinez, P. (1993). The NIMH Community Violence Project: I. Children as victims of and witnesses to violence. *Psychiatry, 56*, 7–21.

Rosario, M., Salzinger, S., Feldman, R.S., & Ng-Mak, D.S. (2003). Community violence exposure and delinquent behaviors among youth: The moderating role of coping. *Journal of Community Psychology, 31* (5), 489–512.

Rosenthal, B.S., & Wilson, W.C. (2008). Community violence and psychological distress: The protective effects of emotional social support and sense of personal control among older adolescents. *Adolescence, 43* (172), 693–712.

Ross, G., & O'Carroll, P. (2004). Cognitive behavioural psychotherapy intervention in childhood sexual abuse: Identifying new direction from the literature. *Child Abuse Review, 13*, 51–64.

Rudolph, K.D., & Hammen, C. (1999). Age and gender as determinants of stress exposure, generation, and reactions in youngsters: A transactional perspective. *Child Development, 70* (3), 660–677.

Ruma, C.D. (1993). Cognitive-behavioral play therapy with sexually abused children. In S.M. Knell (ed.), *Cognitive-behavioral play therapy* (pp. 199–230). Northvale, NJ: Jason Aronson.

Saltzman, W., Pynoos, R., Layne, C., Steinberg, A., & Aisenberg, E. (2001). Trauma- and grief-focused intervention for adolescents exposed to community violence: Results of a school-based screening and group treatment protocol. *Group Dynamics, 5*, 291–303.

Sampson, R.J., & Lauritsen, J.L. (1990). Deviant lifestyles, proximity to crime, and the offender-victim link in personal violence. *Journal of Research in Crime and Delinquency, 32*, 110–139.

Sampson, R.J., Raudenbusch, S.W., & Earls, F. (1997). Neighborhoods and violent crime: A multilevel study of collective efficacy. *Science, 277*, 918–924.

Sampson, R.J., Morenoff, J.D., & Gannon-Rowley, T. (2002). Assessing "neighborhood effects": Social processes and new directions in research. *Annual Review of Sociology, 28*, 443–478.

Scarpa, A., Hurley, J.D., Shumate, H.W., & Haden, S.C. (2006). Lifetime prevalence and socioemotional effects of hearing about community violence. *Journal of Interpersonal Violence, 21* (1), 5–23.

Schiff, M., & McKay, M.M. (2003). Urban youth disruptive behavioral difficulties: Exploring association with parenting and gender. *Family Process, 42* (4), 517–529.

Schwab-Stone, M., Ayers, T., Kasprow, W., Voyce, C., Barone, C., Shriver, T., & Weissberg, R.P. (1995). No safe haven: A study of violence exposure in an urban community. *Journal of the American Academy of Child and Adolescent Psychiatry, 34*, 1343–1352.

Schwab-Stone, M., Chuansheng, C., Ellen, G., Silver, D., Lichtman, J., & Voyce, C. (1999). No safe haven, II: The effects of violence exposure on urban youth. *Journal of the American Academy of Children and Adolescent Psychiatry, 38* (4), 359–367.

Schwartz, D., & Proctor, L. (2000). Community violence exposure and children's social adjustment in the school peer group: The mediating roles of emotion regulation and social cognition. *Journal of Consulting and Clinical Psychology, 68*, 670–683.

Selner-O'Hagan, M.B., Kindlon, D.J., Buka, S.L., Raudenbush, S.W., & Earls, F.J. (1998). Assessing exposure to violence in urban youth. *Journal of Child Psychology and Psychiatry and Allied Disciplines, 39*, 215–224.

Shahinfar, A., Fox, N.A., & Leavitt, L.A. (2000). Preschool children's exposure to violence: Relation of behavior problems to parent and child reports. *American Journal of Orthopsychiatry, 70*, 115–125.

Singer, M.I., Anglin, T.M., Song, L.Y., & Lunghofer, L. (1995). Adolescents' exposure to violence and associated symptoms of psychological trauma. *Journal of the American Medical Association, 273*, 477–482.

Singer, M.I., Miller, D.B., Guo, S., Flannery, D.J., Frierson, T., & Slovak, K. (1999). Contributors to violent behavior among elementary and middle school children. *Pediatrics, 104*, 878–884.

Skinner, E.A., & Wellborn, J.G. (1994). Coping during childhood and adolescence: A motivational perspective. In D. Featherman, R. Lerner, & M. Perlmutter (eds) *Life-span development and behavior, Vol. 12* (pp. 91–133). Hillsdale, NJ: Lawrence Erlbaum Associates.

Skogan, W.G., Hartnett, S.M., Bump, N., & Dubois, J. (2008). *Evaluation of Ceasefire-Chicago.* Grant Number 2005-MU-MU-003. Washington, DC: National Institute of Justice, Office of Justice Programs. Retrieved July 1, 2009, from www.northwestern.edu/ipr/publications/ceasefire_papers/mainreport.pdf.

Slovak, K., & Singer, M.I. (2002). Children and violence: Findings and implications from a rural community. *Child and Adolescent Social Work Journal, 19*, 35–55.

Smith, S.S. (2007). *Lone pursuit: Distrust and defensive individualism among the Black poor.* New York: Russell Sage Foundation.

Snyder, H.N., & Sickmund, M. (1999). *Juvenile offenders and victims: 1999 national report.* Washington, DC: Office of Juvenile Justice and Delinquency Prevention.

Snyder, H.N., & Sickmund, M. (2006). *Juvenile offenders and victims: 2006 national report.* Washington, DC: U.S. Department of Justice, Office of Justice Programs, Office of Juvenile Justice and Delinquency Prevention.

Stein, B.D., Jaycox, L.H., Kataoka, S., Rhodes, H.J., & Vestal, K.D. (2003). Prevalence of child and adolescent exposure to community violence. *Clinical Child and Family Psychology Review, 6* (4), 247–264.

Suglia, S.F., Staudenmayer, J., Cohen, S., & Wright, R.J. (2009). Posttraumatic stress symptoms related to community violence and children's diurnal cortisol response in an urban community-dwelling sample. *International Journal of Behavioral Medicine, 17* (1), 1–6.

Sullivan, T.N., Kung, E.M., & Farrell, A.D. (2004). Relation between witnessing violence and drug use initiation among rural adolescents: Parental monitoring and family support as protectors. *Journal of Clinical Child and Adolescent Psychology, 33*, 488–498.

Sweatt, L., Harding, C.G., Knight-Lynn, L., Rasheed, S., & Carter, P. (2002). Talking about the silent fear: Adolescents' experiences of violence in an urban high-rise community. *Adolescence, 37*, 109–120.

Taylor, L., Zuckerman, B., Harik, V., & Groves, B.M. (1994). Witnessing violence by young children and their mothers. *Journal of Developmental and Behavioral Pediatrics, 15*, 120–123.

Thornton, T.N., Craft, C.A., Dahlberg, L.L., Lynch, B.S., & Baer, K. (2000). *Best practices of youth violence prevention: A sourcebook for community action.* Atlanta, GA: Centers for Disease Control and Prevention.

Tolan, P.H., & Guerra, N.G. (1994). *What works in reducing adolescent violence?: An empirical review of the field.* Boulder, CO: Center for the Study and Prevention of Violence, University of Colorado.

Tolan, P.H., & Henry, D.B. (1996). Patterns of psychopathology among urban poor children: Comorbidity and aggression effects. *Journal of Consulting and Clinical Psychology, 64*, 1094–1099.

Trickett, P.K., Durán, L., & Horn, J.L. (2003). Community violence as it affects child development: Issues of definition. *Clinical Child and Family Psychology Review, 6*, 223–236.

Uehara, E.S., Chalmers, D., Jenkins, E., & Shakoor, B.H. (1996). African American youth encounters with violence: Results from the community mental health council violence screening project. *Journal of Black Studies, 26* (6), 768–781.

Uniform Crime Reports. (2002). Washington, DC: U.S. Government Printing Office.

U.S. Bureau of Justice Statistics. (2008). *Crime and victimization statistics: Trends from 1973–2006.* Retrieved July 6, 2009, from www.ojp.usdoj.gov/bjs/cvict.htm.

U.S. Census Bureau. (2003). *Statistical abstract of the United States, 2002.* Washington, DC: U.S. Census Bureau.

U.S. Department of Education. (1997). *Principal/school disciplinarian survey on school violence. Fast response survey system, 63.* Washington, DC: National Center on Educational Statistics.

U.S. Department of Health and Human Services. (2001). *Youth violence: A report of the Surgeon General.* Rockville, MD: U.S. Department of Health and Human Services, National Institutes of Health, National Institute of Mental Health.

van der Kolk, B.A. (1987). *Psychological trauma.* Washington, DC: American Psychiatric Press.

Vermeiren, R., Schwab-Stone, M., Deboutte, D., Leckman, P.E., & Ruchkin, V. (2003). Violence exposure and substance use in adolescents: Findings from three countries. *Pediatrics, 111* (3), 535–540.

Voisin, D. (2003). Victims of community violence and HIV sexual risk behaviors among African American males. *HIV/AIDS Education and Prevention for Adolescents and Children, 5* (3), 111–121.

Voisin, D., & Guilamo-Ramos, V. (2008). A commentary on community violence exposure and HIV risk behaviors among African American adolescents. *African American Research Perspectives, 12* (1), 83–100.

Vostanis, P., Tischler, V., & Cumella, S. (2001). Mental health problems and social supports among homeless mothers and children victims of domestic and community violence. *International Journal of Social Psychiatry, 47*, 30–40.

Webster, D.W. (1993). The unconvincing case for school-based conflict resolution programs for adolescents. *Health Affirmations, 12*, 126–141.

Weist, M.D., Acosta, O.M., & Youngstrom, E.A. (2001). Predictors of violence exposure among inner-city youth. *Journal of Clinical Child Psychology, 30*, 187–198.

Werner, E.E. (1995). Resilience in development. *Current Directions in Psychological Science, 4*, 81–85.

White, K.S., Bruce, S., Farrell, A., & Kliewer, W. (1998). Impact of exposure to community violence on anxiety: A longitudinal study of family social support as a protective factor for urban children. *Journal of Child & Family Studies, 7*, 187–203.

Widom, C.S. (1989). Child abuse, neglect, and violent criminal behavior. *Criminology, 244*, 160–166.

Widom, C.S. (1999). Posttraumatic stress disorder in abused and neglected children. *American Journal of Psychiatry, 156*, 1223–1229.

Wilson, A.N. (1991). *Understanding black adolescent male violence: Its remediation and prevention.* New York: Afrikan Infosystems.

Wilson, D., Kliewer, W., Teasley, N., Plybon, L., & Sica, D. (2002). Violence exposure, catecholamine excretion, and blood pressure non-dipping status in African-American male versus female adolescents. *Psychosomatic Medicine, 64*, 906–915.

Wilson, S.J., & Lipsey, M.W. (2005). *The effectiveness of school-based violence prevention programs for reducing disruptive and aggressive behavior*. Washington, DC: U.S. Department of Justice. Retrieved July 20, 2009, from www.ncjrs.gov/pdffiles1/nij/grants/211376.pdf.

Wolfe, D.A., Crooks, C.V., Lee, V., McIntyre-Smith, A., & Jaffe, P.G. (2003). The effects of children's exposure to domestic violence: A meta-analysis and critique. *Clinical Child and Family Psychology Review*, *6*, 171–187.

Wright, R.J., Mitchell, H., Visness, C.M., Cohen, S., Stout, J., Evans, R. et al. (2004). Community violence and asthma morbidity: The inner-city asthma study. *American Journal of Public Health*, *94*, 625–632.

Yoshikawa, H. (1994). Prevention as cumulative protection. Effects of early family support and education on chronic delinquency and its risks. *Psychological Bulletin*, *115* (1), 28–54.

Part II
Mental health conditions

12 Autism spectrum conditions

Joseph Walsh and Jacqueline Corcoran

The *Diagnostic and statistical manual of mental disorders* (American Psychiatric Association (APA), 2000) includes three related conditions that comprise the "autism spectrum": autism, Asperger's disorder, and pervasive developmental disorder not otherwise specified. The DSM-IV-TR in fact delineates five distinct *pervasive developmental disorders* (PDDs), the other two being Rett's disorder and childhood disintegrative disorder. All of these are characterized by "severe and pervasive impairment in several areas of development: reciprocal social interaction, communication skills, or the presence of stereotyped behavior, interests, and activities" (APA, 2000, p. 65). They are evident in the first few years of life and are often associated with some degree of mental retardation. First identified by Leo Kanner in 1943, *autism* is the best known of these conditions, but in the past several decades researchers have noted that the three PDDs noted above may in fact represent different disability levels of the same core condition. These have come to be known as the *autism spectrum disorders* (ASDs). For several reasons (noted below) the spectrum conditions have been increasingly diagnosed, and because they require such intensive intervention, often with modest impact, they represent a great challenge for service providers, resource developers, and health care funders.

Definitions of autism spectrum conditions

Autism is characterized by marked abnormal development in social interaction and communication and a stereotypical, repetitive range of ritualized behaviors such as rocking, toe-walking, flapping, clapping, whirling, and an obsessive desire for sameness (Schreibman, Stahmer, & Akshoomoff, 2006). Its DSM-IV criteria include twelve symptoms divided among three categories, including social interaction, communication/play/imagination, and limitations of interests and behaviors (APA, 2000). Still, there is a great variability in possible symptoms among persons with autism. Relatively few such persons (10–40 percent) display any particular behavioral marker, regardless of the diagnostic system being used (there are several). No common neural or cognitive deficits, behavior patterns, or life courses have been found among persons with the condition; nor is there a typical response to behavioral or drug intervention.

Despite differences in individual presentation, the impairments in social relatedness underlie and define the condition (Volkmar, Chwarska, & Klin, 2005). These include a lack of awareness of the feelings of others, an impaired capacity to imitate and express emotion, and the absence of capacity for social and symbolic play. Even in infancy children with autism may lack reciprocal social engagement and are unable to maintain eye contact with others. As the child grows older, these social disabilities persist, as indicated by difficulty in forming friendships, showing empathy, and understanding rules and expectations that are a part of daily social interaction.

Communication deficits in persons with autism include a reliance on non-verbal communication (seen in 50 percent of clients), echolalia (repetition of words or phrases), abnormal prosody (atypical speech rhythm, stress, intonation, and loudness), and pronoun reversal (for instance, the person refers to "you" as him or herself, and the other person as "me"). These impairments are most pronounced in the social aspects of language (Akshoomoff, 2006). Persons with autism may present irrelevant details, inappropriately perseverate on a topic, suddenly shift to a new topic, and ignore others' attempts to initiate conversation. Deficits also involve language comprehension as speech is interpreted in overly concrete and literal ways. In fact, persons with autism have more difficulty understanding language than they do learning the structures necessary to produce language. Thus, half the autistic population does not develop speech and a majority fails to use speech functionally (Peliosa & Lund, 2001). Persons with autism do, however, often possess characteristic "pockets" of ability, such as memorization, visual and spatial skills, and attention to details.

As noted earlier, since the late 1980s researchers have observed that the characteristics of autism are spread across two other spectrum disorders without clear lines of demarcation among them. The core symptoms of autism are less severe in these other two diagnostic categories, and they are sometimes referred to as "high functioning" autism. Assessment and intervention strategies are similar for all three conditions (Akshoomoff, 2006). Children with these other conditions also have varying degrees of impairment in verbal and non-verbal communication skills, and restricted and repetitive behaviors.

In *Asperger's disorder*, early development of cognition and language is apparently normal, but the child often has unusual interests that are pursued with great intensity (Holter, 2004). The child's approaches to peers and new adults may be unusual or idiosyncratic, but attachment patterns to family members are well established. Social deficits become more prominent as the child enters preschool and is exposed to peers. The current criteria for Asperger's disorder emphasize impairments in social interaction and non-verbal communication similar to those found in autism, but without the unusual behaviors and environmental responsiveness. While limited in their repertoire of social skills, persons with Asperger's disorder are better able than those with autism to show interest in peers, experience joy in social interactions, share interests with others, be affectionate with their parents and responsive to other adults, and master basic conversational skills (Macintosh & Dissanayake, 2006). Referral for assessment is usually later than in cases of suspected autism (Smith, Magyar, & Arnold-Saritepe, 2002). Although limited data exist on the course of Asperger's disorder, individuals with the condition generally have a better outcome than those with autism – they are more likely to attain gainful employment, live independently, and establish a family (Howlin, 2005). Still, the social difficulties of Asperger's disorder are apparently lifelong.

The term *pervasive developmental disorder not otherwise specified* (PDD-NOS), sometimes termed atypical PDD or atypical autism, encompasses sub-threshold autism cases in which there is marked impairment in social interaction, communication, or stereotyped behavior patterns or interests, but the full features of autism or of another defined PDD are not met (Koyama, Tachimor, Osada, & Kurita, 2006). This category represents the highest level of functioning within the spectrum. The natural history of PDD-NOS has not been extensively studied. The issue of whether meaningful subtypes might be defined within the broad PDD category remains a topic of debate. PDD-NOS is more commonly seen than autism (Fombonne, 2007). The limited data suggest that individuals with PDD-NOS have a better prognosis than persons with autism, but social, communicative, or adaptive and behavioral problems may be prominent during the school years. In adolescence and adulthood these persons have an increased risk of anxiety and mood disorders although they may function well in a limited social capacity (Towbin, 2005).

Demographics

The reported incidence of ASD has increased at a remarkably high rate around the world since the late 1980s. The causes of this increase include changing diagnostic criteria, service eligibility regulations, knowledge about intervention, political advocacy and the increased diagnosis of very young children (Shattuck & Grosse, 2007). The Centers for Disease Control and Prevention found that the prevalence of autism spectrum conditions was 6.6 per 1,000 children in the United States (Rice, 2007). The number of students aged 6–21 years identified in the ASD reporting category in the United States in special education grew between 1994 and 2005 from 18,540 to 165,552 (Safran, 2008). To put this into context, the ASDs are more common in childhood than cerebral palsy, hearing loss, vision impairment, and diabetes, but less so than mental retardation (Yeargin-Alsopp, Rice, Karapurkar, Doernberg, Boyle, & Murphy, 2003). According to the CDC and others, autism spectrum disorder occurs more often in males than females, with a 4.3 to 1 ratio (Rice, 2007). Autism is represented in all social classes and ethnic groups (Shattuck & Grosse, 2007) with no ethnic differences in prevalence (Liptak, Stuart, & Auinger, 2006).

Children and adolescents with ASD experience a range of co-occurring, or comorbid, conditions. Estimates of the frequency of these comorbid conditions vary widely, with some estimates as high as 81 percent (de Bruin, Ferdinand, Meester, de Nijs, & Verheij, 2007). Several things account for this pattern of high comorbidity. First, the majority of studies rely on clinical rather than epidemiological samples, which tends to inflate comorbidity rates. Second, studies include differences in the way samples are selected, the ages of participants, methods of inquiry, and the clinical experience of the interviewers. Third, different instruments and diagnostic measures are used for assessment (Leyfer et al., 2006). Fourth, the features of ASD can make the diagnosis of other psychiatric conditions difficult. Finally, the high comorbidity is largely due to the broadly debilitating features of the ASDs, their associated medical conditions, and the problematic life experiences related to having autism.

Common co-occurring conditions include mental retardation (severe in 50 percent of cases; mild to moderate in 30 percent of cases), seizure disorders (25–30 percent of cases), depression (4–57 percent of cases), anxiety conditions (7–84 percent of cases), overactivity and attention problems (21–72 percent of cases), and tic disorders (7–29 percent of cases) (Aman & Langworthy, 2000; Bernard, Young, Pearson, Geddes, & O'Brien, 2002; Matson, Nebel-Schwalm, & Matson, 2007; Schopler, 2001). Aggression and self-injury (head-banging, finger or hand-biting, head slapping, and hair pulling) are also common behavioral symptoms for children. These behaviors are due to biological factors (such as seizures), the child's cognitive and emotional impairments (leading to impulsivity and low frustration tolerance), an inability to communicate verbally, difficulty managing change, learned behaviors to avoid certain tasks or situations, and misreading of others' intent as threatening (Gadow, DeVincent, & Schneider, 2008).

Population

Research suggests that the ASDs are genetic, neuro-biological disorders (Maimberg & Vaeth, 2006). There is no association of ASD with any psychological or social influences, including parenting styles. Although about 50 percent of parents believe that vaccinations are the cause of the ASDs (Harrington, Rosen, Garnecho, & Patrick, 2006), the Institute of Medicine (2004) has determined, from reviews of the extant research, that no causal link between autism and childhood vaccines has been established.

Approximately 60 percent to 70 percent of persons with ASD manifest distinct neurological abnormalities and various levels of developmental disability. Although brain abnormalities exist in a majority of diagnosed individuals, 30 percent to 40 percent of the population of persons with ASD possesses an anatomically intact central nervous system (Peliosa & Lund, 2001). Thus, ASD has many etiologies, including the following:

- Genetic conditions (see below)
- Viral infections (such as congenital rubella, a type of mental retardation that results from infection during pregnancy)
- Metabolic conditions (such as abnormalities of purine synthesis, the amino acid that energizes many physical reactions)
- Congenital anomaly syndromes (such as Williams's syndrome, a genetic disability characterized by outgoing behavior and intellectual and developmental deficits).

None of the identified etiologies are invariably associated with ASD, however, and knowledge of these causes has not clarified the neuro-psychological basis of the condition.

Several *brain abnormalities* have been identified in persons with ASD, but which of them are specific and universal to the conditions is unclear. The most consistent findings point to disruptions in the limbic system and the cerebellum and its circuits (Holter, 2004). Structural and functional brain imaging studies have also indicated that ASD may be associated with enlarged overall brain size and decreased size and activity in specific areas of the brain. One of these areas may be the *midsagittal* area of the cerebellum, thought to be involved in the sequencing of motor activities. Another is the lower *hippocampus* (in the midbrain), which is associated with complex learning processes. A third area is the *amygdala* (located in the temporal lobe), which is believed to contribute to the recognition of faces and emotional expression. A final area is the *brain stem*, in a section associated with attention.

With regard to deficits in brain functioning, ASD has been conceptualized in a variety of ways (Volkmar, Lord, Bailey, Schultz, & Klin, 2004). It may be a disorder of *central coherence* in which the person is unable to holistically process information and develops a bias toward part-oriented processing. It may be a disorder of *executive function* in which the person is not able to process bits of information or regulate behavior, and thus is inclined toward rigid, repetitive behaviors and impoverished social interaction. It may be a deficit in *social cognition* in that the internal mental states of other people are not understood. Today, however, most research on brain deficits in autism focuses on *language and communication*, involving the difficulties in using and comprehending words and their meanings.

Children with ASD may have an overgrowth of neurons in some areas of the brain, coupled with an underdeveloped organization of neurons into specialized systems. These findings have not been consistently replicated across studies, however, and therefore must be viewed with caution (Southgate & Hamilton, 2008). Research also indicates that children with ASD may have high levels of the neurotransmitter serotonin in the midbrain and brain stem (Lam, Aman, & Arnold, 2006). Genes that promote serotonin may facilitate the multiple neuron interactions that are prerequisites for developing ASD. Again, any conclusions about these processes are speculative at this time.

In twin studies, the concordance rate for autism spectrum disorder in identical twins ranges from 36 percent to 91 percent (Veenstra-Vanderweele & Cook, 2003). In other family studies, up to 90 percent of siblings are diagnosed with one of the pervasive developmental disorders (Matson et al., 2007). The research suggests that different genes (perhaps between three and ten of them) and the variety of ways they can be manifested contribute to different symptoms of ASD (Liu, Paterson, & Szatmari, 2008). To date, there is some evidence for three loci, in chromosomes 7q, 13q, and 15q (Happe & Ronald, 2008). In the search for causes, researchers have come to appreciate the great complexity of the genetic interactions that appear to produce ASD (Veenstra-Vanderweele & Cook, 2003).

Some children with ASD have experienced identifiable *prenatal or perinatal* (immediately after birth) *events* that are linked to these conditions (Maimberg & Vaeth, 2006). A higher risk of ASD has been seen among children with low birth weight and congenital malformations. Additionally, the risk of the conditions increases for firstborn children and the children of older parents (mothers aged 35 years or older, and fathers aged 40 and older) (Reichenberg et al., 2006). These findings, while tentative, may be related to a firstborn's greater ingestion of maternal toxins in utero, or to the hygiene hypothesis, which suggests that firstborns are exposed to fewer infections from other children early in childhood and thus are more likely to develop autoimmune toxins that affect brain development. Parental age may be associated with age-specific genetic and chromosomal damage in the parents or the effects of environmental toxins.

Autism does not appear any later than the age of three and is usually diagnosed by age four (Smith et al., 2002). The other spectrum conditions may not be diagnosed until several years later because their associated symptoms may not be as prominent. Practice guidelines adopted by the American Academy of Pediatrics call for pediatricians to examine for signs of ASD in all babies and toddlers (Johnson & Myers, 2007). Between the ages of one and three years, when parents are most likely to seek evaluation, differences from peers are readily apparent, and idiosyncratic, self-absorbed behaviors and communication problems are striking. In the first year of life the child with an ASD displays unusual social development, being less likely to imitate the movements and vocal sounds of others, and to exhibit problems with attention and responding to external stimulation. About 90 percent of parents of autistic children recognize a significant abnormality in the child, and parental reports of the child's regression from a higher level of functioning are made in 20–40 percent of cases (Volkmar et al., 2004).

Studies on the course of ASD over time show variable results that depend on the severity of the condition. For autism specifically, a sample of 48 children was followed up in late adolescence (McGovern & Sigman, 2005). Almost all persons were still diagnosed with an ASD, but their parents described improvements in the areas of social interaction, repetitive or stereo-typed behaviors, adaptive behaviors, and emotional responsiveness to others in adolescence compared to middle childhood. In a Swedish prospective study children who had been diag-nosed with autism or atypical autism (N=120) were assessed in adulthood (Billstedt, Gillberg, & Gillberg, 2005). None of the persons from either the autistic or atypical autism groups had a "good" outcome. The majority (57 percent) was categorized as having a very poor outcome. No statistically significant differences existed between the autistic and the atypical autism group. The next common outcome was "poor" (21 percent) followed by "restricted" (13 percent), and "fair" (8 percent).

In another prospective study, Swedish men diagnosed with autism or Asperger's disorders were followed for five years after diagnosis (Cederlund, Hagberg, Billstedt, Gillberg, & Gillberg, 2008). Outcomes were worse for the persons in the autism group compared to the Asperger's group, with the majority (76 percent) having poor to very poor outcome. The intellectual level was much lower among those in the autism study group, where only five (7 percent) persons had a normal intellectual capacity at follow-up.

For the Asperger's group, in the majority of cases the diagnosis was still valid (84 percent), and even those without the ongoing diagnosis showed impairment (Cederlund et al., 2008). About a quarter of the Asperger's sample had a poor outcome, despite their having average IQs. Barnhill (2007) studied the course of Asperger's disorder into adulthood in a U.S. sample and found that those persons who achieved adaptive functioning levels continued to experience some impairment in employment, perception, social isolation, motor skills, and mood, with depression being a common condition.

Certain factors are associated with a more or less favorable adaptation. Early diagnosis of the autism spectrum conditions is important so that intervention can begin as soon as possible, when it is most likely to have a positive impact on the core features of the conditions (Rogers & Vismara, 2008). Parental concern is a more important factor in identifying a child with ASD than pediatric testing (Mandell & Novak, 2005). Parents often voice concerns a year earlier than diagnosis formally takes place, which is, not surprisingly, perceived by parents as a delay (Harrington et al., 2006). Researchers at the Center for Disease Control found that children with ASDs were initially evaluated at a mean age of 48 months, but were not diagnosed until 61 months (with no differences by gender or SES) (Wiggins, Baio, & Rice, 2006). Most practitioners (70 percent) did not use a diagnostic screening instrument in the process, and 24 percent of children were not diagnosed until after entering school. Often neurologists and developmental pediatricians are responsible for diagnosing ASDs with primary pediatricians playing only a small role in diagnosis (12 percent of the time) (Harrington et al., 2006). Some of the reasons cited by Harrington et al. (2006) to explain the low rate of pediatrician contribution to diagnosis include the inability of the physician to feel equipped to do so, time constraints on conducting screens, and fear of labeling a child prematurely.

Certain provider, family, and child factors are associated with the early or later diagnosis of autism. Protective provider influences include a pediatrician referral to a specialist (Landa, Holman, & Garrett-Mayer, 2007), while risk mechanisms involve inconsistency in the provision of primary care (more than four providers), a dearth of knowledge about ASDs, and a lack of screening tools that providers have the time and capability to use (Matson, Nebel-Schwalm, & Matson, 2007). Unfortunately, a pediatrician conducting developmental tests is not correlated with an earlier diagnosis, in part because two-thirds of pediatricians report that they do not feel adequate to conduct such assessments (Dosreis, Weiner, Johnson, & Newschaffer, 2006). Family factors associated with early diagnosis are urban residence and being of middle socioeconomic status (Landa et al., 2007). Child characteristics that promote early diagnosis include severe language deficits, and, in general, a more severe form of the condition (Wiggins et al., 2006), having an IQ of 70 or lower, experiencing developmental regression (Shattuck et al., 2009), and demonstrating particular symptoms (hand flapping and toe walking). Later diagnosis is related to oversensitivity to pain, having a hearing impairment (Landa et al., 2007) and female gender (Shattuck et al., 2009).

Other than the timing of intervention, risk influences for the course of ASD are related to certain child factors – the person's IQ, the acquisition of speech, the presence of co-occurring medical conditions, female gender (Billstedt, Gillberg, & Gillberg, 2007), and the severity of the disorder (McGovern & Sigman, 2005). Children with higher IQs (over 60) are more responsive to intervention. IQ scores usually stabilize after five years and correlate with later academic and work achievement. The acquisition of intelligible speech capacity by the age of five was the most important predictor of outcome in the Billstedt et al. (2007) prospective study.

Risk mechanisms for the course of autism include the child's aggression and self-injury (head-banging, finger or hand-biting, head slapping, and hair pulling), which compromise home and community placements (Gadow et al., 2008). These aggressive behaviors are due to the following:

- Cognitive and emotional impairments, which lead to impulsivity, low frustration tolerance, poor emotional and behavioral regulation, and difficulties with coping skills
- The inability to communicate anger verbally
- Difficulty negotiating change
- Learned behaviors to avoid tasks or certain situations
- Misreading of others' intent as threatening
- Seizures or other biological factors.

Mental health care disparities

The growth in identified cases of ASD, and the financial expense of comprehensive intervention, has created a situation where many such children do not receive adequate medical, educational, and behavioral health care for achieving their highest functional potential. The needs of children with ASD for medical and other services place health care providers and insurers at a high financial risk. It also increases the vulnerability of these children to cost-limiting measures that may affect their quality of care. The U.S. Department of Education has characterized autism as the largest growing relatively low-incidence disability, as 92 percent of those persons experience significant functional impairment (Liptak et al., 2006). The mean total annual expenditures for children with ASD in 2006 was $6,132, 65 percent of which went for outpatient expenses, and $613 of this was out-of-pocket (Liptak et al., 2006). Much of this spending ($2,239 per child in 2006) went to home health care, including personal care attendants and non-skilled home-based workers. By contrast, all children without ASD generated an average of $860 in annual health care costs. When this amount is combined with annual expenditures for educational services ($12,773 per pupil for the 98 percent of ASD persons who require special education), the expense per child is enormous.

Federal legislation designates two programs to provide services to children with disabilities – the Individuals with Disabilities Education Act and Medicaid (Stahmer & Mandell, 2007). Children with autism are more likely than other children to have private insurance (although 46 percent have public insurance) and their parents are more likely to have incomes more than twice the poverty level. These children carry a substantial burden of medical care, averaging 42 outpatient visits (vs. 3.3 for other children) and 22 prescription medications and refills per year (with 24 percent taking psychotropic medications, the most common being Risperdal and Adderall).

Federal law 94–142 mandates the provision of an appropriate educational plan for all children with ASDs in the United States (Holter, 2004). As part of this educational plan, ancillary services are often required, including speech or language therapy, occupational therapy, and physical therapy. Social work professionals should be prepared to consult and collaborate with teachers and other school personnel and have working knowledge of state, as well as federal laws and policies, related to services (Holter, 2004). Depending on the district and the particular school, social workers may provide psychosocial services, including sociocultural assessments, support to the child and family, and skills training. The possibility of new federal mandates for the provision of remedial services beginning in infancy and continuing through the child's life may increase the availability of services for families (Volkmar et al., 2004).

Medicaid is the largest single public payer of behavioral health services, and accounts for 75 percent of all funding for developmentally disabled related services (translating into $29.3 billion) (Beasley & Hurley, 2007). Title XIX of the Social Security Act requires state Medicaid programs to offer certain basic services in order to receive federal matching funds. Because children with disabilities consume more services than those without disabilities, financial incentives to control overall costs have a greater impact on those children. A study of service use by persons with ASD in one state's (Tennessee) Medicaid Managed Care program illustrates the effects of public funding on the problem (Ruble, Heflinger, Renfrew, & Saunders, 2005). The major finding of this study was that, although the number of children who received services increased, this represented only one-tenth of the estimated number of persons with ASD. Additionally, the mean number of services provided per child decreased over a five-year period. While more costly services such as day treatment disappeared, case management and medication management services increased. Cost shifting to other service sectors such as schools adds an additional source of redirection and diffusion of responsibility. Further, parents may choose not to access behavioral health services because children are receiving school-based services. These findings lend support to the claim that service utilization patterns of children with ASDs are sensitive to financial incentives under Medicaid managed care.

Another issue for public policy is what will happen when the large numbers of children with ASDs become adults and leave the school systems, the primary public institutions for the delivery of services. Currently people with disabilities are 15 percent of all Medicaid recipients but account for 37 percent of expenditures (Flanders, Engelhart, Pandina, & McCracken, 2007). The long-term care components of these expenditures will rise significantly if the autistic population of tomorrow requires the same kinds of care as today's population. When these persons reach age 18, many will quality for Supplemental Security Insurance, and will become eligible for Medicaid. For now, private insurers can continue to deny coverage for services such as speech and occupational therapy as well as medications because of a lack of evidence basis for many interventions.

One important factor in service trends is that there is still no consensus as to the causes of the ASDs, whether they are best classified as medical or mental health disorders, and the optimal treatments (Steuernagel, 2005). A basic question for policy makers is: how do stakeholders plan policies and programs for these conditions in which there may be a variety of causes, and in which there may be a variety of potentially promising intervention strategies?

Although autism can be diagnosed between the ages of two and three years, the findings of Shattuck et al. (2009) involving the relatively late age of identification of ASD (5.7 years) and the significant proportion of cases (27.1 percent) that were still not identified at age eight are cause for alarm. They point to limitations in the system for screening and identification of ASDs. Researchers at the Center for Disease Control found that most practitioners (70 percent) did not use a diagnostic screening instrument in the process, and 24 percent of children were not diagnosed until after entering school (Wiggins et al., 2006). Often neurologists and developmental pediatricians are responsible for diagnosing ASDs with primary pediatricians playing only a small role in diagnosis (12 percent of the time) (Harrington et al., 2006). Some of the reasons cited by Harrington et al. (2006) to explain the low rate of pediatrician contribution to diagnosis include inability of the physician to feel equipped to do so, time constraints on conducting screens, and fear of labeling a child prematurely. If parents do not have enough information to pursue a specialist or they do not have access to such, then their child will not be diagnosed in a timely manner and age of diagnosis is related to ultimate prognosis.

Even agencies that specialize in providing early identification services show a striking lack of consistency in how children with ASDs are screened and diagnosed, as well the type of care they receive. Only 20 percent of states utilize formal diagnostic guidelines for assessing ASDs, and only 22 percent required diagnosticians to be experienced with the disorders (Stahmer & Mandell, 2007, as cited in Swiezy, Stuart, & Korzekwa, 2008). This finding is alarming given that early identification and intervention are keys for optimizing long-term positive outcomes for individuals with an ASD (Swiezy et al., 2008). In an effort to improve the timeliness of ASD evaluation, the American Academy of Pediatrics has published specific guidelines, and the Centers for Disease Control and Prevention is involved in the "Learn the Signs, Act Early" campaign (Shattuck et al., 2009).

A final potential disparity is that, thus far, interventions have targeted Caucasian youth, but culture may play an important role in how well programs work with children from ethnic minorities (Rogers & Vismara, 2008). Many potential cultural issues must be taken into account: language and socioeconomic barriers exist, as do different expectations about appropriate child behavior, namely independence, parental authority, and the role of extended family and kin in childcare. Further, different perceptions of the causes of ASDs and the stigma attached to mental conditions may impact receipt of services. Efforts to provide programming that is sensitive to cultural and socioeconomic factors, as well as training for researchers and service providers, are critical (Rogers & Vismara, 2008).

Gender is another disparity that emerged in Shattuck et al. (2009). Females are diagnosed later as having ASDs despite their often being more severely afflicted. This suggests the possibility of disparate clinical practices in terms of referral and screening, as well as gender bias in expectations of behavior that is considered normal in boys and girls (Shattuck et al., 2009).

Most early disability policy in the United States was based on a medical model. As more people have become involved in advocacy efforts for persons with disabilities, a new *social model of disability* (also known as the "recovery" model) has evolved, incorporating a central belief that the experience of people with the disability, not the expertise of professionals, should be the critical factor in policy making (Reindal, 2008). This newer approach emphasizes self-advocacy and a resolve that the world should be altered to accommodate persons with disabilities, rather than altering the people who have chronic disabilities. Since a social model of disability suggests that autism is not a disabling condition per se, but that the problem lies in how society treats people with autism, a case can be made that fewer resources should be devoted to eradicating autism than to understanding the specific educational needs of children with autism. Whether the social model of disability policy best serves the needs of persons with autism is a matter of debate (Reindal, 2008). Reliance on the medical model, for example, might lead to more resources devoted to uncovering the yet-unknown causes of the ASDs and their treatment. Perhaps the best development in social policy would be to promote both the medical and social models of autism. Parents of such children would be able to think about what interventions they need, and a combination of public and private resources would ensure access to those services. At the same time, society would begin to understand the need to embrace all individuals, including those with autism.

The national Mental Health Parity Act, originally passed in 1996, and amended in 2010, was intended to require insurance companies to provide parity coverage for mental health and medical benefits, when both are offered (Kjorstad, 2003). Some insurance companies have argued, however, that mental health coverage under the Parity Act must be provided only for biologically-based severe mental illnesses, and a judgment of which diagnoses qualify can be arbitrary. As long as autism is defined as a mental health issue, it will continue, like all mental health issues, to be under-insured. Ironically, if the ASDs were treated as health issues rather than mental health issues, persons with autism might have greater access to services than they currently do.

Social work programs and social work roles

Social workers can serve as direct practitioners with persons who have ASDs and their families (including as applied behavior analysts), team leaders, and program administrators (Calohan & Peeler, 2007). Still, neither social workers, nor members of any other professional groups, can work exclusively in the assessment and treatment of persons with autism spectrum disorders. Inter-professional teamwork is always required to develop the kinds of comprehensive programs necessary to target the behavioral and systems problems that arise with these conditions.

Assessment of the ASDs is a challenging process because no biochemical tests are available to diagnose them; or does a single behavior or set of behaviors unequivocally denote any of the conditions (Jordan, 2001). A core assessment, therefore, includes the following (Johnson & Myers, 2007; Ozonoff, Goodlin-Jones, & Solomon, 2007):

- Information from parents about mother's pregnancy, labor, and delivery; the child's early neonatal course; the parents' earliest concerns about their child; family history of developmental disorders; symptoms in the areas of social interaction, communication/play, and restricted or unusual interests; the presence of problem behaviors that may interfere with intervention such as aggression, self-injury, and other behavioral oddities; and the child's prior response to educational or behavioral interventions.
- Direct observations in structured (school) and unstructured (home) settings and in interactions with peers, parents, and siblings.
- A medical evaluation, which includes learning about possible seizures, visual and hearing examinations for possible sensory problems, and testing for lead levels.
- Cognitive assessment to establish the level of intellectual functioning.
- An assessment of adaptive functioning and social skill development.
- A speech and language assessment.

Neuropsychological testing might also be indicated for those with some verbal ability in order to gain a sense of their strengths and limitations for treatment and education planning (Ozonoff et al., 2007). Professionals from various disciplines can use formal instruments to assist in their diagnostic assessments. There are a variety of instruments available that can be used for this purpose. Two instruments, both clinician-administered, are considered the "gold standards" for assessment of autism (Ozonoff et al., 2007): the Autism Diagnostic Interview-Revised (Lord, Rutter, & Le Couteur, 1994); and the Autism Diagnostic Observation Schedule (Lord et al., 2000). Another recommended measure is the Social Communication Questionnaire, which is a parent report version of the Autism Diagnostic Interview – Revised (Rutter, Bailey, Lord, & Berument, 2003). The Modified Checklist for Autism in Toddlers (M-CHAT) (Dumont-Mathieu & Fein, 2005) is another parent-report measure designed to screen for autism at the 24-month well child pediatric visit.

The social worker's assessment should include observations of the client in structured and unstructured settings such as the school and home. The social worker should further examine the child's prior response to any educational programs or behavioral interventions, including information from standard rating scales and symptom checklists and narrative reports of teachers and care providers. Observations of the child's interactions with parents and other family members will provide information about the child, the levels of stress experienced by the family in response to the child's symptoms, and the effectiveness of parental interventions. The social worker should note the presence of any client behaviors that may interfere with the delivery of intervention programs, such as aggression and self-injury. Information about family support and stress is critical, as studies have demonstrated that the family stress associated with having a child with ASD is greater than having a child with mental retardation, Down syndrome, or chronic physical illness (Gabriels, Hill, Pierce, Rogers, & Wehner, 2001). *Comprehensive interventions* for children with autism spectrum conditions are defined as small-group or one-on-one behavioral and educational interventions that are delivered for at least 10–15 hours per week for a significant period of time, ranging from months to years (Shattuck & Grosse, 2007). Unfortunately, no intervention has yet been shown to change the core features of ASD to a sufficient extent that the individual is able to achieve normative levels of functioning. After a thorough diagnostic evaluation, however, steps may be taken to help the individual develop and function with significant gains. The range of interventions should include special education, family support, behavioral management, and social skills training for persons with higher functioning ASD. Medications may also be used to control behavioral symptoms, although considerable caution should be exercised when doing so and the child's response should be monitored closely. There are a range of complementary and alternative medicines that are also available and that parents find appealing (Harrington et al., 2006). These will be briefly described, as well.

Applied behavior analysis (ABA) involves the examination of the antecedents of a problem behavior (the event or situation that precedes the behavior) and its consequences (the event or situation that follows the behavior). Any avoidable antecedents for a problem behavior are removed and desirable behaviors are broken down into their component parts. Positive reinforcement is then provided for their performance. The program developed by Lovaas was the first of the structured behavioral modification programs (Lovaas, 1987, 2003). Seida, Ospina, Karkhaneh, Hartling, Smith, and Clark (2009) conducted a review of the meta-analyses and systematic reviews that have been conducted for autism interventions. Support was provided for ABA in terms of improvements in adaptive, cognitive, and language skills, as well as reductions in problem behavior. Although the literature commonly urges parental participation in such programs (Rogers & Vismara, 2008), a Cochrane Collaboration review indicated that only two randomized, controlled studies have been conducted of parent-mediated training, and they could not be synthesized because of methodological differences (Diggle & McConachie, 2002). A more recent systematic review of parent-implemented early intervention for ASD has been undertaken by McConachie and Diggle (2007), with 12 studies located. The authors concluded that randomized and controlled studies of parent training resulted in improved child communication skills for the treatment groups. Parent training also resulted in enhanced maternal knowledge of autism, maternal communication style, and parent child interaction, and reduced maternal depression. However, the studies were analyzed through a vote count method rather than meta-analyzing the results of studies across common domains.

Rogers and Vismara (2008) conducted a review of the previous ten years of research on autism interventions according to the American Psychological Association (APA) Task Force 12 Criteria (Chambless et al., 1998). None was concluded to be "well-established" (meaning that the interventions are represented by treatment manuals and either two independent well-designed control/comparison group studies indicating the benefit of an intervention over placebo or alternative treatment, or that it is at least as effective as another well-established treatment). The intensive behavioral treatment program developed and tested by Lovaas (1987, 1993), involving one-on-one assistance 40 hours a week for two or more years, garnered the categorization of a "probably efficacious" intervention. This means that the test of the intervention involves either of the following: two methodologically sound group studies by the same investigator showing the experimental intervention to be better than placebo or an alternative treatment, or at least three single-subject studies that compare the intervention to another intervention (Chambless et al., 1998).

In Rogers and Vismara's (2008) review, the intervention known as pivotal response training (PRT) earned the categorization of "probably efficacious". PRT is a type of ABA taught to parents that focuses on "pivotal" aspects of the child's functioning: motivation, self-management (to be more independent and less reliant on prompts), initiation (to initiate interactions), and the ability to respond to multiple cues (to select cues that are relevant in a given situation) (Koegel, Kern Koegel, & Carter, 1999). It is distinguished from other behavioral approaches by taking advantage of naturally occurring teaching situations and consequences offered to children. PRT was rated as probably efficacious, based primarily on single-subject studies, although a more recent larger scale study was done on a diverse sample (Baker-Ericzén, Stahmer, & Burns, 2007).

For Asperger's specifically, other studies have suggested the importance of behavioral coping interventions to increase the child's ability to manage negative emotions. An experimental study of a six-week, two-hours weekly anger management session for persons with Asperger's disorder and their parents demonstrated a significant decrease in episodes of anger and an increase in parents' confidence about managing anger in the child (Sofronoff, Attwood, Hinton, & Levin, 2007). Another experimental study found that children with Asperger's disorder experienced a reduction in anxiety after participating in a weekly, six-week program of educational and entertaining small-group sessions that included parent consultation (Sofronoff, Attwood, & Hinton, 2005).

Social skills interventions are typically provided to persons with ASDs because social reciprocity deficits are a core feature of the conditions. These programs can take a variety of forms; most incorporate modeling, coaching, social problem solving, behavior rehearsal, feedback, and reinforcement-based strategies (Bellini & Peters, 2008). There is only modest evidence that skills can be generalized to situations in the child's daily life.

One of the problems with the research on social skills training is the lack of a common definition of social skills. While certain skills appear to be universally included (e.g., greeting, initiating conversations), others appear to be more idiosyncratic and often represent very complex behavior patterns (e.g., problem solving skills, exercising self-control), which makes cross-study comparisons difficult. Further, few investigations utilize group designs to control for the effects of maturation and time over the course of treatment. Only two studies (Ozonoff & Miller, 1995; Solomon, Goodlin-Jones, & Anders, 2004) used a comparative group design.

For *adolescents*, interventions should emphasize the acquisition of adaptive and vocational skills to prepare the individual for independent living. Sexual development in adolescence brings with it some other potential behavioral problems, which may be addressed using sexual education and behavioral techniques (Holter, 2004). Because public school responsibility ends when a person reaches age 22, the identification of community resources and support for adults in planning for long-term care is critical. Options include independent living (or more likely, semi-independent), living at home with parents (sometimes funded by Supplemental Security Income (SSI) and Social Security Disability Insurance (SSA)), foster homes, supervised group living, and institutions (for those who need intensive, constant supervision) (National Institute of Mental Health (NIMH), 2007). In many states adults with pervasive developmental disorders are not eligible for services that provide supported employment and residential living arrangements unless they also have mental retardation.

The symptoms of ASD that respond to *medications* do not represent the basic deficits in social interaction and communication. Rather, drug intervention may help with aggression, self-injury, inattention, and stereotyped movements, and these improvements may help the individual become more amendable to education and other interventions (des Portes, Hagerman, & Hendren, 2003). What follows is a review of medications used to treat these symptoms.

For the client's anxiety, selective serotonin re-uptake inhibitor (SSRI) drugs may be helpful (Leskovec, Rowles, & Findlay, 2008), although behavior programs, desensitization, structure, and steps to minimize stressful situations should be used as first-line interventions.

General attention in ASD children may be improved through the use of stimulants and other medications, but controlled studies are limited and adverse affects may outweigh benefits in some cases (Oswald & Sonenklar, 2007). The response for children with ASD for the stimulants is generally lesser than with non-ASD youth with attention deficit hyperactivity disorder (ADHD) (Aman & Langworthy, 2000). Empirical evidence for significant reductions in hyperactive symptoms is strongest for the antipsychotic drugs (particularly Risperdal), psychostimulants, and naltrexone, an opiate antagonist that is most often used to treat alcohol dependence. For children with ASD who have co-occurring ADHD, the psychostimulant medications produce a positive response rate of 50–60 percent. Some evidence of the benefits of risperidone in irritability (including aggression, deliberate self-injury, and temper tantrums), repetition and social withdrawal were apparent (Jesner, Aref-Adib, & Coren, 2007) but long-term studies have yet to determine the range of possible risks. Weight gain is a noticeable side effect, even at the short term.

For reducing aggression, antipsychotic medications including risperidone may be effective, often without inducing severe adverse reactions (Jesner et al., 2007). This medication has been shown to improve self-injury, aggression, and agitation in 70 percent of children and adolescents, compared to a placebo rate of 11.5 percent. Other antipsychotics, olanzapine and clozapine, have also been recommended for treating aggression. In addition, naltrexone has been posited to block opioids that may be released during self-injurious repetitive behaviors.

Biopterin (a naturally occurring enzyme) supplements appear to elicit small improvements in language and social functioning in some ASD persons, with few side effects reported (Tager-Flusberg, Joseph, & Folstein, 2001). For sleep problems, which are common in children with autism, behavioral measures are applied initially, possibly along with melatonin, light therapy, or chronotherapy (time structuring). For intractable cases of sleep impairments, medication may be useful.

In a constant search for ways to help their children, parents may try various *complementary and alternative medicines* (CAM). The National Center for Complementary and Alternative Medicine groups these therapies into four domains: mind-body medicine, biologically based practices, manipulative and body-based practices, and energy medicine. The most commonly used CAM treatments for ASD fall into the categories of biologically based, and manipulative and body-based practices. Approximately half of families of children with ASD use a biologically based therapy (e.g., dietary supplements), 30 percent use a mind-body therapy (e.g., music therapy), and 25 percent use a manipulation or body-based method (e.g., auditory integration) (Hanson et al., 2007). Hanson et al. (2007) reported that 41 percent of respondents endorsed benefit with dietary and nutritional treatments, whereas Wong and Smith (2006) found that 75 percent of respondents thought their treatments were helpful. Several of these CAM interventions will be briefly discussed here as Cochrane Collaboration reviews have been conducted on them.

Because people with autism spectrum conditions have difficulties with communication, music therapy is sometimes used to facilitate communication and expression of feelings. Three small experimental studies have examined the short-term effect of brief music therapy interventions for autistic children (Gold, Wigram, & Elefant, 2006). Music therapy was shown to be superior to placebo with respect to verbal and gestural communicative skills, but it was uncertain whether there were effects on behavioral outcomes.

Auditory integration therapy and other sound therapies were formulated to counteract the abnormal sound sensitivity in individuals with autism and improve concentration (Levy & Hyman, 2008). Unfortunately, results of most of the studies could not be synthesized because of methodological problems, but for the two studies that could be meta-analyzed, results were positive.

A high-use complementary intervention for ASDs is gluten and/or casein exclusion (e.g., wheat, oat, rye, barley, milk) diets. Current evidence for efficacy of these diets is poor, however (Millward, Ferriter, Calver, & Connell-Jones, 2008). Secretin is a gastro-intestinal hormone, but there is no evidence that it is effective and as such it should not currently be recommended as a treatment for autism (Williams, Wray, & Wheeler, 2005). The use of vitamin B6 for improving the behavior of individuals with autism also cannot currently be supported (Nye & Brice, 2005). In general, the recommendations of these systematic reviews is that large-scale, randomized controlled trials are needed, given the appeal of these interventions to families.

While many interventions help to control symptoms of the autism spectrum conditions, and the early intervention programs may ameliorate some of the core symptoms, most interventions are only effective for 50–70 percent of participants (Howlin, 2005). Efforts to identify types of clients who may respond to specific interventions have been hampered by the small size and heterogeneity of most samples, placebo responses, and the lack of widely agreed-upon standards for rating scales. There is also a lack of generalizability to people and settings external to the treatment environment (Rao, Beidel, & Murray, 2008). Many of the studies are also relatively short term in nature, without follow-up over time. This is a particular concern given the chronicity of the ASDs (Schopler, 2001).

Illustration and discussion

Wesley is a 15-year-old Asian male. An only child, his parents moved from China to the United States 20 years ago. They speak fluent English and are actively involved in Wesley's life. Wesley's parents knew something was wrong with him long before their son was diagnosed with autism. Wesley had no vocal communication, but used gestures to communicate. He also physically guided others to objects and situations in which he was interested. His identified problems at home, at school and in the community included aggression, self-injurious behaviors, property destruction, non-compliance with requests, deficits in personal care skills, and deficits in leisure skills. The manifestations of his aggression were hitting, kicking, scratching, punching, spitting and biting. His self-injurious behavior was characterized by slapping his face, punching his legs, and banging his head on objects, walls, and floors. The features of his property destruction were throwing or breaking objects. He did not babble as a baby, did not talk as a toddler, and he had long, violent tantrums. Wesley often engaged in problem behavior when he was denied access to a desired item or was attempting to gain attention from others.

After frequent visits to the pediatrician, Wesley's parents were told, "he is a late talker," "he will grow out of the tantrums" and "boys develop slower than girls" – a typical first experience for parents of children with autism spectrum disorders. As a last resort, Wesley's parents went to a center that specializes in developmental disabilities. Wesley was seen by a group of professionals including a neurologist, developmental pediatrician, speech pathologist, and occupational therapist. At three and a half years old – two years after his parents first noticed symptoms – he was diagnosed with autism. His multi-axial diagnosis is as follows:

Axis I: Autistic Disorder; Axis II: None; Axis III: Seasonal allergies; Axis IV: Problems with primary support system and academic problems; Axis V: GAF: 20/30 (current/highest in past year).

After the diagnosis, Wesley's parents researched autism and educated themselves about treatment options. Almost immediately, Wesley began receiving speech and occupational therapy services. He also began a preschool program at a nearby hospital that provided early intervention services to children with autism. One of Wesley's few strengths was his excellent physical health. The family was on the right track, but unfortunately Wesley had a severe form of the disorder.

Both parents were excellent advocates for their son, and highly nurturing of him. They were both recently diagnosed with depression, however, and Wesley's mother had an additional diagnosis of a generalized anxiety disorder, the symptoms of which had been present long before Wesley's diagnosis. His parents had very different parenting styles. Wesley's father was reactive when Wesley engaged in problem behaviors; he gave Wesley the item or attention he was trying to obtain. Wesley's mother tried to redirect the problem behavior and limit the attention he received. Both parents clearly loved their son, and were each doing what they felt was best in this difficult family situation. Still, their differences in response to Wesley's problem behaviors caused much tension in the household. When Wesley was 14 years old, his mother moved out of the family home due to the severity of his aggressive behavior.

Since the age of three, Wesley had been placed in special education classes. His most recent middle school placement was in a "varying exceptionalities class" that included children diagnosed with physical, behavioral and developmental disabilities. The intensity and frequency of Wesley's behaviors became so severe that the school was unable to provide an appropriate education under the Individuals with Disabilities Act. Consequently, the school system selected a residential placement in an attempt to stabilize him. The goal of the placement was to reduce Wesley's maladaptive behaviors and increase the adaptive behaviors, to improve his quality of life, and to improve his relationships so that he could return home and to school.

Upon admission to the current residential facility, the social worker, who was also a certified behavior analyst, conducted a functional behavior assessment (FBA). The FBA included interviews with Wesley's parents and teachers and observations of the child. Both the parents and teachers reported that many of Wesley's disruptive behaviors appeared to be maintained by escaping from a demand, access to a tangible item, and attention from others. His parents also reported that he would engage in self-injurious behaviors during non-demand situations or when he was not attempting to access preferred items. During the admission assessment, it was also observed that Wesley engaged in aggression, property destruction and self-injurious behaviors to gain access to preferred activities and to escape settings and activities he found aversive. The behavior analyst also observed Wesley engaging in face slapping when he was alone and not engaged in an activity. This suggested that there was a sensory component to the self-injury that was maintained by automatic reinforcement.

All *interventions* with Wesley were based on the scientific principles of applied behavior analysis (ABA). Staff working with Wesley recorded his maladaptive behaviors on a checklist 24 hours a day. The behavior checklist consisted of diagnostic information including apparent antecedents (the event/situation that preceded the behavior), consequences (the event/situation that proceeded the behavior), and the location, duration, intensity, group size, and time of day when the behaviors occurred. These data were used by the social worker to adjust and refine treatment strategies. It was hypothesized that if his problem behaviors were blocked and ignored, and Wesley was redirected to complete a task, the frequency of his escape maintained behavior (i.e., self-injury and aggression) would decrease in the future. Additionally, as Wesley received continuous positive reinforcement for completing tasks and was taught to request brief breaks appropriately, the frequency of his aggression and self-injury would decrease. It must be emphasized that Wesley's pre-treatment aggressive behaviors were extreme. His self-injurious behaviors were so severe that he was often bloody and bruised within minutes, and his aggressive episodes were at a level that he injured several staff who worked with him.

A token economy system was developed to increase Wesley's communication and decrease his harmful behaviors. Wesley earned tokens for positive, adaptive, and cooperative behavior. These behaviors included following directions (compliance), keeping hands and feet to himself and using them as intended (no aggression or self-injury), using objects as intended (no property destruction) and "bonus" tokens for other positive behaviors (i.e., sharing and using appropriate communication). Back-up reinforcers selected by Wesley and the staff included, but were not limited to, walks, food items (cookies, apples, rice cakes), music, and access to a beanbag chair. The back-up reinforcers were detailed for Wesley and staff on a menu to ensure treatment consistency. Frequently adding novel items and activities, as well as allowing Wesley to select new items enhanced the effectiveness of these reinforcers. By using these tokens, more attention was provided following appropriate behaviors than following inappropriate behaviors. This was a proactive procedure that focused on arranging consequences for Wesley's positive behaviors.

When the token system was first introduced, Wesley was earning tokens every 15–30 seconds due to the high frequency of his aggression and self-injury. Subsequently, Wesley received tokens intermittently based on the above behaviors. Upon earning three tokens, Wesley had opportunity to exchange them for an item or activity from the reinforcer menu.

Another intervention used with Wesley was systematic compliance trials to complete fairly quick and easy tasks throughout the day. Compliance trials consisted of presenting Wesley with pre-selected instructions during the day. In effect, he was presented with trials at which he was likely to succeed so that following directions was reinforced.

All staff working with Wesley were trained in appropriate restraint procedures to ensure he was safe and to reduce the risk of harm to himself or others. Restraint procedures (as defined in the behavior plan) were initiated in the event that Wesley's aggression and self-injury rose to an unmanageable level.

The primary treatment philosophy in working with children with autism is to teach new skills that are incompatible with problem behaviors. For Wesley and most children with autism, verbal behavior is the most efficient replacement behavior: 80 percent of problem behaviors are a response to frustrations with communication (Tager-Flusberg & Caronna, 2007). When Wesley was admitted to the residential facility, he engaged in approximately 400 incidents of aggression and self-injury per day. Since he was a young child, Wesley learned that he could gain access to a desired item, gain access to attention, or escape a task by hitting himself or others. Over the course of ten months Wesley learned that appropriately using his communication device would produce the desired item or activity whereas aggression and self-injury would not.

Communication and various other functional behaviors (including academic goals) were taught to Wesley using Discrete Trial Teaching (DTT), an approach based on principles of applied behavior analysis. DTT is a specific method of teaching that is comprised of an instruction, a response, and a consequence. Within DTT sessions, various prompts, shaping procedures and levels or reinforcement are used. Wesley responded very well to DTT and acquired new skills quickly using this method. He was given clear instructions, prompted when he gave an incorrect response, and provided with positive reinforcement after correct responses.

Another applied behavior analysis approach used to teach Wesley new skills included task analyses. A task analysis consists of breaking up a large behavior into several small behaviors. Wesley required verbal, gestural and physical prompts to complete many of his personal care skills. Instead of teaching showering in its entirety, Wesley learned using a task analysis. Showering, for example, was broken down into 17 steps and each one was taught independently. This is the same approach that was used to teach Wesley several other personal care skills (hand washing, dressing, brushing teeth) and daily living skills (laundry, preparing small snack, making his bed).

At the residential facility where Wesley resided there was a treatment partnership between the psychiatrist and social worker/behavior analyst. In many facilities, medications are prescribed based on anecdotal reports, independent of behavioral data or regard to behavioral treatment component analyses. These sometimes competing strategies have the potential to confound behavioral treatment effects data or, more importantly, a resident's receptiveness and participation in teaching sessions. Adjustments to medication dosages and time of administration are made to coordinate with behavioral treatment plans, schedules, and progress data. The two professionals met weekly to review Wesley's behavior reduction and acquisition data to make any medications changes as indicated.

Since Wesley's FBA and subsequent behavioral observation data suggested that self-injurious behaviors served a self-stimulatory function, psychopharmacology treatment acted as a motivating operation – reducing the natural reinforcement produced by the brain – to enhance the efficacy of his behavioral acquisition of replacement behaviors. Along with the opioid receptor antagonist medication used for self-injury, Wesley was prescribed two antipsychotic and one anticonvulsant medication to improve his mood stability and explosive outbursts.

In the ten months that Wesley received intensive services, the frequency of his aggression decreased by 80 percent and the frequency of self-injury decreased by 75 percent. He learned to independently use his assistive technology device to access desired items and activities. He completed most of his daily living skills with verbal and gestural prompts, rather than physical prompts. Wesley could smile, play, jump, laugh, and successfully go out into the community for leisure activities with staff members and peers. He enjoyed adult and peer attention and was so successful in school that he achieved most of his individualized education program (IEP) goals. Through behavior reduction and skill acquisition procedures, Wesley learned that appropriate behavior produces better outcomes.

A vital part of Wesley's program was family therapy. This was not traditional family therapy in the sense that the child was not involved, but it did affect the entire family system. Wesley's parents experienced a great deal of guilt prior to and immediately after placing him in a residential program. It is often difficult for parents to admit that they cannot care for their child with autism on their own. The social worker investigated some aspects of Chinese family life to better understand the parental subsystem. She learned that there is much shame in Chinese culture when one member is perceived as a "failure" in some way. The mother is considered the primary caregiver, while the father takes a more formal and distant role with the children. This balance of roles was upset when each of the parents developed their own, conflicted means of dealing with their son. They had a cultural resistance to the intensive interventions that were recommended for their son (feeling intimidated by the professionals and unhappy about their perceived loss of parenting respon-sibilities) and tended, in the view of the social worker, to infantilize their son.

The normalcy of humdrum life does not happen for a family with a child with autism. For example, buying groceries becomes a major planned-out event that may end in a catastrophe. For six years, Wesley's parents were trapped in their own home. They could not take him out in the community because he would become aggressive or self-injurious in the car and in the community. He was home-schooled for a year prior to residential treatment because he injured two staff members on his school bus and his classroom teachers could not manage his behavior. This put an enormous strain on Wesley's parents but their relationship became more stressed when the possibility of residential treatment was discussed. When a child is placed in residential treatment, the marriage may either begin to heal and follow normal patterns of growth, or the guilt consumes the parents and they are unable to forgive themselves.

The role of social work was essential in working with Wesley's family. Wesley's parents admitted they did not have a healthy marriage. Wesley's mother had moved out of the home when his aggression became unmanageable. Differences in parenting styles may occur in any marriage, while parents of children with autism have a bigger battle. Wesley's parents stated at admission that they spoke to each other only when they fought, and they only fought over Wesley. A child with autism will pick up subtle cues that a couple is having conflicts thus causing escalating behaviors in the child. Prior to family intervention the issues that the couple was having were never addressed and left unresolved.

After a few months of weekly meetings, Wesley's parents began healing and accepting they made the right decision. Their guilt began to lessen as they observed Wesley making significant progress. During weekly family therapy sessions, the social worker focused much on strengthening the parents' relationship. Wesley's mother moved back into their home. They began communicating about other topics besides Wesley. They engaged in normalized activities together such as shopping, errands, spending time with friends, dates, and even vacations. Wesley's parents stated that they could again enjoy being around one another, and around Wesley. They could enjoy that his repertoire of daily living skills increased, he required less prompting to complete many activities of daily living, and he could sit still for long periods of time, working independently on self-care tasks. The challenges of living with autism persisted, but Wesley and his parents could again share a loving and supportive household.

Conclusion

Persons with autism spectrum conditions represent a client population that experiences significant and long-term functional impairments. While these conditions are primarily biological in origin, clients and their families require intervention and supports targeted at all facets of their lives – the medical, psychological and social. The social work profession's distinct person-and-environment perspective makes those practitioners well suited to practice with persons who have ASDs and their significant others. For example, the functional behavioral assessments described earlier represent an attempt to systematize a review of the social systems with which persons with ASDs interact, as social workers have always been trained to do.

Social workers are not qualified to intervene directly in the medical and health aspects of comprehensive intervention, but they are highly qualified to provide the systems interventions described in this chapter. As the social or recovery model of practice becomes more prominent, social workers will be able to apply their strengths perspective toward natural support system development, and their advocacy perspectives toward helping the larger community adapt to the needs of persons with ASDs. In their case management roles social workers can coordinate the interventions provided by a range of professionals and help clients plan for long-term professional involvement. Finally, social workers who engage in policy and programming activities can have an influence on the nature of professional services available to this client population.

Acknowledgements

The authors acknowledge Amy Wooley, MSW and Certified Behavior Analyst, for her valuable contribution of the case illustration in this chapter.

Web resources

Association for Science in Autism Treatment
www.asatonline.org

Autism National Committee (AUTCOM)
www.autcom.org

Autism Network International (ANI)
www.ani.ac

Autism Research Institute (ARI)
www.autismresearchinstitute.com

Autism Society of America
www.autism-society.org

Autism Speaks, Inc.
www.autismspeaks.org

MAAP Services for Autism, Asperger Syndrome, and PDD
www.maapservices.org

National Dissemination Center for Children with Disabilities, U.S. Dept. of Education, Office of Special
    Education Programs
www.nichcy.org

National Institute of Child Health and Human Development (NICHD)
www.nichd.nih.gov

National Institute on Deafness and Other Communication Disorders Information Clearinghouse
www.nidcd.nih.gov

References

Aman, M., & Langworthy, K. (2000). Pharmacology for hyperactivity in children with autism and other pervasive developmental disorders. *Journal of Autism and Developmental Disorders, 30* (5), 451–459.

American Psychiatric Association (APA). (2000). *Diagnostic and statistical manual of mental disorders* (4th ed., text revision). Washington, DC: APA.

Akshoomoff, N. (2006). Autism spectrum disorders: Introduction. *Child Neuropsychology, 12,* 245–246.

Baker-Ericzén, M.J., Stahmer, A.C., & Burns, A. (2007). Child demographics associated with outcomes in a community-based pivotal response training program. *Journal of Positive Behavior Interventions, 9* (1), 52–60.

Barnhill, G. (2007). Outcomes in adults with Asperger syndrome. *Focus on Autism and Other Developmental Disabilities, 22* (2), 116–126.

Beasley, J.B., & Hurley, A.D. (2007). Public systems supports for people with intellectual disability and mental health needs in the United States. *Mental Health Aspects of Developmental Disabilities, 10* (3), 118–120.

Bellini, S., & Peters, J.K. (2008). Social skills training for youth with autism spectrum disorders. *Child and Adolescent Psychiatric Clinics of North America, 17* (4), 857–873.

Bernard, L., Young, A.H., Pearson, J., Geddes, J., & O'Brien, G. (2002). Systematic review of the use of atypical antipsychotics in autism. *Journal of Psychopharmacology, 16* (1), 93–101.

Billstedt, E., Gillberg, C., & Gillberg, C. (2005). Autism after adolescence: Population-based 13- to 22-year follow-up study of 120 individuals with autism diagnosed in childhood. *Journal of Autism and Developmental Disorders, 35* (3), 351–360.

Billstedt, E., Gillberg, C., & Gillberg, C. (2007). Autism in adults: symptom patterns and early childhood predictors: Use of the DISCO in a community sample followed from childhood. *Journal of Child Psychology and Psychiatry, 48* (11), 1102–1110.

Calohan, C.J., & Peeler, C.M. (2007). Autistic disorder. In B.A. Thyer & J.S. Wodarski (eds), *Social work in mental health: An evidence-based approach* (pp. 53–73). Hoboken, NJ: John Wiley & Sons.

Cederlund, M., Hagberg, B., Billstedt, E., Gillberg, C., & Gillberg, C. (2008). Asperger syndrome and autism: A comparative longitudinal follow-up study more than 5 years after original diagnosis. *Journal of Autism and Developmental Disorders, 38* (1), 72–85.

Chambless, D., Baker, M., Baucom, D., Beutler, L., Calhoun, K., Crits-Cristoph, P. et al. (1998). Update on empirically validated therapies, II. *Clinical Psychologist, 51,* 3–16.

de Bruin, E.I., Ferdinand, R.F., Meester, S., de Nijs, P.F.A., & Verheij, F. (2007). *Journal of Autism and Developmental Disorders, 37,* 877–886.

des Portes, V., Hagerman, R.J., & Hendren, R.L. (2003). Pharmacotherapy. In S. Ozonoff, S.J. Rogers, & R.L. Hendren (eds), *Autism spectrum disorders: A research review for practitioners* (pp. 161–186). Washington, DC: American Psychiatric Association.

Diggle, T.T.J., & McConachie, H.H.R. (2002). Parent-mediated early intervention for young children with autism spectrum disorder. *Cochrane Database of Systematic Reviews,* Issue 2. Art. No.: CD003496. DOI: 10.1002/14651858.CD003496.

Dosreis, S., Weiner, C.L., Johnson, L., & Newschaffer, C.J. (2006). Autism spectrum disorder screening and management practices among general pediatric providers. *Journal of Developmental and Behavioral Pediatrics, 27* (Suppl. 2), S88–S94.

Dumont-Mathieu, T., & Fein, D. (2005). Screening for autism in young children: The Modified Checklist for Autism in Toddlers (M-CHAT) and other measures. *Mental Retardation and Developmental Disabilities Research Reviews, 31,* 253–262.

Flanders, S.C., Engelhart, L., Pandina, G.J., & McCracken, J.T. (2007). Direct health care costs for children with pervasive developmental disorders: 1996–2002. *Administration and Policy in Mental Health and Mental Health Services Research, 34* (3), 213–220.

Fombonne, E. (2007). Epidemiological surveys of pervasive developmental disorders. In F.R. Volkmar (ed.), *Autism and pervasive developmental disorders* (2nd ed., pp. 33–68). New York: Cambridge University Press.

Gabriels, R.L., Hill, D., Pierce, R., Rogers, S., & Wehner, B. (2001). Predictors of treatment outcome in young children with autism. *Autism: International Journal of Research and Practice, 5* (4), 407–429.

Gadow, K., DeVincent, C., & Schneider, J. (2008). Predictors of psychiatric symptoms in children with an autism spectrum disorder. *Journal of Autism and Developmental Disorders, 38* (9), 1710–1720.

Gold, C., Wigram, T., & Elefant, C. (2006). Music therapy for autistic spectrum disorder. *Cochrane Database of Systematic Reviews, 2.* Art. No.: CD004381. DOI: 10.1002/14651858.CD004381.pub2.

Hanson, E., Kalish, L.A., Bunce, E., Curtis, C., McDaniel, S., Ware, J., & Petry, J. (2007) Use of complementary and alternative medicine among children diagnosed with autism spectrum disorder. *Journal of Autism and Developmental Disorders, 37* (4), 628–636.

Happe, F., & Ronald, A. (2008). The "fractionable autism triad": A review of evidence from behavioural, genetic, cognitive and neural research. *Neuropsychology Review, 18* (4), 287–304.

Harrington, J., Rosen, L., Garnecho, A., & Patrick, P. (2006). Parental perceptions and use of complementary and alternative medicine practices for children with autistic spectrum disorders in private practice. *Journal of Developmental and Behavioral Pediatrics, 27* (2 Suppl.), S156–S161.

Holter, M. (2004). Autistic spectrum disorders: Assessment and intervention. In P. Allen-Meares & M. Fraser (eds), *Intervention with children and adolescents: An interdisciplinary perspective* (pp. 205–228). Washington, DC: NASW Press.

Howlin, P. (2005). Outcomes in autism spectrum disorders. In F.R. Volkmar, R. Paul, A. Klin, & D. Cohen (eds), *Handbook of autism and pervasive developmental disorders, Vol. 1: Diagnosis, development, neurobiology, and behavior* (3rd ed., pp. 201–220). Hoboken, NJ: John Wiley & Sons.

Institute of Medicine. (2004). *Immunization safety review: Vaccines and autism.* Retrieved June 15, 2009, from www.nap.edu/catalog.php?record_id=10997#description

Jesner, O.S., Aref-Adib, M., & Coren, E. (2007) Risperidone for autism spectrum disorder. *Cochrane Database of Systematic Reviews 2007,* Issue 1. Art. No.: CD005040. DOI: 10.1002/14651858.CD005040.pub2.

Johnson, C.P., & Myers, S.M. (2007). Identification and evaluation of children with autism spectrum disorders. Council on Children with Disabilities. *Pediatrics, 120* (5), 1183–1215.

Jordan, R. (2001). Multidisciplinary work for children with autism. *Educational and Child Psychology, 18* (2), 5–14.

Kjorstad, M.C. (2003). The current and future state of mental health insurance parity legislation. *Psychiatric Rehabilitation Journal, 27* (1), 34–42.

Koegel, R.L., Kern Koegel, L., & Carter, C.M. (1999). Pivotal teaching interactions for children with autism. *School Psychology Review, 28* (4), 576–594.

Koyama, T., Tachimor, H., Osada, H., & Kurita, H. (2006). Cognitive and symptom profiles in high-functioning Pervasive Developmental Disorder Not Otherwise Specified and Attention-Deficit/Hyperactivity Disorder. *Journal of Autism and Developmental Disorders, 36* (3), 373–380.

Lam, K.S.L., Aman, M.G., & Arnold, L.E. (2006). Neurochemical correlates of autistic disorder: A review of the literature. *Research in Developmental Disabilities, 27* (3), 254–289.

Landa, R.J., Holman, K.C., & Garrett-Mayer, E. (2007). Social and communication development in toddlers with early and later diagnosis of autism spectrum disorders. *Archives of General Psychiatry, 64* (7), 853–864.

Leskovec, T.J., Rowles, B.M., & Findlay, R.L. (2008). Pharmacological treatment options for autism spectrum disorders in children and adolescence. *Harvard Review of Psychiatry, 16* (2), 97–112.

Levy, S.E., & Hyman, S.L. (2008) Complementary and alternative medicine treatments for children with autism spectrum disorders. *Child and Adolescent Psychiatric Clinics of North America, 17* (4), 803–820.

Leyfer, O.T., Folstein, S.E., Bacalman, S., Davis, N.O., Dinh, E., Morgan, J. et al. (2006). Comorbid psychiatric disorders in children with autism: Interview development and rates of disorders. *Journal of Autism and Developmental Disorders, 36,* 849–861.

Liptak, G.S., Stuart, T., & Auinger, P. (2006). Health care utilization and expenditures for children with autism: Data from U.S. national samples. *Journal of Autism and Developmental Disabilities, 36* (3), 871–879.

Liu, X., Paterson, A.D., & Szatmari, P. (2008). Genome-wide linkage analyses of quantitative and categorical autism subphenotypes. *Biological Psychiatry, 64* (7), 561–570.

Lord, C., Rutter, M., & Le Couteur, A. (1994). Autism Diagnostic Interview – Revised: A revised version of a diagnostic interview for caregivers of individuals with possible pervasive developmental disorders. *Journal of Autism and Developmental Disorders, 24* (5), 659–685.

Lord, C., Risi, S., Lambrecht, L., Cook, E.H., Leventhal, B.L., DiLavore, P.C. et al. (2000). The Autism Diagnostic Observation Schedule – Generic: A standard measure of social and communication deficits associated with the spectrum of autism. *Journal of Autism and Developmental Disorders, 30* (3), 205–223.

Lovaas, O.I. (1987). Behavioral treatment and normal education and intellectual functioning in young autistic children. *Journal of Consulting and Clinical Psychology, 55* (1), 3–9.

Lovaas, O.I. (1993) The development of a treatment-research project for developmentally disabled and autistic children. *Journal of Applied Behavioral Analysis, 26* (4), 617–630.

Lovaas, O.I. (2003). *Teaching individuals with developmental delays: Basic intervention techniques.* Austin, TX: PRO-ED.

Macintosh, K., & Dissanayake, C. (2006). Social skills and problem behaviours in school aged children with high-functioning autism and Asperger's disorder. *Journal of Autism and Developmental Disorders, 36* (8), 1065–1076.

Maimberg, R.D., & Vaeth, M. (2006). Perinatal risk factors and infantile autism. *Acta Psychiatrics Scandinavia, 114*, 257–264.

Mandell, D.S., & Novak, M. (2005). The role of culture in families' treatment decisions for children with autism spectrum disorders. *Mental Retardation and Developmental Disabilities Research Reviews, 11* (2), 110–115.

Matson, J.L., Nebel-Schwalm, M., & Matson, M.L. (2007). A review of methodological issues in the differential diagnosis of autism spectrum disorders in children. *Research in Autism Spectrum Disorders, 1* (1), 38–54.

McConachie, H., & Diggle, T. (2007). Parent implemented early intervention for young children with autism spectrum disorder: A systematic review. *Journal of Evaluation in Clinical Practice, 13* (1), 120–129.

McGovern, C.W., & Sigman, M. (2005) Continuity and change from early childhood to adolescence in autism. *Journal of Child Psychology and Psychiatry, 46* (4), 401–408.

Millward, C., Ferriter, M., Calver, S.J., & Connell-Jones, G.G. (2008). Gluten- and casein-free diets for autistic spectrum disorder. *Cochrane Database of Systematic Reviews*, Issue 2. Art. No.: CD003498. DOI: 10.1002/14651858.CD003498.pub3.

National Institute of Mental Health. (2007). *Autism spectrum disorders: Pervasive developmental disorders.* Washington, DC: National Institute of Health.

Nye, C., & Brice, A. (2005). Combined vitamin B6-magnesium treatment in autism spectrum disorder. *Cochrane Database of Systematic Reviews*, Issue 4. Art. No.: CD003497. DOI: 10.1002/14651858.CD003497.pub2.

Oswald, D.P., & Sonenklar, N.A. (2007). Medication use among children with autism-spectrum disorders. *Journal of Child and Adolescent Psychopharmacology, 17* (3), 348–355.

Ozonoff, S., & Miller, J. (1995) Teaching theory of mind: A new approach to social skills training for individuals with autism. *Journal of Autism and Developmental Disorders, 25* (4), 415–433.

Ozonoff, S., Goodlin-Jones, B.L., & Solomon, M. (2007). Autism spectrum disorders. In E.J. Marsh & R.A. Barkley (eds), *Assessment of childhood disorders* (4th ed., pp. 487–525). New York: Guilford Press.

Peliosa, L., & Lund, S. (2001). A selective overview of issues on classification, causation, and early intensive behavioral intervention for autism. *Behavior Modification, 25* (5), 678–697.

Rao, P.A., Beidel, D.C., & Murray, M.J. (2008). Social skills interventions for children with Asperger's syndrome or high-functioning autism: A review and recommendations. *Journal of Autism and Developmental Disabilities, 38*, 353–361.

Reichenberg, A., Gross, R., Weiser, M., Bresnahan, M., Silverman, J., Harlap, S. et al. (2006). Advancing paternal age and autism. *Archives of General Psychiatry, 63* (9), 1026–1032.

Reindal, S.M. (2008). A social relational model of disability: A theoretical framework for special needs education? *European Journal of Special Needs Education, 23* (2), 135–146.

Rice, C. (2007). Prevalence of autism spectrum disorders: Autism and developmental disabilities monitoring network, six sites, United States, 2000. *Morbidity and Mortality Weekly Report, 56* (SS01), 1–11.

Rogers, S.J., & Vismara, L.A. (2008). Evidence-based comprehensive treatments for early autism. *Journal of Clinical Child and Adolescent Psychology, 37* (1), 8–38.

Ruble, L.A., Heflinger, C.A., Renfrew, J.W., & Saunders, R.C. (2005). Access and service use by children with autism spectrum disorders in Medicaid managed care. *Journal of Autism and Developmental Disabilities, 35* (3), 3–13.

Rutter, M., Bailey, A., Lord, C., & Berument, S. (2003). *Social Communication Questionnaire (SCQ) manual*. Los Angeles, CA: Western Psychological Services.

Safran, S.P. (2008). Why youngsters with autistic spectrum disorders remain underrepresented in special education. *Remedial and Special Education, 29* (2), 90–95.

Schopler, E. (2001). Science. In E. Schopler, N. Yirmiya, C. Shulman, & L.M. Marcus (eds), *The research basis for autism intervention* (pp. 9–24). New York: Kluwer Academic/Plenum.

Schreibman, L., Stahmer, A.C., & Akshoomoff, N. (2006). Pervasive developmental disorders. In M. Hersen (ed.), *Clinician's handbook of child behavioral assessment* (pp. 503–524). Burlington, MA: Elsevier Academic Press.

Seida, J.K., Ospina, M.B., Karkhaneh, M., Hartling, L., Smith, V., & Clark, B. (2009) Systematic reviews of psychosocial interventions for autism: An umbrella review. *Developmental Medicine & Child Neurology, 51* (2), 95–104.

Shattuck, P.T., & Grosse, S.D. (2007). Issues related to the diagnosis and treatment of autism spectrum disorders. *Mental Retardation and Developmental Disabilities, 13*, 129–135.

Shattuck, P.T., Durkin, M., Maenner, M., Newschaffer, C., Mandell, D.S., Wiggins, L. et al. (2009). Timing of identification among children with an autism spectrum disorder: Findings from a population-based surveillance study. *Journal of the American Academy of Child and Adolescent Psychiatry, 48* (5), 474–483.

Smith, T., Magyar, C., & Arnold-Saritepe, A. (2002). *Autism spectrum disorder*. New York: John Wiley & Sons.

Sofronoff, K., Attwood, T., & Hinton, S. (2005). A randomized controlled trial of a CBT intervention for anxiety in children with Asperger syndrome. *Journal of Child Psychology and Psychiatry, 46* (11), 1152–1160.

Sofronoff, K., Attwood, T., Hinton, S., & Levin, I. (2007). *Journal of Autism and Developmental Disabilities, 37*, 1203–1214.

Solomon, M., Goodlin-Jones, B.L., & Anders, T.F. (2004) A social adjustment enhancement intervention for high functioning autism, Asperger's syndrome, and pervasive developmental disorder NOS. *Journal of Autism and Developmental Disorders, 34* (6), 649–668.

Southgate, V., & Hamilton, A.F. de C. (2008). Unbroken mirrors: Challenging a theory of autism. *Trends in Cognitive Sciences, 12* (6), 225–229.

Stahmer, A.C., & Mandell, D.S. (2007). State infant/toddler program policies for eligibility and services provision for young children with autism. *Administration and Policy in Mental Health and Mental Health Services Research, 34* (1), 29–37.

Steuernagel, T. (2005). Increases in identified cases of autism spectrum disorders: Policy implications. *Journal of Disability Policy Studies, 16* (3), 138–146.

Swiezy, N., Stuart, M., & Korzekwa, P. (2008). Bridging for success in autism: Training and collaboration across medical, educational, and community systems. *Child and Adolescent Psychiatric Clinics of North America, 17* (4), 907–922.

Tager-Flusberg, H., & Caronna, E. (2007). Language disorders: Autism and other pervasive developmental disorders. *Pediatric Clinics of North America, 54* (3), 469–481.

Tager-Flusberg, H., Joseph, R., & Folstein, S. (2001). Current directions on research on autism. *Mental Retardation and Developmental Disabilities Research, 7* (1), 21–29.

Towbin, K.E. (2005) Pervasive developmental disorder not otherwise specified. In F.R. Volkmar, R. Paul, A. Klin, & D. Cohen (eds), *Handbook of autism and pervasive developmental disorders. Vol. 1: Diagnosis, development, neurobiology, and behavior* (3rd ed., pp. 184–191). New York: John Wiley & Sons.

Veenstra-Vanderweele, J., & Cook, E.H. (2003). Genetics of childhood disorders: XLVI. Autism, part 5: Genetics of autism. *Journal of the Academy of Child and Adolescent Psychiatry, 42* (1), 116–119.

Volkmar, F., Lord, C., Bailey, A., Schultz, R.T., & Klin, A. (2004). Autism and pervasive developmental disorders. *Journal of Child Psychology and Psychiatry, 45* (1), 135–170.

Volkmar, F., Chwarska, K., & Klin, A. (2005). Autism in infancy and early childhood. *Annual Review of Psychology, 56*, 315–336.

Wiggins, L.D., Baio, J., & Rice, C. (2006). Examination of the time between first evaluation and first autistim spectrum disorder diagnosis in a population-based sample. *Journal of Developmental and Behavioral Pediatrics, 27* (2), 79–95.

Williams, K.J., Wray, J.J. Wheeler, D.M. (2005). Intravenous secretin for autism spectrum disorder. *Cochrane Database of Systematic Reviews*, Issue 3. Art. No.: CD003495. DOI: 10.1002/14651858.CD0 03495.pub2.

Wong, H.H.L., & Smith, R.G. (2006). Patterns of complementary and alternative medical therapy use in children diagnosed with autism spectrum disorders. *Journal of Autism and Developmental Disorders, 36* (7), 901–909.

Yeargin-Allsopp, M., Rice, C., Karapurkar, T., Doernberg, N., Boyle, C., & Murphy, C. (2003) Prevalence of autism in a U.S. metropolitan area. *Journal of the American Medical Association, 289* (1), 49–55.

13 Executive function conditions and self-deficits

Joseph Palombo

The efforts to integrate the research findings of the neurosciences into social work practice have gained increased attention in recent years. Works such as those of Applegate and Shapiro (2005), and Schore and Schore (2008) exemplify these efforts. Whereas social workers in school setting have historically been familiar with the challenges that children with learning disabilities and other neurobehavioral problems present, few efforts have been made to provide a conceptual framework for the clinical approaches involved in the treatment of these children (Palombo, 2001, 2006). Even less attention has been given to similar problems that adults confront. At the Chicago Institute for Clinical Social Work, students have generated several dissertations devoted to the study of some of these disorders (Himrod, 1995; Leamy, 2008; McNulty, 2000; Orenstein, 1992; Sclufer, 1996; Segal, 1994; Zummo, 2007). This chapter attempts to fill in the part of the gap between clinical social work practice and recent knowledge derived from the neurosciences.

In his discussion of "executive function," Goldberg (2001, p. 23) compares the frontal lobes of a human being to the CEO of a corporation or an orchestra's conductor. Its functions involve the capacity to impose order among activities, to plan future actions, and to organize the sequence in which those actions should unfold. He suggests that among the talents of those who posses good executive functions are the capacity to be "smart" and "shrewd" (p. 104).

An initial tentative definition states that executive function disorders (EFD) manifest in patients as neuropsychological impairments that reflect frontal lobe dysfunctions. Individuals with these impairments suffer from a range of constraints on their competencies and on their capacity to function; their disorganization interferes with their ability to obtain successful outcomes in the tasks they undertake. They have difficulties initiating steps to implement plans; they are unable to manage time, to organize resources, and to self-monitor and self-regulate their actions to ensure the successful completion of the task. These disruptions may lead to academic underachievement in children and adolescents and to impairments in the capacity to be successful in the pursuit of a career path in adults (Palombo, 2001, pp. 163–190).

Such patients may also display problems in social interactions that disrupt their ability to sustain intimate relationships and emotional problems that lead to self-esteem disturbances and disorders of the self. Depending on the severity of their problems, the disorders of the self may range from mild disruptions in the capacity for self-regulation to serious disorganization in the sense of self. At the emotional level a sense of bewilderment as to why things do not work out overtakes them, resulting in an erosion of their self-esteem. Symptoms of depression, substance abuse, and negativity are common in those affected.

Although many affected by this disability fail to achieve academically or to realize their career aspirations, some, through a variety of strategies, are able to become highly successful in their chosen fields. In part, this is because success or failure is directly linked to the competencies that people bring to the challenges they face. Some succeed merely because they are able to avoid tasks or situations that play into their vulnerabilities; others are able to find compensatory strategies that minimize the effects of their deficits (Anderson, Jacobs, & Anderson, 2008; Bernstein & Waber, 2007; Lyon & Krasnegor, 1996; Meltzer & Krishman, 2007).

The interest in brain function and dysfunction in the past decade has brought to our attention a number of conditions that were previously poorly understood. Among these are the non-verbal learning disabilities (Palombo, 2006), Asperger's disorders (Klin, Volkmar, & Sparrow, 2000, p. 141; Mcdonald, 2008, p. 476), autism (Baron-Cohen & Swettenham, 1997; Ozonoff & Schetter, 2007), and the developmental variant of executive function disorders (Anderson, 2008; Bernstein & Waber, 2007; Borkowski & Burke, 1996; Denckla, 1996; Eslinger, 1996; Lyon & Krasnegor, 1996; Meltzer, 2007; Palombo, 2001; Torgesen, 1994). The challenges these conditions present to psychodynamically informed practitioners are multiple. The first challenge is to establish an adequate *understanding of the effects of the neuropsychological deficits on a patients' development.* Questions arise as to which is the primary contributor to the presenting problem, the neuropsychological deficits or the effects of the environment. Granted that we accept the premise that all development results from the interaction between nature and nurture, how do we calibrate the effects of the constraints that factors related to endowment place on a person's ability to attain an optimal level of development and of functioning over those of the impact of the environment?

The second challenge is that of *formulating the psychodynamics* that structure the psyche of individuals with this disorder. The interplay between factors related to endowment and those related to the environment present a level of complexity that challenges traditional formulations. Since elements of both are intertwined, how do we differentiate whether a set of responses by the individual is the products of the neuropsychological deficits or whether they represent defensive strategies to deal with others' responses to them?

Finally, *conceptualizing the treatment process and modifying traditional modes of interventions* to make those interventions effective present a separate set of challenges. How are we to understand what constitutes transference and what is due to non-transferential factors in how the patient relates to the social worker? What is the role of interpretation in the helping of clients with these life conditions and are didactic formulations necessary adjuncts to the treatment?

Insufficient attention has been given to the psychodynamics that are at play in the symptoms of clients with executive function disorder, the primary focus having been on the nature of the cognitive impairment and its sequelae. Social workers unfamiliar with the effects of the neurobiological deficits of their clients have been at a particular disadvantage in their ability to formulate adequate assessment and diagnostic impression and, consequently, to modify their interventions to take these deficits into account. Any psychodynamic formulation must take into consideration not only the relational dimensions of their clients' experiences and the particular meaning they have assigned to their exposure to their environment but also the neuropsychological strengths and weaknesses that clients bring into the world with them. An illustrative vignette helps visualize how the disorder may appear when encountered by a clinician.

> Cory's mother described him as having been a very active toddler. At times, he would have serious tantrums. He learned the alphabet by 18 months. By age three, he liked to climb and jump off the jungle gym, taking risks and being unafraid. As a student in grade school, his teachers said he always rushed through his work. He made careless mistakes and was poorly organized. They also said he needed to show more control and not speak out so often in class. In fifth grade, Cory's teacher asked his parents to empty his desk into

a garbage bag because it was so messy and unorganized. From grade school through high school, his mother would joke that she was going to tie him to his desk. When he would go to his room to study, he would stay 10 minutes, at most. She would next find him watching TV, or teasing his brother. He seldom brought home his assignments, he would procrastinate getting to work on them; even if he completed them, he would forget to take back to school the work he had done. Cory's mother constantly had to prod him and nag him to do his schoolwork because he had very poor time management skills. In the mornings, after his mother woke him up, she frequently found him lying in bed 15 to 20 minutes later. By the time Cory was in high school, it was a daily battle to get him out of the house and to school on time. They thought he would never graduate from high school. His bedroom and bathroom were cluttered with papers, clothes, and books. At home, Cory never followed through with his chores. It seemed as if he weren't listening and some tasks would take three days of nagging and reminding before he completed them.

With the considerable support of his mother and tutors, Cory was able to place remarkably well on his SATs. He graduated from high school and even qualified for a National Merit Scholarship. A well-respected university accepted him with the anticipation that he would be able to sail smoothly through its curricular demands. However, Cory spent the first semester partying with friends, seldom attending classes, and was asked to take a leave because he was on the verge of flunking out. He came home feeling confused and utterly embarrassed at having to live at home with his parents. In short order, he fell into a significant depression.

In consultation with a clinical social worker who specializes in learning disabilities, his parents accepted a referral for neuropsychological testing, which established that Cory had an executive function disorder and also suffered from a dysthymia disorder. Upon referral for an evaluation, the psychiatrist placed him on an antidepressant. Cory also accepted a recommendation for twice-a-week therapy.

Historically, the association between damage to the frontal lobes and the consequent personality changes that occur was first demonstrated in the famous case of Phineas Gage in the mid-1800s. Gage was a railroad worker who survived an accidental explosion that resulted in a metal rod penetrating his lower left cheek and exiting through his skull. This resulted in damage to his left and partly his right frontal cortical regions (Damasio, 1994, pp. 3–51). The injury left Gage with reasonably intact cognitive faculties but had a devastating effect on his personality. He changed from a valued leader of his crew to an impulsive, argumentative, erratic worker, who was no longer able to perform his job. In time, cases such as those of Gage helped establish an association between frontal lobe lesions and poor performance in the execution of life skills that we now identify as executive function disorders.

Between the 1930s and 1950s, neurologists performed lobotomies to "alleviate the symptoms of some mental disorders" (Solms & Turnbull, 2002, pp. 203–205). The procedure involved the random destruction of prefrontal cortical tissue. This left the person without the anxieties and psychotic symptoms from which they previously suffered but resulted in dramatic changes in the patients' personalities, displaying blunted affect and became zombie-like shadows of their former selves (see El-Hai, 2005; Gazzaniga, Ivry, & Mangun, 2002, pp. 122–123). Milos Forman's (1975) movie version of Ken Kesey's book (1962) *One flew over the cuckoo's nest* dramatically illustrated the devastatingly deleterious effects of the procedure. These procedures provided further confirmation of the association between damage to the frontal regions of the brain and serious personality changes.

In his informative book *The executive brain: Frontal lobes and the civilized mind*, Goldberg (2001) states: "Frontal lobe dysfunction is to brain disease what fever is to bacterial infection" (p. 115). Executive function difficulties are ubiquitous among many conditions, such as Parkinsonism (De Luca & Leventer, 2008, p. 41), Traumatic Brain Injury (Baddeley & Wilson, 1988), and psychiatric disorders such as schizophrenia (De Luca & Leventer, 2008, p. 41). Drug dependence and Obsessive Compulsive Disorder (Green & Ostrander, 2009) may also disrupt executive function capacities. The neuropsychological deficits and psychosocial disturbances from which persons with these conditions suffer are not unlike those with the *developmental variant* of the disorder, who manifest no evidence of brain damage and who do not suffer from a major psychiatric condition, except possibly for ADHD, which is often a comorbid condition (Barkley, 1990, 1996, 1998). In this chapter, the focus is on individuals with the *developmental variant of the disorder of executive function disorders* (Bernstein & Waber, 2007; Harris, 1998, p. 43).

In spite of the apparent correlation between frontal lobe lesions and symptoms of personality changes, current views of brain function caution against attempts to localize specific psychological functions within specific regions of the brain. Whereas in the early days of the history of neurology, localization of the effect of brain damage yielded insights into the relationship between brain dysfunctions and behavioral manifestations, such a modular approach is now brought into question. Neuropsychologists now follow Luria's, the Soviet neuropsychologist's path in viewing a more complex picture (Luria 1973, 1979). Taking issue with localization theories, he proposed three functional interacting units as organizing brain activity: *the unit for regulating arousal, waking, and mental states; the unit for receiving, analyzing, and storing information*; and *the unit for programming, regulation, and verification of activities* (Luria, 1973, p. 43). The last of these is associated with executive function capacities. Luria led the way to conceptualizing brain functions in holistic terms rather than a set of isolated systems that have little impact on one another other. Multiple regions of the brain undergird any specific psychological function. Consequently, it is inaccurate to attempt to establish a direct correlation between executive function disorders and frontal lobe dysfunctions.

In summary, whereas historically executive function disorders were correlated with specific impairments of the frontal lobe, this view proved to be simplistic and imprecise. The brain systems that undergird the psychological functions associated with executive functions turned out to be much more broadly distributed. The personality changes that accompanied brain injuries or lesions present challenges to those who seek a psychodynamic understanding of the psychological makeup of these patients. Furthermore, the recognition that some children and adolescents for whom no evidence of actual brain damage existed but who displayed behavioral symptoms similar to those who had known brain lesions, led to the hypothesis of the existence of a developmental variant to the disorder. Answering those challenges requires a closer examination of the definitions that neuropsychologists propose and an exploration of their limitations.

Definitions of executive function disorders

Executive function disorders (EFD) of developmental origins are defined as learning disorders found in individuals of at least average intelligence, whose neuropsychological deficits are due to genetic, heritable, or environmental disruption in brain function. These deficits must be *unrelated* to brain dysfunctions caused by lesions, head injuries, or other physical impairments (Coplin & Morgan, 1988, p. 614). The dysfunctions interfere with the person's capacity to perform satisfactorily in one or more of the social, academic, occupational, or emotional domains. Learning disabilities are a subcategory of learning disorders. Educators, educational psychologists, and neuropsychologists use the term learning disabilities in their assessments of children eligible for school special education services. Executive function disorders are not officially designated as learning disabilities, consequently children with the condition are not eligible for the school services that are mandated under federal legislation, but may receive accommodations because of the related attentional problems that often coexist with the condition (Cohen, 2009; Ellenberg, 1999).

From a neuropsychological perspective Lezak (1983, Ch. 16; Lezak, Howieson, & Loring, 2004, Ch. 16) describes four behavioral components of executive function: goal formulation, planning, carrying out goal-directed plans, and effective performance. Individuals with executive function problems may have difficulties in one or more of these areas. Goal formulation involves the capacity to conceptualize a plan and the ability to initiate steps to implementing it. Procrastination is probably the most prominent symptom of the failure in this capacity. Planning involves the ability to select and bring to bear a number of resources such as materials and skills that will be necessary to implement the plan. It involves drawing upon a pool of knowledge as well as envisioning the actual steps or obstacles that may lie ahead for the successful completion of the task. Carrying out the activities, or implementing the plan, involves the translation of the conceptual scheme into a set of behaviors or actions. Effective performance requires the person to inhibit responses to distractions so that tangential factors do not interfere with the attainment of the goal. Furthermore, it requires the resourcefulness and flexibility to find alternative paths to the goal if obstacles are met. Self-monitoring and self-regulation are important psychological functions necessary to stay focused on the task.

From an educational perspective, disorganization has frequently been considered a hallmark of EFD. Levine (1994, pp. 138–141) describes four types of persistent organizational failures in school-age children:

1   Material-spatial disorganization, which prevents children from dealing effectively with the equipment needed to be efficient in school. This occurs in such behaviors as losing personal possessions, creating messes among belongings; and not bringing home or returning assignments in a timely way.
2   Temporal-sequential disorganization, in which children display confusion about time and the sequencing of tasks, such as being late, procrastinating; having trouble allocating time, estimating how long a task will take to complete, or knowing the order of steps needed to complete a task.
3   Transitional disorganization, which involves difficulty shifting gears smoothly, and results in rushing from one activity to the next, having difficulty settling down to work, or being slow in preparing to leave home for school in the mornings.
4   Prospective retrieval disorganization, which involves the inability to remember to do something that had been planned in advance, such as forgetting the deadline of a project until the night before, failing to follow through with a promise to finish a task. Adolescents and adults are subject to similar difficulties.

Finally, the condition is not included in the *Diagnostic and statistical manual of mental disorders-IV* (American Psychiatric Association (APA), 1994).

From a neuropsychological perspective, Anderson (2008) states: "While a number of conceptual models of executive function have been proposed no model has been uniformly accepted" (p. 6). In what follows, I briefly summarize two of the major models proposed by investigators of the disorder.

Denckla (1994, 1996, 2007) presents a compelling argument for the relationship between executive function disorders and brain dysfunction. She presents data from neurology that indicates that patients with damage to the prefrontal cortex and its interconnected subcortical regions manifest many of the symptoms associated with executive function disorders. She suggests that executive function disorders are a domain-general impairment as contrasted with the modular or domain-specific impairments, such as dyslexia. By this she means that while researchers hypothesize a direct association between a set of symptoms and a dysfunction in a specific brain system, as in specific learning disabilities, such a direct relationship is too simplistic for our understanding of executive function disorders. The functions subsumed under executive function are broad and probably widely distributed, that is they involve a number of brain systems. Bernstein and Waber (2007) state:

> Developmental abilities and disabilities, therefore, are likely to reflect processes associated with the construction, integration, and the definition of functional networks, rather than the functions of specific brain regions. . . . It follows from this more systemic view that behavioral manifestations of executive functions can reflect the multiplicity of underlying factors that can influence the effectiveness and integrity of the network on which the task execution depends rather than the integrity of the specific region or regions, as a more modular approach would suggest.
>
> (Bernstein & Waber, 2007, p. 45)

Emerging agreement exists among researchers that an overlap exists between the executive function capacities and attentional abilities. Barkley (1996), who is a major advocate for this position, presents a hybrid model that incorporates both sets of functions. This hybrid model combines behavioral inhibition and four separable executive functions: non-verbal working memory; verbal working memory or the internalization of speech; self-regulation of affect, which includes regulation of arousal and motivation; and reconstitution, which includes the analysis and synthesis of the meanings of behaviors. This model of human self-regulation specifies that behavioral inhibition is critical to the proficient performance of executive functions. Behavioral inhibition refers to individuals' ability to inhibit responding to a stimulus. This implies that disorders of attention and executive function are closely intertwined; working memory is one of the most important components of the executive function system (Reader, Harris, Schuerholz, & Denckla, 1994; Sergeant, Geurts, & Oosterlaan, 2002).

Working memory is the term currently used to describe what was formerly classified under short-term memory (Torgesen, 1994). It is a frontal lobe function that has three component parts: a *visual-spatial sketchpad*, a *phonological loop*, and a *central executive* (Anderson, 2008, p. 10). As a short-term perceptual register that retains immediate visual and auditory stimuli, it makes that information available for manipulation and processing by the central executive. The *visual-spatial sketchpad* is the memory store (i.e., buffer) that retains the color and shape of objects or the spatial configuration of one's environment; such as the color of the wall of a room, its dimension and the placement of its contents. Whereas the *phonological loop* retains brief segments of auditory stimuli, such as spoken sentences, musical phrases, or other sounds. The schemas associated with these perceptual stimuli become available for processing by the central executive, which makes use of them to accomplish the immediate task. The *central executive* also has a retrieval function in that it may draw from long-term memory to sequence and organize the information necessary for the person's use. The critical role of working memory in the capacity for executive function becomes evident when we understand that it serves as locus for most cognitive and emotional activities and is a critical component of executive function abilities (Baddeley, 1996; Pennington, Bennetto, McAleer, & Roberts,

1996; Smith & Jonides, 1999; Torgesen, 1994, 1996; Wagner, Bunge, & Badre, 2004; Wong, 1984).

These definitions and explanatory paradigms highlight three central issues that require the attention of psychodynamically informed practitioners. First, by locating the disorder within the individual, they discount the view that, as with all organisms, human beings are the products of their endowments in interaction with the environment. Second, the definitions treat executive function disorders as related to deficits in cognition ignoring the widely held belief among researchers nowadays that cognition and emotions are indissolubly linked together. Third, the definitions leave little room for the psychodynamic elements of motivation as a contributor to the symptoms the patients display.

With regard to the interaction between endowment and the environment, two intertwined facets of this issue require consideration. First, few nowadays question the proposition that our brains require the stimulation of the environment in order to mature. Schore (2000, 2003, 2005a, 2005b) has amply documented in his work on attachment that infants require the timely responses of their caregivers for their orbito-frontal regions to acquire the capacity to regulate their emotional states. Those interactions contribute to the brain's maturation and enhance the capacities for self-regulation, which is an essential component of executive function (Beebe & Lachmann, 1988, 1997; Beebe, Rustin, Sorter, & Knoblauch, 2005a; Beebe, Sorter, Rustin, & Knoblauch, 2005b; Fonagy, 2005; Fonagy & Target, 1998, 2002; Fonagy, Gergely, Jurist, & Target, 2002). As Bernstein and Waber (2007) state: "Executive capacities may be thought of as the interface between the child and the social and physical world within which he or she interacts" (p. 46).

The second facet has been the subject of extensive debate in the psychoanalytic literature, the issue center around two views of psychological development, the so-called "isolated mind" view and the two-person psychology perspective (Leighton, 2004, pp. 169–170; Stolorow, 1992, pp. 7–28). One side of the controversy accuses the other of ignoring our interdependence and conceiving of the psyche as simply the product of its own internal processes. The other side responds by claiming that their opponents distort their perspective since their concern is with the factors that shape a person's internal psychodynamics. The controversy appears to conflate the perspective from which one views people's psyche with the undeniable contention that, as human beings, we are interdependent. Our interdependence is a central tenet of the position that I propose in this chapter, yet there is no denying that we can articulate the processes that are at work within individuals to account for issues such as the sense of agency, the motivations that drive development, and the affect states that accompany their subjective experience. I believe the two views complement one another rather than being antagonistic to each other (Gedo, 2005, pp. 127).

Second, the definitions of executive function also neglect the significance of *emotional factors* in the lives of individuals with the dysfunction. The neurologist, Damasio (1994) was among the first to examine the effects of brain lesions on a person's emotional life. He proposed that reason and feelings are closely enmeshed. Human reason depends on several brain systems, working in concert across many levels of neuronal organization, rather than on a single brain center. Both "high-level" and "low-level" brain centers cooperate in the making of reason. Cognitive functions, such as those involved in executive functions, are not dissociable from feelings. In his work, he details the emotional blunting that often accompanies brain lesions. By proposing the "somatic marker hypothesis," which describes how our body's responses reflect our cognitive states, he concludes that the division between cognition and emotion is an artifact of academic studies. There is now general agreement that we are "embodied" beings for whom mind and brain are indivisible from one another (Barrett & Lindquist, 2008; Klin & Jones, 2007; Semin & Cacioppo, 2008). However, the integration of these innovative views of the neurobiological underpinnings of emotions with a psychodynamic perspective remains a work in progress.

Some neuropsychologists differentiate "cold" cognition, which does not involve affect states from "hot" cognition that does include an affective dimension. With regard to executive function, De Luca and Leventer (2008) state:

> The term "cold" executive abilities generally refers to strategic planning, organization, goal setting, behavior monitoring, problem solving, inhibition, working memory, and cognitive flexibility. The term "hot" executive ability has been applied to empathy, theory of mind, emotional regulation, and affective decision-making.
>
> (De Luca & Leventer, 2008, p. 23)

Finally, the definitions do not give sufficient importance to the *role of motivation* in the lives of these individuals. At the emotional level, individuals with EFD had often been exposed to considerable criticism. Whereas others often perceived them as bright and competent, some found it difficult to understand why they had so much trouble with the simple tasks that others perform with ease. They were berated for being lazy, not trying hard enough, or simply for being defiant of others' directions and expectations. These criticisms led them to feel considerable resentment of others. They felt misunderstood and devalued. These experiences led to the deflection of course of their development from its path. Some internalized the criticism and lost motivation to try to do better. The loss of motivation compounded the problem, as it reinforced others' negative perception of them. Some veered away from the social expectations and values common to their peers. They devalued their community's lifestyle, their career paths, and their moral standards; they embraced an anti-establishment lifestyle, which they found to be more in conformity with their own limitations and the image of themselves as not fitting in. Once again, the integration of this psychodynamic perspective with the neuropsychological data presents further challenges to practitioners (Palombo, 2001).

The *Psychodynamic diagnostic manual* (PDM Task Force, 2006), under Disorders of Mental Functions in children and adolescents, SCA317.5 Executive Function Disorders, provides a more comprehensive definition than those cited above. It can serve as the basis for a psychodynamic perspective. It states:

> Executive function disorders involve a complex set of deficits that include difficulties in the initiation, conception, and implementation of a plan. These difficulties include the inability to manage time, organize resources, self-monitor, and self-regulate so as to translate a plan into productive activity that insures its completion. Generally, children with these disorders know what they have to do but cannot take the initiative or implement their knowledge. Academically, the child underachieves because homework assignments are lost or not turned in. The child has poor study skills, procrastinates, is inefficient in doing class assignments, and is scattered and disorganized. No distinctive emotional problems are associated with this disorder, although a pattern emerges of not being able to keep life occurrences straight and in order. Children with problematic executive function generally achieve developmental milestones on schedule. Problems do not begin to emerge until demands are made of them to undertake tasks whose complexity is greater than their capabilities. Because these demands increase with maturation, they encounter greater difficulties over time. As they get closer to young adulthood, they are generally ineffectual in adapting to social and life situations, perhaps reflecting an inadequacy of psychic structure. No single pattern of affect, thought, somatic state, or relationship characterizes the executive function disorders.
>
> (PDM Task Force, 2006, p. 272)

This definition implies that, whereas all patients with EFD have a range of neuropsychological deficits, the responses to those deficits by those in their environment as well as the individual's emotional responses to those responses and the meanings that they construe from those responses vary enormously. Consequently, no single set of psychodynamics or disorders of the self are associated with the neuropsychological deficits.

These considerations lead to the conclusion that the integration of a neuropsychological perspective with a psychodynamic perspective requires a new clinical model. I call this model the *neuropsychodynamic model*. This model proposes going beyond the use of the constructs of one theory and redefining them in terms applicable to the other. It entails the creation of a new terminology that can encompass neuropsychological, neurological, and psychological phenomena. In what follows, I outline some of the main concepts that inform this model as it applies to issues related to individuals with EFD.

Demographics

No data are available on prevalence rates of these disorders in children or adults. Neither are there any data as to the sex ratio among males and females (Palombo, 2001).

Population

The brain's developmental trajectory sets the course for the maturation of executive function abilities. As previously stated, cognitive psychologists distinguish between two interrelated components those of "cold" cognition that involve the tasks of plan formulation, initiation of activities related to the achievement of a goal, and self-monitory, the process made toward that goal. "Hot" cognition, on the other hand, includes the capacity for empathy, and emotional regulation. De Luca and Leventer (2008) describe developmental stages of these two components. The brief summary that follows is largely based on their chapter.

The maturation of the frontal regions of the brain that are associated with executive function capacities is progressive and continuous into early adulthood – around the third decade of life. The normal aging process brings with it a decline in those capacities. Environmental factors may influence positively or negatively this trajectory, although its bell shaped configuration of increasing and decreasing function remains stable.

Evidence suggests that by the age of two, most neurotypically developing children develop a greater capacity to control their responses and a more sophisticated understanding of others' mental states. Adolescence is a period of major brain reorganization with synaptic and neuronal pruning that impacts executive function abilities directly. In spite of the turmoil associated with this period, adolescents make gains in the areas of working memory, and the ability to plan and problem solve.

By the mid to late twenties, executive function abilities reach their peak when they plateau, before beginning a slow decline that becomes evident by the mid sixties, when the speed at which information is processed decreases, attentional capacities decline, working memory is less reliable than previously, and the capacity for self-monitoring is reduced. These changes may affect selective areas of executive function and may vary from individual to individual, with some retaining greater capacities than others.

There are no comparable data for individuals with deficits in the developmental variant of executive function discussed above. Clinical evidence, based on over 45 years of experience with children, adolescents, and adults, presents a mixed picture. From informal follow-up obtained from the parents of children and adolescents I have seen in psychotherapy, I have reports of remarkable changes in patients with significant executive function disorders identified in childhood and adolescents. To my surprise, the reports indicate that in some of my former patients major positive shifts in functioning occurred towards the end of their junior years in high school or later during their sophomore years in college. A few have gone on to obtain degrees in law or higher education, with comparable achievements in their careers. However, in general, the detrimental effects of EFD that were evident earlier became magnified by the increased demands that adulthood imposes, leading some of my former patients to become totally reliant on their parents for their support and making marginal and spasmodic social adjustments themselves.

Mental health care disparities

Given the absence of data, it is not possible to give an accurate account of the mental health care disparities for the provision of services to individuals with executive function disorders. The following comments are impressionistic based on my clinical experience.

School social workers have traditionally been in the forefront of professionals that provide services for students in schools. There is general agreement that these services vary greatly from district to district across the nation depending on the affluence of the population in those districts. Furthermore, given that EFD are not on the list of learning disabilities or other mental health impairments for which services are mandated, this disorder is seldom identified and no provisions exist for its remediation in those children affected by it. However, since some of these children also suffer from ADHD, which is considered a mental health impairment for which schools must provide accommodations, these children may receive indirectly some services for the condition. This situation is complicated by the fact that the symptoms that children with EFD manifest are often falsely interpreted as being motivated by lack of discipline, poor parenting, or laziness. The children are then found to have behavior problems and sometimes labeled "Oppositional/Defiant" because they fail to comply with expectations. Such labels fail to address the children's problems and compound the difficulties that the service providers face.

Some isolated affluent communities nationally have schools with resources that permit their social workers to attend seminars that inform them of trends and have brought to their awareness the nature of this condition. However, strategies for its remediation are still evolving and their application produce mixed results. In some of those communities, some private practitioners and tutors have developed special techniques to help these students. However, the cost must be borne by the families as no insurance coverage exists for these types of interventions. One center, with which I have been associated for some years, is unique in the United States. It is the Rush Neurobehavioral Center, which is part of a large medical center in the metropolitan Chicago area. It has a department that provides diagnostic and tutorial services to meet the needs of children under 18 years of age, but it charges fees and does not accept insurance reimbursement.

The situation for adults with the disorder is even direr, as few are diagnosed. When assessment is available by a neuropsychologist, the cost generally exceeds $3,000. Furthermore, the availability of services is even more limited than for children and the cost must be carried by the affected individual.

Social work programs and social work roles

As the comments in the prior section indicate, to my knowledge, specific social work programs are nonexistent in spite of the fact that school social workers as well as clinical social worker have a large role to play in the provision of services to this population. What is required is those school social workers begin to advocate for the inclusion of this disorder under the category of

"Other Mental Health Impairments" by the U.S. Department of Education. This would trigger processes that would permit referral for testing of children with the condition and mandate schools to provide both accommodations and remediation to affected students.

As for the role of social work in services for adults, a campaign to publicize the condition and its deleterious effects on the function of those affected should be followed by seminars and programs that educate clinicians to recognize the disorder and to make adequate referral for services.

Professional methods and interventions

The *neuropsychodynamic model* flows out of an evolutionary perspective. It proposes that we are born pre-adapted to survive in our environments. All development results from the interaction between our environment and ourselves. Our brains require exposure to external stimuli in order to grow and function. Both endowment and the environment impose constraints on the extent to which we can develop and mature. Innate differences may limit the extent to which we are able to achieve in our environment and, in turn, the unavailability of resources in our environment may impose limitations on how we mature. Furthermore, our social interactions as well as our emotional communication with others shape our relationships to others. The attachment system brings with it a configuration of secure or insecure bonds to others that we carry with us for a lifetime. A set of patterns of interactions is laid down during development that act as organizers of experience and become predictors of how we expect others to respond to us. These patterns are the product of our unique givens, our experiences within the social system in which we mature, and the unique set of meanings that results from our interpretation of events in our lives.

We are also imperfect beings who require others to sustain us. We search for involvements that will give meaning to our experiences. Our greatest anxiety is the fear of isolation and disconnection from those who are significant to us. The failure to find meaning in our lives leads to despondency and despair. In brief, we live in a world in which we are interdependent and interconnected with one another. What we do or how we act can have consequences that extend far beyond the reach of our imaginations. This view is in contrast to prior views of development that proposed the idea of mature development as consisting of the achievement of separation and individuation. This is not to deny that each of us has his/her own individuality and distinctive personality. We each possess a unique history, a sense of agency, and a capacity to make choices. The concept of being separate from others as an end-point of mature development that Mahler's (1975) developmental framework proposes reflects the frontier mentality and values of prior times when rugged individualism was tied to the idea of self-sufficiency and freed them from reliance on others. Whether the ideal is now outdated or whether it provided an inaccurate vision of human nature might be a matter of debate. What seems undeniable at this time is that our survival as a species is contingent upon assuring the survival of all of our conspecifics.

In what follows, I highlight these two themes of *imperfection* and *interdependence*. I conceptualized our imperfections as self-deficits that interfere with our capacity for self-cohesion. I expand the traditional view of self-deficits as resulting from factors related to nurture to include those that are related to nature, i.e., our endowment. As for our interdependence, it manifests in the psychological functions that we provide each other by filling in the functions that are absent because of our self-deficits, thus complementing each other's sense of self. I refer to *the sense of self* as *the experience of being a self*. I will refer to these as the *complementary functions* that we provide each other. These constructs will provide a bridge between the neuropsychological and the psychodynamic framework, which is central to the neuropsychodynamic model (Kaplan-Solms & Solms, 2002).

The proposal to extend the *concept of self-deficits* originated from my work with children with learning disorders and my familiarity with self-psychology. For self-psychology, deficits result from a developmental failure. Such deficits results from the repeated frustrations associated with an environment that persons experienced as unresponsive to their needs. The deficits denote the absence of the development of a psychological structure. Evidence for the absence of psychic structure appears in the anxiety associated with inability to sustain an integrated sense of self and the manifestation of a desire for the requisite selfobject functions. Selfobject functions are psychological functions that others provide, which are eventually internalized. A pattern ensues that structures situations and provides motives for interactions with others (Kohut, 1971, 1977, 1984; Palombo, 2008b).

This formulation raises the question of the existence of a parallel between neuropsychological deficits and selfobject deficits. We may conceptualize the symptoms that emerge in individuals with executive function disorders also as reflective of deficits in their sense of self. These individuals suffered from failure in the recognition of their need for the missing cognitive functions in a fashion similar to the failures for responses to their selfobject functions needs. Phenomenologically, the effects of both types of deficits on a person's development are categorically the same. Whether we deal with narcissistic personality disorders who suffer from selfobject deficits, or patients with insecure attachments who have not internalized the capacity for self-regulation (Schore, 2001a, 2001b, 2005a), or patients with learning disorders whose neuropsychological deficits interfere with their functioning (Palombo, 1985b, 1987, 1991, 1993, 1995), the sequellae are often associated with disorders of the self. These individuals' sense of self may be either threatened or become unstable.

Elsewhere, I proposed that the process through which complementarity is achieved is what I have called mindsharing. *Mindsharing is a form of intersubjectivity in which one person understands the mental state of another and/or provides psychological functions that complement another's psychological functions. At times, this complementarity is essential to the maintenance of an integrated sense of self. The interchanges between dyads may be reciprocal* (Palombo, 2008a). We distinguish between two senses of the term mindsharing. In one sense of the term, we speak of mindsharing as the set of phenomena in which one person is capable of *understanding what is on another person's mind or his or her mental state*. Examples of this sense of the term are the capacity for empathy, in which one person may apprehend what another person thinks. The second sense of mindsharing is as we have seen that complementary functions are those that I have identified and self-deficits, i.e., neuropsychological deficits, deficits in the capacity for self-regulation, and selfobject deficits (Palombo, 2006).

From an evolutionary perspective, Bowlby (1969) states:

> [B]ecause . . . the survival of populations of higher species is dependent on the co-operation of individuals, much of the equipment of one individual is *complementary to that of another* of different age or sex in the same population. Behaviour patterns mediating attachment of young to adults are *complementary to those mediating care of young by adults*.
>
> (Bowlby, 1969, p. 141, italics added)

The responses from those in the person's context may either heighten or mitigate the effects of a self-deficit. In line with the premise that our connection to others is essential to our survival, the relationship between our psychological strengths and weaknesses and the extent to which we provide supports to others or obtain support from others becomes a critical factor in our ability to maintain a sense of self-cohesion. We can conceptualize that relationship as one of complementarity with those to whom we provide and those from whom we borrow function (Palombo, 2001).

It now becomes possible to carry over the concepts of deficits and complementary to the development of an approach to the treatment of patients with executive function disorders; keeping in mind the three types of deficits, the neuropsychological, the self-regulatory, and the emotional as well as the need for complementarity that patients bring to the clinical setting. The patients' transferences will reflect these psychodynamics. We can conceive of treatment process as a process that involves a measure of mindsharing that includes an empathic understanding of patients' experience of their deficits and a response that addresses those deficits.

In some ways, the processes involved in the neuropsychodynamic model of individual psychotherapy are no different from traditional psychodynamic approaches to psychotherapy; in other ways, as we will see; the model offers strategies that depart from traditional modes of responding to patients. With regard to its similarity to traditional approaches, it consists in understanding patients and explaining their psychodynamics. Patients replicate in the transference the thwarted desires to have their deficits complemented by others. They also re-enact the defenses they have habitually used to deal with the pain of not having their desires satisfied. The differences between the two approaches consist in the explanations that patients require and in the interventions that are necessary to deal with the neuropsychological deficits. These deficits do not represent developmental arrests that the process will repair. As we will see, those deficits require different strategies for patients to benefit from the process.

I conceptualize the treatment process of patients with neuropsychological deficits as a series of moments. Moments in therapy are organizing events that capture the essence of the issues with which the patient is struggling at a given time during the process. These moments do not necessarily arrive sequentially but occur episodically. Moments are activated when specific types of exchanges between the therapist and patient are in the foreground of the interaction. By foreground I mean periods during which the ebb and flow of the process is focused on a set of patterns that emerge in the transference. Such moments activate mindsharing responses on the part of the therapist, that is, they evoke empathy or the desire to complement the patient's deficits. I conceptualize three types of moments, *concordant moments, complementary moments*, and *disjunctive moments* (Racker, 1968, 1972). We can now turn to a more detailed description of the treatment process itself.

Concordant moments are moments during which maintaining empathic contact with the patient's experience is in the foreground of the process. This part of the process involves attempts by therapists to understand their patients. During such moments, therapists become attuned to patients' experiences and their meaning. The therapist can then catch a glimpse of the ways the patient experiences and organizes his or her perceptions. However, fully understanding and empathizing with patients with EFD requires that we go beyond what they can tell us (Gedo, 2005, p. 17). Patients with brain-based deficits, in particularly, require that we digest information included in psychological or neuropsychological reports, reports from speech and language pathologists, occupational therapists, school personnel. Information about the family's dynamics, the patient's relationship with siblings and peers, and other relevant data may enhance our view of the factors that contributed to the patient's self-state. The notion that we can rely exclusively on patients' reports in order to understand them seriously under-estimates the importance of these other sources of information. True empathic understanding cannot be achieved in many cases in the absence of such information. In fact, a danger exists of seriously misunderstanding both the patients' self-state and the motives for their thoughts and behaviors in the absence of such information. Consequently, if some of this information is not available, it is necessary to supplement the history we obtain from patients with a referral for a full neuropsychological evaluation. The completion of an accurate diagnostic assessment can occur only after obtaining a full accounting of the patients' neuropsychological strengths and weakness.

A factor that frequently confounds therapists' understanding of these patients' symptoms is the basic psychoanalytic premise that all thoughts and behaviors are motivated. From a psychodynamic perspective, it may be true that all behaviors or symptoms have reasons that may explain their occurrence. Yet, from a neuropsychological perspective, it is difficult to extend this principle to behaviors that manifest underlying brain-based deficits. In the case of patients with EFD, it is difficult for therapists to attribute motives, particularly unconscious motives, to the manifestation of some of these impairments, as it leads to a misunderstanding of the patient's mental states. These are no more "motivated" than are the expressive language difficulties of patients who suffer aphasia because of a stroke in Broca's area. We cannot say that such patients resist talking to us. The thoughts, feelings, and behaviors of patients with such deficits must be understood differently. They display symptoms that directly or indirectly relate to an underlying impairment. Much like the person with aphasia who cannot speak, these patients evoke in therapists a desire to complement their deficits to help them restore the ability to communicate. The fact that they are unaware of precisely what their needs are does not indicate that they have lost their desire for the function, it is simply that they may have no conscious awareness of what it is that they lack.

Two corollaries follow from this formulation. First, the absence of an awareness of the deficit does not mean that patients have not attached meanings to the manifestations of the deficits, that is, patients provide therapists with what they believe to be the *reasons* for their thoughts and behaviors. Those meanings may or may not have something to do with the impairment itself. As Gazzaniga (1988) states:

> Our interpretative mind is always attributing a cause to felt states of mind, and we now know that these interpretations are frequently irrelevant to the true underlying causes of a felt state. Our mind's explanations become more relevant only as we come to believe our own theories about the cause of a state like anxiety.
>
> (Gazzaniga, 1988, p. 98)

Some patients may believe that they are inept, or may attribute their difficulties to the injustices perpetrated by others, or may attribute difficulties to a number of seemingly rational, inaccurate explanations of objective reality. These meanings become a rich source of exploration during the therapeutic process. However, understanding the meanings helps only to clarify the nature of the deficit, it does not correct it. Understanding and interpretations cannot reverse the brain dysfunction or repair those kinds of self-deficits. As we will see, other intervention will be necessary to circumvent the sequelae of those deficits.

The second corollary is associated with the defenses that patients institute to deal with the sequelae of their deficits. Patients with EFD may have experienced directly or indirectly its effects. Their failures loom large on their horizon. They had felt criticized for their deficits and had frequently been injured by what they felt was unjustified disapproval. They instituted a variety of defenses in the service of avoiding these injuries and protecting themselves for the anxieties that overshadow their lives. They may have suppressed or disavowed the effects of the deficits as a defense against the pain caused by others' responses to them. These defensive styles may become habitual patterns of interaction. It is often necessary to undo the effects of these defenses before patients can move on to develop compensatory functions.

In summary, understanding these patients involves more than simply empathizing with their self-state. Therapists must go beyond those patients' experiences to the underlying factors to appreciate fully the motives behind the overt thoughts and behaviors. Patients are often unaware of their neuropsychological deficits not necessarily because they are dynamically repressed, but rather because they are descriptively unconscious. In their struggles to understand their responses, they attach meanings that are unrelated to the causes of their feelings, thoughts, and behaviors. Furthermore, they institute defenses to deal with the frequent injuries they sustain.

Complementary moments are episodes that occur when the transference occupies the foreground of the interaction. Patients re-enact the needs for complementarity associated with their deficits within the transference. In other words, complementary moments represent episodes during which patients' deficits, whether neuropsychological, self-regulatory, or of selfobject functions become activated and the patient expects the therapist to respond by providing those functions. These are moments when positive or negative transference issues gain ascendancy. During these moments, sorting the patterns that drive the transference from those that simply reflect the EFD may be difficult. Applying our understanding of brain function in the clinical setting requires a reconsideration of our views regarding what constitutes transference and non-transference. Therapists who treat patients with EFD problems find it difficult to distinguish between a patient's responses based on transference and those based on the patients' search for complementary responses to their neuropsychological deficits. While sharp differentiations are difficult to make, some distinctions are possible which would help therapists in making interventions.

These moments offer therapists the opportunity to provide interpretations or explanations to patients of their psychodynamics. Interpretations in this model provide explanations of the psychodynamics associated with the deficits and of the nature of the deficits themselves. Through the process, patients reformulate the meanings they construed from the sequelae of their deficits and rework the associated idiosyncratic views of themselves. They had interpreted their responses and others' responses to them from a particular vantage point that was often critical and negative, filtered through the lens of their deficits. These interpretations and explanations are no different from the traditional forms of interpretation, which involve dealing with the psychodynamics associated with the deficit, that is, to the patterns that have crystallized because of the deficit. They may relate to the erosion in self-esteem that may have occurred, the fantasies surrounding the meaning associated with the effects of the deficits, the effects of the patients' responses to others and others' responses to patients' that led to relational difficulties, and the impact on the sense of self and self-cohesion. These take the form of mutative interpretations.

Clients require a different type of explanation for them to understand the nature of their self-regulatory difficulties, or neuropsychological dysfunctions. These explanations involve the non-conscious functions of the patients' minds. Patients need to understand the ways in which their brains process their experiences. However, these explanations alone do not lead to the internalization of the function or to development of the missing capacity that is due to the neuropsychological deficit. Since such explanations alone cannot heal the neuropsychological deficits, other interventions are indicated.

At this juncture, interventions depart from traditional modes. Therapists may find it necessary to complement the patient's social and cognitive deficits by providing the client with missing functions related to the deficits. Whereas traditional technique frowns upon supplying such "provisions" because it gratifies the client's desires and is thought not to produce growth, in cases of EFD, depriving patients of such interventions would represent failures in empathy that may give rise to negative transferences. Much as some patients need medication to help restore their neurochemical imbalances, these patients require activities that help remediate the deficit.

In order to give up old habits or patterns of behavior and acquire new ones, patients must undertake a particular form of learning to modify their responses to the circumstances they confront; the new learning involves facilitating the transfer of knowledge from episodic memory to procedural memory (Gedo, 2005, pp. 152–155). In essence, what is involved is having clients use conscious information, present in episodic memory, to develop new procedures to guide their conduct and using that information to develop new habitual patterns, which are then stored in procedural memory. The techniques for the attainment of this goal may involve didactic methods that include direct instruction and rehearsal of ways of approaching and solving individual life stressors and problems.

Such clients require instruction so that they may compensate for the deficit. They may require actual modeling of the function or even provision of that function. These interventions are not necessarily "curative" in that the insight does not lead to a repair of the deficit. The explanations open the possibility that they will acquire more effective ways of having others complement the missing functions or that they will develop compensatory structures that bypass the effects of the deficits. At times, a client may develop compensatory structures either spontaneously or through the process, nevertheless some deficits may remain as lifelong impairments; such persons require mindsharing functions for the rest of their lives.

When offered, both the emotional supports and the complementary functions are best provided in the *zone of proximal development* (Vygotsky, 1986, p. 187). This term, used in developmental psychology, refers to a type of scaffolding that others provide to permit the patient to exercise available functions. This term may translate into Tolpin's concept of the "forward edge," although it comes from a different theoretical framework (Tolpin, 2002, 2007). As stated earlier, the dilemma that confronts caregivers of patients with these deficits is how much to do for them and how much to let them struggle to do for themselves, when to praise and when to withhold praise. If too much is done for them, they will be prevented from exerting any effort to do for themselves. They may also regress and develop an inordinate reliance on others. If too little is done, they may become frustrated, fail at a task, give up trying, and lose motivation. Staying within the zone of proximal development means meeting them half way and challenging them even as they are supported to avoid failure. By using this approach, social workers can avoid having clients become overly dependent or failing to develop potential competencies.

Specific types of interventions can be designed to address the requirements for complementary function in patients with EFD. Among others, these interventions may involve, first, providing suggestions that help clients enhance their working memory, second, giving assistance in transferring knowledge from episodic memory to procedural memory thus encouraging the development of new patterns and habits, and third, encouraging the use of assistive devices that compensate deficits.

Given our understanding of *working memory*, we can help clients reinforce the auditory channel or the visual channel. The auditory channel may be reinforced by techniques such as self-talk. We can suggest to clients that they verbalize to themselves what they are doing which helps them focus their attention, allowing them to keep track of the steps in the task. Hearing is one of our strongest senses. Hearing our own voice repeat things assists our memory. By talking to ourselves, we hear what we are about to do. Patients may find it helpful to hear themselves say: "I'll put my key here, so I won't forget it!" By talking to the object they wish to remember, they attach a verbal tag that allows them to remember. Similarly, the visual channel may be reinforced through visual aids. List making or the use of a white board on which to write items that the client must remember may be useful. Keeping a large calendar on a desk or a wall, which cannot be overlooked or ignored, may act to visually refresh the person's memory and recall tasks for which the patient must plan. Such clients' personal space may look like a disaster area to most people with a sense of organization, but when asked, those clients will claim that they know exactly where everything is. This is indeed often the case. They rely on their visual strength to compensate for their disorganization. What a social worker might recommend is that items be placed on an open shelf system rather than in drawers, where out-of-sight is out-of-mind.

Episodic memory is conscious, often verbal memory of events to which a person has been exposed. Autobiographical memory is an example of episodic memory. Procedural memory is non-conscious memory that encodes activities in which we habitually engage or repetitive tasks that require little conscious effort. Procedural memory is not memory of events that have been dynamically repressed. Examples of the manifestation of procedural memory are such activities as driving a car, swimming, dancing or other automatized actions. Less concrete examples are such activities as how we approach complex tasks, implement plans, or monitor our progress to assure the completion of a project.

For individuals with EFD, *substituting habits, by encoding them in procedural memory* in the case of actions that require conscious decision making, clients can bypass a central impediment that they face in their effort to accomplish a task. Given their difficulties in initiation and decision making, and their procrastination as avoidance to undertaking tasks, the development of a set of non-conscious habits may allow them to compensate for their deficits. A precondition to the formation of such habits is the motivation to bring about change in their lives and to persevere and sustain the effort that will be required for them to succeed. We may say, facetiously, that a cure for EFD is the development of a mild form of obsessive compulsive disorder. Therapy directed to the motivational aspects of these patients' difficulties may enhance their abilities to succeed in their efforts to bring about change.

At a more abstract level, dealing with these clients' distractibility and proclivity for the pursuit of tangential thoughts is somewhat more problematic. Nevertheless, some of strategies can be effective, if combined with those of the enhancement of working memory.

What were once simple devices to make phone calls, cell phone have now become accessories that are capable of complementing many functions that we require to live in our complex world. The Global Position System permits us to obtain directions, especially for those who have difficulties with directionality. Its alarm can act as reminder that tasks require our attention. Its thousands of "apps" permit people to enhance their everyday lives. What many fail to realize, however, is that these aids are of greater assistance to those who do not have the deficit than those who do. It requires executive function capacities for the efficient use of these devices.

Among the more complex issues with which social workers must deal with these clients is the issue of procrastination. Most clients with EFD insist that they know exactly what they have to do to accomplish the goals set by a task, however, where they fail is in the initiation of the steps necessary to begin working on the task. Procrastination is a pejorative term that we use for those who appear to willfully avoid undertaking tasks for which they are responsible. They defer taking action, they find excuses, and they may claim to have forgotten they were supposed to, and on and on. What is overlooked is that the *procrastination is part of the syndrome* in that it involves the inability to initiate activities. Decision-making is a major problem for individuals with EFD, consequently, what appears as willful avoidance is very much a part of the deficit. Matters become more convoluted in that often a set of dynamics have evolved that are entwined with the neuropsychological deficit. As a defense against the embarrassment some clients feel regarding their indecisiveness, they have instituted modes of responding that blur the reasons for their inaction. Those dynamics may become part of another set of dynamics, such as the fear of failure or of competition, that make it almost impossible for social workers to determine the motives behind a set of responses. Furthermore, having faced repeated failures and criticism many patients are hesitant to undertake any task that will test their capacities. They appear to be unmotivated to try. Unless the therapist can confront these dynamics and help the client work those through, real changes may not be forthcoming.

An important caveat to undertaking these departures from traditional modes of intervention must now be stated. The initial reason for instituting these interventions was in order to inform clients of the nature of their deficits and to deal with the associated psychodynamics. In the absence of adequate motivation to change, the helping efforts would face defeat. Clients also require a demonstration of the effectiveness of alternative modes of functioning before being able to take the initiative to bring about change on their own. Once such issues have been dealt with, it is possible to make a referral to an appropriate educational specialist who can provide more extensive strategies to compensate for the EFD. Such specialists are found increasingly in some regions of the country and constitute and excellent resource for such patients.

Disjunctive moments: the rupture and repair sequence The imperfections in our capacity to stay connected to others lead inevitably to ruptures in our relationships with clients and their connection to us as social workers. A *disjunction* may occur when the client ceases to feel understood by the social worker. When such disjunctions occur, *the treatment is in crisis*; it is essential that the therapist heal the rupture and reestablish the concordance between himself and the patient. These disjunctions may emanate from negative transference reactions, transferences of the social worker to the client, and non-transferential areas of the social worker's functioning.

If the social worker is unable to fill in the functions required by the client, for whatever reason, the client will experience that incapacity as an intentional assault. In a sense, the therapist's motives are irrelevant; only the effect on the patient is relevant. Such disjunctions become crises in the treatment that require repair to make further work possible. For example, there are moments when the frustration and rage that has accumulated in the client from years of feeling isolated and misunderstood may surface in the relationship with the social worker. The social worker in turn responds with impatience, anger, puzzlement, or distancing. Such moments represent opportunities for the client and social worker to work through an important interaction. The client's rage at others must be distinguished from the frustration and rage the client may feel toward the therapist. While both are understandable, the social worker must be able to look at and acknowledge any contribution he or she has made to provoke the patient's response. That piece of reality must first be addressed before the transference dimensions can be dealt with.

We see then that as the social worker responds differently from the way others have, a new set of experiences is generated for the patient. This new set of experiences lays the groundwork for what is to be curative in the process. In obtaining help, clients experience patterns that are different from those they resorted to in the past, and gain an understanding of the old patterns through the social worker's interpretations. Clients are then in a position to compensate for their deficits. The new patterns include the meanings of past experiences and the new meanings gained through the relationship with the social worker. The understanding clients acquire through this set of shared experiences with the social worker serves to break through their former isolation. Patterns that were central in the configuration of the patient personality are reshaped. New patterns come into play and the patient's expectations are modified. These new patterns give the patient greater hope for success than was possible in the past.

The evidence for the greater integration of the client's experiences is found in the greater sense of cohesiveness clients experience. Themes that formerly reflected the construal of personal meanings now encompass a set of shared meanings that grew out of the client's maturation and experiences in therapy. Specific events or interventions are difficult to specify that produce this greater sense of coherence; it usually results from the cumulative effects of the implementation of the broad service plan. The client's rehabilitation and restoration to better function can be credited to the combination of greater understanding, improved social functioning, enhanced self-esteem, and the social worker's educative, corrective, and interpretive efforts.

It is useful to review briefly some of the kinds of *countertransference* problems clients with EFD present. Therapists at times experience extreme frustration at what they perceive to be a patient's resistance to treatment. They may then resort to power struggles or to punitive measures in an attempt to involve the client. What social workers must keep in mind is that, from the perspective of the client, the environment has felt so hostile that the client cannot allow the social worker to experience the world as the client experiences it (Palombo, 1985a).

Another possible source of countertransference can be the social worker's theoretical orientation. Some social workers do not believe neuropsychological deficits are neurologically based conditions that have a heritable or constitutional basis. In the helping of these clients, such social workers often inadvertently re-create disjunctions similar to the ones the client has experienced already, the consequence being that stalemate occurs. In such instances, it is advisable that social worker seek consultation that would help broaden their theoretical outlook or refer the client to a therapist who can deal with such issues. The stalemate must be brought to a resolution or the therapy will be interrupted.

Illustration and discussion

Mark's mother, Mrs. P, requested a consultation regarding her 18-year-old son, who is a senior in high school. A psychologist who evaluated Mark found that he exhibits aspects of attention deficit disorder without hyperactivity. He had difficulties in particular in the area of activating himself, organizing his work, and sustaining his efforts to complete tasks. She made a diagnosis of a learning disability. Mrs. P's greatest concern was that Mark has not been doing well academically; he was failing sociology and analysis. Part of the problem was that he procrastinated. After seeing a tutor for a while, he decided that he wanted to be on his own and stopped seeing her. In addition, he had stopped seeing a psychologist because he did not find that relationship helpful.

On a day-to-day basis, he was always late for school; at times he would wake up feeling that he did not want to go to school. He was often critical of himself saying, "I can't do anything right." Socially, he had a group of friends with whom he played soccer. Mark reported that he frequently got moody and sad. He considered himself a "huge" procrastinator. Although, he wanted to do well in school, he ended up failing some his tests. He watched too much TV, played computer games, and did not make good choices. His tutor told him that he was too lazy to put any effort into his work, and that he had trouble organizing his thoughts. Now, he was working at a computer store, repairing computers. His major interest was in computer security and he expressed the wish that someday he could work for the security division of the FBI.

Mrs. P reported that in elementary school Mark did well academically because he was so bright. He was an independent learner, who loved to spend time in the library. She never saw him as distractible or as having a short attention span. He read voraciously, was creative, and loved school. When Mark was five years old, his father was diagnosed with leukemia. There was much upheaval as the family relocated temporarily to Seattle, where he had a bone marrow transplant. They were there for approximately six months. Mr. P then had a long remission of six years, at which point he relapsed. Mark, who was at summer camp at the time, was called back home. In the Fall, his father's condition deteriorated; by January, Mr. P went back to Seattle for a second bone marrow transplant. This was not successful and he remained in intensive care for three months. He died in mid-July of that year. Mark was 11 years old.

It was Mrs. P's impression that after his father's death, Mark was never quite the same. She made several attempts at instituting psychotherapy, but for the most part these were unsuccessful. He saw a social worker for a few times, then a school counselor, then a psychiatrist. None of the therapists were successful in engaging him. Although he appeared quite depressed, he had no wish to discuss his feelings about his father's death. Another psychiatrist prescribed medications, none of which were effective. He was tried on Prozac, Wellbutrin, Remeron, Adderall, Ritalin SR, and Celexa. He is now on Paxil and Ritalin SR.

The clinical psychologist who evaluated Mark saw him as an extremely bright young man. His Verbal IQ on the WAIS III was 140, in the Very Superior range, his Performance IQ was 119, in the High Average range, and his Full Scale IQ of 129 was at the very top of the Superior range. Mark's particular strengths were in verbal comprehension, verbal reasoning, acquired knowledge, and logical thinking (both language-based and non-verbal). He showed a relative weakness in perceptual organization, specifically having difficulty in knowing how to approach, analyze, conceptualize, and remember complex visual stimuli, registering important details as well as taking in the whole gestalt. He also had difficulties sorting through facts and ideas he had at his disposal, being unable to pick out what is most salient to the issue at hand. He got bogged down in less relevant details and often did not differentiate these from the main point. These cognitive problems were exacerbated by Mark's emotional response to them. Mark had a strong wish to do well, but his anxiety built up quickly, especially when he was under time pressure and he felt he was not meeting his own very high standards. As his anxiety built up, he was less and less able to think flexibly and productively. He then became frustrated and directed his anger toward the test, the assignment, or the person who imposed it on him. In his wish for a successful outcome, he disregarded external cues that indicated that his approach to the problem was not correct. A major factor was the emotional interferences with his productivity and not a lack of motivation.

After my initial diagnostic session, I referred Mark for a second opinion to a psychiatrist familiar with medications for adolescents with learning disabilities. Her impressions were that Mark was a bright young man whose poor executive functions created much pain and discomfort. He had periods when he succeeded after trying hard but could not sustain the effort over long periods. Mark's difficulty with perceptual organization created internal tension and anxiety when he met external expectations and was disappointed at not meeting his own standards. That left him with anxiety and tension that increased his rigid thinking and interfered with his problem-solving abilities. The intense anxiety and internal pressures that he experienced, as well as the fluctuations in his functioning, made it hard for him to deal with his emotions when faced with situation in which he had to make reasoned, careful judgments about everyday life situations, relationships with others, and solve problems intellectually. She felt that medication to treat his anxiety was appropriate but it would not help the anxiety created by his poor executive skills. Stimulants were generally not helpful in learning to prioritize and follow through, so it was not surprising that stimulants have not worked in the past. Stimulant treatment would only enhance sustained attention once the task was selected. She gave as her diagnosis as Axis I: Dysthymia, Generalized Anxiety Disorder, and ADHD, Inattentive Subtype. She recommended a trial of Paxil.

When I saw Mark, he stated that he felt depressed, burdened by everything, and bored. He believed that his depression may have started with his father's death, but then other problems developed on top, so that now he felt completely overwhelmed and wished to withdraw or distract himself. He was waiting to hear from the colleges to which he had applied. In the meantime, he had started the Paxil prescribed by the psychiatrist. The medication did not seem to improve his mood. We agreed that we would meet twice a week until he left for college, which gave us three months in which to work.

Mark felt some urgency to deal with his organizational problems since he was at risk of not succeeding in college if his current patterns of functioning persisted when he left home. He did not see the relevance of dealing with his father's death, as he did not feel it contributed to his current problems.

Most of these initial sessions were spent discussing practical issues, such as the need for him to develop some regularity in his schedule to avoid the disruptions caused by his lack of organization.

He expressed confidence that once he was out of the house and away from his mother, he would be able to manage his life. He knew what he needed to do and once at school he would implement the plans we had discussed. It seemed unproductive to point out the fact that knowing what he should do was not the same as being able to implement that knowledge.

Before he left for school, we agreed that he and I would keep in touch by phone once a week to make sure that he maintains his functioning. During these initial phone calls, he reported that he was having a great time socially. He had made many friends and was hoping to join a fraternity. However, after a while, he stopped contacting me until he came home during the Christmas break, at which point he made two appointments. We spent these catching me up on his adaptation in college.

I did not hear again from Mark until March of the following year, his sophomore year. He had been asked to take a one-year leave of absence from school because he was failing. He wanted to come and see me, but he also wanted to live at the college to be close to his friends. This meant that he had to drive for six hours each way for his twice a week appointment. I did not challenge these unrealistic plans. He came to the sessions regularly, although he was most often ten to fifteen minutes late. Shortly after we started, he realized that his plans were unrealistic, and with my encouragement, he decided to move back home.

For the next nine months, I saw Mark twice a week for approximately 60 sessions. Three major themes organized the material of these sessions: the use of medication to help alleviate his depression, the problems with organization, and the loss of his father.

Mark would generally begin each session with a discussion of the *medication* he was taking. He complained bitterly about not feeling well. He kept hoping that the psychiatrists would find the right medication to alleviate his depression. He described feeling sad and depressed, feeling disconnected from the world. At times, when he became deeply depressed, he had paranoid thoughts that his food was being poisoned by his mother, which he acknowledged could not be true. His psychiatrist found him difficult to medicate. Mark complained about his medications' many side effects and the weird feelings that they produced in him. When he had to have an EKG to check his heart before he could begin a new medication, he expressed concern that he might die. At one point the psychiatrist, hearing of the severity of the symptoms, became convinced that Mark was manifesting pre-schizophrenic symptoms – a diagnosis with which I disagreed. He worried about an eventual breakdown. He put Mark on Geodon. Mark stopped taking that medication within two days, claiming that it made him feel weird. None of the medications were effective. In fact, he felt much better off medications than on them. Eventually, he settled on Effexor since it helped with his anxiety but not with the depressive symptoms. I remained convinced that those symptoms reflected his defenses against the intense feeling associated with the unresolved grief over his father's death, and emphasized the need to address those feelings.

A central focus of our discussion was on his desire to deal with the problem of his *poor time management and his disorganization*, which he now recognized were responsible for his failure in school. As I mentioned earlier, Mark consistently came late to his sessions. At first, he joked about it, stating that his appointments really began ten minutes after the hour. He then became more self-conscious about his lateness, and gave excuses, such as a train at the crossing stopped him, or that his mother had insisted that he take care of some chores, or that he had to make an urgent phone call. In an effort to break the pattern, I even offered to change his appointments from 10 AM to 4 PM because it was difficult for him to get up in the mornings. He never succeeded in coming on time, in spite of my calling him to wake him up so that he could come on time. Eventually, I pointed out to him that he was playing games with himself and defeating his own determination to develop different habits. This led him to start coming precisely on time, something in which he took great pride and of which he kept asking for my affirmation of his improvement.

Another issue centered on his desire to complete a difficult advanced computer course that he had not completed the previous summer. To obtain the degree, Mark had to pass five exams covering sections of the course. His efforts were half-hearted. He had taken and passed one of the five exams. My efforts to help him structure his studies were unsuccessful. Instead of studying, he found himself playing games online until three or four in the morning, and sleeping until one or two in the afternoon.

Mark became increasingly concerned that he would be a failure in life. He talked about his pattern of beginning tasks with much enthusiasm and preparation. He always felt confident that he would do well. However, after about three to four weeks, his interest would wane; he would get distracted and lose his sense of direction. He would get behind in the work and not be able to catch up to get a passing grade. He felt considerable shame that his image was already tarnished. How could he face his friends and relatives who always thought of him of becoming as successful as his father had been? He expressed his determination to overcome the difficulties in his path, although, he did not know what he had to do to avoid further failure.

In a final effort to break the pattern of disorganization, I enlisted his cooperation in choosing a simple task in which we could be assured that he would succeed. He decided that he wanted to clean up his room, which was in total disarray. I coached him into breaking down the task and estimating how long each activity would take. First, he suggested that he would get all his clothing off the floor, and then he would clean some drawers that he had not cleaned since high school, and then he would clean his desk, and finally, his closet. He estimated that each task would take three to four hours, and decided he would work for two hours two days a week until he got everything done. According to this plan, it would have taken six weeks for him to finish. I agreed to the plan. The first three weeks, he came and proudly informed me of the progress he was making. His mother was impressed. Then, I stopped hearing about it. When I finally inquired what was happening, he said he had run into a problem. Our plan had not included maintenance and upkeep of the areas already covered. After three weeks, his floor was as messy as it had been. He finally gave up.

These issues were always accompanied with discussion of dynamic factors that also intruded into his desire to be successful. In this connection, we dealt at length with the meaning of the loss of his father.

Mark experienced *delayed grief and mourning*. His father had been a highly successful producer of music videos. He had started his own business after he was first diagnosed with leukemia, and managed to reach national prominence in his area. Mark's fantasy was that, had his father lived, his life would have taken an entirely different course. Not only would he not have had his current problems, but also he would have had a mentor who would have taught him the ins and outs of the computer business so that he could have followed in his father's footsteps. In addition, the family would not be as financially constrained as it is now. He was convinced that his father would have bought him his dream car – a $75,000 Porsche. With this car and his father's support, Mark felt that he would be on top of the world. He would not be depressed, he would be encouraged to complete his work, and his future would be assured.

Mark talked about how he felt a year ago when he was dating a girl who was the daughter of a CEO of a multinational corporation. The girl's father liked him very much, as did her mother. They welcomed him warmly into their house and took him on vacations with them. He felt on top of the world. The problem was that he felt that the girl was shallow and superficial, which eventually contributed to their breakup. He now wished he could recapture that old feeling. He was tempted to call her to see if they could get back together again. However, he knew it would be wrong; he had a new girlfriend and could not do that to her. The new girlfriend's parents were divorced and he could not get the same feeling from them that he got from his old girlfriend's parents.

I commented on the parallel between how he must have felt when his father was alive, and how he felt after his father died. It is as though something within him died with the death of his father. He now wished he could recapture how he felt before. He asked how he could do that. I respond by saying that he needed to recover his ability to feel and to recapture some of the sadness he felt after the loss. He had suppressed many of those feelings and they were now disconnected from the loss. He responded that even if he could go back it would be too painful and he wanted to avoid doing that.

Mark could recover few memories of his experiences with his father. He could not remember specifics. His memories were global and hazy. His father was around in the evenings; he was not working as hard after he became successful. He used to help him with his written work. I asked if he had any feelings about the relationship but he remembered none. He did remember that when his father was away during the first bout of his illness, his mother said that his father tried to fight hard so he could get back to be with the family. At this point, Mark became tearful for the first time. He remembered sitting in the living room on the couch with his father; he had asked his father if he was afraid that he might die. His father said that he was afraid but he felt he could conquer his illness. At this point, Mark stopped and said that in the past, therapists tried to get him to talk about these things, but he had always refused. He wondered why that was so. I said that as a kid he was probably in great pain; the feelings were intolerable for him. He probably suppressed them and now it is hard for him to get in touch with them. That was probably why he gets those feelings of being disconnected.

Such sessions would be followed by sessions in which he would come and say that he was feeling depressed, he did not see how therapy was helping. His coming to see me had become ritualized; he felt that he just repeated the same stories but seemed to go around in circles. He did not seem to see any progress. I commented on how hard this kind of work is for him, but that his avoidance was also reflective of his pattern of starting new things but not hanging in long enough to get results. He gets discouraged, loses interest, and eventually drops out. His response was to ask how he could get out of repeating this pattern. In addition, he just wanted to feel better. I suggested that therapy is hard work, it would eventually yield results but he needed to stay with it.

When we could return to that topic, I asked what makes it so hard to talk about his feelings. He responded that he gets overwhelmed; he feared that he might die and abandon his mother just as his father had. There was so much he had not said to her that he would now like to tell her. If he were to die, these would be left unsaid. He felt much guilt about the way he had treated her, and had been mean to her when she asked him to help around the house. On the other hand, he thought about the possibility of his mother dying; he would have so many regrets about things he had done and said to her. He would feel terrible. He realized that he got angry at her for no reason. He remembered a scene when his father was in the hospital in the intensive care unit. He had asked his mother if he could see his father, but she said he could not. He was enraged at her, but said nothing. Now he realized that he had been carrying a lot of anger at her and directed his resentment for his father's death toward her.

I said that he feels she deprived him of the opportunity to get close to his dad. He responded by saying that he needed to see his father; it was a chance for him to be with him. There were times, when he was at the hospital, that she told him that he could go home if he wanted to. She was giving him permission to leave. However, he felt that she was depriving him of the opportunity of being with his father. Now he understands her motives; she was trying to protect him from seeing how sick his father was, she wanted him to have good memories, but instead she caused more pain in the long run for him.

He described a dream in which he was sitting in a field of dark green grass, the sun was setting, and it was getting dark. He felt all alone. I suggested that the loneliness that he experienced was related to what happened to him. It may mean that when his father died his mother was also unavailable because of her grief; that left him all by himself to deal with his sadness. He responded that he had always felt alone, he did not feel connected to anyone. It is as though he stood next to himself and watched events, even when there were people around. There always was a feeling of distance between him and others.

During another session, I explained to him the mourning process: grieving, the pain associated with the loss, and morning that lasts a much longer period. Then there are the anniversaries usually associated with "Yortzeit," the Jewish yearly revisiting of the period of mourning. This process included working through old memories. He responded by saying that he could not locate himself in this process. He did not see things that way, because his mind did not work in a sequential manner. This is like his room; there is no orderly way to proceed. I agreed that he was unable to have a map before him that plots where he started and where he is going. It was more like being in a jungle where he felt lost. He got discouraged seeing that there was no path to follow. He gave up or backtracked, telling himself that he would do better by starting over. He agreed and said this problem got in his way in so many areas. It affected his entire life. What could he do? He needed to establish some kind of template that would guide him through the process.

During our discussion of his organizational problems, the issue of his lack of motivation to try harder came up frequently. I asked if he could remember when he lost his motivation to do well in school. He thought it happened in sixth grade. He had done very well until then. His father got sick and they moved to Seattle so that he could be treated. When he came back to seventh grade, he did poorly and became a behavior problem. He then went on to talk about how discouraged he had felt. Now he saw no point in making any effort to achieve, because his life might be cut short at any time, just as his father's was.

He reiterated, as he had numerous times before, that he has the knowledge, the means to be successful, but simply could not act on that knowledge. He listed three reasons for not trying harder. First, why should he give up the pleasure he gets from playing his computer games, if there is no certainty of a future. Second, he will die young in any case, as did his father. Third, if he tried, he might fail. If he failed, he could not live with himself. The threat of death hung over his head. That's why he could not get over his feelings; if he is certain to die, he might as well enjoy the moment, and get as much pleasure as he can! He went on to say that even if he lived and worked hard, even if he made millions, what good would that do if he were to die at 25 or 30. His father got sick at 35 and died when he was 42. As he reflected about this, he said, on the other hand, he might live to be 80 and then he would look back and feel he had accomplished nothing. That would be weird!

I responded by saying that his father did not give up, even though he knew the illness might have been fatal. Why did he think his father did that? He responds that it was true; not only did his father conquer the illness the first time, but also he went on to build a very successful business after the first bone marrow transplant. He left the family quite comfortable from the proceeds of that business. The second time, he did not succeed. He went on to say that there were moments when he did get fired up, he could then take the initiative and work hard and do very well, like the time when he spent an entire week devising a business plan. Not only did he write out the plan, but also he designed stationery, business cards, invoices, everything. He did not feel discouraged; he was swept up by flow of energy.

I said that the difference was that he had started therapy; he had someone whom he could consider to be a mentor, a teacher who was by his side. He responded that when he has someone like that, it is as though his father was there helping him. He wished that his father could be by his side, teaching him and urging him on. He would not feel the sadness and despair he now felt. He was silent for a while, then said, "Yes, but he is not!" I said it is hard for him to see me in that role, it does not feel to him as it would if his father was alive. My encouraging and cheering him on simply does not do it. He agreed. I responded, saying that he might think of how proud his father would be to see him be successful.

At this point, our work had to be interrupted because it was time for him to go back to school. Once more, we agreed to stay in touch, although the contacts were erratic. He reported that he was doing well in his classes, had not been late or missed a single class. He felt very proud, considering it a great accomplishment. His girlfriend was a young woman who was well organized and was happy to help him with his organizational problems.

The following summer, he returned home for a few weeks. This gave us the opportunity to meet for a few sessions. I noticed a perceptible change in his demeanor and attitude at this time. The lack of concern that was habitual was no longer there. What he had to say was moving and encouraging. He had managed to get good grades during the last semester. However, his overall grade point average was brought down by the grades he had received in the first year at college. This meant that he would not be accepted in the internship to which he intended to apply as part of pursuing his career goal to be an FBI agent. He complained that no matter how hard he worked during the next three years, he could never raise his grade sufficiently to get the government job to which he aspired. He blamed himself for having wasted that first year in college and once more reverted to wishing that his father had been alive. Had his father been alive, he felt sure that would never have happened. I commented that he continues to grieve that loss and is able to draw strength from memories he had of the time when his father was alive. He responded that without the work we had done together, he would never have been able to succeed in college as he did the past semester; but, he added poignantly, "It's not the same as if my father were alive!"

This case illustrates, first, how intertwined psychodynamics and neuropsychological deficits can be in an adolescent with an executive function disorder. Second, it illustrates the type of explanations that an adolescent can give himself to understand the nature of his difficulties. Third, it illustrates the modifications that were introduced into the therapeutic process in order to bring about a beneficial result.

Understanding the intertwined nature of the psychodynamics and the executive function disorder required taking a closer look at the unfolding transference. Mark's executive function disorder was partly responsible for his failure to achieve at the level at which he was capable. The other set of deficits were related to the failures to develop self-regulatory and selfobject functions. Although self-regulatory disruptions are ubiquitous in adolescence, the fact that in Mark's case these included and impairment in self-organization indicated that these were related to his EFD. At the selfobject level, the loss of his father interfered with the ontogenetic development of a specific aspect of the idealizing selfobject functions that would have provided him with the inner strength to confront the adversities he faced. The cognitive impairments may also have contributed to these selfobject deficits. In the therapeutic context, these deficits manifested as transferences and non-transferences.

In the initial phase, Mark did not wish to deal directly with his father's loss. This led us to focus on the contribution his neural psychological deficits made to the problems he faced. The non-transference dimensions that manifested in his behavior were his lateness for his appointments, his cognitive style, and his inability to order his thoughts sufficiently to track his location in the process, and to organize aspects of his personal space.

The central organizing theme that Mark had drawn from his experiences did not include the contributions of his neuropsychological deficits to his life's problems. In spite of the fact that the psychologist and psychiatrist had given him cognitive explanations regarding his executive function difficulties, the explanations were not fully integrated. His inability to function in accordance with his expectations contributed to his depression and demoralization.

I have found it necessary to modify the model of interventions to accommodate my under-standing of the contributions of neuropsychological deficits to his psychodynamics. In part, the modification involves demonstrating directly within the context of the therapeutic relationship the precise way in which the deficits interfere in the patient's day-to-day functions. My attempt at mentoring him through the process of organizing his room was an educational effort that was meant to demonstrate to him how he could use complementary functions that others can provide. He became aware of the self-discipline that is necessary to complete an assigned task. Mark found the exercise instructive although it did not alleviate his problem; in part, it was because he found it difficult to sustain the effort involved in persevering with the task. However, when he returned to college he was able to make better use of his girlfriend's organizational abilities and with some effort develop the self-discipline to undertake successfully the school tasks that faced him.

It is notable that no major rupture occurred between Mark and me. My understanding of the causes of his symptoms forestalled my becoming impatient with him or irritated at him. Others, without an understanding of EFD, might have interpreted his behavior as representing a resistance to the process or as provocative intended to get a response. Such a misunderstanding of the psychodynamics would not only have triggered a rupture but also have set the stage for the emergence of a negative transference.

In closing, Mark came into adolescence saddled with problems that forestalled his ability to consolidate an integrated sense of self. The combination of the loss of his father during early adolescence as well as his executive function deficits was partly responsible for this failure. The responses he got from others in his context did not or could not complement his deficits sufficiently for him to compensate for them. In addition, his own distress interfered with his ability to use others who were available to complement his needs. As he integrated an understanding of his EFD and worked through the loss of his father, Mark was able to begin to exercise the self-discipline necessary to complete tasks within the context of a supportive relationship. He developed a greater sense of self-cohesion and greater self-understanding. However, he remains at risk for blaming future failures to the loss of his father and would lead him to perceive himself as a victim of circumstances.

Conclusion

Executive functions are psychological functions associated with the development of the frontal lobes. These functions, however, are more broadly distributed and not strictly localized to that region of the brain. Although executive function disorders were initially associated with injuries to that region, the existence of a developmental variant with similar symptoms was discovered in individuals without specific brain impairments. This variant may be classified among the learning disorders, but has not been categorized as a specific learning disability.

Current neuropsychological definitions and explanatory theories of EFD have not paid sufficient attention to the psychodynamics associated with this disorder. These conceptualizations have neglected the significance of the social context on those affected and of the responses by those affected to their context. Furthermore, they did not give sufficient consideration to the role of emotional and motivational factors.

Individuals filter their experiences through their endowment. Because of their executive function deficits, these clients cannot adequately regulate their thought processes, affect states, and/or behaviors. They respond to events based on their experience, but the responses are not congruent with the expectations of those in the context. The efforts of both patients and others to continue the dialogue lead to confusion and to a derailment of the dialogue. The consequence is that patients cannot avail themselves of the obtainable selfobject functions. Others, in the patients' context, misinterpret the motives behind the patients' responses and perceive the behavior to be defiant, oppositional, or negativistic. A set of patterns of interactions is established in which patients expect to be misunderstood, and are made anxious because of their failure to understand. Their frustration increases and eventually leads to rage or to withdrawal. Overlaid over this set of patterns are the selfobject deficits that result from the primary neuropsychological deficits.

This chapter attempts to bridge the gap between the developments in the neurosciences and clinical social work practice. It highlights school social workers, who provide services to children and adolescents, and practitioners, who provide services to adults, unfamiliarity with the disorder as a major impediment to the provision of services to these populations. These problems are compounded by the economic disparities that exist in school districts and the failure of insurance companies to reimburse for diagnostic and treatment services.

From the perspective of a clinician who provides individual therapy to clients of all ages, I proposed a neuropsychodynamic model that permits the formulation of some of the psychodynamics of individuals with the disorder. Two major components of those dynamics were those associated with the self-deficits the disorder produces and the complementary functions that individuals with the disorder require others to perform for them to avoid the development of a disorder of the self. These complementary functions include those associated with the neuropsychological, the social, and the emotional deficits from which persons with the disorder suffer. When others provide those functions, those with the deficits are able to sustain an integrated sense of self. Given these formulations, the model offers a set of treatment approaches that are more likely to produce a therapeutic outcome than those that neglect to take into consideration the neuropsychological deficits.

The treatment approach conceives of the process as a set of moments during which one of three different aspects of the relationship between the client and the therapist is in the foreground, the concordant, the complementary, or the disjunctive. During concordant moments, the focus of the interaction centers on the therapist's efforts to understand the patient's experience and the factors such as the neuropsychological, the social, and personal meanings that contribute to the patient's interpretations of those experiences. To arrive at an accurate diagnosis, the therapist needs to supplement the information gathered through empathy with that of other sources, such as neuropsychological testing, or reports from significant others in the patient's social context.

During complementary moments, the positive and negative transferences are in the foreground, activated by the patient's expectations that the therapist will either gratify the need for the complementary function or disappoint that expectation as others have in the patient's past. Whereas in traditional forms of therapy providing for the missing function is not considered necessarily therapeutic, a different approach is indicated with these patients. Interpretations involve not only unconscious repressed contents but also the non-conscious functions of our minds. Patients need to understand the way in which their brains process information just as they need to understand how they relate to people. For some patients with these types of deficits, understanding is not enough. Interpretations alone do not lead to the internalization of the function or to development of the missing capacity. Some patients require scaffolding or instruction so that they may compensate for the deficit. Other clients may require actual modeling of the function or even provision of that function. Others still may need medication to help restore their neurochemical balance.

The implications for practice of these modifications are numerous and remain to be fully explored. As we begin to apply these newer ways of thinking to clients with such disorders, many of the formerly problematic technical issues, such as whether the provision of functions is contra-indicated, fade and no longer need to burden our work with such patients.

Web resources

Dyslexia
www.dyslexia.wordpress.com/2007/11/09/exercise-and-executive-function-in-the-brain/

Learning Disabilities
www.learningdisabilities.about.com/od/eh/a/executive_funct.htm

References

American Psychiatric Association (APA). (1994). *Diagnostic and statistical manual of mental disorders* (4th ed.). Washington, DC: APA.

Anderson, P.J. (2008). Towards a developmental model of executive function. In V. Anderson, R. Jacobs, & P. J. Anderson (eds), *Executive functions and the frontal lobes: A lifespan perspective* (pp. 3–21). New York: Taylor & Francis.

Anderson, V., Jacobs, R., & Anderson, P.J. (eds). (2008). *Executive functions and the frontal lobes: A lifespan perspective*. New York: Taylor & Francis.

Applegate, J.S., & Shapiro, J.R. (2005). *Neurobiology for clinical social work: Theory and practice*. New York: W.W. Norton.

Baddeley, A.D. (1996). Exploring the central executive. *Quarterly Journal of Experimental Psychology, 49A* (1), 5–28.

Baddeley, A.D., & Wilson, B. (1988). Frontal amnesia and the dysexecutive syndrome. *Brain and Cognition, 7*, 212–230.

Barkley, R.A. (1990). *Attention-deficit hyperactivity disorder: A handbook for diagnosis and treatment*. New York: Guilford Press.

Barkley, R.A. (1996). Linkages between attention and executive function. In G.R. Lyon & N.A. Krasnegor (eds), *Attention, memory, and executive function* (pp. 307–325). Baltimore, MD: Paul H. Brookes.

Barkley, R.A. (1998). *Attention-deficit hyperactivity disorder: A handbook for diagnosis and treatment* (2nd ed.). New York: Guilford Press.

Baron-Cohen, S., & Swettenham, J. (1997). Theory of mind in autism: Its relationship to executive function and central coherence. In D.J. Cohen & F.R. Volkmar (eds), *Handbook of autism and pervasive developmental disorders* (pp. 880–893). New York: John Wiley & Sons.

Barrett, L.F., & Lindquist, K.A. (2008). The embodiment of emotion. In G.R. Semin & E.R. Smith (eds), *Embodied grounding: Social, cognitive, affective, and neuroscientific approaches* (pp. 237–262). New York: Cambridge University Press.

Beebe, B., & Lachmann, F.M. (1988). Mother-infant mutual influence and precursors of psychic structure. In A. Goldberg (ed.), *Progress in self psychology* (Vol. 3, pp. 3–25). Hillsdale, NJ: Analytic Press.

Beebe, B., & Lachmann, F.M. (1997). Mother-infant structures and presymbolic self and object representations. *Psychoanalytic Dialogues, 7*, 30–182.

Beebe, B., Rustin, J., Sorter, D., & Knoblauch, S. (2005a). An expanded view of forms of intersubjectivity in infancy and their application to psychoanalysis. In B. Beebe, S. Knoblauch, J. Rustin, & D. Sorter (eds), *Forms of intersubjectivity in infant research and adult treatment* (pp. 55–88). New York: Other Press.

Beebe, B., Sorter, D., Rustin, J., & Knoblauch, S. (2005b). Forms of intersubjectivity in infant research: A comparison of Melzoff, Trevarthen, and Stern. In B. Beebe, S. Knoblauch, J. Rustin, & D. Sorter (eds), *Forms of intersubjectivity in infant research and adult treatment* (pp. 29–54). New York: Other Press.

Bernstein, J.H., & Waber, D.P. (2007). Executive capacities from a developmental perspective. In L. Meltzer (ed.), *Executive function in education: From theory to practice* (pp. 77–105). New York: Guilford Press.

Borkowski, J.G., & Burke, J.E. (1996). Theories, models, and measurements of executive functioning: An information processing perspective. In G.R. Lyon & N.A. Krasnegor (eds), *Attention, memory, and executive function* (pp. 235–261). Baltimore, MD: Paul H. Brookes.

Bowlby, J. (1969). *Attachment and loss: Vol. 1, Attachment*. New York: Basic Books.

Cohen, M. (2009). *A guide to special education advocacy: What parents, clinicians and advocates need to know*. London: Jessica Kingsley Publishers.

Coplin, J.W., & Morgan, S.B. (1988). Learning disabilities: A multidimensional perspective. *Journal of Learning Disabilities, 21* (10), 614–622.

Damasio, A.R. (1994). *Descartes' error: Emotion, reason, and the human brain*. New York: G.P. Putnam's Sons.

De Luca, C.R., & Leventer, R.J. (2008). Developmental trajectories of executive functions across the lifespan. In R. Jacobs, V. Anderson, & P.J. Anderson (eds), *Executive functions and the frontal lobes: A lifespan perspective* (pp. 23–56). New York: Taylor & Francis.

Denckla, M.B. (1994). Measurement of executive function. In G.R. Lyon (ed.), *Frames of reference for the assessment of learning disabilities* (pp. 117–142). Baltimore, MD: Paul H. Brookes.

Denckla, M.B. (1996). A theory and model of executive function: A neuropsychological perspective. In G.R. Lyon & N.A. Krasnegor (eds), *Attention, memory, and executive function* (pp. 263–278). Baltimore, MD: Paul H. Brookes.

Denckla, M.B. (2007). Executive function: Binding together the definitions of attention-deficit/hyperactivity disorder and learning disabilities. In L. Meltzer (ed.), *Executive function in education: From theory to practice* (pp. 5–18). New York: Guilford Press.

El-Hai, J. (2005). *The lobotomist: A maverick medical genius and his tragic quest to rid the world of mental illness.* New York: John Wiley & Sons.

Ellenberg, L. (1999). Executive functions in children with learning disabilities and attention deficit disorder. In J.A. Incorvia, B.S. Mark-Goldstein, & D. Tessmer (eds), *Understanding, diagnosing, and treating AD/HD in children and adolescents: An integrative approach* (pp. 197–219). Northvale, NJ: Jason Aronson.

Eslinger, P.J. (1996). Conceptualizing, describing, and measuring components of executive function: A summary. In G.R. Lyon & N.A. Krasnegor (eds), *Attention, memory, and executive function* (pp. 367–395). Baltimore, MD: Paul H. Brookes.

Fonagy, P. (2005). Attachment, trauma and psychoanalysis: When psychoanalysis meets neuroscience. IPA 44th Conference on Trauma: Developments in psychoanalysis, Rio de Janeiro.

Fonagy, P., & Target, M. (1998). Mentalization and the changing aims of child psychoanalysis. *Psychoanalytic Dialogues, 8* (1), 97–114.

Fonagy, P., & Target, M. (2002). Early intervention and the development of self-regulation. *Psychoanalytic Inquiry, 22* (3), 307–335.

Fonagy, P., Gergely, G., Jurist, E.L., & Target, M. (2002). *Affect regulation, mentalization, and the development of the self.* New York: Other Press.

Gazzaniga, M.S. (1988). *Mind matters: How mind and brain interact to create our conscious lives.* Boston, MA: Houghton Mifflin.

Gazzaniga, M.S., Ivry, R.B., & Mangun, G.R. (2002). *Cognitive neuroscience: The biology of the mind* (2nd ed.). New York: W.W. Norton.

Gedo, J.E. (2005). *Psychoanalysis as biological science: A comprehensive theory.* Baltimore, MD: Johns Hopkins University Press.

Goldberg, E. (2001). *The executive brain: Frontal lobes and the civilized mind.* New York: Oxford University Press.

Green, R.L., & Ostrander, R.L. (2009). *Neuroanatomy for students of behavioral disorders.* New York: W.W. Norton.

Harris, J.C. (1998). *Developmental neuropsychiatry.* Oxford: Oxford University Press.

Himrod, L.K. (1995). Protective vigilance: The experience of parenting an adolescent who has learning disabilities. Ph.D. dissertation, Institute for Clinical Social Work, Chicago, IL. Retrieved February 3, 2010, from ProQuest Digital Dissertations database (Publication No. AAT DP11762).

Kaplan-Solms, K., & Solms, M. (2002). *Clinical studies in neuro-psychoanalysis: An introduction to a depth neuropsychology* (2nd ed.). New York: Karnac.

Kesey, K. (1962). *One flew over the cuckoo's nest.* New York: Penguin.

Klin, A., & Jones, W. (2007). Embodied psychoanalysis? Or, on the confluence of psychodynamic theory and developmental science. In L. Mays, P. Fonagy, & M. Target (eds), *Developmental science and psychoanalysis: Integration and innovation* (pp. 5–38). London: Karnac.

Klin, A., Volkmar, F., & Sparrow, S.S. (eds). (2000). *Asperger syndrome.* New York: Guilford Press.

Kohut, H. (1971). *The analysis of the self.* New York: International Universities Press.

Kohut, H. (1977). *The restoration of the self.* New York: International Universities Press.

Kohut, H. (1984). *How does analysis cure?* Chicago, IL: University of Chicago Press.

Leamy, D. (2008). The lived experience of young adolescents with learning disabilities. Ph.D. dissertation, Institute for Clinical Social Work, Chicago, IL. Retrieved February 3, 2010, from ProQuest Digital Dissertations database (Publication No. AAT 3334415).

Leighton, J. (2004). The analyst's sham(e): Collapsing into a one-person system. In W.J. Coburn (ed.), *Transformations in self psychology: Progress in self psychology* (Vol. 20, pp. 169–188). Hillsdale, NJ: Analytic Press.

Levine, M. (1994). *Educational care: A system for understanding and helping children with learning problems at home and in school.* Cambridge, MA: Educators Publishing Service.

Lezak, M.D. (1983). *Neuropsychological assessment.* New York: Oxford University Press.

Lezak, M.D., Howieson, D.B., & Loring, D.W. (2004). *Neuropsychological assessment* (4th ed.). New York: Oxford University Press.

Luria, A.R. (1973). *The working brain: An introduction to neuropsychology*. New York: Basic Books.

Luria, A.R. (1979). *The making of mind: A personal account of Soviet psychology*. Cambridge, MA: Harvard University Press.

Lyon, G.R., & Krasnegor, N.A. (eds). (1996). *Attention, memory, and executive function*. Baltimore, MD: Paul H. Brookes.

Mahler, M.S. (1975). *The psychological birth of the human infant*. New York: Basic Books.

Mcdonald, S. (2008). Social information processing difficulties in adults and implications for treatment. In R. Jacobs, V. Anderson, and P.J. Anderson (eds), *Executive functions and the frontal lobes: A lifespan perspective* (pp. 471–499). New York: Taylor & Francis.

McNulty, M.A. (2000). Dyslexia and the life course. Ph.D. dissertation, Institute for Clinical Social Work, Chicago, IL. Retrieved February 3, 2010, from ProQuest Digital Dissertations database (Publication No. AAT 9979953).

Meltzer, L. (ed.). (2007). *Executive function in education: From theory to practice*. New York: Guilford Press.

Meltzer, L., & Krishman, K. (2007). Executive function difficulties and learning disabilities: Understandings and misunderstandings. In L. Meltzer (ed.), *Executive function in education: From theory to practice* (pp. 5–18). New York: Guilford Press.

Orenstein, M. (1992). Imprisoned intelligence: The discovery of undiagnosed learning disabilities in adults. Ph.D. dissertation, Institute for Clinical Social Work, Chicago, IL. Retrieved February 3, 2010, from ProQuest Digital Dissertations database (Publication No. AAT 9816334).

Ozonoff, S., & Schetter, P. L. (2007). Executive dysfunction in autism spectrum disorders: From research to practice. In L. Meltzer (ed.), *Executive function in education: From theory to practice* (pp. 133–159). New York: Guilford Press.

Palombo, J. (1985a). Self psychology and countertransference in the treatment of children. *Child and Adolescent Social Work Journal, 2* (1), 36–48.

Palombo, J. (1985b). The treatment of borderline neurocognitively impaired children: A perspective from self psychology. *Clinical Social Work Journal, 13* (2), 117–128.

Palombo, J. (1987). Selfobject transferences in the treatment of borderline neurocognitively impaired children. In J.S. Grotstein, M.F. Solomon, & J.A. Lang (eds), *The borderline patient* (pp. 317–346). Hillsdale, NJ: Analytic Press.

Palombo, J. (1991). Neurocognitive differences, self cohesion, and incoherent self narratives. *Child and Adolescent Social Work Journal, 8* (6), 449–472.

Palombo, J. (1993). Neurocognitive deficits, developmental distortions, and incoherent narratives. *Psychoanalytic Inquiry, 13* (1), 85–102.

Palombo, J. (1995). Psychodynamic and relational problems of children with nonverbal learning disabilities. In B.S. Mark & J.A. Incorvaia (eds), *The handbook of infant, child, and adolescent psychotherapy: A guide to diagnosis and treatment* (Vol. I, pp. 147–176). Northvale, NJ: Jason Aronson.

Palombo, J. (2001). *Learning disorders and disorders of the self in children and adolescents*. New York: W.W. Norton.

Palombo, J. (2006). *Nonverbal learning disabilities: A clinical perspective*. New York: W.W. Norton.

Palombo, J. (2008a). Mindsharing: Transitional objects and selfobjects as complementary functions. *Clinical Social Work Journal, 36*, 143–154.

Palombo, J. (2008b). Self psychology theory. In B.A. Thyer (ed.), *Comprehensive handbook of social work and social welfare: Human behavior in the social environment* (Vol. 2, pp. 163–205). Hoboken, NJ: John Wiley & Sons.

PDM Task Force. (2006). *Psychodynamic diagnostic manual*. Silver Spring, MD: Alliance of Psychoanalytic Organizations.

Pennington, B., Bennetto, F.L., McAleer, O., & Roberts, R.J. (1996). Executive functions and working memory. In G.R. Lyon & N.A. Krasnegor (eds), *Attention, memory, and executive function* (pp. 327–348). Baltimore, MD: Paul H. Brookes.

Racker, H. (1968). *Transference and countertransference*. New York: International Universities Press.

Racker, H. (1972). The meaning and uses of countertransference. *Psychoanalytic Quarterly, 41*, 487–506.

Reader, M.J., Harris, E.L., Schuerholz, L.J., & Denckla, M.B. (1994). Attention deficit hyperactivity disorder and executive dysfunction. *Developmental Neuropsychology, 10* (4), 493–512.

Schore, A.N. (2000). Attachment and the regulation of the right brain. *Attachment and Human Development, 2* (1), 23–47.

Schore, A.N. (2001a). Effects of a secure attachment relationship on right brain development, affect regulation, and infant mental health. *Infant Mental Health Journal, 22* (1–2), 7–66.

Schore, A.N. (2001b). The effects of early relational trauma on right brain development, affect regulation, and infant mental health. *Infant Mental Health Journal, 22* (1–2), 201–269.

Schore, A.N. (2003). Minds in the making: attachment, the self-organizing brain, and developmentally-oriented psychoanalytic psychotherapy (Seventh Annual John Bowlby Memorial Lecture). In J. Corrigall and H. Wilkinson (eds). *Revolutionary connections: Psychotherapy and neuroscience* (pp. 7–51). London: Karnac.

Schore, A.N. (2005a). Attachment, affect regulation, and the developing right brain: Linking developmental neuroscience to pediatrics. *Pediatrics in Review, 26* (6), 204–217.

Schore, A.N. (2005b). A neuropsychoanalytic viewpoint: Commentary on paper by Steven H. Knoblauch. *Psychoanalytic Dialogues, 15* (6), 829–854.

Schore, J.R., & Schore, A.N. (2008). The central role of affect regulation in development and treatment. *Clinical Social Work Journal, 36* (1), 9–20.

Sclufer, A. (1996). Social-emotional disturbances in children with learning problems and a 15-point Wechsler Performance IQ deficit. Ph.D. dissertation, Institute for Clinical Social Work, Chicago, IL. Retrieved February 3, 2010, from ProQuest Digital Dissertations database (Publication No. AAT DP11784).

Segal, E. (1994). Mothering a child with attention-deficit hyperactivity disorder: Learned mothering. Ph.D. dissertation, Institute for Clinical Social Work, Chicago, IL. Retrieved February 3, 2010, from ProQuest Digital Dissertations database (Publication No. AAT 9612115).

Semin, G.R., & Cacioppo, J.T. (2008). Grounding social cognition: Synchronization, coordination, and co-regulation. In G.R. Semin & E.R. Smith (eds), *Embodied grounding: Social, cognitive, affective, and neuroscientific approaches* (pp. 119–147). New York: Cambridge University Press.

Sergeant, J.A., Geurts, H., & Oosterlaan, J. (2002). How specific is a deficit of executive functioning for attention-deficit/hyperactivity disorder? *Behavioural Brain Research, 130*, 3–28.

Smith, E.E., & Jonides, J. (1999). Storage and executive processes in the frontal lobes. *Science, 283* (5408), 1657–1661.

Solms, M., & Turnbull, O. (2002). *The brain and the inner world: An introduction to the neuroscience of subjective experience.* New York: Other Press.

Stolorow, R.D. (1992). *Contexts of being: The intersubjective foundations of psychological life.* Hillsdale, NJ: Analytic Press.

Tolpin, M. (2002). Doing psychoanalysis of normal development: Forward edge transferences. In A. Goldberg (ed.), *Progress in self psychology, Vol. 18: Postmodern self psychology* (pp. 167–190). New York: Analytic Press.

Tolpin, M. (2007). The divided self: Shifting an intrapsychic balance the forward edge of a kinship transference: To bleed like everyone else. *Psychoanalytic Inquiry, 27* (1), 50–65.

Torgesen, J.K. (1994). Issues in the assessment of executive function: An information-processing perspective. In G.R. Lyon (ed.), *Frames of reference for the assessment of learning disabilities: New views on measurement issues* (pp. 143–162). Baltimore, MD: Paul H. Brookes.

Torgesen, J.K. (1996). A model of memory from an information processing perspective: The special case of phonological memory. In G.R. Lyon & N.A. Krasnegor (eds), *Attention, memory, and executive function* (pp. 157–184). Baltimore, MD: Paul H. Brookes.

Vygotsky, L. (1986). *Thought and language* (A. Kozulin, Trans.). Cambridge, MA: MIT Press.

Wagner, A.D., Bunge, S.A., & Badre, D. (2004). Cognitive control, semantic memory, and priming: Contribution from prefrontal cortex. In M.S. Gazzaniga (ed.), *The cognitive neurosciences* (Vol. 3, pp. 709–725). Cambridge, MA: MIT Press.

Wong, B.Y.L. (1984). Metacognition and learning disabilities. In T.G. Waller, D. Forrest-Pressley, & E. MacKinon (eds), *Metacognition, cognition and human performance.* New York: Academic Press.

Zummo, J.C. (2007). Measuring the impact of milieu therapy for students excluded from public schools. Ph.D. dissertation, Institute for Clinical Social Work, Chicago, IL. Retrieved February 3, 2010, from ProQuest Digital Dissertations database (Publication No. AAT 3267061).

14 Oppositional defiant and conduct conditions

Amanda N. Barczyk and David W. Springer

Externalizing conditions (also referred to as disruptive behavior conditions) include conduct disorder (CD), oppositional defiant disorder (ODD), and attention deficit/hyperactivity disorder (ADHD) (Stubbe, 2007). A diagnosis of one of these conditions may lead to a diagnosis of another. For example, ADHD has been found to put children at risk for ODD in part due to children with ADHD often being corrected by authority and having difficulty conforming to rules. Due to repeated negative interactions with authority, ODD may develop (Kronenberger & Meyer, 2001). Youth diagnosed with CD are likely to have met the criteria for ODD at an earlier age while CD is likely to predict a diagnosis of antisocial personality disorder in adulthood (Loeber, Lahey, & Thomas, 1991).

This chapter focuses on ODD and CD, two very similar conditions that display similar characteristics such as the breaking of societal norms, disruptive behavior, and disobedient behavior. Adolescents with CD or ODD usually exhibit anger, distrust, problems with authority, family problems, and often rebel against expectations (Kronenberger & Meyer, 2001). CD is the more severe of the two conditions (Burke, Loeber, & Birmaher, 2002). Both conditions are highly prevalent in children (American Psychiatric Association (APA), 2000).

In recent years, significant advances have been made in the treatment of children and adolescents with ODD and CD (Springer & Lynch, 2008). This chapter not only provides an overview of oppositional defiant and conduct conditions but also covers the social worker's role in working with youth with these conditions and in evidenced-based practices including videotape modeling parent program, problem-solving skills training (PSST), parent management training (PMT), functional family therapy (FFT), and family behavior therapy (FBT). Some of these evidence-based practices will be applied to the case illustration of Oneil towards the end of the chapter. For purposes here, Rosen and Proctor's (2002) definition of evidence-based practice (EBP) has been adopted, whereby "practitioners will select interventions on the bases of their empirically demonstrated links to the desired outcomes" (p. 743).

Definitions of oppositional defiant and conduct condition

Conduct disorder first appeared in the *Diagnostic and statistical manual II* (APA, 1968). Twelve years later, the DSM-III (APA, 1980) included oppositional disorder, which was considered the milder version of CD. It was not until the DSM-III-R (APA, 1987) that the disorder named oppositional defiant disorder was identified (Mash & Barkley, 1996). The most current version, DSM-IV-TR, states that the essential diagnostic feature of CD is the persistent and repetitive display of behaviors that violate age-appropriate social rules or norms or violate of the basic rights of others (APA, 2000). These behaviors are categorized into four main groupings. The first is labeled aggressive conduct which refers to causing physical harm or threatening to harm other people or animals (i.e. physical fights, using a weapon to harm another individual, rape, and assault). The second is non-aggressive conduct leading to the damage or loss of property (i.e. deliberately setting a fire or destroying another person's property). The third is theft or deceitfulness (i.e. lying or breaking promises frequently to acquire something or avoid debts, shoplifting, and forgery). The final grouping is serious violations (i.e. staying out late, running away, and truant from school) (APA, 2000).

Two subtypes of conduct disorder have been identified by the DSM-IV-TR, the first being the childhood-onset type. This subtype is defined by having a minimum of one behavior that characterizes conduct disorder before the child is 10 years old. Typically, individuals with childhood-onset type are male, are physically aggressive towards others, have poor peer relationships, have had ODD prior to CD, and usually meet the full criteria for CD before they reach puberty. In addition, some children exhibiting the aggressive behaviors associated with CD have been shown to have low self-esteem (Sadock & Sadock, 2007). These children also often suffer from attention deficit/hyperactivity disorder. These children are also more likely to develop antisocial personality disorder in adulthood when compared to those with adolescent-onset type (APA, 2000).

Adolescents with the adolescent-onset type begin to show at least one of the behaviors characterizing CD after the age of 10. Adolescents over 18 years of age may also be diagnosed with CD if the criteria for antisocial personality disorder are not met. When compared with the childhood-onset type, these individuals are less likely to be aggressive toward others, have poor peer relationships, and develop antisocial personality disorder in adulthood (APA, 2000).

Children and adolescents with ODD or CD exhibit similar symptoms. However, ODD does not include the persistent pattern of behaviors that violate age-appropriate social rules or norms or the violation of the basic rights of others (APA, 2000). The essential diagnostic features of ODD include the persistent pattern of disruptive behaviors that are hostile, disobedient, defiant, and negativistic toward authority figures known by the child or adolescent (APA, 2000). ODD behaviors that may be exhibited by the child include the following: being easily annoyed by others or touchy, defying the rules set by an adult, feeling anger and resentment toward others, losing his or her temper, doing things to annoy others deliberately, blaming others for his or her mistakes or misbehavior, acting in a spiteful or vindictive manner, and arguing with adults (APA, 2000).

ODD is likely to interfere with school performance and the interpersonal relationships of the child resulting in poor grades and few friends. In addition, low self-esteem, depression, frustration, temper outburst and substance use is likely (Sadock & Sadock, 2007). ODD symptoms have also been shown to lead to an increased risk of substance use conditions and risk of developing conduct conditions as the child ages (Sadock & Sadock, 2007). ODD often does not continue into late adolescence. In fact, approximately one-quarter of children and adolescents who are diagnosed with ODD do not continue to meet the diagnostic criteria as they age and while this is the case, the reasoning is unknown (Sadock & Sadock, 2007). However, this may in part be due to the fact that the severity of ODD symptoms increases over time with age and can result in a diagnosis of CD.

As shown, CD and ODD have many similar traits, CD being more severe. Another similarity between CD and ODD is that they are both likely to have comorbidities with other conditions. However, the specific conditions with which they are comorbid do differ. Children and adolescents with severe CD are more vulnerable to comorbid conditions when they are older such as substance use and mood conditions (Sadock & Sadock, 2007). Children with ODD have been found to be comorbid with internalized conditions such as anxiety and depression (Boylan, Vaillancourt, Boyle, & Szatmari, 2007). Social workers should be aware of these comorbidities and keep them in mind while assessing their clients.

In addition, social workers should be aware that while the child or adolescent suffers from having CD or ODD, the individuals around the child including family, friends and teachers are most severely affected and upset by the displayed behaviors of CD and ODD (Sadock & Sadock, 2007; Stubbe, 2007). The behavioral patterns of the child are often displayed in a variety of settings (i.e. school, home and community) and often the child will minimize their own behavior to others. Symptoms of ODD are more often observed when the child or adolescent is interacting with peers or adults they know well and may not occur during clinical examination (APA, 2000). Therefore, it is important for social workers to rely on additional informants including the child's parents and teachers in order to assess the severity and onset of the condition (APA, 2000).

Social workers may also have difficulty when working with a child or adolescent with CD and ODD due to the disruptive behaviors displayed. The child may be provocative, uncooperative and hostile. Often the youth will also deny any problem and will justify their behavior. It is also possible that the child may become angry with the social worker and resent the examination by acting belligerently or withdrawing from the session (Sadock & Sadock, 2007). Social workers should be aware to the likelihood of these behaviors and learn skills and intervention strategies to successfully work with these children and adolescents. Examples of such skills and intervention strategies will be discussed later in this chapter.

Demographics

Approximately between 2 and 16 percent of school-aged children meet the DSM-IV-TR criteria for ODD and/or CD (Stubbe, 2007). Prevalence rates for CD and ODD have been exceptionally high in certain populations. For example, ODD and CD have been found to be two of the most common conditions for male and females in juvenile detention (Teplin, Abram, McCelland, Dulcan, & Mericle, 2002). In addition, when looking at students receiving special educational services for behavioral difficulties, evidence has shown high prevalence rates of ODD (one-half) and CD (one-third) (Déry, Toupin, Pauzé & Verlaan, 2004). The prevalence rate of CD has increased over the past decades and is now one of the most frequently diagnosed conditions for children. Currently, the prevalence of CD ranges from 1 to 10 percent; however, these numbers are widely dependent on the research study (APA, 2000). The prevalence of ODD ranges from 2 to 16 percent (APA, 2000). While ODD has no distinct family patterns, CD is more prevalent in children who have parents diagnosed with antisocial personality disorder and alcohol dependence (Sadock & Sadock, 2007).

In a review of the literature, no conclusions were reached in terms of the prevalence rates of CD or ODD as a function of age. While some researchers found CD increased from middle childhood to adolescents, others found CD had no age difference (Loeber, Burke, Lahey, Winters & Zera, 2000). Some researchers have reported prevalence of CD being higher in adolescents aged 12–16 (7 percent) when compared to children aged 4–11 (4 percent) (Stubbe, 2007). Lahey et al. (2000) found in a household survey of 1,285 youth aged 9 to 17 years that there was no significant age difference in ODD or CD. However, younger children had greater levels of oppositional behavior whereas property and status offenses were more prevalent in adolescents who were older (Lahey et al., 2000). These data are consistent with the DSM-IV-TR findings that number of symptoms exhibited by the child or adolescent tends to increase with age (APA, 2000).

Gender differences have been shown to not emerge for ODD and CD until after age 6 (Loeber et al., 2000). Numerous studies have found CD to be more prevalent in boys than girls; however, the prevalence rates of ODD between genders has been inconsistent (APA, 2000; Lahey, Miller, Gordon & Riley, 1999; Lahey et al., 2000; Lumley, McNeil, Herschell & Bahl,

2002; Stubbe, 2007). The estimated ratios for this difference in prevalence rates of CD in males and females range from 4 to 1, to as high as 12 to 1 (Sadock & Sadock, 2007). For ODD, most studies suggest no sex difference or a slightly higher rate of ODD for boys during middle childhood and adolescence (Lahey et al., 2000; Loeber et al., 2000). Others studies have shown that ODD is more prevalent in males as compared to females before puberty; however, this difference appears to fade after puberty (APA, 2000; U.S. Department of Health and Human Services, 1999).

While the symptoms of CD and ODD are similar between genders, males tend to have more persistent and confrontational behaviors than females (APA, 2000). Researchers have also debated that the higher prevalence of males with CD may in part be due to the CD symptoms not representing the problem behaviors exhibited by females. For example, rather than physical aggression displayed by males, females are more likely to use verbal, indirect and relational aggression such as lying, truancy and substance use (APA, 2000; Loeber et al., 2000).

Studies have shown weak and inconsistent racial and ethnic differences in the rates of individuals with CD and ODD (Lahey et al., 1999). Non-Hispanic Whites have a higher lifetime risk of ODD and CD when compared to Hispanics (Breslau, Aguilar-Gaxiola, Kendler, Su, Williams, & Kessler, 2006; Teplin et al., 2002). When compared to African Americans, non-Hispanic white males have been shown to have higher rates of CD, whereas non-Hispanic white females have been shown to have higher rates of CD and ODD. Hispanic females have also been shown to have higher rates of ODD and CD compared to African Americans (Teplin et al., 2002). In the Hispanic population, Puerto Ricans were found to have the lowest prevalence rate of CD and ODD when compared to mainland Hispanics, African Americans and non-Hispanic Whites (Bird, Canino, Davies, Zhang, Ramirez, & Lahey, 2001). More rigorous studies are needed to support this evidence; however, these findings show that overall non-Hispanic Whites have the highest prevalence rates of these disruptive conditions followed by Hispanics. African Americans have been found to have the lowest risk of developing CD or ODD.

Population

Disruptive behavioral conditions are considered stable, not transient. ODD is often considered a precursor to CD and CD can evolve into antisocial personality disorder in adulthood. However, this may not be the case in girls given that late onset of CD is more common in girls than boys (Burke et al., 2002). As a child matures, a major shift occurs in the manifestation of the disruptive behavior they display (Burke et al., 2002). Typically, at a younger age the less severe behaviors emerge such as lying and shoplifting. As the youth ages, more severe behaviors may emerge such as burglary. Severe behaviors such as rape and assault are usually the last to emerge (APA, 2000). While some youth exhibit the most severe disruptive behaviors of CD at an early age, typically the severity of their behaviors develops over time (APA, 2000). However, one study found that while non-aggressive conduct such as status violations increased as the child or adolescent grew older, aggressive symptoms such as physical fights decreased (Maughan, Rowe, Messer, Goodman, & Meltzer, 2004).

As ODD and CD usually go into remission or develop into the more serious diagnosis of antisocial personality disorder at approximately 18 years of age, the developmental course for these conditions is brief. While the onset of ODD may occur as early as 3 years of age, it often occurs before the age of 8 and typically no later than the child's early adolescence (APA, 2000; Sadock & Sadock, 2007). The onset is usual gradual, with the disruptive behaviors of ODD occurring at home and then over time occurring in other settings. It may take a few months or even years for the onset to occur. ODD will then typically develop into CD; however, this is not always the case and it may remit as the child ages (APA, 2000).

The onset of CD in a child may take place as early as the child's preschool years. However, typically the more significant disruptive behaviors will emerge at some time between middle childhood and middle adolescence. After age 16, it is rare for the onset of CD to occur (APA, 2000). On average, boys meet the diagnostic criteria for CD by 10 to 12 years of age, while girls often meet the diagnostic criteria at an older age, between 14 and 16 years (Sadock & Sadock, 2007). For many children, CD will remit during adulthood. However, adults who continue to display disruptive behaviors likely meet the criteria for antisocial personality disorder. The earlier the onset, the more likely the child will develop antisocial personality disorder and substance-related disorders in adulthood (APA, 2000).

While less than half of children diagnosed with CD continue to suffer with CD through adulthood, 80 percent of adults who had CD as a child are diagnosed with some type of psychiatric condition in adulthood (Stubbe, 2007). Adults diagnosed with CD as a child have been shown to demonstrate poorer physical health, poorer social relationships and marital relationships, lower occupational and academic achievement and higher rates of criminality, substance abuse and psychiatric conditions than their non-diagnosed peers (Stubbe, 2007).

Etiological factors – such as school, peer, and familial factors – may play a role in the development of CD and ODD (Finch, Nelson, & Hart, 2006; Pardini & Lochman, 2006; Searight, Rottnek, & Abby, 2001). For example, an inadequate school environment (e.g., poor facilities/workspace, infrequent use of positive feedback from the teacher, unavailability of staff, including teachers, to deal with difficulties of the student) have been found to place youth at greater risk of CD or ODD (Stubbe, 2007). In terms of peer factors, children who have CD have been found to be rejected more by their peers (Finch et al., 2006). In addition, one study found that externalizing problems were predicted by children who befriended more aggressive peers. However, if a child was liked by aggressive peers, it did not predict the development of externalizing problems (Mrug, Hoza, & Bukowski, 2004).

Various parenting and familial factors have been shown to be substantially influential to the development of CD and ODD (Holmes, Slaughter, & Kashani, 2001; Loeber & Stouthamer-Loeber, 1986; Pardini & Lochman, 2006). Parental neglect, abuse (Finch et al., 2006; Widom, 1989), criminality, and absence have all been reported as being related to conduct problems (Loeber & Stouthamer-Loeber, 1986). In a meta-analysis of the relationship between familial factors and conduct problems/delinquency in juveniles, parental rejection, the lack of parental supervision, and low parent-child involvement (e.g., intimate communication, sharing of activities, confiding) were among the highest predictors of conduct problems and delinquency (Loeber & Stouthamer-Loeber, 1986).

Poor parental physical and mental health has also been shown to relate to children's conduct problems (Loeber & Stouthamer-Loeber, 1986). One study of clinic-referred boys found high rates of substance abuse and antisocial personality disorder in the parents of children with CD and ODD, with those who had ODD showing the highest rates (Frick, Lahey, Loeber, Stouthamer-Loeber, Christ, & Hanson, 1992).

Marital relations are yet another factor associated with conduct problems (Loeber & Stouthamer-Loeber, 1986). Jouriles, Murphy, and O'Leary (1989) found that marital aggression was related to the development of conduct conditions and clinical levels of problematic behavior in children.

Other parental factors, including the disciplining styles of the parent, also relate to conduct problems. Strict parents, as well as those who have erratic and lax discipline styles, have been found to be related to the development of conduct problems (Loeber & Stouthamer-Loeber, 1986). Moreover, Rey and Plapp (1990) found that adolescents with CD or ODD perceived their parent as less caring and more overprotective.

Mental health care disparities

While prevalence rates have shown that boys are more likely to have the CD diagnosis than girls, this difference may be due to the diagnostic patterns of service providers. Girls are more likely to receive the ODD diagnosis; boys typically are diagnosed with CD (Sadock & Sadock, 2007). As previously mentioned, the disruptive behaviors displayed by girls and boys differ, with girls exhibiting more indirect and relational aggression and boys exhibiting more physical aggression (APA, 2000; Loeber et al., 2000). However, the severity and impact relational aggression has on a female victim may be just as traumatizing as physical aggression would be for a male victim. While this is unknown, possibly CD is being under-diagnosed in females and, therefore, undertreated.

When looking at the environment the child or adolescent lives in, various other disparities are apparent. The risk for CD and ODD has been consistently found to be higher among children from lower income families. In addition, the prevalence of disruptive behavioral conditions, including CD and ODD, has also been found to be related to other measures of socioeconomic status. For example, a diagnosis of CD or ODD has been shown to be inversely related to parental occupational status, parental employment and parental education (Lahey et al., 1999; Loeber et al., 2000). Conduct conditions may also be predicted by the lack of a supportive social network or participation in positive community activities (Sadock & Sadock, 2007).

Studies have shown neighborhood characteristics (e.g., neighborhood crime rates, use of public assistance, mean income, quality of housing, safety and rates of unemployment) to be associated with CD behaviors but not ODD behaviors (Lahey et al., 1999). The prevalence of CD may be highest in inner-city neighborhoods considered to be the worst (Loeber et al., 2000). However, disadvantaged and advantaged inner-city neighborhood comparisons have not been sufficiently documented and mixed results have been found for CD and ODD prevalence differences in urban and rural areas (APA, 2000; Lahey et al., 1999; Loeber et al., 2000).

While differences have been noted, service providers should consider the social and economic context of the disruptive behaviors. Understanding the environment the child or adolescent grew up in may help with both deciding the suitable diagnosis and choosing the most effective services for the individual. For example, children and adolescents from impoverished areas, high-crime areas, or those that have emigrated from a country at war may have exhibited aggressive behaviors as a means of survival (APA, 2000). Therefore, while the child or adolescent's behaviors fit the DSM-IV-TR criteria, a diagnosis of CD or ODD may be inappropriate.

Social work programs and social work roles

Social workers have important and unique roles in helping children with CD or ODD. Not only are social workers providing services to the youth and their family, but also they must advocate for their clients. Given the variety of negative behaviors that youth with these disruptive conditions can display such as lying, fighting, destroying property, or defying rules (APA, 2000), teachers, community members, and even their parents may begin to label these youth as delinquent or "bad." If these youth are labeled as delinquent, the adults in their lives are less likely to assist them in receiving the proper help, believing them to be a "lost cause." Teachers are also likely to treat these youth differently, holding lower standards of achievement and ultimately leading the youth to receive a poorer education. Therefore, social workers must advocate for their clients, helping them to negotiate their families, schools and communities.

Engaging these youth in a professional relationship requires advanced practice skills. As will be discussed in the case illustration below, professionals must obtain thorough assessments of the youth, including a biopsychological interview, in order to acquire information about the youth's background. The social worker must engage the youth and his/her family in order to implement the most beneficial individualized services. Including the parents and the children in the intervention is crucial, as a review of the literature found this to result in a lasting improvement in the behavioral problems of children (Farmer, Compton, Burns, & Robertson, 2002).

Detailed information about the specific evidence-based intervention strategies that can be effectively utilized by social workers is discussed below.

Professional methods and interventions

Helping children and adolescents with oppositional defiant and conduct conditions can be challenging, even for the most seasoned clinician. Fortunately, in recent years, significant advances in psychosocial treatments have been made in helping youth with disruptive behavior conditions, such as ODD and CD. Some of these evidence-based practices are applied in the case example of Oneil, presented a little later in this chapter. First, some of the interventions with the strongest evidence-base supporting their effectiveness in helping youth with ODD and CD are presented below.

Among the effective interventions for children with conduct problems, two have been found to be "well-established," according to the Division 12 (Clinical Psychology) Task Force on Promotion and Dissemination of Psychological Procedures (Brestan & Eyberg, 1998). One of these is the *Incredible Years Parents, Teachers and Children's Training* series developed by Webster-Stratton, which is based on a trained leader using videotape modeling to trigger group discussion. The second well-established approach is parent-training programs based on Patterson and Gullion's (1968) manual *Living with children* (Alexander & Parsons, 1973; Bernal, Klinnert, & Schultz, 1980; Wiltz & Patterson, 1974).

First we review Webster-Stratton's approach, which is geared toward helping younger oppositional youth. This will be followed by an overview of other approaches with a strong evidence-base supporting their effectiveness in treating conduct-disordered youth, including problem-solving skills training (PSST), parent management training (PMT), functional family therapy (FFT), and family behavior therapy (FBT). It is worth noting that all of the interventions reviewed in this chapter and supported by outcome research, with the exception of PSST, are heavily family-oriented in their approach.

Webster-Stratton's Videotape Modeling Parent Program, part of the *Incredible Years* training series, was developed to address parent, family, child, and school risk factors related to childhood conduct conditions. The series is a result of Webster-Stratton's own research, which suggested that comprehensive videotape training methods are effective interventions for early-onset ODD/CD. The training series includes the *Incredible Years Parent Interventions*, the *Incredible Years Teacher Training Intervention*, and the *Incredible Years Child Training Intervention*, each of which relies on performance training methods, including videotape modeling, role play, practice activities, and live therapist feedback (Webster-Stratton & Reid, 2003b).

The parent component aims to promote competencies and strengthen families by increasing positive parenting skills, teaching positive discipline strategies, improving problem solving, and increasing family supports and collaboration, to name a few. The teacher component of the training series aims to promote teacher competencies and strengthen home–school relationships by increasing effective classroom management skills, increasing teachers' use of effective discipline and collaboration with parents, and increasing teachers' abilities in the areas of social skills, anger management, and problem solving. The child component aims to strengthen children's social and play skills, increase effective problem-solving strategies and emotional awareness, boost academic success, reduce defiance and aggression, and increase self-esteem.

Webster-Stratton and Reid (2003b) assert that the most proactive and powerful approach to the problem of escalating aggression in young children is to offer their programs using a school-based prevention/early intervention model designed to strengthen *all* children's social and emotional competence. Their reasons are threefold: first, offering interventions in schools makes programs more accessible to families and eliminates some of the barriers (i.e., transportation) typically encountered with services offered in traditional mental health settings; second, offering interventions in schools integrates programs before children's common behavior problems escalate to the point of needing intense clinical intervention; and third, offering a social and emotional curriculum such as the Dinosaur School program to an entire class is less stigmatizing than a "pullout" group and is more likely to produce sustained effects across settings and time.

There are a number of supporting randomized control group studies using the program as a treatment program for parents of children ages 3 to 8 years with conduct problems and as a prevention program for high-risk families (see studies by Reid, Webster-Stratton, & Baydar, 2004; Reid, Webster-Stratton, & Hammond, 2003; Spaccarelli, Cotler, & Penman, 1992; Webster-Stratton, 1984, 1990, 1994, 1998; Webster-Stratton, Kolpacoff, & Hollinsworth, 1988; Webster-Stratton, Reid, & Hammond, 2001a).

Problem-solving skills training (PSST) (Spivak & Schure, 1974) is a cognitively based intervention that has been used to treat aggressive and antisocial youth (Kazdin, 1994). The problem-solving process involves helping clients learn how to produce a variety of potentially effective responses when faced with problem situations. Regardless of the specific problem-solving model used, the primary focus is on addressing the thought process to help adolescents address deficiencies and distortions in their approach to interpersonal situations (Kazdin, 1994). A variety of techniques are used, including didactic teaching, practice, modeling, role-playing, feedback, social reinforcement, and therapeutic games (Kronenberger & Meyer, 2001). The problem-solving approach typically includes five steps for the practitioner and client to address: (1) defining the problem; (2) brainstorming; (3) evaluating the alternatives; (4) choosing and implementing an alternative; and (5) evaluating the implemented option (Corcoran & Springer, 2005; Kazdin, 1994).

Several randomized clinical trials have demonstrated the effectiveness of PSST with impulsive, aggressive, and conduct-disordered youth (Baer & Nietzel, 1991; Durlak, Furhman, & Lampman, 1991; Kazdin, 2000, 2002). Webster-Stratton and colleagues have developed a small-group treatment program that teaches problem solving, anger management, and social skills for children ages 4 to 8 years, and two randomized control group studies demonstrate the efficacy of this treatment program (Webster-Stratton & Hammond, 1997; Webster-Stratton & Reid, 2003a; Webster-Stratton, Reid, & Hammond, 2001b; Webster-Stratton, Reid, & Hammond, 2004). Problem-solving training produces significant reductions in conduct symptoms and improvements in pro-social behavior among antisocial youth.

Parent management training (PMT) is a summary term that describes a therapeutic strategy in which parents are trained to use skills for managing their child's problem behavior (Kazdin, 1997), such as effective command-giving, setting up reinforcement systems, and using punishment, including taking away privileges and assigning extra chores. While PMT programs may differ in focus and therapeutic strategies used, they all share the common goal of enhancing parental control over children's behavior (Barkley, 1987; Cavell, 2000; Eyberg, 1988; Forehand & McMahon, 1981; Patterson, Reid, Jones, & Conger, 1975; Webster-Stratton & Reid, 2003a).

To date, parent management training is the best treatment for youth with oppositional defiant condition, such as Oneil's brother Alex (see case example below). Yet, studies examining the effectiveness of PMT with adolescents are equivocal, with some studies suggesting that adolescents respond less well to PMT than do their younger counterparts (Dishion & Patterson, 1992; Kazdin, 2002).

Functional family therapy (FFT) (Alexander & Parsons, 1973, 1982), grounded in learning theory, is an integrative approach that relies on systems, behavioral, and cognitive views of functioning. Clinical problems are conceptualized in terms of the function that they serve for the family system and for the individual client. The goal of treatment "is the achievement of a change in patterns of interaction and communication, in a manner that engenders adaptive family functioning" (Fonagy, Target, Cottrell, Phillips, & Kurtz, 2002, p. 158).

FFT has clinically significant and lasting effects on juvenile recidivism. In nine studies conducted on FFT between 1973 and 1997, a 25 percent to 80 percent improvement was found in recidivism, out-of-home placement, or future offending by siblings of the treated youth (Fonagy et al., 2002).

Family behavior therapy (FBT) was developed to treat substance-abusing clients in the early 1990s by Nathan Azrin, Brad Donohue, and their colleagues (Azrin, Donohue, Teichner, Crum, Howell, & DeCato, 2001; Donohue, Allen, & LaPota, 2009). FBT includes more than 20 behavioral interventions delivered over the course of about 6 months, and is capable of addressing a wide array of problem behaviors associated with, and including, substance abuse and dependence. Along these lines, FBT intervention plans often target coexisting mood, anxiety and conduct conditions.

FBT was the first comprehensive behavioral therapy to demonstrate positive outcomes in adolescent drug abusers utilizing controlled methodology and objective biological measures of drug use (see National Institute on Drug Abuse, 1998). Moreover, Bender, Springer, and Kim (2006) systematically reviewed randomized clinical trials of interventions for dually diagnosed adolescents. Results examining both between-group effect sizes and within-group changes indicated the efficacy of several treatment modalities in improving specific aspects of social, emotional, learning needs, but the findings from their meta-analysis highlighted individual cognitive problem-solving therapy (presented above) and family behavior therapy as showing large effect sizes across externalizing, internalizing, and substance abuse outcomes in dually diagnosed youth. In short, FBT would be just right for a dually diagnosed client like Oneil, who we present below.

Illustration and discussion

Here, we present a case exemplar of a social worker who is helping a court-referred dually diagnosed adolescent, Oneil, and his family. We use the case of Oneil to help the reader work through how one might select the appropriate intervention for a client presenting with multiple problems. At the end of the case, we offer our own observations about clinical- and policy-related themes that emerge in the case, and that warrant broader consideration by practitioners and policy makers. We begin with a brief case description.

Oneil is a 15-year-old Cuban male, recently arrested and taken to a local juvenile assessment center for truancy, possession of marijuana, and busting mailboxes in his neighborhood with a baseball bat. On one occasion, he threatened a youth at school with a tire-iron. This was Oneil's second time being arrested in six months; he was adjudicated through the juvenile court six months ago for breaking into a neighbor's house and vandalizing their property. Because this was Oneil's second arrest in the last six months, the judge extended his probation and required Oneil to receive counseling and assured him that if he was arrested again he would be sentenced to a juvenile hall or residential treatment. Oneil lives with his mother, three brothers, and one sister. Oneil never met his biological father and was physically abused by his stepfather, who was stabbed to death three years ago in a bar fight. Oneil has consistently been getting into trouble since the age of 12 years. He ran away from home twice, each time for one week, when he was 12 and 13. Several of Oneil's close friends have been arrested for drug possession, truancy, robbery, or assault. Oneil often disrespects his mother by cursing at her and disobeying her rules. He shows little remorse for this behavior. Oneil's IQ falls within the normal range and his medical history is uncomplicated. It is worth noting that Oneil's mom did not have reliable transportation (the car was often not running well), that the family lived in an impoverished inner-city neighborhood that was marked by violence, and that Oneil's mom had tried in the past to access services for Oneil but was unsuccessful in her attempt to navigate the county's complex service system.

The first phase of helping is a thorough *assessment,* and a *biopsychosocial history* often serves as the cornerstone of a solid treatment plan (Springer & Bender, 2009). During their initial session together, the social worker conducted a complete biopsychosocial assessment with Oneil and his family (for a more detailed exposition of the biopsychosocial interview, see, for example, Austrian, 2002; Springer & Tripodi, 2009).

Oneil was also referred for psychological testing as part of the juvenile court's assessment process. After ruling out medical causes, and based upon the collective results of the bio-psychosocial assessment, standardized scales, and psychological testing the social worker used the DSM-IV-TR (APA, 2000) to diagnose Oneil as follows: Axis I. 312.82 (Conduct Disorder, Adolescent-Onset Type, Moderate); Alcohol Abuse 305.20 (Cannabis Abuse); Axis II. V71.09 (No diagnosis); Axis III. (None) Axis IV. V61.20 (Parent-Child Relational Problem); V62.3 (Academic Problems; Involvement with juvenile justice system).

Now that the initial assessment had been conducted, the social worker began working collaboratively with Oneil and his mother to decide the best course of action. Through a search of the literature and key databases (see list of Web resources and References at the end of this chapter), the social worker was able to determine that interventions with the strongest evidence-base (as demonstrated in meta-analyses and randomized controlled clinical trials) for helping children and adolescents with conduct conditions include those reviewed earlier in this chapter: videotape modeling, parent management training (PMT), cognitive problem-solving skills training (PSST), and functional family therapy (FFT) (Baer & Nietzel, 1991; Brestan & Eyberg, 1998; Durlak, Furhman, & Lampman, 1991; Fonagy et al., 2002; Hanish, Tolan, & Guerra, 1996; Henggeler, Schoenwald, Borduin, Rowland, & Cunningham, 1998; Kazdin, 2002). Moreover, family behavior therapy (FBT) was found to be especially effective for adolescents with comorbid conditions, such as substance abuse and conduct conditions (Bender et al., 2006).

The social worker shared as much as she knew about all of these approaches back with Oneil and his mother, with the collaborative decision-making taking place as follows. Given that Oneil was 15 years old, that the outcome findings on PMT with adolescents were equivocal, and that his pattern of behavior was rather entrenched, the social worker and Oneil's mother decided against PMT as a primary service option for Oneil. However, given that Oneil's 6-year-old brother, Alex, had been diagnosed with oppositional defiant disorder, the social worker and mother agreed that she would benefit from PMT. Oneil's intervention package included both PSST and FBT, as well as group therapy. To help Oneil's mother and brother Alex, PMT was also part of the treatment plan. Nevertheless, here we focus on Oneil to illustrate the treatment of a conduct-disordered youth. Recall that Oneil presented with both conduct disorder and with substance (alcohol and marijuana) use. Given its effectiveness with dually diagnosed adolescents, the social worker used FBT techniques to enable Oneil and his mother to reduce substance use and maintain behavioral/ cognitive changes. Given their car troubles, FBT was also chosen because it promotes home-based therapy, especially when children are involved (Donohue et al., 2009).

In the first two sessions, as is common with FBT, a structured program orientation was completed and behavioral goals established, primarily focused on the elimination and management of cues to substance use and problematic behavior. Additionally, the social worker and Oneil's mom focused on parenting and home safety skills training. Treatment goals were reviewed at the start of each session. Moreover, the social worker modeled all of the intervention skills and engaged Oneil's mom in rehearsing these skills. They started with easy scenarios first, and increased the difficulty of the scenarios over the course of their work.

The social worker and Oneil's family agreed to implement the individualized treatment plan that they collaboratively developed, change the concerning behavior, and improve relational skills such as communication and parenting. The sessions were structured, which allowed the social worker to implement the service plan effectively.

During individual sessions (with Oneil) and family sessions, techniques commonly used in PSST (e.g., role-playing, feedback, and *in-vivo* practice) were used to help Oneil generate alternative solutions to interpersonal problems that triggered his alcohol and drug use. PSST was used to help Oneil think of alternatives to getting into fights at school and arguments with his mom. To do this, the social worker and Oneil used the five self-statements in problem solving:

1 What am I supposed to do?
2 I have to look at all my possibilities.
3 I'd better concentrate and focus in.
4 I need to make a choice.
5 I did a good job (or) Oh, I made a mistake.

The social worker engaged Oneil in multiple role-plays, repeatedly practicing how he might respond to perceived provocation using these five self-statements as a guide. The social worker effusively praised Oneil's quick recall of the self-statements and his efforts to use a "stop and think" technique that he modeled and prompted. Additionally, they practiced how to respond to mistakes and failure without exploding at others or destroying property. Oneil's mother was instructed to praise and reward his efforts to avoid conflicts and employ the problem-solving steps in everyday situations at home. As counseling progressed, Oneil was encouraged to use the steps in increasingly more difficult and clinically relevant, real-life situations (Kazdin, 2003).

As the end of treatment neared, the social worker also implemented effective relapse prevention techniques (e.g., role-playing, discussing how to cope with emotions without using drugs, and how to socialize and have fun while staying sober) when Oneil's substance use significantly declined. The social worker also served as a family case manager, helping the family find resources such as Alcoholics Anonymous (AA), al-anon, al-ateen, and the National Alliance for the Mentally Ill (NAMI).

As termination approached, the social worker introduced longer intervals between sessions, treating the final sessions as once-a-month maintenance sessions where the family reported on how things were going. Oneil and his family made considerable progress on their treatment goals, as evidenced across several areas of functioning (e.g., improved grades in school, producing clean urinalyses as part of his probation, not being rearrested).

Oneil's progress was also *monitored* using the Child and Adolescent Functional Assessment Scale (CAFAS: Hodges, 2000), a standardized scale that is used to measure the degree of impairment in youth. It is a clinician-rated measure that covers eight areas of functioning: school/work; home; community; behavior toward others; moods/emotions; self-harmful behavior; substance use; and thinking. The adolescent's level of impairment in functioning in each of these eight domains is scored as severe (score of 30), moderate (20), mild (10), or minimal (0). Additionally, an overall score can be computed. These scores were graphed on a one-page scoring sheet that provided Oneil with a profile of his functioning. The CAFAS was completed by the social worker at intake and termination, and the scores from the CAFAS demonstrated an overall improvement in Oneil's level of functioning.

Additionally, the *timeline follow-back* (TLFB) procedure (Sobell & Sobell, 1992) was used to assess Oneil's substance abuse history (his primary drugs of choice were alcohol and marijuana). This procedure, a structured interview technique that samples a specific period of time, may offer the most sensitive assessment for adolescent substance abusers (Leccese & Waldron, 1994). A monthly calendar and memory anchor points were used to help Oneil reconstruct daily use during the past month.

Finally, the Family Environment Scale (FES: Moos & Moos, 1984) was used to measure family conflict and family cohesion. This assessment provided the social worker with a sense of family functioning in terms of family conflict and cohesion, family support, and problem behaviors exhibited by Oneil and Alex.

Standardized scales such as the CAFAS, TLFB, and FES should be used to guide and monitor client functioning, and to evaluate the effectiveness of interventions (Springer & Tripodi, 2009).

Of course, there are a number of important *assessment and intervention themes* that we could address here, as cases like Oneil's are rich with complexity and opportunity for change. Nevertheless, we focus on four important issues.

First, it is a truism that *families should play a critical role* in a juvenile offender's treatment much like Oneil's family did. Research has demonstrated that involving families in the treatment of young offenders decreases the likelihood of further criminal behavior and reduces adolescent incarceration rates. In order to systematically analyze the literature on the effects of including family counseling to services for young offenders, Latimer (2001) conducted a meta-analysis with 35 experimental research studies. Compared to young offender programs that do not include family involvement, Latimer (2001) found that family interventions significantly reduce the recidivism rate of young offenders.

There are many forms of family therapy from which to choose. For example, functional family therapy (FFT), presented earlier in this chapter, has been found to reduce a juvenile's recidivism rates by 15.9 percent (Aos, Miller, & Drake, 2006).

Second, Oneil, like many ODD adolescents, presents with multiple problems and comorbid conditions. The terms *comorbid disorders* and *coexisting disorders* are frequently used interchangeably to describe adolescents who have two or more coexisting diagnoses on Axis I or Axis II of the DSM-IV-TR (APA, 2000), while the term *dual diagnosis* is often reserved to refer to clients with at least one Axis I diagnosis and a substance abuse problem. Findings from the National Comorbidity Study indicate that 41 to 65 percent of individuals with substance abuse conditions also meet criteria for a mental disorder, and approximately 43 to 51 percent of those with mental disorders are diagnosed with a substance use condition (Kessler, Berglund, Demler, Jin, Merikangas, & Walters, 2005; Tripodi, Kim, & DiNitto, 2006). Roberts and Corcoran (2005) assert that dually diagnosed adolescents are in fact not a special subpopulation of adolescents but the norm. Given the prevalence of coexisting conditions in clinical settings and the seriousness of making false-positive or false-negative diagnoses, social work practitioners must assess for the presence of comorbid conditions in a deliberate manner; otherwise, we run the risk of letting clients like Oneil and his brother Alex fall through the cracks of service delivery.

Third, when presenting with multiple needs and problems (legal, school, intrapersonal, interpersonal, substance use, familial), clients like Oneil and his family easily fall through the cracks of service delivery. There has been an amplified call, especially since the late 1990s, for agencies to engage in "boundary-spanning" activities. Basically, boundary-spanning activities are those which bridge "turf" issues to enable organizations to work together toward a common goal (in this case, treating Oneil and his family) (Radin, 1996; Springer, Stokes Sharp, & Foy, 2000). This is one of the hallmark characteristics of the system-of-care approach, now widely adopted in communities across the country. As a natural extension of the movement started under the Child and Adolescent Service System Program (VASSP) initiated in 1984 by the National Institute of Mental

Health (NIMH), many communities across the states have received large pots of federal funding through the Substance Abuse and Mental Health Services Administration (SAMHSA), Center for Mental Health Services (CMHS) to implement a community-based, wraparound approach to service delivery within a system-of-care. In this approach, practitioners gather together many community supports that interact with the youth to determine the best ways to support a youth to adopt pro-social behaviors (Aguilar & Springer, 2008; Flash, 2003). In short, a system-of-care makes it easier for families like Oneil's to navigate the mental health care system, because once they enter the system through one agency (e.g., juvenile court), they should have more ready access to other services delivered through other agencies that are a part of that system-of-care. When this is not the case, it is critical that we continue to build community action structures that allow for ease of access to needed care. In other words, when communities do not have a structure that allows local citizens to identify health care/mental health needs and to make decisions relevant to these issues, action structures must be developed or revitalized (Poole, 1997). Action structures provide channels through which responsible citizens can take part in community health and mental health decision-making through local planning and voluntary social action (Springer et al., 2000).

Fourth, Oneil and his family, like many others, are affected by many of the social and economic based *mental health care disparities* discussed earlier in this chapter. For example, Oneil and his siblings were at a higher risk of CD and ODD due to their low socioeconomic status and the fact that they lived in an inner-city neighborhood (Lahey et al., 1999; Loeber et al., 2000).

A variety of parental factors may have also contributed to Oneil's CD diagnosis. For example, research has shown that parents who use severe physical and verbal aggression may lead to their child developing similar aggressive behaviors. A chaotic home life, severe parental disharmony, negligence, child abuse and parental pathology (including psychotic conditions) may also contribute (Sadock & Sadock, 2007). Therefore, the physical abuse Oneil experienced from his stepfather was likely a contributing factor to his disruptive behavior. This demonstrates the importance of conducting thorough assessments in order for social workers to be informed of the various mental health care disparities their clients, like Oneil and his family, have faced.

Conclusion

Conduct disorder and oppositional defiant disorder though different conditions have many similar characteristics including similar disruptive behaviors. In addition, CD and ODD are both challenging conditions. However, recently, some evidence-based interventions are available for practitioners to utilize to effectively help youth with these conditions.

While there is no one approach that can assist all individuals with CD or ODD, social workers have several options from this chapter to reference when selecting the best treatment approach for their clients. Webster-Stratton's Videotaped Modeling Parent Program has a number of randomized control trials supporting its efficacy for parents of children with conduct problems aged 3 to 8 years old and its efficacy as a prevention program for high-risk families. Several randomized clinical trials show problem-solving skills training's effectiveness with conduct-disordered youth. For youth with ODD, parent management training is currently the best option, however, it has not shown to be as effective with adolescents. Functional family therapy has shown lasting clinically significant effects on juvenile recidivism. Finally, family behavioral therapy appears effective for dually diagnosed clients such as Oneil in the case illustration. Social workers should work with the parents and client in order to assess the appropriate evidence-based intervention.

Given the multiple roles that social workers play (i.e. advocate, case manager, therapist), social workers should assist youth with ODD and CD in a variety of ways. Social workers must advocate for youth with ODD or CD to receive assistance. Social workers need to guide the youth and their parents through service delivery to ensure they do not fall through the cracks of the system. Finally, social workers must implement the appropriate evidence-based practices by working with the youth and their parents in order to reduce the disruptive behaviors presented by the youth.

Web resources

American Academy of Child and Adolescent Psychiatry (AACAP)
www.aacap.org

Center for the Study and Prevention of Violence (CSPV)
www.colorado.edu/cspv/blueprints

Children's Mental Health Facts: Children and Adolescents with Conduct Disorder
www.mentalhealth.samhsa.gov/publications/allpubs/Ca-0010/default.asp

ConductDisorders.com
www.conductdisorders.com

Family Behavior Therapy
www.unlv.edu/centers/achievement/index.html

Helping America's Youth
www.guide.helpingamericasyouth.gov/programtool-ap.cfm

National Center for Mental Health and Juvenile Justice (NCMHJJ)
www.ncmhjj.com

National Guideline Clearinghouse: "Practice parameter for the assessment and treatment of children and adolescents with oppositional defiant disorder"
www.guideline.gov/summary/summary.aspx?ss=15&doc_id=10550&nbr=5513

National Youth Violence Prevention Resource Center
www.safeyouth.org/scripts/index.asp

Office of Juvenile Justice and Delinquency Prevention (OJJDP)
www.ojjdp.ncjrs.org

Prevention of Youth Violence
www.cdc.gov/ncipc/dvp/bestpractices/chapter2a.pdf

Promising Practices Network on Children, Families, and Communities
www.promisingpractices.net/programs.asp

Report of the Surgeon General on Youth Violence
www.surgeongeneral.gov/library/youthviolence

Substance Abuse and Mental Health Services Administration (SAMHSA)
www.samhsa.gov/

World Health Organization Report on Violence
www.who.int/violence_injury_prevention/violence/world_report/en/index.html

References

Aguilar, J.P., & Springer, D.W. (2008). Assessment, classification, and treatment with juvenile delinquents. In A.R. Roberts (ed.), *Correctional counseling and treatment* (pp. 25–40). Upper Saddle River, NJ: Prentice Hall.

American Psychiatric Association (APA). (1968). *Diagnostic and statistical manual of mental disorders* (2nd ed.). Washington, DC: APA.

American Psychiatric Association (APA). (1980). *Diagnostic and statistical manual of mental disorders* (3rd ed.). Washington, DC: APA.

American Psychiatric Association (APA). (1987). *Diagnostic and statistical manual of mental disorders* (3rd ed., revised). Washington, DC: APA.

American Psychiatric Association (2000). *Diagnostic and statistical manual of mental disorders* (4th ed., text revision). Washington, DC: APA.

Alexander, J.F., & Parsons, B.V. (1973). Short-term behavioral intervention with delinquents: Impact on family process and recidivism. *Journal of Abnormal Psychology, 81*, 219–225.

Alexander, J.F., & Parsons, B.V. (1982). *Functional family therapy.* Monterey, CA: Brooks/Cole.

Aos, S., Miller, M., & Drake, E. (2006). *Evidence-based public policy options to reduce future prison construction, criminal justice costs, and crime rates.* Olympia, WA: Washington State Institute for Public Policy. Retrieved July 5, 2007, from www.wsipp.wa.gov/rptfiles/06-10-1201.pdf

Austrian, S.G. (2002). Guidelines for conducting a biopsychosocial assessment. In A.R. Roberts & G.J. Greene (eds), *Social workers' desk reference* (pp. 204–208). New York: Oxford University Press.

Azrin, N.H., Donohue, B., Teichner, G.A., Crum, T., Howell, J., & DeCato, L.A. (2001). A controlled evaluation and description of individual-cognitive problem solving and family-behavioral therapies in dually-diagnosed conduct disordered and substance-dependent youth. *Journal of Child and Adolescent Substance Abuse, 11* (1), 1–22.

Baer, R.A., & Nietzel, M.T. (1991). Cognitive and behavioral treatment of impulsivity in children: A meta-analytic review of the outcome literature. *Journal of Clinical Child Psychology, 20*, 400–412.

Barkley, R.A. (1987). *Defiant children: A clinician's manual for parent training.* New York: Guilford Press.

Bender, K., Springer, D.W., & Kim, J.S. (2006). Treatment effectiveness with dually diagnosed adolescents: A systematic review. *Brief Treatment and Crisis Intervention, 6* (3), 177–205.

Bernal, M.E., Klinnert, M.D., & Schultz, L.A. (1980). Outcome evaluation of behavioral parent training and client-centered parent counseling for children with conduct problems. *Journal of Applied Behavior Analysis, 13*, 677–691.

Bird, H., Canino, G., Davies, M., Zhang, H., Ramirez, R., & Lahey, B. (2001). Prevalence and correlates of antisocial behaviors among three ethnic groups. *Journal of Abnormal Child Psychology, 29* (6), 465–478.

Boylan, K., Vaillancourt, T., Boyle, M., & Szatmari, P. (2007). Comorbidity of internalizing disorders in children with oppositional defiant disorder. *European Child and Adolescent Psychiatry, 16* (8), 484–494.

Breslau, J., Aguilar-Gaxiola, S., Kendler, K., Su, M., Williams, D., & Kessler, R. (2006). Specifying race-ethnic differences in risk for psychiatric disorder in a USA national sample. *Psychological Medicine, 36* (1), 57–68.

Brestan, E.V., & Eyberg, S.M. (1998). Effective psychosocial treatments of conduct-disordered children and adolescents: 29 years, 82 studies, and 5,272 kids. *Journal of Clinical Child Psychology, 27* (2), 180–189.

Burke, J.D., Loeber, R. & Birmaher, B. (2002). Oppositional defiant disorder and conduct disorder: A review of the past 10 years, part II. *Journal of the American Academy of Child and Adolescent Psychiatry, 41* (11), 1275–1293.

Cavell, T.A. (2000). *Working with parents of aggressive children: A practitioner's guide.* Washington, DC: American Psychological Association.

Corcoran, J. & Springer, D. (2005). Work with adolescent conduct problems. In J. Corcoran (ed.), *Building strengths and skills: A collaborative approach to working with clients.* London: Oxford Press.

Déry, M., Toupin, J., Pauzé, R., & Verlaan, P. (2004). Frequency of mental health disorders in a sample of elementary school students receiving special educational services for behavioural difficulties. *Canadian Journal of Psychiatry. Revue Canadienne De Psychiatrie, 49* (11), 769–775.

Dishion, T.J., & Patterson, G.R. (1992). Age effects in parent training outcomes. *Behavior Therapy, 23*, 719–729.

Donohue, B., Allen, D.N., & LaPota, H.B. (2009). Family behavior therapy for substance abuse and associated problems. In D.W. Springer & A. Rubin (eds), *Substance abuse treatment for youth and adults: Clinician's guide to evidence-based practice*, Hoboken, NJ: John Wiley & Sons.

Durlak, J., Fuhrman, T., & Lampman, C. (1991). Effectiveness of cognitive-behavior therapy for maladapting children: A meta-analysis. *Psychological Bulletin, 110*, 204–214.

Eyberg, S. (1988). Parent-child interaction therapy: Integration of traditional and behavioral concerns. *Child and Family Behavior Therapy, 10*, 33–45.

Farmer, E.M.Z., Compton, S.N., Burns, J.B., & Robertson, E. (2002). Review of the evidence base for treatment of childhood psychopathology: Externalizing disorders. *Journal of Consulting and Clinical Psychology, 70* (6), 1267–1302.

Finch, A.J., Jr., Nelson, W.M., III, & Hart, K.J. (2006). Conduct disorder: Description, prevalence, and etiology. In W.M. Nelson, III, A.J. Finch, Jr., & K.J. Hart (eds), *Conduct disorders: A practitioner's guide to comparative treatments.* (pp. 1–13). New York: Springer.

Flash, K. (2003). Treatment strategies for juvenile delinquency: Alternative solutions. *Child and Adolescent Social Work Journal, 20,* 509–527.

Fonagy, P., Target, M., Cottrell, D., Phillips, J., & Kurtz, Z. (2002). *What works for whom? A critical review of treatments for children and adolescents.* New York: Guilford Press.

Forehand, R.L., & McMahon, R.J. (1981). *Helping the noncompliant child: A clinician's guide to present training.* New York: Guilford Press.

Frick, P.J., Lahey, B.B., Loeber, R., Stouthamer-Loeber, M., Christ, M.A.G., & Hanson, K. (1992). Familial risk factors to oppositional defiant disorder and conduct disorder: Parental psychopathology and maternal parenting. *Journal of Consulting and Clinical Psychology, 60* (1), 49–55.

Hanish, L.D., Tolan, P.H., & Guerra, N.G. (1996). Treatment of oppositional defiant disorder. In M.A. Reinecke, F.M. Dattilio, & A. Freeman (eds), *Cognitive therapy with children and adolescents* (pp. 62–78). New York: Guilford Press.

Henggeler, S.W., Schoenwald, S.K., Borduin, C.M., Rowland, M.D., & Cunningham, P.B. (1998). *Multisystemic treatment of antisocial behavior in children and adolescents.* New York: Guilford Press.

Hodges, K. (2000). *The Child and Adolescent Functional Assessment Scale self training manual.* Ypsilanti, MI: Eastern Michigan University, Department of Psychology.

Holmes, S.E., Slaughter, J.R., & Kashani, J. (2001). Risk factors in childhood that lead to the development of conduct disorder and antisocial personality disorder. *Child Psychiatry and Human Development, 31* (3), 183–193.

Jouriles, E.N., Murphy, C.M., & O'Leary, K.D. (1989). Interspousal aggression, marital discord, and child problems. *Journal of Consulting and Clinical Psychology, 57* (3), 453–455.

Kazdin, A.E. (1994). Psychotherapy for children and adolescents. In A.E. Bergin & S.L. Garfield (eds), *Handbook of psychotherapy and behavior change* (4th ed., pp. 543–594). New York: John Wiley & Sons.

Kazdin, A.E. (1997). Parent management training: Evidence, outcomes, and issues. *Journal of the American Academy of Child and Adolescent Psychiatry, 36,* 1349–1356.

Kazdin, A.E. (2000). *Psychotherapy for children and adolescents: Directions for research and practice.* New York: Oxford University Press.

Kazdin, A.E. (2002). Psychosocial treatments for conduct disorder in children and adolescents. In P.E. Nathan & J.M. Gorman (eds), *A guide to treatments that work* (2nd ed., pp. 57–85). New York: Oxford University Press.

Kazdin, A.E. (2003). Problem-solving skills training and parent management training for conduct disorder. In A.E. Kazdin & J.R. Weisz (eds), *Evidence-based psychotherapies for children and adolescents* (pp. 241–262). New York: Guilford Press.

Kessler, R.C., Berglund, P., Demler, O., Jin, R., Merikangas, K.R., & Walters, E.E. (2005). Lifetime prevalence and age-of-onset distributions of DSM-IV disorders in the National Comorbidity Survey replication. *Archives of General Psychiatry, 62* (6), 593–605.

Kronenberger, W., & Meyer, R. (2001). *The child clinician's handbook.* Needham Heights, MA: Allyn & Bacon.

Lahey, B., Miller, T., Gordon, R., & Riley, A. (1999). Developmental epidemiology of the disruptive behavior disorders. *Handbook of disruptive behavior disorders* (pp. 23–48). Dordrecht, Netherlands: Kluwer Academic.

Lahey, B., Schwab-Stone, M., Goodman, S., Waldman, I., Canino, G., Rathouz, P. et al. (2000). Age and gender differences in oppositional behavior and conduct problems: A cross-sectional household study of middle childhood and adolescence. *Journal of Abnormal Psychology, 109* (3), 488–503.

Latimer, J. (2001). A meta-analytic examination of youth delinquency, family treatment, and recidivism. *Canadian Journal of Criminology, 43,* 237–253.

Leccese, M., & Waldron, H.B. (1994). Assessing adolescent substance abuse: A critique of current measurement instruments. *Journal of Substance Abuse Treatment, 11,* 553–563.

Loeber, R., & Stouthamer-Loeber, M. (1986). Factors as correlates and predictors of juvenile conduct problems and delinquency. In M. Tonry & N. Morris (eds), *Crime and justice: An annual review of research* (Vol. 7, pp. 29–149). Chicago, IL: University of Chicago Press.

Loeber, R., Lahey, B.B., & Thomas, C. (1991). Diagnostic conundrum of oppositional defiant disorder and conduct disorder. *Journal of Abnormal Psychology, 100* (3), 379–390.

Loeber, R., Burke, J.D., Lahey, B.B., Winters, A. & Zera, M. (2000). Oppositional defiant and conduct disorder: A review of the past 10 years, part I. *Journal of the American Academy of Child and Adolescent Psychiatry, 39* (12), 1468–1484.

Lumley, V., McNeil, C., Herschell, A., & Bahl, A. (2002). An examination of gender differences among young children with disruptive behavior disorders. *Child Study Journal, 32* (2), 89–100.

Mash, E., & Barkley, R. (1996). *Child psychopathology*. New York: Guilford Press.

Maughan, B., Rowe, R., Messer, J., Goodman, R., & Meltzer, H. (2004). Conduct disorder and oppositional defiant disorder in a national sample: Developmental epidemiology. *Journal of Child Psychology and Psychiatry, 45* (3), 609–621.

Moos, R., & Moos, B. (1984). *Family environment scale*. Palo Alto, CA: Consulting Psychologists Press.

Mrug, S., Hoza, B., & Bukowski, W. M. (2004). Choosing or being chosen by aggressive-disruptive peers: Do they contribute to children's externalizing and internalizing problems? *Journal of Abnormal Child Psychology, 32* (1), 53–65.

National Institute on Drug Abuse (National Institutes of Health) (1998). *Principles of drug addiction treatment: A research based guide*. (Publication No. 99–4180). Retrieved August 25, 2008, from NIDA NIH Reports Online via: www.nida.nih.gov/PDF/PODAT/PODAT.pdf.

Pardini, D.A., & Lochman, J.E. (2006). Treatments for oppositional defiant disorder. In M.A. Reinecke, F.M. Dattilio, & A. Freeman (eds), *Cognitive therapy with children and adolescents: A casebook for clinical practice* (2nd ed., pp. 43–69). New York: Guilford Press.

Patterson, G.R., & Gullion, M.E. (1968). *Living with children: New methods for parents and teachers*. Champaign, IL: Research Press.

Patterson, G.R., Reid, J.B., Jones, R.R., & Conger, R.E. (1975). *A social learning approach to family intervention. Vol. 1: Families with aggressive children*. Eugene, OR: Castalia.

Poole, D. (1997). Achieving national health goals in prevention with community organization: The "bottom up" approach. *Journal of Community Practice, 4* (2), 77–92.

Radin, B.A. (1996). Managing across boundaries. In D.F. Kettl & H.B. Milward (eds), *The state of public management*. Baltimore, MD: Johns Hopkins University Press.

Reid, M.J., Webster-Stratton, C., & Hammond, M. (2003). Follow-up of children who received the incredible years intervention for oppositional defiant disorder: Maintenance and prediction of 2-year outcome. *Behavior Therapy, 34* (4), 471–491.

Reid, M.J., Webster-Stratton, C., & Baydar, N. (2004). Halting the development of conduct problems in Head Start children: The effects of parent training. *Journal of Clinical Child and Adolescent Psychology, 33* (2), 279–291.

Rey, J.M., & Plapp, J.M. (1990). Quality of perceived parenting in oppositional and conduct disordered adolescents. *Journal of the American Academy of Child and Adolescent Psychiatry, 29* (3), 382–385.

Roberts, A.R., & Corcoran, K. (2005). Adolescents growing up in stressful environments, dual diagnosis, and sources of success. *Brief Treatment and Crisis Intervention, 5* (1), 1–8.

Rosen, A. & Proctor, E.K. (2002). Standards for evidence-based social work practice: The role of replicable and appropriate interventions, outcomes, and practice guidelines. In A.R. Roberts & G.J. Greene (eds), *Social workers' desk reference* (pp. 743–747). New York: Oxford University Press.

Sadock, B., & Sadock, V. (2007). *Kaplan & Sadock's synopsis of psychiatry: Behavioral sciences/clinical psychiatry* (10th ed.). Philadelphia, PA: Lippincott Williams & Wilkins.

Searight, H.R., Rottnek, F., & Abby, S.L. (2001). Conduct disorder: Diagnosis and treatment in primary care. *American Family Physician, 63* (8), 1579–1588.

Sobell, L.C., & Sobell, M.B. (1992). Timeline follow-back: A technique for assessing self-reported alcohol consumption. In R.Z. Litten & J.P. Allen (eds), *Measuring alcohol consumption: Psychosocial and biochemical methods* (pp. 41–72). Totowa, NJ: Humana Press.

Spaccarelli, S., Cotler, S., & Penman, D. (1992). Problem-solving skills training as a supplement to behavioral parent training. *Cognitive Therapy and Research, 16*, 1–18.

Spivak, G., & Shure, M.B. (1974). *Social adjustment of young children*. San Francisco, CA: Jossey-Bass.

Springer, D.W., & Bender, K. (2009). Treatment planning with adolescents: ADHD case application. In A.R. Roberts (ed.), *Social workers' desk reference* (2nd ed., pp. 526–530). New York: Oxford University Press.

Springer, D.W., & Lynch, C.J. (2008). Effective interventions for students with conduct disorder. In C. Franklin, M.B. Harris, & P. Allen-Meares (eds), *The school practitioner's concise companion to mental health.* (pp. 3–18). New York: Oxford University Press.

Springer, D.W., & Tripodi, S.J. (2009). Assessment protocols and rapid assessment instruments with troubled adolescents. In A.R. Roberts (ed.), *Social workers' desk reference* (2nd ed., pp. 385–389). New York: Oxford University Press.

Springer, D.W., Stokes Sharp, D., & Foy, T.A. (2000). Coordinated service delivery and children's well-being: Community Resource Coordination Groups of Texas. *Journal of Community Practice, 8* (2), 39–52.

Stubbe, D. (2007). *Child and adolescent psychiatry: A practical guide.* Philadelphia, PA: Lippincott Williams & Wilkins.

Teplin, L.A., Abram, K.M., McClelland, G.M., Dulcan, M.K., & Mericle, A.A. (2002). Psychiatric disorders in youth in juvenile detention. *Archives of General Psychiatry, 59* (12), 1133–1143.

Tripodi, S.J., Kim, J.S., & DiNitto, D.M. (2006). Effective strategies for working with students who have co-occurring disorders. In C. Franklin, M.B. Harris, & P. Allen-Meares (eds), *School social work and mental health workers training and resource manual.* London: Oxford University Press.

U.S. Department of Health and Human Services (1999). *Mental health: A report of the Surgeon General.* Rockville, MD: U.S. Department of Health and Human Services, Substance Abuse and Mental Health Services Administration, Center for Mental Health Services, National Institutes of Health, National Institute of Mental Health.

Webster-Stratton, C. (1984). Randomized trial of two parent-training programs for families with conduct-disordered children. *Journal of Consulting and Clinical Psychology, 52,* 666–678.

Webster-Stratton, C. (1990). Enhancing the effectiveness of self-administered videotape parent training for families with conduct-problem children. *Journal of Abnormal Child Psychology, 18,* 479–492.

Webster-Stratton, C. (1994). Advancing videotape parent training: A comparison study. *Journal of Consulting and Clinical Psychology, 62,* 583–593.

Webster-Stratton, C. (1998). Preventing conduct problems in Head Start children: Strengthening parenting competencies. *Journal of Consulting and Clinical Psychology, 66* (5), 715–730.

Webster-Stratton, C., & Hammond, M. (1997). Treating children with early-onset conduct problems: A comparison of child and parent training interventions. *Journal of Consulting and Clinical Psychology, 65* (1), 93–109.

Webster-Stratton, C., & Reid, M.J. (2003a). Treating conduct problems and strengthening social emotional competence in young children (ages 4–8 years): The Dina Dinosaur treatment program. *Journal of Emotional and Behavioral Disorders, 11* (3), 130–143.

Webster-Stratton, C., & Reid, M. J. (2003b). The incredible years parents, teachers, and children training series: A multifaceted treatment approach for young children with conduct problems. In A.E. Kazdin & J.R. Weisz (eds), *Evidence-based psychotherapies for children and adolescents* (pp. 224–240). New York: Guilford Press.

Webster-Stratton, C., Kolpacoff, M., & Hollinsworth, T. (1988). Self-administered videotape therapy for families with conduct-problem children: Comparison with two cost effective treatments and a control group. *Journal of Consulting and Clinical Psychology, 56,* 558–566.

Webster-Stratton, C., Reid, M.J., & Hammond, M. (2001a). Preventing conduct problems, promoting social competence: A parent and teacher training partnership in Head Start. *Journal of Clinical Child Psychology, 30* (3), 283–302.

Webster-Stratton, C., Reid, M.J., & Hammond, M. (2001b). Social skills and problem solving training for children with early-onset conduct problems: Who benefits? *Journal of Child Psychology and Psychiatry, 42* (7), 943–952.

Webster-Stratton, C., Reid, M.J., & Hammond, M. (2004). Treating children with early onset conduct problems: Intervention outcomes for parent, child, and teacher training. *Journal of Clinical Child and Adolescent Psychology, 33* (1), 105–124.

Widom, C.S. (1989). The cycle of violence. *Science, 244* (4901), 160–166.

Wiltz, N.A., & Patterson, G.R. (1974). An evaluation of parent training procedures designed to alter inappropriate aggressive behavior of boys. *Behavior Therapy, 5,* 215–221.

15 Mood conditions

Ellen Smith

Mood conditions are one of the most common mental health issues, and are among the top ten causes of disability worldwide (United States Public Health Service, n.d.). In the United States, major depressive disorder is the leading cause of disability among people aged 15–44 (National Institutes of Health, n.d.). Although mood conditions are quite treatable, many people who suffer from them – as many as 80 percent – do not receive care (Public Broadcasting Service, n.d.).

Mood conditions have a significant impact on the individuals affected, and on their family members. Depression is more common than bipolar disorder, and can have serious negative effects on an individual's functioning. In adolescents, academic performance and peer relationships can be affected (Gallagher, 2005). The consequences of depression over time include poor social relationships, increased substance abuse, interference with long-term cognitive functioning, increased use of medical services, major health problems, and younger ages of death (Commission on Adolescent Depression and Bipolar Disorder, 2005). Bipolar disorder is less common than major depression, but it is even more impairing (Kessler, Merikangas, & Wang, 2007). Most individuals with bipolar disorder – approximately 75 percent – are not able to function at the level that they did before the onset of the illness (Keck et al., 1998), and many experience significant deterioration of their relationships and careers (Zaretsky, 2003). Bipolar disorder can also lead to substance abuse and to extremely risky behaviors (Lewis, 2005), and poses major challenges for family members (Mueser, Webb, Pfeiffer, & Gladis, 1996). Finally, suicide is probably the most disturbing consequence of mood conditions, with rates of completed suicide among individuals with bipolar disorder about 15 times those of the general population (Barnes & Mitchell, 2005), higher than those of any other mental illness (Kupfer, Frank, Grochocinski, Houck, & Brown, 2005). For all these reasons, social workers must develop an understanding of mood conditions and of effective means of intervening.

Definitions of mood conditions

Mood conditions can take a range of forms and manifestations, and there are a variety of ways in which they are conceptualized. Some fluctuations in mood are a basic element of human experience, and are not a sign of a diagnosable disorder. When these changes go beyond ordinary feelings of sadness or being "down," and begin to impact a person's functioning, then they may be considered problematic. One commonly used perspective on mood conditions comes from the *Diagnostic and statistical manual*, or DSM-IV-TR (American Psychiatric Association (APA), 2000), which describes and establishes criteria for a number of mood disorders, including major depressive disorder, dysthymic disorder, adjustment disorder with depressed mood, bipolar disorder I, and bipolar disorder II.

According to the DSM-IV-TR, major depressive disorder is defined by the presence of a major depressive episode, which is characterized by a number of symptoms that are present over a period of at least two consecutive weeks. A depressive episode is marked by significant distress or by some impairment in functioning, either socially, occupationally, or in another important area. Perhaps the most important criterion is the individual's mood, which is marked by sadness or hopelessness, and sometimes by irritability as well. In children and adolescents, depressed mood may manifest more as irritability than sadness. Another defining feature is anhedonia, or loss of interest or pleasure in activities that were previously enjoyable. In order to meet criteria for a major depressive episode, the individual must also experience at least four of the following additional symptoms. Physical changes may include increased or decreased appetite, insomnia or increased need for sleep, and psychomotor agitation or retardation. Decreased energy is also common, as are difficulties with memory or concentration. Finally, depressed individuals often have intense and unrealistic feelings of guilt or worthlessness, and they may have thoughts of death or suicide.

Dysthymic disorder can be considered a low-grade, long-term form of depression. Individuals with dysthymia do not meet the full criteria for a major depressive episode. Instead, they suffer from depressed mood most of the time for a period of at least two years. In addition to feelings of sadness, they also experience at least two of the following symptoms: increased or decreased appetite, sleep disturbance, low energy, and low self-esteem, problems with concentration or decision-making, and feelings of hopelessness. Other signs of dysthymia include anhedonia, social withdrawal, and feelings of guilt or inadequacy. For children, as with major depression, dysthymia may present as irritability, and symptoms must be present for only one year. Because the symptoms of dysthymia are so chronic and long-lasting, they are often experienced as part of the individual's identity.

In contrast, an adjustment disorder with depressed mood is a relatively time-limited period of depressive symptoms that occurs in response to a specific stressor. The symptoms of this condition must begin with three months of the beginning of the stressor, and must conclude within six months of the resolution of the stressor. Individuals with an adjustment disorder with depressed mood do not meet the criteria for a depressive episode, but they do experience marked distress or significant impairment in functioning, characterized by feelings of sadness or hopelessness.

Several issues can complicate the diagnosis of a depressive disorder. First, the signs of bereavement are often quite similar to those of depression. In order to meet the criteria for major depressive disorder, however, the symptoms must last longer than two months, or they must include marked impairment in functioning, feelings of worthlessness, and thoughts of suicide, psychotic symptoms, or psychomotor retardation. If these criteria are not met, then bereavement is the appropriate diagnosis. Another issue is the tendency of individuals with depressive conditions simultaneously to experience other mental health problems (Reinecke & Ginsburg, 2008). In children, for example, depression often coexists with attention deficit disorder, and adults may have anxiety or panic conditions, substance abuse, an eating condition, or borderline personality disorder condition in addition to depression. This tendency is known as comorbidity. Finally, as is the case with many mental health diagnoses, ruling out any medical issues or substance use that may be underlying the depressive symptoms is essential.

Bipolar conditions are characterized by extremes of mood. Bipolar I disorder is defined by the presence of at least one manic or mixed episode. A manic episode is a period of at least one week in which the individual's mood is unusually elevated, expansive, or irritable. In order to meet the criteria for a manic episode, the symptoms must significantly impair the individual's functioning, or there must be some evidence of psychosis. In addition, the individual must experience at least three of the following symptoms (APA, 2000). Inflated self-esteem and grandiosity are common features of a manic episode, as is a decreased need for sleep. Both speech and thought processes may be accelerated; speech may have a pressured quality, and the person's thinking may jump quickly from one topic to the next. He or she may also be easily distracted or agitated. Finally, there is frequently an increase in social, sexual, or occupational activity, and particularly in engagement in pleasurable activities, which may result in reckless behavior that has the potential for negative consequences, and that the individual later regrets.

A mixed episode is a period of at least one week in which the individual meets the criteria for both a manic episode and a depressive episode. Again, the episode must cause impaired functioning or be marked by psychotic features. The individual's mood may fluctuate quickly from sadness or irritability to euphoria. The presence of either a mixed episode or a manic episode allows for a diagnosis of bipolar I disorder, though individuals with bipolar disorder often experience depressive episodes as well. Moreover, they may have ongoing symptoms in between acute episodes that are disruptive and difficult, even if they do not meet the criteria for a full-blown mood episode.

Bipolar II disorder is similar to bipolar I disorder, but requires the presence of at least one depressive episode, as well as a hypomanic episode. A hypomanic episode is like a manic episode, but it is shorter lived and not severe enough to impair functioning or to require hospitalization. The episode is defined as a period of at least four days of elevated, expansive, or irritable mood. The other criteria are the same as those of a manic episode, though the symptoms tend to be somewhat milder. If there are any signs of psychosis, then the episode is considered to be manic. Individuals with bipolar II disorder are more likely than those with bipolar I disorder to suffer from rapid cycling, which is defined as the presence of at least four mood episodes in the course of one year (Curtis, 2005).

The diagnosis of bipolar conditions can be difficult. Bipolar I disorder is often initially misdiagnosed (Bowden, 2001; Lewis, 2005), which can create a significant barrier to care. One study, for example, found that clients saw an average of four providers before being correctly diagnosed, delaying the beginning of appropriate treatment (Bhugra & Flick, 2005). Providers tend to be even less knowledgeable about bipolar II disorder, and frequently mistake it for bipolar I disorder or for major depression (MacQueen & Young, 2001). As with major depression, the diagnosis of both bipolar I and bipolar II can be complicated by the presence of coexisting mental health issues, such as substance abuse, anxiety, eating disorders, and personality disorders. Moreover, the criteria for bipolar conditions in children are somewhat unclear, which may contribute to a recent increase in the number of children being diagnosed with the illness. This issue will be discussed in greater depth below.

The DSM is helpful in describing and establishing diagnostic criteria for various mood disorders, but does not provide an explanation for the reasons that an individual might develop a mood disorder. Our understanding of this question has evolved over time, and there are different explanations proposed for different mood disorders. Freud (1917) offered an early conceptualization of depression in his classic paper, "Mourning and melancholia." Noting the similarities between depression, or melancholia, and bereavement, he attempted to clarify the distinction between them. He suggested that both are a reaction to loss, but postulated that melancholia develops when an individual has negative feelings, such as anger or resentment, toward the person who has died. Following the loss, the individual no longer has the opportunity to express these feelings directly to the deceased person, or lost object. Instead, these negative emotions are kept inside and directed inward. In Freud's (1917) words, "the shadow of the object falls upon the ego" (p. 119). From this perspective, melancholia, or depression, can be understood as unexpressed anger that is turned against the self.

While Freud's work remains relevant, current thinking about depression is that its etiology is complex and multi-determined. Depression exists on a continuum; endogenous, meaning it comes from within, or reactive, a response to environmental factors and its cause is usually a combination of both. Psychological, social, environmental, and biological factors are all involved, and these factors mutually influence one another (Reinecke & Ginsburg, 2008). Biological factors include inheritability, neurobiology, and hormonal differences between men and women. Depression tends to run in families, and at least part of this family transmission of depression can be explained by genetic factors. Estimates of hereditability range from 30 percent to 80 percent (Avenevoli, Knight, Kessler, & Merikangas, 2008). Moreover, the first episode of depression lays down pathways in the brain that are difficult to overcome and are likely to endure, placing the individual at risk for future bouts of depression (Commission on Adolescent Depression and Bipolar Disorder, 2005).

These biological factors make a person more vulnerable to mood conditions, such that stressful life events are likely to trigger depression. Stressful life events may have occurred in the distant past, in which case they are referred to as predisposing events, setting the stage for a future mood disorder. More recent triggers for a depressive episode are referred to as pre-cipitating events. In children, these life events may include loss, abuse, divorce of parents, academic problems, and poor psychosocial functioning (Watts & Markham, 2005). In adults, stressors such as loss, divorce, housing problems, or work-related difficulties may trigger a depressive episode (Sloan & Kornstein, 2003).

Another important contribution to the understanding of depression comes from cognitive theory. Cognitive theory emphasizes the role of an individual's thought patterns in creating and maintaining his or her difficulties. Depression is thought to be the result of negative attitudes and beliefs about the self, the world, and the future, which distort a person's ability to process information in an unbiased way. Instead, he or she focuses only on the negative aspects of experiences, and tends to interpret all experience in a negative way, paying little attention to the positive. From this perspective, the symptoms of depression – hopelessness, loss of motivation, self-criticism – are a product of an individual's selective focus on the negative. These symptoms themselves are then perceived through the person's distorted lens, creating a negative feedback loop (Beck, 2008).

More recent cognitive models of depression take into account the importance of stressful life events and biological factors, emphasizing the interaction of these forces with a person's attitudes and beliefs (Reinecke & Ginsburg, 2008). In particular, stressful events during childhood, especially the loss of a parent, may be interpreted in ways that crystallize into cognitive schemas, categories used to organize information that generally contain negative beliefs about the self and the world. These schemas can then be activated by subsequent nega-tive life events, a pattern which serves to further reinforce dysfunctional thoughts and attitudes. The more these cognitive schemas are activated, the more entrenched and automatic they become. Moreover, a genetic predisposition to depression may affect a person's neurobiological functioning, making him or her more sensitive to negative experiences (Beck, 2008).

A final way of conceptualizing depression suggests that certain personality traits may make a person vulnerable, particularly if he or she experiences a life stressor that poses a challenge to that trait (Lewinsohn, Pettit, Joiner, & Seeley, 2003). One such trait is perfectionism, which is associated with what Blatt (1995) calls introjective or self-critical depression. Perfectionist individuals tend to set impossibly high standards for themselves, and are very oriented toward achievement and competition. When faced with criticism or failure, they may experience profound feelings of unworthiness, inferiority, failure, and guilt, which can lead to depression. Another potentially problematic trait is called sociotropy, which is characterized by high levels of dependence, an excessive need to please others, and a longing to be loved and nurtured. In the face of abandonment or rejection, such individuals may struggle with feelings of loneliness, helplessness, or weakness. The depression that can result is referred to as anaclitic or dependent depression (Blatt, 1995). Thus, the nature of the depression is consistent with the type of stressor that triggers the episode (Lewinsohn et al., 2003).

Depression, then, can be understood from several perspectives, and is best understood as the product of multiple factors that all interact with one another. Bipolar conditions are also affected by both biological and environmental factors, but genetics play a larger role than they do with unipolar depression (Watts & Markham, 2005). Estimates of the risk of bipolar among first-degree relatives of someone with the illness range from 1.5 to 10.2 percent, and the risk is higher for children of parents with early-onset bipolar (Curtis, 2005). As with depression, however, stressful life events may increase the risk of bipolar disorder for individuals who are biologically vulnerable (Miklowitz & Chang, 2008).

Cognitive-behavioral theory elaborates upon the idea that the etiology of bipolar conditions lie in the interaction of biological and environmental factors. This perspective suggests that biological vulnerability to the disorder leads to unstable circadian rhythms of sleeping and waking, which over time cause prodromal symptoms of mild hypomania or depression. Eventually, these mood symptoms may be made worse by poor coping skills, leading to a full-blown manic or depressive episode. These episodes are usually quite disruptive to an individual's work life and relationships, causing more stress. The cycle then continues, with social difficulties and sleep deprivation exacerbating the individual's biological vulnerability (Zaretsky, 2003).

Another factor that may play a role in bipolar conditions is "expressed emotion," which refers to the emotional attitudes of family members toward the person with mental illness. High levels of expressed emotion can manifest as a critical or hostile stance toward the individual with bipolar disorder, or as an over-involvement, in which family members are overprotective or self-sacrificing in relation to the ill person. Families with high levels of expressed emotion also tend to attribute any problems to the individual, rather than to the illness. While expressed emotion does not cause bipolar conditions, it is an environmental factor that may interact with biological vulnerability to cause poor outcomes and higher rates of relapse for the ill individual (Morris, Miklowitz, & Waxmonsky, 2007).

Demographics

Mood conditions are among the most common mental health conditions in the United States. Among children, rates of major depression are approximately 1 percent; among adolescents, estimates range from 4 percent to 24 percent (Avenevoli et al., 2008). Among adults, major depression affects approximately 8 percent of the population in any given year (Public Broadcasting Service, n.d.).

Gender is a significant factor in determining one's risk of major depression. Prior to adolescence, rates of depression are similar in boys and girls. By mid-adolescence, however, rates are higher in girls (Avenevoli et al., 2008; Watts & Markham, 2005), probably due to both hormonal and psychosocial changes (Sloan & Kornstein, 2003). These gender differences continue into adulthood. Women experience higher rates of depression than men (Ialongo et al., 2004; Ohayon, 2007; Sachs-Ericsson & Ciarlo, 2000), with some estimates suggesting that the prevalence among women is twice as high as it is in men, especially during their childbearing years (Sloan & Kornstein, 2003). Depression may also look different in women than it does in men; these differences will be discussed below. Finally, depression in women is sometimes linked to the female reproductive cycle, as is the case with postpartum depression and premenstrual dysphoric disorder, and there is some question as to whether these manifestations of depression are different in some way from mood disorders that affect both men and women (Freeman, 2006).

An individual's racial or ethnic identity also plays a role in his or her risk of depression, in complex ways. One study, for example, found that whites have higher lifetime prevalence rates of major depression, but African Americans and Mexican Americans have higher lifetime prevalence rates of dysthymia (Riolo, Nguyen, Greden, & King, 2005). Another study determined that lifetime rates of depression were higher for whites than for Caribbean American blacks and African Americans, but the chronicity and severity of symptoms were higher for both black groups than for whites (Williams et al., 2007). A meta-analysis of multiple studies indicated that Latinos had similar or lower rates of major depression, as compared to Whites, but higher rates of depressive symptoms (Mendelson, Rehkopf, & Kubzansky, 2008). Chinese Americans, too, may have lower rates of depression than those found among the general population (Yeung et al., 2004), though other studies have suggested otherwise (Hsu et al., 2005). While being a member of a minority group may be a risk factor, then, cultural factors can also promote resilience, protecting people of color from the stressors associated with their minority status (Mendelson et al., 2008).

For others, however, membership in a vulnerable group appears to increase the risk of depression. People of low socioeconomic status have higher rates of depression (Riolo et al., 2005), and these depressive symptoms are more likely to persist over time (Mendelson et al., 2008). Individuals with physical disabilities have been found to have elevated rates of depression (Turner & Beiser, 1990), as have lesbians and gays, especially during adolescence and young adulthood (Cochran, 2001). For both these groups, the social stigma associated with their sexual orientation or disability is a likely contributing factor to the increased risk of depression.

Bipolar conditions are somewhat less common than unipolar depression, affecting approximately 3 percent of adults in the United States in any given year (Public Broadcasting Service, n.d.). The lifetime prevalence of bipolar conditions is thought to be as high as 4 percent of the population (Curtis, 2005). Pediatric bipolar conditions were previously thought to be rare, but since 2000, the number of children diagnosed with bipolar disorders has more than tripled (Youngstrom, Meyers, Youngstrom, Calabrese, & Findling, 2006). There are several ways of understanding this dramatic increase. As noted earlier, there is some lack of clarity about the diagnostic criteria for bipolar disorder in children, so it is possible that it was under-diagnosed in the past, and is now being over-diagnosed (Miller & Barnett, 2008).

Other explanations for the apparent rise of pediatric bipolar conditions lie more in the system of mental health service delivery. One theory suggests that problems in children are often complex and multifaceted, and that the symptoms associated with bipolar conditions in children may in fact be attributable in part to difficult family dynamics, including abuse or neglect. Mental health providers may be tempted to overlook these challenging issues, and to focus instead on a diagnosis of bipolar disorder, which, as a biologically based condition, appears to provide a clear-cut explanation for the child's difficulties. It also has relatively straightforward treatment implications, usually involving psychiatric medication, which is likely to be covered by medical insurance. However, the tendency to diagnose children with bipolar disorder can prevent providers from recognizing and intervening with problems that have a significant impact on the child. Moreover, it can lead to the use of potent medications, which should be used with caution (Harris, 2005). Another theory about the rise of pediatric bipolar conditions relates to the psychiatric medications that are prescribed to children for depression or attention deficit hyperactivity disorder. These medications can trigger symptoms that are characteristic of pediatric bipolar disorder. Children are then diagnosed with bipolar and are prescribed with even more powerful medications, which can have a long-term impact on their neurobiological functioning (Whitaker, 2007).

Among adults, bipolar disorder I appears to affect men and women equally (Rasgon et al., 2005). There is a lack of consensus in the literature about bipolar II, however. Some studies have suggested that bipolar II is more common in women (Baldassano et al., 2005; Curtis, 2005), with estimates of lifetime prevalence ranging from 5 to 10 percent (Barnes & Mitchell,

2005). Other researchers have found no gender differences in the prevalence of bipolar II, among youth (Duax, Youngstrom, Calabrese, & Findling, 2007) or among adults (Kawa et al., 2005). The illness may present differently in men and women; these differences will be discussed below.

Population

Mood conditions can occur at any time during the life cycle, but there are some variations in the ways that they manifest, depending on the age of the individual. The core symptoms of major depression are similar in children and adults, but there are also developmental differences. Somatic complaints, for example, tend to decrease with age (Avenevoli et al., 2008). Depressed children and adolescents are also more likely to experience other conditions at the same time, including anxiety, behavior disorders, eating disorders, and substance abuse (Avenevoli et al., 2008). In general, the symptoms of depression in adolescents are similar to those in young adults, so it appears that the diagnostic criteria identified in the DSM-IV-TR are appropriate for adolescents (Lewinsohn et al., 2003).

There are a number of factors that place children and adolescents at risk of developing depression, including early experience, parent–child interaction patterns, biological factors, and life events (Reinecke & Simons, 2005). Individuals who experience their first depressive episode early in life are likely to have a recurrence of the illness (Avenevoli et al., 2008), and this risk is increased if the child has a family history of depression, a negative cognitive style, exposure to stressful life events, or other conditions such as dysthymia or anxiety (Birmaher, Arbelaez, & Brent, 2002). Some research has also found that the relationship between depressed children and their mothers can be problematic, with lack of engagement on the mother's part and negativity on the child's part, placing the child at higher risk of future depressive episodes (Dietz et al., 2008). Moreover, those who suffer from early onset chronic major depression have higher rates of negative outcomes, such as recurrent depressive episodes, personality disorders, lifetime substance use disorders, and psychiatric hospitalization (Dietz et al., 2008). Among individuals who first experience depression as children or adolescents, factors that are associated with a more difficult course of illness include being female, increased guilt, prior episodes of depression, and parental psychopathology (Birmaher et al., 2004).

Depression among elderly people tends to manifest somewhat differently than it does in younger people. Older adults experience less depressed mood, but have higher rates of anxiety and psychotic symptoms (Gottfries, 1998). They are at greater risk of recurrence than are younger people (Mueller et al., 2004). They are also more likely to develop bereavement-related depression, a response to the many personal and interpersonal losses that are often experienced later in life (Shear, 2005). In addition, the medical problems that frequently accompany aging contribute to depression in elderly people in several ways. First, medical issues such as neurological changes can be a direct biological cause of depression (Gottfries, 1998). Second, the stress associated with medical problems, and third, the impairment in functioning that they may cause, place elderly people at higher risk of depression (Lenze, 2005). Not surprisingly, then, there are high rates of medical conditions among depressed older adults.

While age is clearly an important influence on the way that depression is experienced, issues of gender and culture also play roles. Through adolescence, gender differences in the features and course of depression do not seem to be significant (Kovacs, 2001). Among adults, however, some differences begin to emerge. One study, for example, found that women appear to have more somatic symptoms of depression, especially changes in appetite (Wenzel, Steer, & Beck, 2005). They also report more sleep disturbance, psychomotor retardation, anxiety, and feelings of guilt or worthlessness (Sloan & Kornstein, 2003). Women seem to have a younger age of onset of depression (Marcus et al., 2005), and there is some evidence that they are more likely to experience chronic and recurrent depression (Sloan & Kornstein, 2003). Among older adults with depression, one study found that women had more appetite disturbances, and men had more agitation (Kockler & Heun, 2002).

An individual's cultural background may also affect the way that depression is expressed and experienced. Depression may look different in different cultures, so the diagnostic criteria established in the DSM may not apply cross-culturally (Bass, Bolton, & Murray, 2007). Chinese Americans, for example, tend to understand mental disorders in physical, embodied terms, and so they are more likely to seek help for somatic symptoms than for depression (Kung & Lu, 2008). Social and environmental factors that are associated with race or ethnicity, such as oppression, also have an impact on the experience of depression. One study found that the African Americans and Hispanics in a sample of depressed adults were more socially disadvantaged and had more coexisting mental disorders than whites, suggesting that the experience of depression for vulnerable populations may be complicated by other mental health conditions (Lesser et al., 2007).

Bipolar conditions also may be expressed differently, depending on the individual's age, gender, and cultural background. As mentioned earlier, rates of bipolar disorder in children have dramatically increased since 2000, and there are several possible reasons for this. One important issue is the lack of clarity about the ways that bipolar disorder manifests in children. It is not apparent that children who are diagnosed with bipolar disorder will go on to have the condition as adults; in fact, most children who exhibit symptoms of bipolar disorder do not develop adult bipolar, though they do have high rates of other mental health problems (Harris, 2005). Moreover, among adults with bipolar disorder, only 15–18 percent had signs of the illness before age 13, and 50–66 percent before age 19 (Morris et al., 2007). A significant percentage of adults with bipolar condition, then, would not have been diagnosed with the condition as children, suggesting that there may be little correlation between pediatric bipolar and adult bipolar.

The symptoms of bipolar conditions in children, a related issue, are not identical to those of the condition in adults. Some signs of bipolar conditions in children resemble those of adult bipolar disorders, including decreased need for sleep and reckless behaviors (McIntosh & Trotter, 2006), as well as mood lability, episodic elation or irritability, depression, inattention, and psychosocial impairment (Miklowitz & Chang, 2008). However, while the mood episodes of adults tend to last several weeks or longer, research indicates that children may experience rapid and pronounced mood changes, even over the course of a day, and that these fluctuations may occur in a chronic and continuous fashion (Birmaher & Axelson, 2006; Leibenluft & Rich, 2008; McIntosh & Trotter, 2006; Miller & Barnett, 2008). Children also seem to experience more irritability than euphoria, so their manic symptoms are different from those of adults (Leibenluft & Rich, 2008; McIntosh & Trotter, 2006). Further complicating the situation, the symptoms that characterize pediatric bipolar disorder are similar to those of developmental disorders, reactive attachment disorder, and post-traumatic stress disorder (Harris, 2005), as well as attention deficit/hyperactivity disorder and conduct disorder (McIntosh & Trotter, 2006).

There are a number of factors that place children at risk of developing bipolar conditions, most notably a family history of the illness. Among children with depression, several symptoms suggest that they are at greater risk of bipolar conditions, including psychosis, psychomotor retardation, and medication-induced mania or hypomania (Birmaher et al., 2002). The age of onset of the condition also has implications for its developmental course. Individuals who develop bipolar conditions at a young age tend to have higher rates of anxiety and substance abuse, more recurrences of the illness, and more suicide attempts and violence (Perils et al.,

2004), as well as increased risk of rehospitalization (Perlick, Rosenheck, Clarkin, Sirey, & Raue, 1999). Among children and adolescents with bipolar conditions, several factors are associated with poor outcomes, including low socioeconomic status, long duration of illness, rapid mood changes, mixed presentations, psychosis, comorbid disorders, and family psychopathology (Birmaher & Axelson, 2006).

Both of the bipolar conditions present as very difficult throughout the life cycle, and adults with the condition experience symptoms approximately half of the time. Sub-syndromal symptoms tend to be present for more of this time than are major depressive or manic symptoms, and depressive symptoms are present significantly more than manic symptoms (Paykel, Abbott, Morriss, Hayhurst, & Scott, 2006). Among elderly people, bipolar disorder is nearly as common as it is among other age groups, accounting for approximately 5–19 percent of mood disorders in this cohort (Sajatovic, 2002). Older adults with bipolar conditions tend to have more functional and cognitive impairments than their younger counterparts, but have lower rates of substance abuse (Depp et al., 2005). As with major depression, then, bipolar conditions manifest differently across the life cycle.

Gender is another factor that affects the way that an individual may experience bipolar conditions. Little consensus exists in the literature about this issue, however. Some research has suggested that there are no gender differences in the symptoms of bipolar in children and adolescents (Biederman et al., 2004), while another study found that girls were more likely to experience depressive symptoms, and boys were more likely to be manic (Duax et al., 2007). Among adults, too, the research has been inconclusive. Several studies have indicated that women have higher rates of depression, mixed episodes, and rapid cycling than men (Amsterdam, Brunswick, & O'Reardon, 2002; Barnes & Mitchell, 2005; Curtis, 2005). Other research, however, has not found significant gender differences in these areas (Baldassano et al., 2005; Kessing, 2004). It appears that men with bipolar conditions may have higher rates of substance abuse than women (Kawa et al., 2005; Kessing, 2004). The course of bipolar conditions in women may be affected by hormonal changes linked to the female reproductive cycle, with mood fluctuations across the menstrual cycle (Rasgon et al., 2005) and changes in symptoms during pregnancy, in some women for the better and in others for the worse (Curtis, 2005). The symptoms of bipolar disorder may also significantly worsen in the postpartum period (Curtis, 2005).

Just as gender may affect the way that either bipolar condition is manifested, cultural factors may also have an impact on the experience of the illness. Little evidence exists that the symptoms of bipolar disorder vary by racial or ethnic background. However, socioeconomic factors linked to race and ethnicity may affect the experiences of people living with the condition. For example, minorities with bipolar conditions seem to have higher rates of both substance abuse and homelessness, which may have implications for their functioning (Kilbourne, Bauer, Pincus, Williford, Kirk, & Beresford, 2005). At the same time, one study found that African Americans hospitalized for bipolar disorder scored higher in an assessment of coping resources than did whites, especially internal resources, which were defined as cognitive, emotional, and spiritual/psychological (Pollack, Harvin, & Cramer, 2000). It appears, then, that cultural factors may play a protective role, even in the face of increased psychosocial stressors associated with minority status.

Mental health care disparities

Despite the high rates of depression in the United States, many people do not receive appropriate treatment for the condition. Overall, as many as 40 percent of individuals with major depression receive no care at all (Ford, Pincus, Unützer, Bauer, Gonzalez, & Wells,

2002). Among children and adolescents with mental health conditions, including depression, only 25–50 percent receive some kind of services, and few of these services are from mental health specialists (Avenevoli et al., 2008). Elderly people are also less likely to receive adequate care for depression (Ohayon, 2007). One study, for example, found that fewer than half of older adults seen in primary care settings obtained successful care (Blasinsky, Goldman, & Unützer, 2006). Women, too, are less likely to receive services for major depression, with only 22 percent obtaining adequate treatment (Sinha & Rush, 2006).

Rates of treatment for depression among non-white individuals are even lower than they are among the general population (Ohayon, 2007). African American youth, for example, are less likely to receive mental health services than are white youth (Avenevoli et al., 2008); one study of urban African American young adults with major depression found that less than 10 percent of the sample had received treatment (Ialongo et al., 2004). This disparity continues throughout the life cycle. Among adults, Caribbean American blacks and African Americans are less likely to receive any form of mental health services (Williams et al., 2007), and a study of elderly homecare patients found that blacks were significantly less likely than whites to be prescribed antidepressant medication, though their rates of depression were similar (Fyffe, Sirey, Heo, & Bruce, 2004). Another study indicated that Chinese Americans, too, seem to have similar rates of depression to other ethnic groups, but few were prescribed medication by their primary care physician (Hsu et al., 2005).

Among individuals with bipolar conditions, rates of treatment appear to be somewhat higher, perhaps because the illness leads to more significant impairment of functioning. Among children with bipolar disorder who receive outpatient mental health services, however, many do not receive family therapy, which is an important component of services (Rizzo et al., 2007). Parents of children with bipolar conditions have identified several barriers to treatment, including the provider's lack of knowledge about the illness, poor communication with providers, and the tendency of providers to blame parents for the child's condition (Mackinaw-Koons & Fristad, 2004). Older adults with bipolar conditions tend to underuse mental health services (Sajatovic, 2002), particularly acute psychiatric services (Depp et al., 2005), but nevertheless use more services than do older adults with unipolar depression, and are more likely to be psychiatrically hospitalized (Bartels, Forester, Miles, & Joyce, 2000).

When it comes to race and ethnicity, there are significant disparities in terms of both accurate diagnosis and access to appropriate mental health services. Throughout the life cycle, African Americans with bipolar conditions are more likely than other groups to be misdiagnosed, most often with schizophrenia (Kilbourne, Haas, Benoit, Bauer, & Pincus, 2004; Lawson & Strickland, 2004). Interestingly, Hispanic adolescents with bipolar disorder were found in one study to be frequently misdiagnosed with major depression. The sample, many of whom were involved with the juvenile justice system, had high rates of mixed states and psychotic symptoms, but no euphoric mania (Dilsaver & Akiskal, 2005).

The tendency of providers to misdiagnose people of color clearly has implications for the services received by these individuals. African Americans with bipolar disorder are more likely to be prescribed antipsychotic medication, both as adolescents (DelBello, Soutullo, & Strakowski, 2000) and as adults (Lawson & Strickland, 2004). They are also likely to receive higher doses of these medications, and for longer periods of time, than other groups (Lawson & Strickland, 2004; Patel, DelBello, Keck, & Strakowski, 2005). Moreover, African Americans with bipolar conditions tend to have more psychiatric hospitalizations (Kupfer, Frank, Grochocinski, Houck, & Brown, 2005), and are less likely to receive psychotherapy (Lawson & Strickland, 2004). African Americans are also more likely to have their medications switched, and to be prescribed multiple medications, both of which are associated with higher rates of emergency room visits and psychiatric hospitalizations (Garver et al., 2006). Finally, people of color overall have higher rates of involuntary commitment than do whites (Kilbourne et al., 2005).

In addition to these disparities in the adequacy of services provided, other barriers to care affect African Americans with bipolar disorder. This population is less likely to seek mental health services because of stigma or fear of hospitalization, which is problematic because primary care providers are not usually able to offer appropriate care (Lawson & Strickland, 2004). Medication non-adherence is an issue for many individuals with bipolar conditions, but one study found that African Americans were more likely to attribute this to factors such as fear of addiction and medication as a symbol of mental illness (Fleck, Keck, Corey, & Strakowski, 2005). African Americans also tend to be underrepresented in research studies, in part because they are often mistrustful of research and in part because efforts are not made to recruit them (Lawson & Strickland, 2004).

Social work programs and social work roles

Social workers play a central role in intervening with individuals who suffer from mood conditions. They are involved at every level of care, providing counseling and support to clients and their families. However, empirical research on different kinds of interventions tends to come more from the field of psychology than from social work (Holosko, Jean-Baptiste, Le, Eaton, & Power, 2007). This literature will be discussed in the following section.

The treatment of mood disorders occurs in the context of the mental health service delivery system. The least restrictive level of care is outpatient services, in which clients are seen in clinics for therapy and possibly for medication management. These clinics may be based in hospitals, community-based organizations, or other settings such as schools or employee assistance programs. Social workers often provide the services, meeting with clients on a regular basis to assist them in reducing symptoms, improving coping, and helping with life stressors. If the client is prescribed medication, a primary care physician, psychiatrist, or clinical nurse specialist, depending on the complexity of the case and the severity of symptoms, generally does this. The social worker works in collaboration with the prescribing provider. If the client is a child, the social worker may also have contact with the family, school personnel, and members of other systems involved in the child's life.

Some clients may require a higher level of care than can be provided in an outpatient setting. These clients are often referred to intensive outpatient programs, which are usually located in hospitals. Here, clients may attend groups several hours each day, several times a week, for a fairly short-term period of several weeks or months. They are also assigned an individual clinician, with whom they work to address program goals. The clinician, who is often a social worker, coordinates the client's care and attends to discharge planning, ensuring that the client has appropriate services in place when he or she completes the program. Social workers may also lead groups and work individually with clients. They may also have collateral contact with families, outpatient providers, and other relevant parties.

The next level of care consists of partial hospitalization programs, which also tend to be located in hospital settings. Partial hospitalization programs are similar to intensive outpatient programs, but clients usually spend more time each week at these programs, for a shorter duration. Clients may come to these programs as a step up from outpatient treatment, generally because they do not meet criteria for inpatient hospitalization, but are in crisis or have needs that cannot be met in outpatient treatment. The programs aim to help stabilize clients, and may also provide diagnostic clarity or medication adjustment in a setting in which clients can be closely monitored. Clients may also attend partial hospitalization programs as a step down from inpatient hospitalization, in which case the program allows them to transition more gradually and to gain further stability before moving into outpatient services. As in intensive outpatient programs, clients attend groups and are assigned an individual clinician. Again, these services are often provided by social workers.

The highest level of care is inpatient hospitalization, which is appropriate for clients who are at risk of harming themselves or others. Suicidality is a significant clinical issue in working with people with mood conditions; rates of completed suicide in individuals with major depression have been estimated to be as high as 15 percent, and range from 10 to 15 percent in people with bipolar I and II disorders (APA, 2000). Suicidal ideation must be carefully and routinely assessed by the social worker, and clients should be referred for inpatient care if necessary (Sach, Yan, Swann, & Allen, 2001). Clients with bipolar conditions may also require hospitalization because of the psychosis that sometimes accompanies a manic episode. Inpatient programs tend to be very short term, a matter of days or possibly weeks, and are designed to stabilize clients through careful assessment, medication management, and discharge planning. Clients attend groups and see an individual clinician, who works collaboratively with families and other providers to put services in place that will help to support the client after he or she is discharged from the hospital. Social workers in inpatient settings function as part of an interdisciplinary team that may include psychiatrists, nurses, psychologists, and paraprofessionals. They are generally responsible for the coordination of care and discharge planning for the clients on their caseload.

At each level of care, then, social workers work directly with clients and their families, providing individual and group counseling. Consistent with social work's emphasis on the person-environment fit (Gitterman & Germain, 2008), social workers also tend to coordinate the various systems that may be involved in a client's life. They work to mobilize these systems to create a network of supports for the client that will help him or her to cope with the challenges of living with a mood condition.

Professional methods and interventions

Within the larger system of mental health services, in which social workers play a critical role, there are many more specific approaches to working with people with mood conditions. Empirical studies have indicated that there are a number of promising interventions, both for major depression and for bipolar disorder. While these interventions are not social work interventions per se, many of them do reflect social work's biopsychosocial perspective, and social workers may be centrally involved in the provision of services.

Because depression is multi-determined, a combination of biological and psychosocial interventions is most effective. Antidepressant medication is often helpful, for both adolescents and adults (Gallagher, 2005). However, medication is not effective for everyone. Over 30 percent of people in research studies of antidepressant medications are non-responsive, and that number increases to 50 percent among individuals with chronic depression (Sinha & Rush, 2006). Moreover, women may respond differently to medication than men (Yonkers & Brawnman-Mintzer, 2002), perhaps because of hormonal changes across the reproductive life cycle (Sinha & Rush, 2006). Another biological intervention, which may be appropriate for chronic, intractable depression, is electroconvulsive therapy (ECT). While ECT is still considered a treatment of last resort, recent advances have made it easier to tolerate, and less likely to have negative side effects, than it has been in the past (Keltner & Boschini, 2009). While social workers cannot administer these biological treatments, they play an important role in educating clients about their usage.

Antidepressant medication tends to be most effective when combined with psychosocial intervention, and there are several approaches to helping with depression and its associated stressors. One is cognitive-behavioral intervention, which draws upon the cognitive theory of depression and adds a behavioral emphasis on teaching skills. Cognitive techniques assist the client in monitoring the negative thoughts that often underlie depression, and in disproving these automatic thoughts. A method called Socratic questioning challenges clients to identify the evidence that supports their thinking, and to generate alternative ways of thinking. Clients are often asked to complete a dysfunctional thought record at home between sessions, on which they record the times that they feel most distressed and their thoughts at those times. They may also be asked to rate their level of belief in the dysfunctional thought and to write a rational response to the thought. The work, then, is about challenging negative thoughts about the self, the world, and the future, and replacing them with more hopeful cognitions. Behavioral techniques aim to teach the client skills in areas such as problem-solving, coping, affect regulation, or relaxation, depending on his or her individual needs. Cognitive-behavioral approaches tend to be relatively short term and structured, with the worker playing an active, directive role. Aspects of the cognitive-behavioral approaches are frequently used by social workers in direct practice.

In contrast, psychodynamic approaches to helping people suffering from depression are often longer term and less structured, though short-term psychodynamic models exist as well. Psychodynamic thinking about depression is based on Freud's idea that depression is an indication of anger that is turned against the self. The focus tends to be on the expression of affect, and on the analysis of the relationship between the worker and the client. Within social work, research by Goldstein (1995) has elaborated the relevance of psychodynamic theory, particularly ego psychology, to social work practice. Ego psychology emphasizes the development of capacities, known as ego functions, which determine the extent to which an individual is able to adapt to his or her environment. Goldstein's work suggests that these strengths and weaknesses develop in the context of environmental resources and gaps, and that difficulties may occur in the individual's capacities, the surrounding environment, or the interaction between them. From this perspective, ego psychology provides a helpful framework that is highly consistent with social work values for intervening with many kinds of mental health problems, including mood disorders.

The Life Model of Social Work Practice, a distinctively social work approach, focuses on the triggers for and the consequences of a life condition such as depression (Gitterman, 2008, 2010; Gitterman and Germain, 2008). In this model, the social work function is to help clients and their families to adapt and cope with the tasks and struggles in day-to-day living with depression. Living with depression is a stressful and painful experience. The stress and associated pain emerges from an imbalance between a person's perceived life demands and self-perceived capability to meet the demands (e.g., job, intimate relationship, deal with loss). These perceived transactional imbalances create life stressors in three interrelated areas: life transitions and traumatic events, environmental pressures, and dysfunctional interpersonal processes.

Little research is available on the effectiveness of psychodynamic therapy and life modeled practice, in part because these approaches are more difficult to quantify than more structured approaches like cognitive-behavioral approaches. However, one psychodynamic model, interpersonal psychotherapy, has been shown to be effective in empirical studies (de Mello, de Jesus Mari, Bacaltchuk, Verdeli, & Neugebauer, 2005). Interpersonal therapy is premised on the idea that depression is caused or maintained by problems in relationships, and so the work focuses on a number of potential areas of interpersonal difficulty.

Similar approaches can be used with children and adolescents with depression, though they must be adapted to the developmental level of the client. In recognition of the importance of families in the lives of children, all of these approaches involve some element of family work. One is cognitive-behavioral treatment, which generally includes a combination of cognitive techniques, skills training, psychoeducation, and family intervention (Gallagher, 2005). Behavioral approaches aim to teach skills in several areas: regulating emotions, problem-solving, relaxation, and social skills such as communication, assertiveness, and negotiation (Gallagher, 2005; Reinecke & Ginsburg, 2008). Family interventions may include training for the parents in such areas as positive reinforcement, empathic listening, family problem-solving, and conflict resolution skills (Stark, Hargrave, Hersh, Greenberg, Herren, & Fisher, 2008).

In addition to cognitive-behavioral, psychosocial treatment, and life modeled practice, several other approaches have been shown to be effective with depressed youth. Interpersonal therapy looks at five areas of interpersonal interactions: separation from parents, authority problems with parents, dyadic relationships, loss of relatives and friends, and relationships in single-parent families. The intervention focuses on the most problematic of these areas for the particular client, and it includes training in problem-solving, negotiation, communication, and relationship maintenance skills (Gallagher, 2005). Another approach that emphasizes the role of relationships is called systemic-behavioral family therapy, which is appropriate when family conflict is the main cause of stress for the adolescent. The treatment aims to change these conflictual relationships, and contains elements of cognitive-behavioral treatment and parenting skills (Gallagher, 2005).

Some specialized approaches also take into account the particular needs of the depressed elderly. One such intervention, called Project IMPACT, is a collaborative team approach that takes place in primary care settings, where older adults often present for treatment. The team consists of a primary care provider, a psychiatrist, and a depression clinical specialist who coordinates the treatment, which may include medication, brief structured psychotherapy, and psychoeducation (Blasinsky et al., 2006). Another approach, designed for low-income depressed older adults, is premised on the idea that depression in this population should be conceptualized and treated as both a social and psychological issue. It combines cognitive-behavioral group treatment with clinical case management, which provides an assessment of the client's needs in several areas – including health, finances, and housing – and links him or her to appropriate services (Arean, Gum, McCulloch, Bostrom, Gallagher-Thompson, & Thompson, 2005). These models are consistent with social work's holistic approach to mental health problems.

Just as there are approaches that are particularly helpful with depression, there are specific approaches to the treatment of bipolar conditions. Bipolar has a stronger biological base than does unipolar depression, and so medication is often a critical element of treatment. Clients are generally prescribed mood stabilizers, and they may be given antipsychotic medications as well. There is limited research on the treatment of bipolar disorder in children, and not all medications are approved for pediatric use (McIntosh & Trotter, 2006). However, it appears that medications can be helpful for young people, particularly mood stabilizers or anti-psychotics (Jerrell, 2008; Leibenluft & Rich, 2008). There are also special considerations for women with bipolar conditions. Again, women may respond differently to medications than men, though there is little research in this area. The medications prescribed for bipolar disorder may also have an impact on fertility, and they are not safe during pregnancy (Curtis, 2005). However, providers need to balance any potential risk to the child with the mental health of the mother, which will also be critical to the child's well-being (Barnes & Mitchell, 2005).

Despite the importance of medications in the treatment of bipolar conditions, many clients do not take their medications consistently, in part because the symptoms of mania can sometimes be enjoyable. Several interventions have been developed to promote medication adherence, including interpersonal group work, cognitive-behavioral treatment, group sessions for partners, and client and family psychoeducation (Sajatovic, Davies, & Hrouda, 2004). Social workers may be involved in the provision of all of these services.

It appears that the psychoeducational component may be particularly important in dealing with the issue of medication compliance (Zaretsky, 2003). In fact, psychoeducation has been shown to be a critical element in the treatment of bipolar disorder, leading to improvements in clients' knowledge about the illness, medication adherence, self-esteem, and overall functioning, as well as fewer hospitalizations and fewer recurrences of the illness (Clarkin, Carpenter, Hull, Wilner, & Glick, 1998; Soares, Stintzig, Jackson, & Skoldin, 1997; Zaretsky, 2003). Another important benefit of psychoeducation is that it allows clients to participate as full partners in their care (Toprac et al., 2000), which has been identified as a key aspect of effective treatment (Davies, McBride, & Sajatovic, 2008; Lewis, 2005), allowing clients to establish more positive working relationships with their providers (O'Connor, Gordon, Graham, Kelly, & O'Grady-Walshe, 2008). A psychoeducational intervention for family members was found to result in improvements in knowledge about the illness, level of distress, attributions of client behavior, and ways of coping (Bland & Harrison, 2000). Even if psychoeducation does not directly affect the symptoms of bipolar disorder, then, it has been shown to have many positive outcomes (Clarkin et al., 1998).

An approach called the collaborative care model aims to involve clients in their own care, engaging clients and families in treatment planning and giving them the skills to manage the illness (Morris, Miklowitz, & Waxmonsky, 2007). This model is clearly consistent with social work's emphasis on client empowerment and self-determination. It promotes collaboration between providers, which has been shown to be important to the effective treatment of bipolar disorder. Individuals with bipolar disorder may have multiple providers, in the fields of both medical and mental health, and at different levels of care. Coordination between these various providers has been shown to improve both medical and mental health outcomes for individuals with bipolar disorder (Williams & Manning, 2008). The goals of the collaborative care model are to enhance access to care, continuity of care, and the flow of information between the various parties involved in the client's treatment (Bauer et al., 2006a). Care coordination is often provided by a nurse, whose role may include performing an initial assessment, engaging in treatment planning, and providing monthly telephone monitoring and group psychoeducation for clients, as well as coordination with the mental health team (Simon, Ludman, Unützer, Bauer, Operskalski, & Rutter, 2005). Several studies of this model have found that it may reduce the length of time of the mood episode, decrease the frequency and severity of manic symptoms, and improve the client's social role function, mental quality of life, and treatment satisfaction (Bauer et al., 2006b).

In addition to these approaches, several other interventions have been shown to be effective in working with individuals with bipolar disorder. Support groups in general help to reduce the stigma and isolation that clients often experience, and also appear to improve treatment adherence and reduce hospitalization (Lewis, 2005). Client-run groups seem to be particularly helpful in improving social functioning (Yanos, Primavera, & Knight, 2001). Another approach, interpersonal and social rhythm therapy, focuses on helping clients recognize the impact of interpersonal events on their social and circadian rhythms. In an effort to address the disruptions in sleep patterns that often accompany bipolar disorder, the treatment emphasizes maintenance of structure and routine despite mood fluctuations. This approach has been used for depression, but there is little research on its effectiveness with bipolar disorder (Zaretsky, 2003). Finally, an approach called family-focused treatment is based on the idea that the level of expressed emotion in a family can influence the functioning of the individual with bipolar disorder. The treatment aims to decrease expressed emotion and negative interactions, and to help clients and families to come to a similar perspective on the role of the disorder. It includes psychoeducation and communication and problem-solving skills to change family interactions, and also draws upon the collaborative care approach described above (Morris et al., 2007).

The treatment of bipolar conditions in children and adolescents uses similar approaches to those used with adults, though there has been less research with this population (Leibenluft &

Rich, 2008; McIntosh & Trotter, 2006). Areas that should be addressed in helping include symptom management, coping skills, social and family relationships, academic functioning, and relapse prevention (Leibenluft & Rich, 2008). Psychoeducation for parents is important, and can be provided either to the individual family unit or in multifamily groups (Fristad, 2006; Leibenluft & Rich, 2008). Given the importance of school functioning in the lives of children, it is also beneficial to provide psychoeducation to teachers and other school personnel (McIntosh & Trotter, 2006). Finally, the collaborative care model can be adapted to work with children and adolescents (Morris et al., 2007).

Illustration and discussion

Judy is a 53-year-old white heterosexual woman who presented for individual therapy at a community mental health center in a small, economically depressed city. In the initial session, Judy reported that she had recently lost her job of 29 years. She had worked as an aide at a nursing home for elderly people. However, she had severe arthritis in her knees that had become progressively more debilitating. When it became difficult for her to perform her job duties, she was given a temporary position in the activities department, but was soon informed that she could not continue in this position. She had been involuntarily placed on medical leave several weeks earlier. Since then, she had been feeling depressed, crying often, and had experienced a panic attack that had sent her to the emergency room. She described the loss of her employment as "traumatic" and stated that she felt "deserted, thrown out to pasture." She had decided to get help at the advice of her daughter, who had been in therapy herself in the past. Judy had never received professional help before, and she denied any history of anxiety or depression. She did report some difficulty following the deaths of her mother and father, which occurred when she was young. However, she had been able to manage these losses on her own, whereas her current situation seemed to have overwhelmed her abilities to cope.

Consistent with her description of herself, Judy appeared sad and anxious during the initial session. She had a nervous, tentative manner, and she was tearful at times. She was soft-spoken, with a somewhat high-pitched voice, and she had an almost childlike quality about her. She had short silvery-blond hair, blue eyes, and a round face, and she was significantly overweight. She walked slowly, with evident difficulty, and she used a cane. She reported little motivation to do anything, excessive sleeping and eating, and difficulty concentrating. She was diagnosed with major depressive disorder, and the worker noted the possibility of a panic disorder as well.

In addition to the arthritis in her knees, Judy reported a number of other medical problems. She had a stomach ulcer, and a condition that affected her urinary tract. She was prescribed several medications, including oxycontin for the pain in her legs. She had received physical therapy, and was exploring the possibility of knee replacement surgery. Several additional medical problems arose in the course of her time in therapy.

Judy was the middle of three children. She was somewhat vague about the details of her early life. Her parents divorced when she was young, and she and her siblings initially lived with her father. He was in the military, and so she reported moving frequently during this time of her life. When Judy was seven, the children went to live with their mother, a nurse, and for several years, she had little contact with her father, whom, she says, "drank" and "had some mental problems," including depression. He came to her home on occasion and was physically abusive to her mother during some of these visits. When Judy was 15, he became ill with heart disease and went to live with his brother. Judy began to re-establish a connection with him, visiting him at her uncle's house during his illness. He died when she was 16. She stated, "I took it badly, even though I didn't really know him. I had just gotten closer to him."

Judy married at age 18, and had been with her husband for 35 years. She had her first child at age 19, and her second at age 20, both girls. When she was 23, her mother died of stomach cancer. Judy reported praying for her mother to die: "She was so sick, I didn't want her to suffer any more." She described a close relationship with her mother, and had difficulty with her death. She had another child, a boy, when she was 25. She reported a particularly close relationship with her younger daughter, Emma, who was usually a source of support and advice. However, Emma was pregnant with twins when Judy began therapy and had been less emotionally available to Judy. It is Emma who encouraged Judy to get help.

Judy's loss of her job represented a major stressor as well as a traumatic event, at several levels. Her work had been a source of significant meaning for her. She had worked in the same place for 29 years, nearly her entire adult life. She enjoyed her work and derived much satisfaction from her relationships with the residents and co-workers at the facility. Her loss of employment had also created financial hardship for the couple, as Judy had been the primary breadwinner. Her husband was severely dyslexic, which limited his employment options. He had previously done construction work, and had a seasonal business when Judy lost her job. Judy reported that they had been in debt in the past, and that her husband was "controlling" about money. While she was receiving disability payments, the decrease in her income had created some conflict between them. The couple owned their own home, so their housing was stable. As Gitterman and Germain (2008, p. 72) note, "When a life stressor strikes and is not successfully managed, additional stressors can erupt in other areas of life." The accumulation of life stressors overwhelmed Judy.

The beginning phase of the work with Judy focused primarily on developing a mutual agreement about focus on her life stressors, gathering information, and on helping her to manage her symptoms of depression and anxiety. Behavioral strategies were used to teach relaxation techniques, and she did not report any additional panic symptoms. The social worker also offered support in coping with the uncertainty of Judy's medical situation. She had been scheduled for a double knee replacement with a local doctor, but this doctor then decided that her case was too complex and referred her to a specialist in the nearest large city. During this phase of the work, Judy saw the agency's nurse practitioner and was prescribed an antidepressant medication. She also expressed ambivalence about being in therapy. "I'm not sure if this is helping, coming and seeing you every week. It's not like I feel any better afterwards," she stated.

> But I know I should be talking about it. I mean, it's there all the time anyway. I can try not to think about it, but it doesn't go away. It's like I can put it away in the corner, and try to pretend it's not there, but it's still there in the corner.

After six weeks, Judy began to open up a bit more to the social worker, and some problems in her marriage emerged as another issue. She shared that her husband was very concerned about their daughter's pregnancy, but was less attentive to Judy and did not know how best to support her (interpersonal). She also reported conflict between them about finances, stating that at times he threatened to leave her, which she found very upsetting. "You know," she stated, "I may seem independent, but I really rely on him." At the same time, she expressed a bit more willingness to depend on the social worker, asking if she could call between sessions if necessary.

This phase of the work also continued to deal with Judy's two primary issues: her feelings about the loss of her employment, and the stress generated by her medical issues. She continued to mourn the loss of her work, and struggled with the feeling that her former colleagues had forgotten her (life transitional stressors). It also became increasingly apparent that she would not be able to return to work, as several new medical problems surfaced during this time. She was diagnosed with kidney stones, and a lesion was identified on her liver. She consulted with a specialist, who was willing to perform a double knee replacement, but he wanted to wait to schedule the surgery until the issue with her liver was resolved. He also recommended that she consider a gastric bypass to help her with weight loss. The social worker helped her to cope with her feelings of discouragement and her sense of powerlessness in negotiating the health care system, helped her negotiate the system (environmental) and explored how her family could support her during this challenging time. Judy had some discomfort with the idea of her husband and children providing support to her, and discussed her tendency to play a caretaking role in relationships, both personally and in her previous place of work. She felt that the antidepressant was helping with her depressive symptoms, but was troubled by her lack of energy and motivation. "It's like I have no ambition to do anything. It's like I have nothing to look forward to," she stated.

After approximately six months of counseling, Judy learned that the lesion on her liver was benign, and her knee replacement surgery was scheduled for two months later. This development marked a new phase in the work. Judy was quite anxious about the surgery, so the social worker addressed ways for her to manage her anxiety about the upcoming procedure. In preparation for the surgery, Judy decided to ask her daughter Emma to be her health care proxy. As she engaged in this process, feelings related to her mother's death emerged, and the social worker helped her with issues of grief and loss. Judy noted during this stage that she was feeling much more resolved about the loss of her employment. As the surgery approached, she also grew more able to handle her anxiety, and by the last session before the procedure, she was feeling fairly calm. As she and the social worker discussed plans for continuing their work together after the surgery, Judy acknowledged her increasing connection to the social worker, stating, "I feel comfortable talking to you. It was hard in the beginning, but it's easier for me now."

Judy and the social worker agreed to a planned break in their work while Judy was in the hospital and then in a rehab facility. When Judy returned after a number of weeks, she was recovering well and feeling less depressed, though she wanted to continue on her antidepressant. The work shifted to an exploration of how she would spend her time, given that she would not be returning to work. Soon after, Judy announced that she and her husband had decided to move to a different part of the country, where her husband's family lived. She was uncertain about this plan, as it would mean being far from her children, but was willing to go along with it on a trial basis. The last several sessions were spent on termination, processing Judy's feelings about the ongoing significant life changes that had resulted from the loss of her work and reflecting upon the year that Judy and the social worker had spent working together.

Practice with Judy illustrates several key issues in helping a person dealing with depression. First, her depression was clearly multidetermined, a result of several interacting factors. She had some family history of depression, so it is likely that there was a genetic component to her mood condition. This biological vulnerability combined with the early loss of both parents, which acted as a predisposing factor in the depressive episode that emerged later in life. The loss of her employment as an adult precipitated her depression, triggering feelings related to these early losses. The significance of loss in the etiology of depression has been discussed both by Freud (1917) and by cognitive theorists such as Beck (2008). In order to be responsive to these multiple underlying causes of Judy's depression, the social worker drew upon several different approaches. The work was primarily supportive, exploring Judy's experiences of loss and helping her to cope with past and present life stressors. Antidepressant medication was another useful tool in decreasing her symptoms of depression.

The social worker drew upon behavioral strategies to help Judy manage her anxiety. It is important to note that Judy suffered from another mental health condition in addition to depression. Comorbidity is common among individuals with mood conditions, and workers must be able to use a range of interventions in order to effectively address all the problems with which their clients are struggling.

Another important theme that emerged in helping Judy relates to her issues with dependency. Judy initially was hesitant to engage with the social worker, and directly expressed her doubts about the possibility of her being helpful. Over time, she became more connected to the social worker, allowing herself to rely on the social worker for support, validation, and environmental interventions. Though this theme was not explored in depth, it appears likely that Judy's outward presentation – her reluctance to depend on others, and her tendency to play a caretaking role in relationships – was a means of protecting herself from an intense longing to be nurtured and taken care of. This pattern is common among individuals with a history of significant loss. When faced with later experiences of abandonment or rejection, they are likely to suffer from anaclitic depression, which is often characterized by feelings of helplessness and loneliness (Blatt, 1995). Indeed, Judy struggled primarily with feeling "forgotten" by her co-workers and powerless in the face of the health care system. From this perspective, it is not surprising that Judy's loss of employment was a key factor both in the onset of her depression and in the way that she experienced her depression.

Finally, the social worker's approach to working with Judy is a clear illustration of a social work approach with people suffering from depression. Judy's difficulties were rooted not just in the individual or the environment, but also in the transactions between them. At the individual level were her genetic predisposition, her history of loss, and her medical issues. At the environmental level were her loss of employment and the stress of negotiating the health care system, both of which were exacerbating her depression. The worker was careful to take into account all of these factors, focusing upon the ways that Judy could build upon the resources that were available to her in order to improve the person-environment fit (Gitterman & Germain, 2008).

Conclusion

Mood conditions are among the most common mental health problems in the United States, and they take a significant toll on the lives of many individuals. While there are differences in the experience of depression or bipolar disorder on the basis of age, race, ethnicity, socio-economic status, and gender, there is no group that is immune to the risk of developing a mood disorder. Fortunately, mood disorders are treatable, and should be approached from a perspective that takes into account the multiple factors that may be underlying the disorder. Mood disorders are best understood as a product of biological, psychological, and social factors that are all mutually interactive. While the relative importance of each type of factor varies from one individual to the next, it is important to consider the role that each may play in causing and maintaining depression or bipolar disorder, and to intervene accordingly.

It is here that social work makes its most important contribution to the understanding and helping with mood disorders. The holistic person-environment perspective that defines social work is particularly helpful both in conceptualizing an individual's difficulties and in creating a framework for intervention. In their efforts to help a client with a mood disorder, social workers may provide support, enhance coping skills, offer psychoeducation, work with families, coordinate services, and intervene with environmental stressors. Moreover, their commitment to social justice demands that these services are offered to all who need them, and so social workers strive to eliminate the disparities in access to care that currently affect many individuals with mood disorders.

The importance of a biopsychosocial approach in the treatment of mood disorders is beautifully articulated by Kay Redfield Jamison (1995) in her discussion of her own experience of living with bipolar disorder. While she refers to psychotherapy, it is clear that she is describing the critical role of the kinds of psychosocial interventions that are often provided by social workers. In Jamison's words:

At this point in my existence, I cannot imagine a normal life without both taking lithium and having had the benefits of psychotherapy. Lithium prevents my seductive but disastrous highs, diminishes my depressions, clears out the wool and webbing from my disordered thinking, slows me down, gentles me out, keeps me from ruining my career and relationships, keeps me out of a hospital, alive, and makes psychotherapy possible. But, ineffably, psychotherapy *heals*. It makes some sense of the confusion, reins in the terrifying thoughts and feelings, returns some control and hope and possibility of learning from it all ... Psychotherapy is a sanctuary; it is a battleground; it is a place I have been psychotic, neurotic, elated, confused, and despairing beyond belief. But, always, it is where I have believed – or learned to believe – that I might someday be able to contend with all of this.

(Jamison, 1995, pp. 88–89)

Web resources

American Psychological Association
www.apa.org

Depression and Bipolar Support Alliance
www.dbsalliance.org/site/PageServer?pagename=home

International Foundation for Research and Education on Depression
www.ifred.org/

Mental Health America
www.nmha.org/

Mental Health: A Report of the Surgeon General
www.surgeongeneral.gov/library/mentalhealth/chapter4/sec3.html

National Alliance on Mental Illness
www.nami.org/

National Institute of Mental Health
www.nimh.nih.gov/index.shtml

Postpartum Support International
www.postpartum.net/

SAMHSA's National Mental Health Information Center
www.mentalhealth.samhsa.gov/publications/allpubs/ken98-0049/default.asp

Web MD
www.DepressionResources.webmd.com

References

American Psychiatric Association (APA). (2000). *Diagnostic and statistical manual of mental disorders* (4th ed., text revision). Washington, DC: APA.

Amsterdam, J., Brunswick, D., & O'Reardon, J. (2002). Bipolar disorder in women. *Psychiatric Annals, 32* (7), 397–404.

Arean, P., Gum, A., McCulloch, C., Bostrom, A., Gallagher-Thompson, D., & Thompson, L. (2005). Treatment of depression in low-income older adults. *Psychology and Aging, 20* (4), 601–609.

Avenevoli, S., Knight, E., Kessler, R., & Merikangas, K. (2008). Epidemiology of depression in children and adolescents. In J. Abela & B. Hankin (eds), *Handbook of depression in children and adolescents* (pp. 6–32). New York: Guilford Press.

Baldassano, C., Marangell, L., Gyulai, L., Ghaemi, S., Joffe, H., Kim, D. et al. (2005). Gender differences in bipolar disorder: Retrospective data from the first 500 STEP-BD participants. *Bipolar Disorders, 7,* 465–470.

Barnes, C., & Mitchell, P. (2005). Considerations in the management of bipolar disorder in women. *Australian and New Zealand Journal of Psychiatry, 39,* 662–673.

Bartels, S., Forester, B., Miles, K., & Joyce, T. (2000). Mental health service use by elderly patients with bipolar disorder and unipolar major depression. *American Journal of Geriatric Psychiatry, 8* (2), 160–166.

Bass, J., Bolton, P., & Murray, L. (2007). Do not forget culture when studying mental health. *The Lancet, 370* (9591), 918–919.

Bauer, M., McBride, L., Williford, W., Glick, H., Kinosian, B., Altshuler, L. et al. (2006a). Collaborative care for bipolar disorder: Part I. Intervention and implementation in a randomized effectiveness trial. *Psychiatric Services, 57* (7), 927–936.

Bauer, M., McBride, L., Williford, W., Glick, H., Kinosian, B., Altshuler, L. et al. (2006b). Collaborative care for bipolar disorder: Part II. Impact on clinical outcome, function, and costs. *Psychiatric Services, 57* (7), 937–945.

Beck, A. (2008). The evolution of the cognitive model of depression and its neurobiological correlates. *American Journal of Psychiatry, 165* (8), 969–977.

Bhugra, D., & Flick, G. (2005). Pathways to care for patients with bipolar disorder. *Bipolar Disorders, 7,* 236–245.

Biederman, J., Kwon, A., Wozniak, J., Mick, E., Markowitz, S., Fazio, V. et al. (2004). Absence of gender differences in pediatric bipolar disorder: Findings from a large sample of referred youth. *Journal of Affective Disorders, 82* (2–3), 207–214.

Birmaher, B., & Axelson, D. (2006). Course and outcome of bipolar spectrum disorder in children and adolescents: A review of the existing literature. *Development and Psychopathology, 18* (4), 1023–1035.

Birmaher, B., Arbelaez, C., & Brent, D. (2002). Course and outcome of child and adolescent major depressive disorder. *Child and Adolescent Psychiatric Clinics of North America, 11* (3), 619–638.

Birmaher, B., Williamson, D., Dahl, R., Axelson, D., Kaufman, J., Dorn, L. et al. (2004). Clinical presentation and course of depression in youth: Does onset in childhood differ from onset in adolescence? *Journal of the American Academy of Child and Adolescent Psychiatry, 43* (1), 63–70.

Bland, R., & Harrison, C. (2000). Developing and evaluating a psychoeducation program for caregivers of bipolar affective disorder patients: Report of a pilot project. *Research on Social Work Practice, 10* (2), 209–228.

Blasinsky, M., Goldman, H., & Unützer, J. (2006). Project IMPACT: A report of barriers and facilitators to sustainabililty. *Administration and Policy in Mental Health and Mental Health Services Research, 33,* 718–729.

Blatt, S. (1995). The destructiveness of perfectionism: Implications for the treatment of depression. *American Psychologist, 50* (12), 1003–1020.

Bowden, C. (2001). Strategies to reduce misdiagnosis of bipolar depression. *Psychiatric Services, 52* (1), 51–55.

Clarkin, J., Carpenter, D., Hull, J., Wilner, P., & Glick, I. (1998). Effects of psychoeducational intervention for married patients with bipolar disorder and their spouses. *Psychiatric Services, 49* (4), 531–533.

Cochran, S. (2001). Emerging research on lesbians' and gay men's mental health: Does sexual orientation really matter? *American Psychologist, 56,* 931–947.

Commission on Adolescent Depression and Bipolar Disorder. (2005). Prevention of depression and bipolar disorder. In D. Evans, E. Foa, R. Gur, H. Hendin, & D. O'Brien (eds), *Treating and preventing adolescent mental health disorders: What we know and what we don't know. A research agenda for improving the mental health of our youth* (pp. 55–67). New York: Oxford University Press.

Curtis, V. (2005). Women are not the same as men: Specific clinical issues for female patients with bipolar disorder. *Bipolar Disorders, 7* (Suppl. 1), 16–24.

Davies, M., McBride, L., & Sajatovic, M. (2008). The collaborative care practice model in the long-term care of individuals with bipolar disorder: A case study. *Journal of Psychiatric and Mental Health Nursing, 15* (8), 649–653.

DelBello, M., Soutullo, C., & Strakowski, S. (2000). Racial differences in treatment of adolescents with bipolar disorder. *American Journal of Psychiatry, 157* (5), 837–838.

de Mello, M., de Jesus Mari, J., Bacaltchuk, J. Verdeli, H., & Neugebauer, R. (2005). A systematic review of research findings on the efficacy of interpersonal therapy for depressive disorders. *European Archives of Psychiatry and Clinical Neuroscience, 255* (2), 75–82.

Depp, C., Lindamer, L., Folsom, D., Gilmer, T., Hough, R., Garcia, P. et al. (2005). Differences in clinical features and mental health service use in bipolar disorder across the life span. *American Journal of Geriatric Psychiatry, 13* (4), 290–298.

Dietz, L., Birmaher, B., Williamson, D., Silk, J., Dahl, R., Axelson, D. et al. (2008). Mother-child interactions in depressed children at high risk and low risk for future depression. *Journal of the American Academy of Child and Adolescent Psychiatry, 47* (5), 574–582.

Dilsaver, S., & Akiskal, H. (2005). High rate of unrecognized bipolar mixed states among destitute Hispanic adolescents referred for "major depressive disorder." *Journal of Affective Disorders, 84* (2–3), 179–186.

Duax, J., Youngstrom, E., Calabrese, J., & Findling, R. (2007). Sex differences in pediatric bipolar disorder. *Journal of Clinical Psychiatry, 68* (10), 1565–1573.

Fleck, D., Keck, P., Corey, K., & Strakowski, S. (2005). Factors associated with medication adherence in African Americans and white patients with bipolar disorder. *Journal of Clinical Psychiatry, 66* (5), 646–652.

Ford, D., Pincus, H., Unützer, J., Bauer, M., Gonzalez, J., & Wells, K. (2002). Practice-based interventions. *Mental Health Services Research, 4* (4), 199–204.

Freeman, M. (2006). Depression: What's sex got to do with it? *Journal of Clinical Psychiatry, 67* (10), 1610–1611.

Freud, S. (1917). Mourning and melancholia. In J. Strachey (ed.), *The standard edition of the complete psychological works of Sigmund Freud* (Vol. 14, pp. 237–258). London: Hogarth Press.

Fristad, M. (2006). Psychoeducational treatment for school-aged children with bipolar disorder. *Development and Psychopathology, 18* (4), 1289–1306.

Fyffe, D., Sirey, J., Heo, M., & Bruce, M. (2004). Late-life depression among Black and White elderly homecare patients. *American Journal of Geriatric Psychiatry, 12* (5), 531–535.

Gallagher, R. (2005). Evidence-based psychotherapies for depressed adolescents: A review and clinical guidelines. *Primary Psychiatry, 12* (9), 33–39.

Garver, D., Lazarus, A., Rajagopalan, K., Lamerato, L., Katz, L., Stern, L. et al. (2006). Racial differences in medication switching and concomitant prescriptions in the treatment of bipolar disorder. *Psychiatric Services, 57* (5), 666–672.

Gitterman, A. (2008). Ecological framework. In Y. Mizrahi and L. Davis (eds), *Encyclopedia of social work* (20th ed.). New York: Oxford University Press.

Gitterman, A. (2010). Advances in the life model of social work practice. In F. Turner (ed.), *Social work treatment, interlocking theoretical approaches*. New York: Oxford Press.

Gitterman, A., & Germain, C.B. (2008). *The life model of social work practice: Advances in knowledge and practice* (3rd ed.). New York: Columbia University Press.

Goldstein, E. (1995). *Ego psychology and social work practice*. New York: Free Press.

Gottfries, C. (1998). Is there a difference between elderly and younger patients with regard to the symptomatology and aetiology of depression? *International Clinical Psychopharmacology, 13* (Suppl. 5), S13–S18.

Harris, J. (2005). The increased diagnosis of "juvenile bipolar disorder": What are we treating? *Psychiatric Services, 56* (5), 529–531.

Holosko, M., Jean-Baptiste, N., Le, T., Eaton, A., & Power, L. (2007). Major depressive disorder. In B. Thyer & J. Wodarksi (eds), *Social work in mental health: An evidence-based approach* (pp. 289–306). Hoboken, NJ: John Wiley & Sons.

Hsu, G., Wan, Y., Adler, D., Rand, W., Choi, E., & Tsang, B. (2005). Detection of major depressive disorder in Chinese Americans in primary care. *Hong Kong Journal of Psychiatry, 15* (3), 71–76.

Ialongo, N., McCreary, B., Pearson, J., Koenig, A., Schmidt, N., Poduska, J. et al. (2004). Major depressive disorder in a population of urban, African-American young adults: Prevalence, correlates, comorbidity and unmet mental health service need. *Journal of Affective Disorders, 79* (1–3), 127–136.

Jamison, K. R. (1995). *An unquiet mind: A memoir of moods and madness*. New York: Vintage.

Jerrell, J. (2008). Pharmacotherapy in the community-based treatment of children with bipolar I disorder. *Human Psychopharmacology: Clinical and Experimental, 23*, 53–59.

Kawa, I., Carter, J., Joyce, P., Doughty, C., Frampton, C., Wells, J. et al. (2005). Gender differences in bipolar disorder: Age of onset, course, comorbidity, and symptom presentation. *Bipolar Disorders, 7*, 119–125.

Keck, P., McElroy, S., Strakowski, S., West, S., Sax, K., Hawkins, J. et al. (1998). Twelve-month outcome of patients with bipolar disorder following hospitalization for a manic or mixed episode. *American Journal of Psychiatry, 155* (5), 646–652.

Keltner, N., & Boschini, D. (2009). Electroconvulsive therapy. *Perspectives in Psychiatric Care, 45* (1), 66–70.

Kessing, L. (2004). Gender differences in the phenomenology of bipolar disorder. *Bipolar Disorders, 6*, 421–425.

Kessler, R., Merikangas, K., & Wang, P. (2007). Prevalence, comorbidity, and service utilization for mood disorders in the United States at the beginning of the twenty-first century. *Annual Review of Clinical Psychology, 3*, 137–158.

Kilbourne, A., Haas, G., Benoit, M., Bauer, M., & Pincus, H. (2004). Concurrent psychiatric diagnoses by age and race among persons with bipolar disorder. *Psychiatric Services, 55* (8), 931–933.

Kilbourne, A., Bauer, M., Pincus, H., Williford, W., Kirk, G., & Beresford, T. (2005). Clinical, psychosocial, and treatment differences in minority patients with bipolar disorder. *Bipolar Disorders, 7*, 89–97.

Kockler, M., & Heun, R. (2002). Gender differences of depressive symptoms in depressed and nondepressed elderly persons. *International Journal of Geriatric Psychiatry, 17*, 65–72.

Kovacs, M. (2001). Gender and the course of major depressive disorder through adolescence in clinically referred youngsters. *Journal of the American Academy of Child and Adolescent Psychiatry, 40* (9), 1079–1085.

Kung, W., & Lu, P. (2008). How symptom manifestations affect help seeking for mental health problems among Chinese Americans. *Journal of Nervous and Mental Disease, 196* (1), 46–54.

Kupfer, D., Frank, E., Grochocinski, V., Houck, P., & Brown, C. (2005). African-American participants in a bipolar treatment registry: Clinical and treatment characteristics. *Bipolar disorders, 7*, 82–88.

Lawson, W., & Strickland, T. (2004). Racial and ethnic issues affect treatment for bipolar disorder. *Psychiatric Annals, 34* (1), 17–20.

Leibenluft, E., & Rich, B. (2008). Pediatric bipolar disorder. *Annual Review of Clinical Psychology, 4*, 163–187.

Lenze, E. (2005). Recognizing late-life depression comorbid with medical illness. *CNS Spectrums, 10* (8), 8–9.

Lesser, I., Castro, D., Gaynes, B., Gonzalez, J., Rush, J., Alpert, J. et al. (2007). Ethnicity/race and outcome in the treatment of depression: Results from STAR*D. *Medical Care, 45* (11), 1043–1051.

Lewis, L. (2005). Patient perspectives on the diagnosis, treatment, and management of bipolar disorder. *Bipolar Disorders, 7* (Suppl. 1), 33–37.

Lewinsohn, P., Pettit, J., Joiner, T., & Seeley, J. (2003). The symptomatic expression of major depressive disorder in adolescents and young adults. *Journal of Abnormal Psychology, 112* (2), 244–252.

Mackinaw-Koons, B., & Fristad, M. (2004). Children with bipolar disorder: How to break down barriers and work effectively together. *Professional Psychology: Research and Practice, 35* (5), 481–484.

MacQueen, G., & Young, T. (2001). Bipolar II disorder: Symptoms, course, and response to treatment. *Psychiatric Services, 52* (3), 358–361.

Marcus, S., Young, E., Kerber, K., Kornstein, S., Farabaugh, A., Mitchell, J. et al. (2005). Gender differences in depression: Findings from the STAR*D study. *Journal of Affective Disorders, 87* (2–3), 141–150.

McIntosh, D., & Trotter, J. (2006). Early onset bipolar spectrum disorder: Psychopharmacological, psychological, and educational management. *Psychology in the Schools, 43* (4), 451–460.

Mendelson, T., Rehkopf, D., & Kubzansky, L. (2008). Depression among Latinos in the United States: A meta-analytic review. *Journal of Consulting and Clinical Psychology, 76* (3), 355–366.

Miklowitz, D., & Chang, K. (2008). Prevention of bipolar disorder in at-risk children: Theoretical assumptions and empirical foundations. *Development and Psychopathology, 20* (3), 881–897.

Miller, L., & Barnett, S. (2008). Mood lability and bipolar disorder in children and adolescents. *International Review of Psychiatry, 20* (2), 171–176.

Morris, C., Miklowitz, D., & Waxmonsky, J. (2007). Family-focused treatment for bipolar disorder in adults and youth. *Journal of Clinical Psychology, 63* (5), 433–445.

Mueller, T., Kohn, R., Leventhal, N., Leon, A., Solomon, D., Coryell, W. et al. (2004). The course of depression in elderly patients. *American Journal of Geriatric Psychiatry, 12* (1), 22–29.

Mueser, K., Webb, C., Pfeiffer, M., & Gladis, M. (1996). Family burden of schizophrenia and bipolar disorder: Perceptions of relatives and professionals. *Psychiatric Services, 47* (5), 507–511.

National Institutes of Health (n.d.). Fact sheet: Mood disorders. Retrieved June 15, 2009, from www.nih.gov/about/researchresultsforthepublic/MoodDisorders.pdf

Ohayon, M. (2007). Epidemiology of depression and its treatment in the general population. *Journal of Psychiatric Research, 41* (3–4), 207–213.

O'Connor, C., Gordon, O., Graham, M., Kelly, F., & O'Grady-Walshe, A. (2008). Service user perspectives of a psychoeducation group for individuals with a diagnosis of bipolar disorder: A qualitative study. *Journal of Nervous and Mental Disease, 196* (7), 568–571.

Patel, N., DelBello, M., Keck, P., & Strakowski, S. (2005). Ethnic differences in maintenance antipsychotic prescription among adolescents with bipolar disorder. *Journal of Child and Adolescent Psychopharmacology, 15* (6), 938–946.

Paykel, E., Abbott, R., Morriss, R., Hayhurst, H., & Scott, J. (2006). Sub-syndromal and syndromal symptoms in the longitudinal course of bipolar disorder. *British Journal of Psychiatry, 189* (2), 118–123.

Perils, R., Miyahara, S., Marangell, L., Wisniewski, S., Ostacher, M., DelBello, M. et al. (2004). Long-term implications of early onset in bipolar disorder: Data from the first one thousand participants in the Systematic Treatment Enhancement Program for Bipolar Disorder (STEP-BD). *Biological Psychiatry, 55* (9), 875–881.

Perlick, D., Rosenheck, R., Clarkin, J., Sirey, J., & Raue, P. (1999). Symptoms predicting inpatient service use among patients with bipolar affective disorder. *Psychiatric Services, 50* (6), 806–812.

Pollack, L., Harvin, S., & Cramer, R. (2000). Coping resources of African-American and White patients hospitalized for bipolar disorder. *Psychiatric Services, 51* (10), 1310–1312.

Public Broadcasting Service (n.d.). Depression out of the shadows: Statistics. Retrieved January 7, 2009, from www.pbs.org/wgbh/takeonestep/depression/pdf/dep_stats.pdf

Rasgon, N., Bauer, M., Grof, P., Gyulai, L., Elman, S., Glenn, T. et al. (2005). Sex-specific self-reported mood changes by patients with bipolar disorder. *Journal of Psychiatric Research, 39* (1), 77–83.

Reinecke, M., & Ginsburg, G. (2008). Cognitive-behavioral treatment of depression during childhood and adolescence. In J. Abela & B. Hankin (eds), *Handbook of depression in children and adolescents* (pp. 179–206). New York: Guilford Press.

Reinecke, M., & Simons, A. (2005). Vulnerability to depression among adolescents: Implications for cognitive-behavioral treatment. *Cognitive and Behavioral Practice, 12* (2), 166–176.

Riolo, S., Nguyen, T., Greden, J., & King, C. (2005). Prevalence of depression by race/ethnicity: Findings from the National Health and Nutrition Examination Survey III. *American Journal of Public Health, 95* (6), 998–1000.

Rizzo, C., Esposito-Smythers, C., Swenson, L., Birmaher, B., Ryan, N., Strober, M. et al. (2007). Factors associated with mental health service utilization among bipolar youth. *Bipolar Disorders, 9,* 839–850.

Sach, G., Yan, L., Swann, A., & Allen, M. (2001). Integration of suicide prevention into outpatient management of bipolar disorder. *Journal of Clinical Psychiatry, 62* (Suppl. 25), 3–11.

Sachs-Ericsson, N., & Ciarlo, J. (2000). Gender, social roles, and mental health: An epidemiological perspective. *Sex Roles, 43* (9–10), 605–628.

Sajatovic, M. (2002). Aging-related issues in bipolar disorder: A health services perspective. *Journal of Geriatric Psychiatry and Neurology, 15* (3), 128–133.

Sajatovic, M., Davies, M., & Hrouda, D. (2004). Enhancement of treatment adherence among patients with bipolar disorder. *Psychiatric Services, 55* (3), 264–269.

Shear, K. (2005). Bereavement-related depression in the elderly. *CNS Spectrums, 10* (8), 3–5.

Simon, G., Ludman, E., Unützer, J., Bauer, M., Operskalski, B., & Rutter, C. (2005). Randomized trial of a population-based care program for people with bipolar disorder. *Psychological Medicine, 35* (1), 13–24.

Sinha, R., & Rush, J. (2006). Treatment and prevention of depression in women. In C. Mazure & G. Keita (eds), *Understanding depression in women: Applying empirical research to practice and policy* (pp. 45–70). Washington, DC: American Psychological Association.

Sloan, D., & Kornstein, S. (2003). Gender differences in depression and response to antidepressant treatment. *Psychiatric Clinics of North America, 26,* 581–594.

Soares, J., Stintzig, C., Jackson, C., & Skoldin, B. (1997). Psychoeducation for patients with bipolar disorder: An exploratory study. *Nordic Journal of Psychiatry, 51* (6), 439–446.

Stark, K., Hargrave, J., Hersh, B., Greenberg, M., Herren, J., & Fisher, M. (2008). Treatment of childhood depression: The ACTION treatment program. In J. Abela & B. Hankin (eds), *Handbook of depression in children and adolescents* (pp. 224–229). New York: Guilford Press.

Toprac, M., Rush, J., Conner, T., Crismon, M., Dees, M., Hopkins, C. et al. (2000). The Texas Medication Algorithm Project and Patient and Family Education Program: A consumer-guided initiative. *Journal of Clinical Psychiatry, 61* (7), 477–486.

Turner, J., & Beiser, M. (1990). Major depression and depressive symptomatology among the physically disabled: Addressing the role of chronic stress. *Journal of Nervous and Mental Disease, 178* (6), 343–350.

United States Public Health Service (n.d.). Mental health: A report of the Surgeon General. Mood disorders. Retrieved June 15, 2009, from www.surgeongeneral.gov/library/mentalhealth/chapter4/sec3.html

Watts, S., & Markham, R. (2005). Etiology of depression in children. *Journal of Instructional Psychology, 32* (3), 266–270.

Wenzel, A., Steer, R., & Beck, A. (2005). Are there any gender differences in frequency of self-reported somatic symptoms of depression? *Journal of Affective Disorders, 89* (1–3), 177–181.

Whitaker, R. (2007). Creating the bipolar child: How our drug-based paradigm of care is fueling an epidemic of disabling mental illness in children. In S. Olfman (ed.), *Bipolar children: Cutting-edge controversy, insights, and research* (pp. 46–63). Westport, CT: Praeger.

Williams, D., Gonzalez, H., Neighbors, H., Nesse, R., Abelson, J., Sweetman, J. et al. (2007). Prevalence and distribution of major depressive disorder in African Americans, Caribbean Blacks, and Non-Hispanic Whites: Results from the National Survey of American Life. *Archives of General Psychiatry, 64* (3), 305–315.

Williams, J., & Manning, J. (2008). Collaborative mental health and primary care for bipolar disorder. *Journal of Psychiatric Practice, 14* (Suppl. 2), 55–64.

Yanos, P., Primavera, L., & Knight, E. (2001). Consumer-run service participation, recovery of social functioning, and the mediating role of psychological factors. *Psychiatric Services, 52* (4), 493–500.

Yeung, A., Chan, R., Mischoulon, D., Sonawalla, S., Wong, E., Nierenberg, A. et al. (2004). Prevalence of major depressive disorder among Chinese-Americans in primary care. *General Hospital Psychiatry, 26* (1), 24–30.

Yonkers, K., & Brawnman-Mintzer, O. (2002). The pharmacologic treatment of depression: Is gender a critical factor? *Journal of Clinical Psychiatry, 63* (7), 610–615.

Youngstrom, E., Meyers, O., Youngstrom, J., Calabrese, J., & Findling, R. (2006). Diagnostic and measurement issues in the assessment of pediatric bipolar disorder: Implications for understanding mood disorder across the life cycle. *Development and Psychopathology, 18*, 989–1021.

Zaretsky, A. (2003). Targeted psychosocial interventions for bipolar disorder. *Bipolar Disorders, 5* (Suppl. 2), 80–87.

16 Anxiety conditions

Nina Rovinelli Heller and Lisa Werkmeister Rozas

Linda, a 52-year-old white woman, presented to her local hospital emergency department saying "I'm dying." Indeed, she was in significant distress, complaining of heart palpitations, dizziness, clammy hands and a pervasive feeling of dread. She further stated that "this keeps happening now." When her medical tests all came back negative, the emergency department social worker was called to talk with her. By this time, the physical symptoms had subsided but Linda expressed her fears that she really was having a heart attack but that the "doctors didn't know it," that she was "going crazy," and that this would "just keep happening." In an effort to obtain a medical and family history, the social worker asked Linda if she had ever felt this way before or had she any family member who seemed to feel this way. Linda responded that she'd "had a spell" in college, when she'd first left home which later subsided, and that she had been "really, really nervous" for a time after the birth of her first child. She also stated that her mother used to get "so worried about the kids' safety," that "she'd always insisted on picking us up at school herself, even when we were older and it was embarrassing." As they talked, the social worker learned that Linda's only child had very recently left for college and she was now alone because her husband had left her the previous spring. She further described herself as "a very competent person" and could not understand how she could fall apart this way. She said she'd had two previous episodes in the last several months wherein she "felt I was dying." Upon further questioning, she revealed that she'd received a second notice of foreclosure in the mail, immediately prior to the onset of the symptoms that led to her coming to the emergency department. Linda was suffering with anxiety and struggling to make sense of its debilitating symptoms and her decreased functioning while worrying that "it would happen again."

In human evolution, anxiety in its many manifestations – fears, worries, panics and obsessions – began as a normal and essentially adaptive human response. Anxiety and classically, the fight or flight response, allows a person to perceive, identify, and respond to a range of conditions of danger. This initial perception of danger is biologically based, signaling the individual to prepare for battle or to retreat. In so doing, a complex array of hormonal and behavioral responses are set into motion. There is ample support for cross-species parallels to both the organism's response to danger and the underlying brain mechanisms; we are hard-wired to both experience and importantly, to deal with anxiety. However, we need not be confronted with danger that threatens our very survival in order to experience significant anxiety; signal anxiety itself can also prod us to utilize important coping strategies to deal with both intra-personal and interpersonal stress.

However, when a client presents to a social worker or other professional with symptoms of anxiety, usually, the normal strategies the person employs to manage the anxiety are no longer working. When anxious, we typically appraise the danger, use cognitive strategies to "talk ourselves down" or "reality test" our fears or to problem solve, use behavioral means such as diversion, use our social support systems (talk to a friend), or employ self-soothing strategies, such as using forms of relaxation. When these attempts to quell our anxiety fail and when this occurs over time, our anxiety is no longer adaptive or useful. Maladaptive anxiety tends to overwhelm the individual, resulting in diminished functioning over discrete or pervasive domains and may result in the development of distressing symptoms. Linda, for example, described herself generally as a competent person, but she was now clearly overwhelmed. Her usual coping strategies were no longer working, perhaps under the stress of marital separation, a child leaving home, the threat of foreclosure of her home and an underlying propensity for anxiety. Behaviorally, the person may avoid distressing stimuli or compulsively confront or seek those stimuli. Cognitively, the person may see danger lurking around every corner and Linda was certainly concerned that she was at imminent risk. Like Linda, the person with anxiety may experience discomforting physiological symptoms which can be both frightening and painful. Affectively, anxiety is distressing, frightening, exhausting and confusing for clients and for the people around them.

If anxiety conditions are initially triggered by environmental factors (though there may exist underlying biological propensities) we must understand the conditions of the environment which also serve to maintain, exacerbate or mediate those symptoms. At the extreme, exposure to the perceived and real dangers of community and interpersonal violence and war, place individuals and groups of individuals at significant and elevated risk. At the more moderate (but perhaps no less distressing) end of the spectrum, fears related to loss of others, or of physical integrity and to life transitions and stressors may produce a range of anxiety symptoms. Racism, oppression and discrimination in all domains present both acute and chronic challenges which can create significant anxieties. At the same time, individual, community and cultural influences may provide factors for resilience as well as vulnerability. The biopsychosocial perspective (Woods & Hollis, 2000) in general and the life model of social work (Gitterman & Germain, 2008) familiar to social workers, provide a framework for understanding the etiology, main-tenance, course, and alleviation of the full range of anxiety conditions.

Definitions of anxiety conditions

Anxiety conditions are most commonly explained *descriptively*, as in the *Diagnostic and statistical manual* (DSM-IV-TR: American Psychiatric Association, 2000) and *phenomenologically*. Limitations of the former, a disease-based classification system which pays scant attention to environmental and cultural considerations, are well documented in the social work literature (Kirk & Kutchins, 1992; Kutchins & Kirk, 1988). The DSM-IV-TR (APA, 2000) classification does not address issues of etiology and has been described as atheoretical. What the manual does provide us is a common language for the description of the symptoms of anxiety conditions which can be useful for initial diagnosis and intervention, and for research purposes. The latter, the phenomeno-logical approach, conveys a greater sense of the *experience* of the specific condition. Taken together, the definitions provide a more comprehensive picture. For example, in the case of Linda, if we were to focus entirely on her symptoms of anxiety, including their duration, degree and frequency and the criterion of impaired functioning, we might well arrive at a DSM-IV-TR diagnosis which would help us to focus in on a specific anxiety condition. From the stand point of beginning interventions and referral for medication evaluation, that would be helpful. However, if that were our exclusive focus, we would miss critical information about the meaning of Linda's symptoms to her and in her life context. We would leave unspoken questions about her experiences and responses to the loss of her husband, her son, and the impending loss of her home. We would have little understanding of her own narrative of her anxious responses to these life events and how she reconciles that with her general sense of herself as a "competent" person. All of Linda's own narratives about her own life can be utilized in the service of the work of restoring her to her usual adaptive functioning and to helping her with her significant life transitions, status and role changes, and environmental stressors. At the same time, a person experiencing debilitating symptoms of anxiety wants rapid relief, which can be aided in part by the identification of the nature of the specific condition. For example, if we were to decide that Linda was suffering with panic disorder, our interventions would be quite different than if she were struggling with generalized anxiety disorder. Those distinctions, in both theory and practice are important. The anxiety in panic disorder is discrete with a focus in a particular area; interventions are targeted for specific symptoms which occur under specific conditions. People struggling with generalized anxiety disorder, with "free floating" feelings of anxiety will require a much broader range of interventions.

In this chapter, we focus on the most prevalent anxiety conditions: generalized anxiety disorder (GAD); panic disorder (PD); phobias; agoraphobia; post-traumatic stress disorder; acute stress disorder; obsessive compulsive disorder and social anxiety disorder.

Generalized anxiety is characterized by the core phenomenon of chronic worry. The person who struggles with generalized anxiety is concerned about nearly everything. This worry involves verbal-linguistic thought rather than imagery and tends to be "free-floating" rather than concrete (Hazlett-Stevens, Pruitt, & Collins, 2009) and may include obsessions and depressive ruminations. A diagnosis of GAD is made when an individual experiences at least six months of excessive anxiety or worry about a number of events of activities; the person finds it difficult to control this worry; and experiences three of the following symptoms: restlessness, easily fatigued, difficulty concentrating, irritability, muscle tension, and sleep disturbance. Furthermore, the anxiety, worry or physical symptoms must cause significant stress or impair social, familial, or occupational functioning. Finally, the condition cannot be the result of a response to another psychological, medical, or substance abuse condition (APA, 2000). The person with generalized anxiety disorder will feel anxious most of the time, about most anything.

Panic disorder, of all the anxiety conditions, engenders strong physiological responses and consists of recurrent, unexpected panic attacks. A panic attack (to be distinguished from panic disorder as described below) occurs in about a ten minute period during which an individual experiences four or more of the following symptoms: palpitations, pounding heart or accelerated heart rate; sweating; trembling or shaking; sensations of shortness of breath or smothering; feeling of choking; chest pain or discomfort; nausea or abdominal distress; feeling dizzy or faint; derealization or depersonalization; fear of losing control or going crazy; fear of dying; numbness or tingling sensations; and chills or hot flushes. Clearly, having a panic attack is a frightening experience and like Linda, many clients first present at hospital emergency departments where they turn for help when they are afraid that they are having a heart attack, respiratory problem or stroke. A diagnosis of *panic disorder* is made when in addition to a series of panic attacks, the individual has for a period of a month or more, had persistent concerns about having another attack or of the consequences of having future attacks, and/or has significantly modified their behavior in reaction to having had the attacks (APA, 2000). Goodwin et al. (2005), noting the prevalence of panic attacks, suggests that isolated panic attacks may, in fact, represent a core psychopathological marker rather than a subthreshold form of panic disorder as it is implicated in a wide range of psychological conditions.

According to the DSM-IV-TR, *specific phobias* involve excessive and persistent or unreasonable fear which is cued by the presence or anticipation of a specific object or situation. This can include exposure to animals, heights, flying, or blood, etc. which provokes an instantaneous anxiety response. The person is aware that their response is excessive and takes steps to avoid the situation or endures it with great distress. This reaction and distress must also cause significant impairment in one or more spheres of functioning or normal routine. Clients with phobias are most likely to seek help when strategies of avoiding the stimuli which cue their specific phobia are thwarted. For example, a woman who has a phobia of flying and has successfully managed to avoid airplanes may seek help when her job necessitates frequent travel. *Agoraphobia* can occur with or without a history of panic disorder and is generally characterized by anxiety about being in situations in which escape may be difficult and usually involve a cluster of symptoms (e.g., fears of being outside the home alone, being in a crowd, or on a bridge, etc.) (APA, 2000). Typically the individual avoids these situations or endures them at great cost.

Social phobia, also known as *social anxiety disorder* (SAD), is characterized by a marked and persistent fear of one or more social or performance situations in which the individual fears they will be exposed to unfamiliar people or open to scrutiny by others. Exposure to the situation must invariably result in significant anxiety and the person must recognize that the fear is excessive or unreasonable. Furthermore, the individual either tries to avoid the social or performance situation or when unable to, endures it with significant anxiety and distress. Finally, the avoidance, anxious anticipation, or distress associated with the feared situation interferes significantly with the individual's functioning and causes significant distress (APA, 2000). Brook and Schmidt (2008), in their review of the literature, identify parenting and family factors, adverse life events, sociocultural factors and gender roles as implicit in the development and prevalence of social anxiety disorder.

An understanding of environmental influences and events is particularly important in the discussion of both post-traumatic stress disorder (PTSD) and acute stress. Unlike the other DSM diagnoses, etiology for these conditions is important in the DSM classification system. For both *stress disorder* and *post-traumatic stress disorder* a prior, precipitating event is required. In PTSD, an individual will have been exposed to a traumatic event in which both of the following were present: experiencing, witnessing or being confronted with events that involved serious threat to life, serious injury or physical integrity; and the person's response of intense fear, helplessness, or horror. It should be noted that exposure to such events are unfortunately not uncommon, that the majority of those exposed to trauma do not go on to develop PTSD and that further conditions must be met to meet the criteria for the diagnosis. The event must have "staying power", i.e., the individual must reexperience the event via recurrent or intrusive recollections; recurrent distressing dreams; acting or feeling the event is reoccurring (e.g., hallucinations, delusions or flashbacks); intense distress at real or symbolic reminders; or physiological reactivity on exposure to internal or external cues. There must also be persistent avoidance of stimuli associated with the event, as indicated by three or more of the following: efforts to avoid thoughts or feelings associated with the trauma; efforts to avoid places, people or activities associated with the trauma; inability to recall a pertinent details of the trauma; marked diminished interest or participation in significant activities; feelings of detachment or estrangement from others; a restricted range of affect; or a sense of a foreshortened future or possibilities. Additionally, the person must have symptoms of hyperarousal associated with the trauma as evidenced by two of the following: difficulty falling asleep or staying asleep; irritability or outbursts of anger; difficulty concentrating; hypervigilance; or exaggerated startle response. Finally, the symptoms must have been present for more than a month and cause significant distress and decrease in functioning (APA, 2000). Clearly, a client struggling with the effects of PTSD suffers significant psychological distress and diminished functioning.

Acute stress disorder describes a similar exposure and reaction to trauma, within a different temporal framework. The major differentiating criteria between acute stress disorder and PTSD is that the former refers to problems which last for a minimum of two days and a maximum of four weeks, and occurs within four weeks of the traumatic event.

The obsessions associated with *obsessive compulsive disorder* are characterized by recurrent and persistent thoughts, impulses, or images that are experienced at some point, as intrusive and inappropriate and cause significant distress; they are not simply excessive worry about real life situations; the person attempts to suppress or ignore or neutralize them; and the person is aware that they are a product of their own mind, rather than externally imposed. While obsessions represent thoughts, compulsions refer to behaviors or mental acts which the person feels compelled to perform in response to the obsessions. These compulsions are typically carried out according to very specific and rigid rituals. Furthermore, there is a cognitive belief that carrying out these compulsions will prevent a specific "worse" thing from happening. The childhood rhyme, "Don't step on a crack, you'll break your mother's back" often elicits among children the compulsion to avoid sidewalk cracks. The child who becomes "obsessed" with this rhyme will find it difficult to stop thinking about it and will feel "compelled" to avoid the cracks, in order to "protect" their mother. As in this situation, the compulsion in OCD bears little realistic relationship to the obsession; avoiding the cracks has no logical effect upon their mother's back health. In order to meet the criteria for the DSM diagnosis, the individual must see both the obsessions and compulsions as excessive or unreasonable and must cause marked distress, be time consuming (typically an hour or more per day), interfere with normal routines and cause significant occupational, social or personal decrease in functioning (APA, 2000).

Genetics have also been implicated in the development of several of the anxiety conditions. Recent research has focused upon the protein, stathmin, the peptide, GRP, and a gene which controls levels of serotonin in the brain. It is likely that these genes work in concert with each other to create certain conditions. In terms of brain structure, the amygdale seems to be active in both fear acquisition and fear extinction. While an understanding of the role of genetics and the brain in the development, maintenance and resolution of anxiety conditions will be helpful, the work remains in its infancy (National Institute of Mental Health (NIMH), 2007). In fact, individual differences in genes and the brain may only serve to lay fertile ground for the development of PTSD and that environmental factors such as brain injuries, childhood trauma and a history of mental illness may affect the early growth of the brain. Furthermore, optimism and a tendency to view challenges as positive or negative may influence adaptation to traumatic events (NIMH, 2007).

Demographics

The epidemiology of anxiety conditions is measured by reports of *lifetime prevalence, 12-month prevalence, age-of-onset, persistence, comborbidity, subtypes* and *course*. Kessler, Chiu, Demier, and Walters (2005), reporting on the National Comorbidity Survey Replication Study (NCS-R), found that 31.2 percent of the general population reported a lifetime occurrence of one or more of the anxiety conditions while 18.7 percent reported the presence of an anxiety condition within the last 12 months. In a review of this literature, Kessler, Ruscio, Shear, and Wittchen (2009) reported three stable patterns in the lifetime prevalence of anxiety disorders. First, the anxiety conditions as a group are more prevalent than any other class of psychiatric conditions, including mood disorders and schizophrenia. Second, specific phobia is the most prevalent of these at 6–12 percent. Third, obsessive compulsive disorder is the least prevalent at below 3 percent. Kessler et al. (2009) on the basis of the National Comorbidity Survey Replication Study reported the following 12-month prevalence rates for these subtypes of anxiety: general anxiety disorder, 3.1 percent of adults; social phobia, 6.8 percent; specific phobia, 8.7 percent; panic disorder, 2.7 percent; obsessive compulsive disorder (OCD), 1.0 percent; post-traumatic stress disorder (PTSD), 3.5 percent. Additionally, *comorbidity* is high for anxiety and depressive conditions and more than half of all individuals with one anxiety condition also have another.

Age of onset (AOA) is a particularly important measure as it yields data pertinent to the importance of early identification and intervention, and of the course of the conditions. In the case of anxiety conditions, specific phobia is always found to have a modal age of onset in childhood; social phobia and obsessive compulsive disorder have modal onset in adolescence or early adulthood. Panic disorder, agoraphobia and generalized anxiety disorder have later and more scattered age of onset. Post-traumatic stress disorder on the other hand, has a highly variable distribution, secondary to the fact that trauma exposure occurs throughout the life course. In addition, Zimmermann, Wittchen, Hofler, Pfistger, Kessler, and Lieb (2003) reported significant associations between early-onset anxiety conditions and the subsequent first onset of other psychiatric and substance abuse conditions. These are important findings for the argument that early treatment of child and adolescent anxiety conditions may prevent the development of secondary conditions which are not uncommon following pediatric onset of anxiety (Kendall & Kessler, 2002). Furthermore, Christiana et al. (2000) reported that treatment for anxiety conditions does not usually occur until adulthood, often a decade or more beyond the onset of symptoms. This has particular relevance for those adolescents who may attempt to "treat" conditions of anxiety with substances with which there is high comorbidity throughout the life course.

Of equal concern are the findings that anxiety conditions are *persistent* through the life course. However, the course of these conditions does not seem to be consistent; rather, it is recurrent-intermittent, characterized by increasing and decreasing episodes of the various anxiety conditions (Angst & Vollrath, 1991; Bruce et al., 2005; Kessler et al., 2009). This suggests that there is high comorbidity across the spectrum of anxiety conditions (Kessler et al., 2009). In practice, the high comorbidity indicates a need for a careful assessment of prior experiences with feelings of anxiety, how they have manifested, and how they have been helped. In the case of Linda, it is pertinent to know that she appeared to have some form of postpartum anxiety prior to her isolated panic attack and more currently to a possible panic disorder.

The prevalence rates for post-traumatic stress disorders are of particular interest to social workers who help clients in the aftermath of exposure to many kinds of trauma including childhood sexual and physical abuse, domestic and community violence, natural disaster and war. The diagnosis of PTSD requires trauma exposure so the general population studies of this exposure are important in understanding the social and environmental contexts which can give rise to PTSD. Kessler, Sonnega, Bromet, Hughes, and Nelson (1995) reported that in a national U.S. household survey, 60.7 percent of men and 51.2 percent of women reported exposure to at least one lifetime traumatic event, with the majority reporting more than one type of trauma. Furthermore, U.S. crime statistics for murder and rape are considerably higher than in other developed countries (Langan & Farrington, 1998). This is an important consideration because all traumas are not alike and therefore risk is conditional for developing PTSD. Breslau, Kessler, Chilcoat, Schultz, Davis, and Andreski (1998) reported that the conditional risk of PTSD after a representative trauma was 9.2 percent while conditional risk associated with assaultive violence was 20.9 percent. These statistics and trends have very real life implications for our clients. These data suggest that a biopsychosocial assessment should include questions regarding exposure to a wide range of events known to have high conditional risk for the development of PTSD. A the same time, social workers should be aware of the factors which appear to provide some mediating effect, or protective factors to developing PTSD following exposure to a traumatic event. Factors promoting resilience include: the ability to both seek out and receive support from others; finding a support group after a traumatic event; feeling good about one's own conduct in the face of danger; having a coping strategy and learning from the event; and being able to act with agency even while being afraid (Charney, 2004).

Populations

While each of the anxiety conditions (except separation anxiety) can manifest at any point during the life course, specific ones pose particular challenges at certain developmental points and we highlight those here. *Anxiety in children and adolescents* has received increasing attention in the last few years (Albano, Chorpita, & Barlow, 2003; Beesdo, Knappe, & Pine, 2009; Furr, Tiwari, Suveg, & Kendall, 2009), in part because of research findings that suggest that anxiety conditions have an early age of onset (Kessler, Amminger, Aguilar-Gaxiola, Alonso, Lee, & Üstün, 2007), that early age of onset is associated with the development of other psychiatric conditions, and that there is typically a delay of ten or more years between onset of symptoms and first intervention. While children can present with any of the symptoms of the anxiety conditions, *separation anxiety disorder* is specific to children and included in DSM-IV with the conditions first diagnosed in childhood. Children suffering with this condition manifest excessive anxiety about separation from their primary attachment figures, fearing that harm will result to either because of the experience of separation. Separation anxiety disorder can be acute and short-lived or chronic and has a prevalence rate of 3–5 percent (Lewinsohn, Holm-Denoma, Small, Seeley, & Joiner, 2008). Lewinsohn et al. (2008) further report an association between separation anxiety disorder and future development of panic disorder and depression, although the nature of that association is unclear. Prevalence rates for the subgroups of anxiety conditions in children range from 2 percent to 27 percent, suggesting the importance of early identification and intervention.

For children, PTSD and the traumatic events that cause it, pose particular challenges, largely because of their adverse effects on biological, psychological, and social development (Davis & Siegel, 2000). Furthermore, Davis and Siegel (2000) report that the development of PTSD by the age of 18 has been significantly correlated with anxiety, suicidal ideation, attention deficit hyperactivity disorder, and psychotic and mood conditions. Children also have a higher vulnerability than their adult counterparts for developing PTSD following trauma exposure (Fletcher, 1996). There is also ample evidence that an earlier age of onset, greater length of abuse, and greater severity of symptoms of PTSD are associated with smaller brain volume (DeBellis & Keshavan, 2003). Perhaps even more disturbing, DeBellis (2001) found that childhood maltreatment of the interpersonal kind can override the certain factors typically associated with resiliency – genetic, constitutional, social and psychological – and heighten the risk for developing PTSD in response to that trauma. While early trauma exposure and the PTSD which may follow are clearly deleterious, the resultant brain abnormalities can play causal roles in a range of cognitive and developmental deficits (DeBellis, Hooper, & Sapia, 2005). For social workers, this is a sober reminder of our dual mission in the profession. While we are often providing direct services to children with trauma caused anxiety conditions, we must maintain our responsibility to identify and prevent social injustices which so negatively impact vulnerable children. We must also be aware of the significant factors which promote resiliency in these children – *and make use of them.* For example, a supportive family and community both prior to and following the trauma can significantly ameliorate the effects of the experience. Caregivers can model prosocial and strong coping skills and at the same time help the child with his cognitive processing of the trauma (Brown, 2005). A child's attributions about what has happened to him can determine the lens through which he may confront future adversity and triumphs. Providing the child with the development of a realistic sense of agency can be protective in many situations (Gitterman, 2001).

Another condition, identified in the late 1990s, that has been associated with *obsessive compulsive disorder* in children is pediatric autoimmune neuropsychiatric disorders associated with streptococcal infections (PANDAS). This condition underscores both the physical underpinnings of anxiety conditions and the need for comprehensive medication evaluation in all people with psychiatric conditions. PANDAS has been implicated in abrupt onset obsessive compulsive disorders in children which are accompanied by facial and/or motor tics, separation anxiety and moodiness and irritability. The disorder is not yet fully understood, but occurs in some subset of children who contract streptococcal infections. The condition typically has an episodic course of symptom severity with dramatic variance followed by a slow gradual improvement. Interventions include treatment for the streptococcal infection and help for the obsessive compulsive symptoms. Serious, persistent tics are often treated with medication (NIMH, 2009). Social workers should always be certain that clients who present with psychiatric conditions have had a recent full medical work up to rule out any medical origins of their symptoms.

Adolescents with anxiety conditions are at particular risk of being overlooked as these symptoms often belong to the class of internalizing behaviors. Whereas their peers with externalizing behaviors are often "identified" and provided services within school and community settings, they themselves may "fly under the radar," which is troubling in light of the evidence that anxiety can adversely affect aspects of social and personal development (Kaufman, 2005) and can later lead to employment and financial difficulties in young adulthood (Last, Hansen, & Franco, 1997). While the developmental course of the anxiety conditions is fairly well understood in children, it is much less understood in adolescents. Van Oort, Greaves-Lord, Verhulst, Ormel, and Huizink (2009) reported that in a general population study, symptoms of anxiety follow an unusual trajectory, first decreasing (from higher rates in childhood) during early adolescence and then increasing between mid and late adolescence. They also found that the substantially higher incidence of anxiety in girls than in boys could be explained by the comorbidity of depression in girls.

One of the more disturbing and potentially dangerous manifestations of anxiety can occur in the *postpartum period for women*. While postpartum depression is fairly well known, postpartum anxiety has not been thoroughly investigated (Reck et al., 2008). Matthey, Barnett, and White (2003) reported that 16.2 percent of mothers were diagnosed with "pure" anxiety disorders six weeks postpartum. Postpartum women are adjusting to significant hormonal, environmental, role status and life transition changes, all of which can be implicated in the development of anxiety symptoms. A confluence of these changes, particularly in someone who may be prone to anxiety spectrum conditions can likely result in a temporary, and in some cases, prolonged and dangerous anxiety. Women in the postpartum period, because they are at elevated risk for developing such a condition, even if transitory, should have access to psychological screening at the six-week postpartum appointment, sufficient resources at home, and prompt intervention if symptoms of either depression or anxiety are present. Anxiety and depression in new mothers can have a deleterious effect on the mother, the infant, and their developing relationship.

A substantial literature examines the relationship between *anxiety and medical illness*. This relationship is particularly pertinent to *older adults* who disproportionately suffer with medical conditions. Being diagnosed with an illness, being either sure or unsure of the course of the illness, and of its outcome, is anxiety producing in itself. Marshalling the resources (psychological, social, financial, family, and otherwise) to manage the medical condition creates stress of its own. In addition, chronic medical conditions often result in significant role impairment, work loss, and financial losses and these have been well documented in the literature related to comorbid depression and medical illness (Evans & Charney, 2003; Stein, Cox, Afifi, Belik, & Sareen, 2006). In their review of the bidirectional relationships between anxiety disorders and medical illness, Roy-Byrne et al. (2008) report strong evidence for the relationship between anxiety and irritable bowel syndrome, cardiovascular disease, and chronic pain. They conclude that the presence of anxiety conditions may exacerbate the symptoms of the medical condition and negatively affect outcomes. A clear role for social workers is suggested, particularly in inpatient and outpatient medical settings, to screen for and identify symptoms of anxiety, which may be related to chronic medical conditions. Social workers can then work with their medical colleagues and their mutual clients to alleviate both symptoms and sources of anxiety, leading to enhanced abilities to cope with related medical conditions and their related stressors.

Likewise, late life anxiety has been implicated with physical disability (Lenze et al., 2001). Anxiety is a risk factor generally (regardless of age) for physical disability (described as inability, difficulty or reliance on others for performing activities of daily living or ADLs). Beekman, de Beurs, van Balkom, Deeg, van Dyck, and van Tilberg (2000) found that anxiety is common in depressed elderly patients and that the pathways by which both anxiety and depression lead to disability are similar. These authors strongly suggest the importance of treating the medical and psychiatric conditions simultaneously in order to ameliorate the effects of each and decrease the likelihood of further deterioration or relapse.

The incidence and experience of post-traumatic stress disorder in older adults has largely been overlooked in the empirical and clinical literature. This is problematic for many reasons. First, the United States has an increasingly "graying" population, and second, increasing age is more frequently associated with higher risk of victimization (Pillemer & Finkelhor (1988). Most of the research on PTSD and elderly people has been focused upon Holocaust survivors and war veterans. In support of a psychosocial understanding of trauma, Elder and Clipp (1989) identify the life events and processes related to aging as potential precipitants or complications from earlier trauma, while they acknowledge that for many the aging process provides an opportunity for adaptation. Furthermore, the cognitive, perceptual and memory changes associated with aging can complicate the management of anxiety and trauma symptoms. Busuttil (2004) argues strongly that older adults in a variety of settings should be screened for chronic, delayed and acute stress disorders and that research should target the best practices for interventions with clients with PTSD and complications of older age.

Findings regarding *gender differences* in the occurrence of anxiety conditions are significant and consistent, though underresearched. Wittchen, Zhao, Kessler, and Eaton (1994) reported that like with the depressive conditions, generalized anxiety disorder is diagnosed twice as often in women as in men. Additionally, Spitzer, Kroenke, Williams, and Lowe (2006) found that women score more highly on self-report measures of anxiety than men, confirming prior findings. Numbers related to DSM criteria symptoms do not tell the whole story though. Armstrong and Khawaja (2002) found gender differences in the manifestation of anxiety in a small non-clinical sample. Specifically, they found that women experienced anxiety-related cognitions as personally more catastrophic and dangerous than their male counterparts, reported higher anxiety sensitivity, and had higher expressions of physiological hyperarousal. These findings too suggest the importance of understanding the anxiety conditions as conditions of the whole person, including the body and its mechanisms, cognitions, and affects or feelings. Leach, Christensen, Mackinnon, Windsor, and Butterworth (2008), in one of the first studies to examine the roles of gender in anxiety, also examined psychosocial mediators, previously ignored in the literature. They concluded that women are disproportionately affected with both anxiety and depression and suggest the following psychosocial variables which may account for this: women had lower physical health, do less physical activity, had lower levels of mastery, have higher levels of behavioural inhibition, a ruminative style and neuroticism and higher interpersonal problems – all at higher levels than men. This study lends further support for a psychosocial model of etiology. It also suggests to social workers the importance of both understanding the macro and gender influences on this area of mental health, while suggesting pathways for supporting better functioning, which may include lifestyle changes on both macro and micro levels.

Some *gays and lesbians* may be at increased risk for anxiety conditions, in direct response to the stress of keeping a stigmatized identity secret, contending with bullying, threats of violence or alienation, and about managing decisions about disclosure to family, friends and work colleagues. Hart and Heimberg (2001) identify the development of social anxiety as a particular risk for gay, lesbian and bisexual youth. These stressors are largely externally driven and can become more problematic when they are internalized. This is a sobering example about the impact of socially constructed values, norms and prohibitions on the development of psychological conditions in individuals who are vulnerable to those pervasive influences. Less research is available that examines the prevalence of anxiety in other gender spectrum identities, however, transgendered people for example, who are subjected to significant external stress and threats, may be considered to be at elevated risk of developing anxiety-related conditions.

Mental health care disparities

Race, ethnicity and culture play critical roles in the identification, interpretation and treatment of many of the anxiety conditions. Unfortunately, little consensus exists among researchers about conceptualizing the elusive aspects of race, ethnicity and culture as they pertain to the anxiety conditions. Due to the different and sometimes discordant definitions researchers use, contrasting findings are often evidenced. We cannot control for this here, but we have taken care to identify studies that utilize similar understandings of these terms.

For the purposes of this chapter, *race* is defined as a social group identity that is created around an individual's physical characteristics (i.e. skin color, phenotype) as well as an identification based on a sense of group affiliation. One's *ethnicity* is defined as a person's sense of affiliation with individuals from common cultural heritages. *Culture* is a set of norms, values and beliefs that are attributable to a distinct social group. Most researchers rely on an individual's self-report of racial affiliation using the federal standards: White, Black/African American, Asian, or Native American, and asking if an individual identifies as Hispanic or not.

A health disparity is generally recognized as an inequality in health that exists due to "social factors or allocation of resources" (Miranda, McGuire, Williams, & Wang, 2008, p. 1102). The same applies for mental health. Miranda et al. (2008) state that with the exception of Latin@s[1] from Puerto Rico, Latin@ Americans, Black Americans, and Asian Americans have lower incidence of mental health issues than their White counterparts. Rates of mental disorders increase in immigrants from Africa, the Caribbean, and Mexico the longer they reside in the United States. Native Americans have a greater risk for PTSD and substance abuse. However, whether the lower rates in these populations are because of fewer mental health issues or because they go under-diagnosed, is unknown. Knowing that the rates of mental illness are lower for the non-white population can cause providers to assume a disorder does not exist. This, along with communication barriers due to language and cultural differences, can lead to differential and/or discriminatory treatment. It is not unusual for providers to miss the severity for individuals who are non-white because the presentation may be different in different racial/ethnic groups. However, the main cause of mental health disparities tends to center around underutilization of services which may have to do with "access, use, and quality of care" (Miranda et al., 2008, p. 1105).

In general the literature supports the assumption that internalized symptoms of anxiety are more prevalent in a collectivist culture (i.e. non-Western) rather than an individualistic culture (i.e. United States) (Varela & Hensley-Maloney, 2009). However, there is an inherent bias in this perspective since the presentation of anxiety tends to be defined from a Western perspective. When a condition falls outside what is familiar to Western norms and behaviors, it generally gets defined as a culture bound syndrome. Culture bound syndromes are said to primarily affect individuals from non-Western countries. Many are expressions of distress or stress as a result of a life circumstance. Like many Western reactions to similar life events, anxiety tends to be a primary symptom. The difference, however, lies in the form in which the anxiety is expressed. Most syndromes are identified with somatic symptoms and behavioral expressions that may be more culturally syntonic to a non-Western population (Varela & Hensley-Maloney, 2009). In many culture bound syndromes, anxiety is the basis of the individual's condition but its expression, either somatic or behaviorally volatile, is not recognized as such from a Western diagnostic framework. For example, most Asian culture bound syndromes get diagnosed with GAD, PD, or PTSD (Hinton, Park, Hsia, Hofmann, & Pollack, 2009), but should they be treated the same way?

Great care must be taken to assess each individual with respect to the population with which they affiliate. What is important is not just the individual's relationship to his/her culture but the culture's relationship to the individual. In other words, how do their multiple identities interact with their culture's dominant values, norms, and behaviors? The answer to this question can explain the amount or type of anxiety an individual may be experiencing.

When examining the rates of *generalized anxiety disorder* across race and ethnicity, culture plays an important role in how symptomatology is interpreted. In the United States, the risk for GAD is higher for non-Latinas Whites than for African Americans, Latin@s, or Asian Americans. Even when compared to a non-Western sample (native born Asians or Africans), those from European descent had much higher rates of GAD (Lewis-Fernández et al., 2010). Although individuals all over the world have experience with worry, how worry is assessed can be very culturally prescribed. Concepts such as quantity, intensity, or length of time may vary on environmental as well as cultural exposure to difficult circumstance. Also, language can play a role in the diagnosing of GAD among Latin@s. A mono-lingual Spanish speaking Latin@ is more likely to use somatic symptom rather than psychological symptom language, making it less likely for her to receive a diagnosis of GAD if psychological aspects of GAD criteria are stressed upon assessment. Another limitation is the cross-cultural validity of assessment scales that may be used to measure these concepts. Culture is embedded in language and direct translation for concepts that involve fear, locus of control, or time is extremely difficult if not impossible in some instances (Lewis-Fernández et al., 2010).

Reporting on multiple studies Lewis-Fernández et al. (2010) described lower rates of *panic disorder* (PD) among US Latin@s, African Americans, Caribbean Blacks, and Asians in comparison to non-Latin@ Whites. American Indians on the other hand have higher rates, as do Puerto Ricans in comparison to other Latin@ subgroups. Lewis-Fernández goes on to question the suitability of the proposed DSM-V criterion of qualifying the attack as "unexpected" citing this as a possible reason for the rates of PD being lower among non-White populations. He argues that individuals with culture bound syndromes are more likely to expect their panic attack because it is something with which they are culturally familiar. He provides the example of the Cambodian culture's experience with Khyâl, a threatening wind that enters into a person's body causing symptoms similar to those found in PD, shortness of breath, dizziness, and tinnitus. However, if the person goes out on a windy day, the *panic attack* (PA) may be expected, or at the very least expected in retrospect. Also, in many cultures panic attacks are almost always expected after experiencing some sort of trauma. An example of this is a woman from Puerto Rico who, after experiencing the death of her husband, is likely to expect that she will have an ataque de nervios. This includes screaming, yelling, fainting, and crying. Expecting an attack does not meet criteria for panic disorder. Therefore, maintaining the DSM-IV criterion that the attack must be unexpected may greatly reduce the likelihood of individuals from cultures that have identifiable culture bound syndromes to be diagnosed with PD.

While it may be important to understand how the inclusion or exclusion of certain diagnostic criteria may raise or lower the prevalence for panic disorder for particular groups, Lewis-Fernández, Guranaccia, Martinez, Salman, Schmidt, and Liebowitz (2002) assert that the lived-experience of ataque de nervios is distinct from what is defined as PD and PA. First, the attack does not necessarily peak within minutes, and second, there tends to be autonomic arousal symptoms not currently listed in the DSM-IV-TR criteria. However, depending on the diagnosing worker these criteria can be ignored or seen as insignificant to the current client condition. Rather than relegating a condition that centers around anxiety as a culture bound syndrome because it does not meet criteria that was created by researching a Western population, it may be more effective to describe how PA can have a cross-cultural variation.

According to the NCS-R, non-Latin@ Whites have higher lifetime rates for panic attack than their African American and Latin@ counterparts. Regarding people of color, according to the Collaborative Psychiatric Epidemiological Studies dataset, there are no differences in lifetime rates among Latin@s, African Americans, or Asian Americans. With regard to how panic attacks are realized, results from the same study report that physical symptomatology differs somewhat across race/ethnicity. Some examples include Whites reporting more trembling and shaking than African Americans and more heart racing than Latin@s, African American reported more heart racing than Latin@s, and Latin@s reported more shortness of breath and nausea than Asian Americans and more sensations of choking than Whites or African Americans (Asnaani, Gutner, Hinton, & Hofmann, 2009). The different manifestations of anxiety symptoms can be ascribed to worries embedded in particular cultural frameworks. Whites may have more heart palpitations considering that heart disease is the leading cause of death for Whites. Similarly, African Americans are at higher risk of heart disease than their Latin@ or Asian counterparts. Lewis-Fernández et al. (2010) found higher rates of skin sensations, such as numbness, in African Americans which could relate to their higher incidence of diabetes and the consequences of limb amputation (Asnaani et al., 2009).

One might imagine that the occurrence and types of *phobias* may be particularly culture bound and that their prevalence or lack thereof may be culturally relevant. Lewis-Fernández et al. (2010) explain that much of the research on cross-racial and ethnic comparisons is conflicting and as a whole is not conclusive. Although particular phobias may be more prevalent in certain cultures, for example, fear of blood injections/injury appear more in a White population, whereas African Americans have great fear of animals, they are not exclusive to any culture. Fears that may be more endemic to a particular country may result from environmental circumstances to culturally socialized norms. For example, people in Western countries with large urban populations may have greater fears of being a victim of a crime as opposed to those in non-Western countries which stress self-control, restraint, and compliance to social norms, the latter may fear personal injury as a result of a non-human interaction such as electric shock or dog bite (Lewis-Fernández et al., 2010).

Although agoraphobia is an independent universal phenomenon (Wittchen et al., 2008) the variability across race and ethnicity has been somewhat ignored. The few cross-cultural studies that have examined this condition found that rates are higher in Blacks than both Latin@s and non-Latin@ Whites, with a significant likelihood of teenage onset (Horwarh & Wiessman, 1997; Lewis-Fernández et al., 2010). However, among Latin@s, Puerto Ricans have a higher rate than other Latin@ subgroups (Alegria et al., 2008). Interestingly, rates are much higher in women than in men, and higher for women who have been socialized in a country that subscribes to stricter gender conforming norms of femininity (Arrindell et al., 2003).

Most research on PTSD has been conducted on male war veterans. Researching solely this population can be particularly problematic when examining a diverse population since African American and Latin@s are disproportionately represented in combat positions compared to their White counterparts. This affects the degree to which individuals are exposed to traumatic experiences, thus placing them at increased conditional risk for the development of PTSD. Some argue that there may even be a difference in severity, asserting that Latin@s report greater severity of symptoms than their non-Latin@ white counterparts (Marshall, Schell, & Miles, 2009). However, some studies have purported that with similar risk factors, prevalence rates for African Americans and Whites are virtually the same, although severity was not discussed (Alim, Charney & Mellman, 2006; Pole, Gone & Kulkarni, 2008). In their review of the literature Marshall et al., (2009) reported that some of the ethnic disparities that exist in symptom manifestation between Latin@s and non-Latin@ Whites are considered by many to be culturally based. For example, Latin@s' tendency to exaggerate health symptoms and to somatasize, their exposure to discrimination, differential use of resources, and disadvantages based on certain sociodemographics, are all worker perceptions that may affect assessment. Determining whether or not the PTSD experienced by Latin@s differs in severity or by phenomenon, has great implications for practice (Marshall et al., 2009).

Hunter and Schmidt (2010) explain that among African Americans there is some concern about measurement validity of paranoia and psychosis. The overarching sense of cultural mistrust that exists within the African American population, due to perceived racism and discrimination may alter the client–social worker interaction and cause a social worker to misdiagnose the client's apprehension and suspicion as evidence of psychosis.

Obsessive compulsive disorder (OCD) can often present a complex picture, particularly because there tends to be high comorbidity of mood and other anxiety disorders. While the NCS-R suggests that there is a trend towards lower lifetime rates of OCD in African Americans and non-Latina Whites than Latin@s, findings were not significant (Breslau, Aguilar-Gaxiola, Kendler, Su, Williams, & Kessler, 2006). Overall, distribution in gender, age onset, and comorbidity show no variability (Fontanelle & Hasler, 2008). Lewis-Fernández et al. (2010) note that regardless of cultural settings, OCD is generally more prevalent in women while early onset is more common in male children. In cross-national studies variation on obsession and compulsion, though existent was not great. Themes for obsessive symptoms predominate around issues of cleanliness whereas those for compulsions emphasize on checking. Many cultural themes may exist in the presentation of obsessions and compulsions but some are also culturally dystonic. Although many obsessive and compulsive symptoms are similar across cultures, in countries that have a strong religious value of cleansing and purification symptomotology tends to be more severe and may go undiagnosed because of its connection to religious ritual (Matsunaga & Seedat, 2007).

A rather complex picture emerges from the data on lifetime rates of social anxiety disorder (SAD), also known as social phobia. It is clear that there is higher prevalence in the United States than in most non-European countries and that women are diagnosed at greater rates than men (Lewis-Fernández et al., 2010). Most people who develop SAD develop it at an early age, when females appear to be particularly vulnerable (Caballo, Salazar, Irurtia, Arias, & Hofmann, 2008; Horwath & Weissman, 1997). Interestingly some protective factors are being over 20, of color, having lower educational level, living in an urban setting (Lewis-Fernández et al., 2010) and having lower socioeconomic status (Horwath & Weissman, 1997). One exception is Native Americans of lower socioeconomic status, who tend to be at higher risk. What actually constitutes a protective factor is difficult to determine since definitions of educational level and urban setting may vary between countries (Lewis-Fernández et al., 2010). Differences in defining protective and risk factors may also explain lower rates for both Latin@ and non-Latin@ White immigrants (Alegria et al., 2008). Although people of color maybe at higher risk at a younger age, non-Latin@ whites have a greater risk of developing SAD throughout their lifetime (Lewis-Fernández et al., 2010).

Kim, Rapee, & Gaston (2008) discuss how Taijin-Kyofusho (TKS), offensive type, a culture-bound syndrome, is often diagnosed as a type of social phobia. Originally this condition was thought to exist exclusively in Japan, however, a review of the literature by Kim et al. (2008) reveals that there have been some documented cases among American university students. This condition is evidenced by the excessive fear of giving offense to others by virtue of one's physical attributes such as appearance or body odor. This condition meets criteria that are identical to a type of SAD (or social phobia) such as avoiding social situations out of fear of negative evaluations by others; however, the fear of offending through a personal physical attribute or flaw is what delineates this as a culture-bound syndrome. In the United States, this culturally related condition is often diagnosed as GAD, SAD, and in some cases given an Axis II diagnosis of avoidant personality disorder (Lewis-Fernández et al., 2010).

As mentioned above, cultural expressions of anxiety can vary and the measures that exist in a typical worker's lexicon are biased towards expressions common in a Western population. Therefore, social workers must refrain from assuming a culture-bound syndrome because the client originates from a particular country where the syndrome exists. Rather, the client should be assessed on an individual basis, with knowledge of the culture and its distinctive expressions as a guide. What we learn about assessing and diagnosing culture-bound syndromes we must utilize when assessing all clients for anxiety disorders (Flaskerud, 2009). As social workers, we must be very conscious of our own cultural framework from which we conceptualize a client's condition. In the cases of TKS and ataque de nervios individuals are diagnosed with often stigmatizing Axis II diagnoses because of a lack of understanding of an individual's cultural reality.

It is important for social workers to have knowledge of cultural idioms that may reference particular symptoms common in what we consider culture-bound syndromes. Although these conditions may be more acceptable or familiar within a particular population, they are nonetheless debilitating, and helping the client to "reframe" their experience can assist them in developing a stronger capacity to cope with difficult situations (Kirmayer, 1997, p. 246).

Social work programs and social work roles

Social workers work with people with anxiety disorders in a wide range of settings, including inpatient and outpatient medical and psychiatric settings, schools, and agency-based practices. As we are increasingly aware of the prevalence of post-traumatic conditions in people across the life course, social workers work with people at elevated risk for developing these conditions. Here, we identify a few areas where opportunities for social work services are critical and increasingly prevalent.

Since the Iraq and Afghan wars there has been a significant increase in the development of intervention services for military soldiers and their families. Multiple deployments with brief returns home, high numbers of injured soldiers and traumatic brain injuries secondary to improvised explosive devices, and increased demands on the Veterans Administration Health Services combine to create extremely stressful post-combat experiences. Social workers are increasingly working in Veterans Administration facilities and in a wide range of community settings with these populations. Because war veterans and particularly those with PTSD are at increased risk for substance use problems, social workers may work in these facilities as well.

As indicated earlier, because anxiety conditions usually manifest as internalizing behaviors in children and adolescents, they are less likely to be identified. However, social workers in school settings can certainly screen for anxiety symptoms and intervene where necessary. Moreover, children in child protection services become clients because of severe neglect and abuse, which generally involves acute and chronic direct trauma or trauma exposure. In these settings, social workers intervene in direct practice with children, biological families and foster families. In the work with any of the anxiety conditions, social workers must help children manage over-whelming worries and fears, promote prosocial skills, develop strategies for determining one's own safety, mediate organizational and network stressors, increase problem-solving skills and in the most extreme situations, manage intrusive fears and flashbacks related to PTSD.

Even when PTSD is not present in a child in state protective custody, consider the range of normative fears that may be present and need attention. If we use a non-clinical definition of anxiety as "a painful or apprehensive uneasiness of mind usually over an impending or anticipated ill" (Merriam Dictionary, Webster 2000) we can certainly expect that children who are removed from their home and replaced, sometimes multiple times, will experience "anxiety" about conditions over which they have neither control nor knowledge. Even a child with no diagnosed psychological conditions is likely to experience apprehension, fear, and worry, sometimes accompanied by somatic complaints. These cognitions, affects and behaviors may not rise to the "diagnosable" but we can consider both the circumstances and the symptoms risk factors.

Social workers play significant roles in the full range of medical facilities, the "first stop" for many people who are struggling with symptoms of anxiety. Like Linda, many clients present to emergency rooms and primary health care facilities. Certainly oncology social workers work with clients who are at every stage of cancer treatment – from first diagnosis, through surgery, radiation and chemotherapy and follow-up. Indeed, given the high prevalence of the range of anxiety conditions, social workers in every practice setting will work with clients, especially those under the extreme stresses of homelessness, domestic violence, poverty and trauma.

While the social worker intervenes on the direct services level as described above, macro-interventions are at least as critical. For example, child protective service agencies must design policies that increase factors promoting resiliency, while taking into account a given child's developmental and cultural needs. Medical facilities must develop policies which help to demystify frightening procedures and provide a range of resources to help clients navigate complicated health systems.

Professional methods and interventions

A vast 30-year literature provides strong empirical support for cognitive, cognitive-behavioral and behavioral interventions for the full range of anxiety conditions (Butler, Chapman, Forman, & Beck, 2006). While cognitive-based approaches have gained preeminence in the last several decades in the treatment of many psychiatric conditions, they are particularly well suited for the alleviation of the symptoms of anxiety. This may be so, in part, because these symptoms represent easily definable and discrete behaviors, well-defined cognitions, clear affective states and somatic manifestations. They are readily targeted. Outcome studies of cognitive-behavioral approaches are relatively easy to research, for many of the same reasons. Most of the comparative approach outcome literature examines medication approaches with cognitive-behavioral ones. However, more recently, exercise and physical activity have been identified as promising interventions for alleviation of anxiety symptoms (Strohle, 2009) though this has not been well researched. Interestingly, Chu, Coudhury, Shortt, Pincus, Creed, and Kendall (2004), while recognizing the importance of cognitive techniques in the alleviation of anxiety in children, also stress the importance of the therapeutic alliance, along with the use of technology. It is important for social workers to implement any cognitive-behavioral techniques within a strong and responsive working alliance with the client of any age.

A *cognitive* understanding of the anxiety conditions focuses primarily upon the cognitions and schemas, which form the basis for the etiology, development, maintenance and eventual altering of symptoms of anxiety. Beck and Emery (1985), the ?????, the "father" of cognitive therapy, believes that when there is a disturbance in cognition, there are resultant disturbances in both feelings and behaviors. In this model, descriptions of cognitive symptoms are as important in both assessment and intervention as the accompanying behavioral, affective, and somatic symptoms. These cognitive symptoms include the sensory-perceptual, thinking difficulties and conceptual ones which include fears and distortions. The targets of intervention therefore are the cognitive symptoms (faulty assumptions, catastrophizing, "irrational beliefs," all or nothing thinking, overgeneralizing, etc.), which may need to be identified, confronted, examined, and modified. The theory holds that once the cognitive processing and structures are modified, the symptoms of anxiety will diminish.

A considerable overlap exists in the interventions for the various anxiety conditions and we describe the primary ones here. People with most anxiety conditions are best helped with a combination of interventions. All clients presenting with anxiety conditions should first be assessed using a biopsychosocial approach which provides a context for their symptoms, distress and impaired functioning. For example, a recent onset of extreme night-time fears of a child would be differentially understood if the family had recently been robbed during the night. Likewise, it would be important to know if there is a family history of anxiety conditions. Each of these data provides critical information in understanding the condition (if there is one), the experience of the child, and possible intervention strategies. Family members should also be involved in select stages of the assessment and intervention process. Long before an individual seeks professional help, they have tried to use their own coping skills and strategies to manage their symptoms. Oftentimes family members have attempted to help as well. Many times this help has been effective and often involves an alteration of family roles and patterns. As a client's symptoms decrease, the compensatory behaviors of family members may no longer be needed. For example, a family with a person struggling with agoraphobia will often assume the client's responsibilities for errands and activities out of the home, because the client is unable to do so. As this client, through professional help, is able to resume some of those activities, a shift must take place in the family. Oftentimes, the client and family can benefit with help readjusting to "normal" life and routines.

Psychoeducation is appropriate for each of the anxiety conditions; simply experiencing uncomfortable anxiety symptoms is anxiety provoking and having a cognitive understanding of "what is happening to me" can be very helpful. When clients and their families have a clear understanding of the biological, social, psychological, and transactional underpinnings and manifestations of their conditions, they are more able to mobilize themselves to address them (Hatfield, 1988).

Many of the behavioral interventions involve *exposure*, which in principal is simply exposing the client to the source of their fear. *In vivo exposure* is a technique in which the social worker gradually exposes the client to the feared situation which is producing unmanageable anxiety. In the case of a postal worker with a specific phobia of dogs, the social worker might begin by showing the client pictures of a dog, eventually introducing them to a therapy dog. *Systematic desensitization, or graduated exposure therapy* is often instituted following the mastery of relaxation skills which reduce anticipatory fear and anxieties to phobias. These interventions have been found to be useful in both symptom reduction and relapse prevention for people with phobias, generalized anxiety disorder and obsessive compulsive disorders (Fava, Grandi, Rafanelli, Ruini, Conti, & Belluardo, 2001).

Applied relaxation techniques involve *guided imagery* or *induced relaxation* to reduce muscular tension and induce symptom relief. Breathing techniques can be taught to clients to induce feelings of calm and to manage or prevent hyperventilation, which often occurs in panic attacks (Sadock & Sadock, 2007).

Cognitive restructuring can be very effective with clients whose expressions of anxiety reveal prominent cognitive distortions. In this intervention, the worker and client examine both dysfunctional schemata and thinking patterns. For example, a client with *panic disorder* can be helped with cognitive therapy which focuses upon the examination and correction of false beliefs, applied relaxation, respiratory training, in vivo exposure and psychopharmacology. The correction of false beliefs typically centers on the client's beliefs about impending doom. For the person with social phobia (social anxiety disorder), the client and worker can examine operative beliefs such as "Everybody's looking at me"; "I'm never good enough"; "I'll make a fool of myself" – all self-schema which result in the person's distress and/or avoidance of social situations. The social worker can help the client to examine the origin and strength of those beliefs, look for confirming and disconfirming evidence, consider alternative explanations, and "try on" other possibilities.

In the more serious case of a client with post-traumatic stress disorder, a rape survivor might struggle with the dysfunctional beliefs and attributions that, "If I hadn't dressed that way, he wouldn't have raped me" or "I knew that if I'd just been nicer to him things wouldn't have turned out that way." Each of those statements conveys the client's erroneous beliefs that men rape because of sexual attraction (rather than out of violence) and that "niceness" can prevent the violent attack of a rapist. Furthermore, the social worker would need to understand the defensive function that those dysfunctional cognitions serve. These beliefs allow the client to think she had some modicum of control over a horrible incident. At some points, that may be preferable to feeling the full effect of her powerlessness. So, as with any social work intervention, examination of dysfunctional beliefs needs to be done within the context of the meaning of the symptoms and the client's life situation. Tact and timing are critical, especially with the more "manualized" interventions.

In the aftermath of trauma, people often struggle with affect dysregulation and behavioral control problems and interventions must be focused upon increasing coping strategies. In their review of the literature on trauma, PTSD and resilience, Agaibi and Wilson (2005) propose an integrative, Person X Situation model which requires interaction among the following variables: personality, affect, regulation, coping, ego defenses and the utilization and mobilization of protective factors and resources to aid coping (p. 195).

In a meta-analysis of cognitive-behavioral interventions for anxiety conditions, Butler et al. (2006) reported the following: for *generalized anxiety disorder* cognitive therapy was substantially superior to no treatment, wait list or drug placebo with persistent effects; for *panic disorder*, the combination of cognitive restructuring and interoceptive exposure showed the strongest effect and cognitive-behavioral treatments had the highest effects compared to pharmacological interventions or combination interventions, with virtually no "slippage"; for social phobia, cognitive therapy was superior to both wait list and placebo and similar to exposure interventions without cognitive restructuring and their combination and superior to benzodiazepines; and for obsessive compulsive disorder, cognitive-behavioral therapy and exposure with response prevention were both effective. In the treatment of post-traumatic stress disorder both trauma-based cognitive-behavior therapy and eye movement desensitization and reprocessing (EMDR) demonstrated clinically significant effects in groups of survivors of assault, combat, sexual assault, accidents and refugees (Butler et al., 2006, pp. 24–26).

All of these interventions can be useful in targeting the specific symptoms of anxiety. However, there is an inherent danger in a narrow focus. Changes in role status, life transitions and a range of environmental stressors frequently create anxiety for people. Often, this anxiety is expectable and people may need support in managing the complexities of change. An intervention designed to facilitate a more positive response from the environment, for example, may result in a decrease in a client's anxiety. In this way, the experience of anxiety can be understood as transactional and a positive change in the environment can mediate that experience.

Sometimes environmental and psychological interventions on their own or in combination, are not sufficient to reduce debilitating symptoms of anxiety. Psychopharmacological interventions are frequently used for all of the anxiety conditions. Social workers must be aware of the medications, their usages, side effects, and efficacies and dangers. Benzodiazepines are often used for rapid symptom relief and can be quite effective, however, social workers and clients should be aware that they have significant sedative properties, potential for cognitive impairment, dependence and abuse, and discontinuation can result in withdrawal syndrome. Selective serotonin reuptake inhibitors (SSRI), antidepressants with some anti-anxiety action, are also used for panic disorder and generalized anxiety disorder. The efficacy of pharmacotherapy in obsessive compulsive therapy is high and drug therapy usually begins with a trial of an SSRI. Other medications used include clomipramine and valproate, lithium or carbamazepine as adjunctive medications (Sadock & Sadock, 2007, pp. 581–627).

Far less attention has been focused on "lifestyle" approaches to preventing and managing anxiety conditions. This is troubling, particularly as we have begun to see positive effects of lifestyle changes on the prevention, management, and course of medical illnesses such as diabetes and cardiovascular disease. Strohle (2009) notes that while there is a general consensus that physical activity and exercise have positive effects on anxiety, there has been scant research to examine it. She suggests that it is insufficient to simply tell patients to exercise, and that exercise prescription must be specific, individualized to both the client and the condition. Furthermore, the client should be educated about the mechanisms by which certain physical exercise might positively and negatively affect their anxiety condition.

Illustration and discussion

Ingrid, a 32-year-old woman from Colombia, presented to a social worker (LWR) at a college counseling center complaining of headaches, an inability to concentrate, and uncontrollable trembling. Ingrid was in her final year of her Bachelor's program where she was a non-traditional student. She had tried to attend community college when she first came to the United States but was unable to continue because of chronic headaches and dizzy spells. Shortly after coming to the United States she became a nanny for the three children in the Billings family. Although at the time of her contact, the Billings no longer had young children (the youngest was 6) she still provided intermittent care for them. She was very close to this family and they provided some financial support for her college education.

In Colombia Ingrid lived with her mother. Her father left the family when she was 13 and had no further contact with the family. She had an older brother who was studying at the local university. Ingrid also had wanted to study but her mother could pay for only one child to attend. Ingrid had moved to the United States ten years earlier with her boyfriend, against her mother's wishes. Shortly after arriving, she discovered she was pregnant. Her boyfriend insisted she have an abortion which she did, even though, as a Catholic, it completely conflicted with her religious beliefs. She explained that she "went through with it" because she was afraid that he would leave her and she would be all alone. She described this as a difficult time but felt she couldn't complain because she held herself to blame. She was very emotional, had difficulty leaving the house, and gave her boyfriend a hard time whenever he went out. She blamed the abortion for her headaches and nausea even though there was nothing medically wrong with her. One year later the boyfriend left her, telling her that he was in love with someone else. To this day she explains, "I was completely selfish and heartless, I can't believe I didn't keep my baby—men cannot be trusted."

Ingrid's relationship with her mother had been strained for many years. Two years previously, with the help of the Billings, she returned to Colombia for her brother's wedding. Communication between her and her mother became more frequent and Ingrid was feeling positive about their relationship. Her brother had agreed to send their mother to the United States for Ingrid's graduation. Unfortunately, her mother suddenly died from undiagnosed deep vein thrombosis. She blames herself for not being there, for being a selfish and careless daughter who did not tell her mother to go to the doctor when she complained of pain in her leg. Ingrid went through a difficult time and almost dropped out of school. She was able to attend the funeral with the financial help of her brother and the Billings family. When she talked about the funeral she said it was very emotional and at times found it difficult to breathe during the burial service. She said she experienced headaches and nausea but thought it was because she hadn't been able to sleep very much because of the flight and time change.

Ingrid was then living in residential housing on campus, which in some respects she enjoyed because of the company of other older women with whom she became friends. She studied with them and they often ate meals together in the cafeteria. Ingrid often complained of feeling as though she was "behind in life" because she was 32 and most of the people she knew at her age had a family and a home of their own. Besides providing some childcare for the Billings family and a professor, she tutored people in Spanish. Ingrid was ambivalent about graduating in a few months. She liked the idea of getting on with her life but was terrified that she would not be successful and in the end, after everything, need to move back to Colombia with her brother. Ingrid faced many life transitions and role status changes as she prepared to graduate, assume independent living and embark on a career. As a non-traditional student, by age, experience, and background, she had to make multiple adaptations to her environment.

The night before Ingrid presented to the counseling center, she had been out on a date with a boyfriend she had seen for a few months. He had been married and she was always worried that he might go back with his former wife because they had a child together. After weeks of worrying about whether her boyfriend would leave her because she did not feel ready to have sex with him yet, she decided to "take the risk" stating that she both wanted to and was afraid he'd leave if she didn't. Ingrid had not been in a sexual relationship with a man since her boyfriend of nine years earlier, although she had dated occasionally. She stated that the sex was consensual and that he was very gentle with her. Although she had used protection she was petrified that she might become pregnant. A week after she had slept with her boyfriend, he announced that he and his former wife were going to try to reconcile.

The first few sessions with Ingrid focused on her fear of graduating and finding a job and figuring out where to live. She had a job opportunity in a different state, which she was considering. We discussed what it would be like to leave the comfort of the small community she had formed at college and we began to focus on her ability to adapt to a variety of situations. I reminded her about how well she was able to adapt when she first came from Colombia and formed positive relationships with the various families for which she had provided childcare. I also encouraged her to talk to career services on campus, anticipating that the large national alumni network could assist her in her transition to another locale. The mutual focus on her strengths and the resources available to her through her community seemed to reduce some of her anxiety; however, she remained "worried" about not having the Billings family in her life.

Ingrid also mentioned that she had a fear of becoming pregnant and had mixed emotions about it. Her brother who always seemed to be ambivalent about having children, had just announced that his wife was pregnant and Ingrid seemed to be very excited for him. She stated that she knew she wanted to have children "but at the right time." She knew she could not afford to have a baby at this point in her life and she also knew she could not have another abortion. She was also keenly aware of her age, given that her older sister-in-law had had difficulty becoming pregnant.

Before the sixth session one of the women on Ingrid's floor brought her into the counseling center in crisis after she found her screaming, crying, and trembling on the floor of their bathroom. Ingrid was calm but appeared tired and depressed. When asked what happened Ingrid said that she had gotten her period but was afraid that it was a miscarriage. She had thought she was pregnant because of some nausea and headaches she had been experiencing. When asked what happened Ingrid said, "It just all suddenly came over me – all the worry, all of the pain, all of the dread – my nerves couldn't take it. I felt like the room was closing in on me and all I saw where dead babies." She explained that her mother had had an ataque de nervios when her father left her but that Ingrid was too young to remember how it began. All she remembered was her aunt running to her mother's side to make sure she didn't fall and her uncle taking Ingrid out of the room.

What followed was an examination of Ingrid's desire to have a baby in order to have something to love that wouldn't leave her and a way to forgive herself for the previous abortion. She talked about how she always felt alone, even when she was in a group of people she calls her friends. She didn't believe that people really wanted to be with her but that they socialized with her because they felt sorry for her. She wondered if the miscarriage was a punishment from God for having had the abortion and she was afraid she'd never be able to have children. Although it was terrifying to her to think of raising a baby on her own, she felt that if she stayed in town she would have the support of the Billings family and with a college degree could figure out how to care for the baby financially.

Understanding the complex issues of loss, panic, and cultural connections to somatic symptoms were all key elements to helping Ingrid. The early experience of abandonment by her father which was repeated by her boyfriends were key to understanding the sense of loss she felt when she found out she was not pregnant. Following her recent losses, including her mother's death, and the impending loss of a structured, supportive college environment and the Billings family, she was reluctant to take a job in another state.

The work with Ingrid centered on a combination of a psychodynamic understanding of her development and cognitive-behavioral interventions to restructure her dysfunctional beliefs that she was selfish, destined to be alone, and unlovable. Addressing Ingrid's cognitive schemas was an important aspect our work together. We began exploring her belief that she was all alone in the world. She had many memories of her brother being the favored one, even as a child. His needs always came before hers. She relayed memories of herself in school in Colombia. Because her father had left the family, they had a great deal of financial difficulty. What money they did have generally went to pay for her brother's schooling. Even though everyone in her school wore uniforms, others made fun of her shoes, coat, and book bag. She explained that the only person with whom she was really friends was a U.S. American girl who was made fun of because of her accent. We spent time restructuring her cognitive schema of isolation and alienation by focusing on the relationships she had with the Billings family and several friends in college. She had difficulty in calling up these caring relationships when she felt alone, so a plan was made for her to keep a journal of the times she felt that all alone and undesirable. By writing down the situation, how she felt, what her automatic thoughts were and replacing those thoughts with a different (rational) response Ingrid was able to recognize what contributed to her belief that she was alone. Most of the situations where she felt this way were when she was in a large group of people whom she felt were of a higher social standing. She stated that these feelings would even come up when she was around the Billings family. Modifying her belief that she was a very selfish person had to be done with an understanding of her cultural background. In many Latin@ cultures daughters are taught to take on the responsibility of their parents as they age. With this in mind, we talked about how she may have gone against cultural tradition but that another cultural value was to follow your heart, which is what she was doing by immigrating to the United States with her boyfriend. She had always planned on bringing her mother later but her mother was never interested.

Ingrid also had an "irrational belief" (Ellis, 1994) of abandonment. Although there was quite a bit of abandonment in her history, she really believed that God was making her suffer for the abortion and her selfishness. So, she believed that God's way of punishing her was to take away people who were important to her. As we explored the different times in her life when she felt abandoned and the fear she had of being abandoned again, Ingrid was able to see differences in her current situation and ability to make choices. We also examined how this belief connected to her distrust of men and how as an older more mature woman she could make different choices than she and her mother had made in the past. Working through the irrational belief that God was punishing her took more time and had roots in her cultural/religious beliefs. Although we explored what kind of God she believed in (a loving or punishing God) it seemed important to respect the belief that God had the power to punish and reward people. Instead we worked on restructuring her understanding of what it means to be selfish.

The week before we were scheduled to end, Ingrid experienced one more "ataque" although she felt that it was not as severe as the one prior. This time she felt dizzy, nauseous, was crying, had difficulty breathing and said she heard her mother's voice. We discussed what it meant for her to experience another incident where she felt overwhelmed. She said that having had a previous episode helped her to understand what was happening to her. She then began to talk about how after her mother's "ataque" she remembers her mother talking about her despondency and sadness related to her failed marriage. "My mother was a very strong and stoic woman so for her to talk about that, for her to be able to feel what she felt must have come from the 'ataque.' I don't think I would have been able to feel all that I felt if it hadn't happened again." Ingrid felt connected to her mother and at the same time was able to manage the feelings that had come up for her; feelings around loss and abandonment due to our termination.

Since culture has profound influence on a person's thoughts, emotions, and behaviors, cultural understanding is imperative in the assessment and treatment of any individual. This was important not only in how she related to the culture but also in how the culture related to her. She had values and beliefs that were syntonic to her Latin@ culture but she also expressed behaviors that would be dystonic. For example I had to understand how her religion may characterize her choice to have an abortion and how that portion of her culture's relationship to her played a tremendous role in how she perceived herself. Just as important was for me to be aware of my own cultural background, biases and awareness. Ingrid may have been diagnosed very easily with panic disorder or generalized anxiety disorder and her "ataques" may have been defined as psychotic episodes. She may even have been diagnosed with an Axis II diagnosis of histrionic personality disorder. Had I not had the knowledge of the Latin@ culture and the meaning of "ataque de nervios" Ingrid may have been given something for her "nerves", and her irrational beliefs would never have been explored, through her changed cognitions, she was able to gain an understanding of herself as a woman who has survived many things and is still able to feel.

Conclusion

Like all mental health conditions, the experience of anxiety poses many challenges for individuals and their families. While there is a common human evolutionary history to the manifestation of adaptive anxiety, certain genetic, environmental, biological, cognitive and transactional influences can combine in the creation of maladaptive thoughts, feelings and behaviors. However, as in the cases of Linda and Ingrid, the symptoms of anxiety are best understood in the broad context of the client's life. Cognitive and behavioral interventions, psychodynamic and sociocultural understandings, along with an appreciation of the complex relationship between mind and body provide the best means of mediating complex human responses to stress.

Note

1 The @ sign is used to represent individuals whose heritage is from Latin American or Caribbean descent through inclusive and non-sexist language: www.sociologistswithoutborders.org/essays/LATINOS.pdf

Web resources

Anxiety Disorders Association of America
www.adaa.org

National Institute of Mental Health
www.nimh.nih.gov

Substance Abuse and Mental Health Services Administration
www.samhsa.gov

References

Agaibi, C.E., & Wilson, J.P. (2005). Trauma, PTSD, and resilience: A review of the literature. *Trauma, Violence, and Abuse, 6* (3), 195–216.

Albano, A.M., Chorpita, B.F., & Barlow, D.H. (2003). Childhood anxiety disorders. In R.A. Barkley (ed.), *Child psychopathology* (2nd ed., pp. 279–329). New York: Guilford Press.

Alegria, M., Canino, G., Shrout, P., Woo, M., Duan, M., Vila, D. et al. (2008). Prevalence of mental illness in immigrant and non-immigrant US Latino groups. *American Journal of Psychiatry, 165,* 359–369.

Alim, T., Charney, D., & Mellman, T., (2006). An overview of posttraumatic stress disorder in African Americans. *Journal of Clinical Psychology, 62,* 801–813.

American Psychiatric Association (APA). (2000). *Diagnostic and statistical manual of mental disorders* (4th ed., text revision). Washington, DC: APA.

Angst, J., & Vollrath, M. (1991). The natural history of anxiety disorders. *Acta Psychiatrica Scandinavica, 84,* 446–452.

Armstrong, K.A., & Khawaja, N.G. (2002). Gender differences in anxiety: An investigation of the symptoms, cognitions, and sensitivity towards anxiety in a non clinical population. *Behavioral and Cognitive Psychotherapy, 30,* 227–231.

Arrindell, E., Eisemann, M., Richter, J., Oei, T., Caballo, V., van der Ende, J. et al. (2003). Masculinity-femininity as a national characteristic and its relationship with national agoraphobic fear levels: Fodor's sex role hypothesis revitalized. *Behavior Research Therapy, 41,* 795–807.

Asnaani, A., Gutner, C.A., Hinton, D.E., & Hofmann, S.G. (2009). Panic disorder, panic attacks and panic attack symptoms across race-ethnic groups: Results of the collaborative psychiatric epidemiology studies. *CNS Neuroscience and Therapeutics, 15* (3), 249–254.

Beck, J., & Emery, G. (1985). *Anxiety disorders and phobias: A cognitive perspective.* New York: Basic Books.

Beekman, A., de Beurs, E., van Balkom, A., Deeg, D., van Dyck, R., & van Tilberg, W. (2000). Anxiety and depression in later life: Co-occurrence and communality of risk factors. *American Journal of Psychiatry, 157,* 89–95.

Beesdo, K., Knappe, S., & Pine, D.S. (2009). Anxiety and anxiety disorders in children and adolescents: Developmental issues and implications for DSM-V. *Psychiatric Clinics of North America, 32* (3), 483–524.

Breslau, N., Kessler, R.C., Chilcoat, H.D., Schultz, L.R., Davis, G.C., & Andreski, P. (1998). Trauma and posttraumatic stress disorder in the community: The 1996 Detroit Area Survey of Trauma. *Archives of General Psychiatry, 55,* 626–632.

Breslau, J., Aguilar-Gaxiola, S., Kendler, K., Su, M., Williams, D., & Kessler, R. (2006). Specifying race-ethnic differences in risk for psychiatric disorder in the USA national sample. *Psychological Medicine, 3,* 657–668.

Brook, C.A., & Schmidt, L.A. (2008). Social anxiety disorder: A review of environmental risk factors. *Neuropsychiatric Disease and Treatment, 4* (1), 123–143.

Brown, E.J. (2005). Correlates and treatment of stress disorder in children and adolescents. *Psychiatric Annals, 35* (9), 759–765.

Bruce, S.E., Yonkers, K.A., Otto, M.W., Eisen, J.L., Weisberg, R.B., Pagano, M. et al. (2005). Influence of psychiatric comorbidity on recovery and recurrence in generalized anxiety disorder, social phobia, and panic disorder: A 12-year prospective study. *American Journal of Psychiatry, 162*, 1179–1187.

Busuttil, W. (2004). Presentations and management of post-traumatic stress disorder and the elderly: A need for investigation. *International Journal of Geriatric Psychiatry, 19*, 429–439.

Butler, A.C., Chapman, G.E., Forman, E.M., & Beck, A.T. (2006). The empirical status of cognitive-behavioral therapy: A review for meta-analyses. *Clinical Psychology Review, 26*, 17–31.

Caballo, V., Salazar, I., Irurtia, M., Arias, B., & Hofmann, S. (2008). Social anxiety in 18 nations: Sex and age differences. *Behavioral Psychology, 16*, 163–187.

Charney, D.S. (2004). Psychobiological mechanisms of resilience and vulnerability: Implications for successful adaptation to extreme stress. *American Journal of Psychiatry, 161* (2), 195–216.

Christiana, J.M., Gilman, S.E., Guardino, M., Mickelson, K., Morselli, P.L., Olfson, M. et al. (2000). Duration between onset and time of obtaining initial treatment among people with anxiety and mood disorders: An international survey of members of mental health patient advocate groups. *Psychological Medicine, 30*, 693–703.

Chu, B., Coudhury, M.S., Shortt, A.L., Pincus, D.B., Creed, T.A., & Kendall, P.C. (2004). Alliance, technology, and outcome in the treatment of anxious youth. *Cognitive and Behavioral Practice, 11*, 44–55.

Davis, L., & Siegel, L.J. (2000). Posttraumatic stress disorder in children and adolescents: A review and analysis. *Clinical Child and Family Psychology Review, 3* (3), 135–154.

DeBellis, M. (2001). Developmental traumatology: The psychobiological development of maltreated children and its implications for research, treatment, and policy. *Development and Psychopathology, 13*, 539–564.

DeBellis, M., & Keshavan, M.S. (2003). Sex differences in brain maturation in maltreatment-related pediatric posttraumatic stress disorder. *Special Edition of Neurosciences and Biobehavioral Reviews: Brain development, sex differences, and stress; Implications for psychopathology, 27*, 103–117.

De Bellis, M.D., Hooper, S.R., & Sapia, J.L. (2005). Early trauma exposure and the brain. In C.R. Brewin (ed.), *Neuropsychology of PTSD: Biological, cognitive, and clinical perspectives* (pp. 153–177). New York: Guilford Press.

Elder, G.H., & Clipp, E.C. (1989). Combat experience and emotional health: Impairment and resilience in later life. *Journal of Personality, 57*, 311–341.

Ellis, A. (1994). *Reason and emotion in psychotherapy*. New York: Birch Lane Press.

Evans, D.L., & Charney, D.S. (2003). Mood disorders and medical illness: A major public health problem. *Biological Psychiatry, 54*, 178–180.

Fava, G.A., Grandi, S., Rafanelli, C., Ruini, C., Conti, S., & Belluardo, P. (2001). Long term outcome of social phobia treated by exposure. *Psychological Medicine, 31*, 899–905.

Flaskerud, J. (2009). What do we need to know about culture bound syndromes? *Issues in Mental Health Nursing, 30* (6), 406–407.

Fletcher, K.E. (1996). Childhood posttraumatic stress disorder. In E.J. Mash & R.A. Barkely (eds). *Child psychopathology* (pp. 242–276). New York: Guilford Press.

Fontanelle, L., & Hasler, G. (2008). The analytical epidemiology of obsessive compulsive disorder: Risk factors and correlates. *Progress in Neuro-Psychopharmacology and Biological Psychiatry, 32*, 1–15.

Furr, J.M., Tiwari, S., Suveg, C., & Kendall, P.C. (2009). Anxiety disorders in children and adolescents. In M.B. Stein (ed.), *Oxford handbook of anxiety and related disorders* (pp. 636–656). New York: Oxford University Press.

Gitterman, A. (2001). Social work practice with vulnerable and resilient populations. In A. Gitterman (ed.), *Social work practice with vulnerable and resilient populations* (2nd ed., pp. 1–38). New York: Columbia University Press.

Gitterman, A., & Germain, C.B. (2008). *The life model of social work: Advances in theory and practice*. New York: Columbia University Press.

Goodwin, R.D., Faravelli, C., Rosi, S., Cosci, F., Truglia, E., de Graaf, H. et al. (2005). The epidemiology of panic disorder and agoraphobia in Europe. *European Neuropsychopharmacology, 15*, 435–443.

Hart, T.A., & Heimberg, R.G. (2001). Presenting problems among treatment seeking gay, lesbian and bisexual youth. *Cognitive and Behavioral Practice, 17* (1), 55–65.

Hatfield, A. (1988). Issues in psychoeducation for families of the mentally ill. *International Journal of Mental Health 17* (1), 48–64.

Hazlett-Stevens, H., Pruitt, L.D., & Collins, A. (2009). Phenomenology of generalized anxiety disorder. In M.B. Stein (ed.), *Oxford handbook of anxiety and related disorders* (pp. 47–55). New York: Oxford University Press.

Hinton, D.E., Park, L., Hsia, C., Hofmann, S., & Pollack, M.H., (2009). Anxiety disorder presentations in Asian populations: A review. *CNS Neuroscience and Therapeutics, 15*, 295–303.

Horwath, E., & Weissman, M.M. (1997). Epidemiology of anxiety disorders across cultural groups. In S. Friedman (ed.), *Cultural issues in the treatment of anxiety* (pp. 21–39). New York: Guilford Press.

Hunter, L.R., & Schmidt, N.B. (2010). Anxiety psychopathology in African American adults: Literature review and development of an empirically informed sociocultural model. *Psychological Bulletin, 136* (2), 211–235.

Kaufman, J.M. (2005). *Characteristics of emotional and behavioral disorders of children and youth* (7th ed.). Upper Saddle, NJ: Merrill/Prentice Hall.

Kendall, P.C., & Kessler, R.C. (2002). The impact of childhood psychopathology interventions on subsequent substance abuse: Policy implications, comments, and recommendations. *Journal of Consulting and Clinical Psychology, 70*, 1303–1306.

Kessler, R.C., Sonnega, A., Bromet, E., Hughes, M., & Nelson, C.B. (1995). Postraumatic stress disorder in the National Comorbidity Study. *Archives of General Psychiatry, 52* (12), 1048–1060.

Kessler, R.C., Chiu, W.T., Demier, O., & Walters, E.E. (2005). Prevalence, severity, and comorbidity of twelve month DSM-IV disorders in the national comorbidity survey replication (NCS-R). *Archives of General Psychiatry, 62* (6), 617–627.

Kessler, R.C., Amminger, G.P., Aguilar-Gaxiola, S., Alonso, J., Lee, S., & Üstün, T.B. (2007). Age of onset of mental disorders: A review of recent literature. *Current Opinion in Psychiatry, 20* (4), 359–364.

Kessler, R.C., Ruscio, A.M., Shear, K., & Wittchen, H. (2009). Epidemiology of anxiety disorders. In M.B. Stein (ed.), *Oxford handbook of anxiety and related disorders* (pp. 19–33). New York: Oxford University Press.

Kim, J., Rapee, R., & Gaston, J. (2008). Symptoms of offensive-type Taijin-Kyofusho among Austrialian social phobics. *Depression and Anxiety, 25*, 601–608.

Kirk, S.A., & Kutchins, H. (1992). *The selling of the DSM: The rhetoric of science in psychiatry*. New York: Aldine de Gruyter.

Kirmayer, L., (1997). Culture and anxiety: A clinical and research agenda. In S. Freidman (ed.). *Cultural issues in the treatment of anxiety* (pp. 225–246). New York: Guilford Press.

Kutchins, H., & Kirk, S.A. (1988). The business of diagnosis: DSM-III and clinical social work. *Social Work, 33* (3), 215–220.

Langan, P.A. & Farrington, D.P. (1998). *Crime and justice in the United States and in England and Wales: 1981–1996*. Washington, DC: Office of Justice Programs, Bureau of Justice Statistics, U.S. Department of Justice.

Last, C.G., Hansen, C., & Franco, N. (1997). Anxious children in adulthood: A prospective study of adjustment. *Journal of the American Academy of Child and Adolescent Psychiatry, 36* (5), 645–652.

Leach, L., Christensen, H., Mackinnon, A., Windsor, T., & Butterworth, P. (2008). Gender differences in depression and anxiety across the adult lifespan: The role of psychosocial mediators. *Social Psychiatry and Psychiatric Epidemiology, 43*, 983–998.

Lenze, E., Rogers, J., Martire, L., Mulsant, B., Rollman, B., Dew, M. et al. (2001). The association of late life depression and anxiety with physical disability: A review of the literature and prospectus for future research. *American Journal of Geriatric Psychiatry, 9* (2), 113–135.

Lewinsohn, P., Holm-Denoma, J., Small, J., Seeley J., & Joiner, T. (2008). Separation anxiety disorder in childhood as a risk factor for future mental illness. *Journal of the American Academy of Child and Adolescent Psychiatry, 47* (5), 548–555.

Lewis-Fernández, R., Guranaccia, P.J., Martinez, I.E., Salman, E., Schmidt, A., & Liebowitz, M. (2002) Comparative phenomenology of ataques de nervios, panic attacks, and panic disorder. *Culture, Medicine, and Psychiatry, 26*, 199–223.

Lewis-Fernández, R., Hinton, D.E., Laria, A.J., Patterson, E.H., Hofmann, S.G., Craske, M.G. et al. (2010). Culture and the anxiety disorders: Recommendations for DSM-V. *Depression and Anxiety, 27* (2), 212–229.

Marshall, G.N., Schell, T.L., & Miles, J.N.V. (2009). Ethnic differences in posttraumatic distress: Hispanics' symptoms differ in kind and degree. *Journal of Consulting and Clinical Psychology, 77* (6), 1169–1178.

Matsunaga, H., & Seedat, S. (2007). Obsessive compulsive spectrum disorders: Cross-national and ethnic issues. *CNS Spectrums, 12* (5), 392–400.

Matthey, S., Barnett, B., & White, T. (2003). The Edinburgh Postnatal Depression Scale. *British Journal of Psychiatry, 182* (4), 368.

Miranda, J., McGuire, T., Williams, D.R., & Wang, P. (2008). Mental health in the context of health disparities. *American Journal of Psychiatry, 165* (9), 1102–1108.

National Institute of Mental Health. (2007). *Post-traumatic stress disorder research fact sheet.* Retrieved from www.nimh.nih.gov/health/publications/post-traumatic-stress-disorder-research-fact-sheet/index.shtml.

National Institute of Mental Health. (2009). *PANDAS: Frequently asked questions about Pediatric Autoimmune Neuropsychiatric Disorders Associated with Streptococcal Infections.* Retrieved from www.nimh.nih.gov/health/publications/pandas/pandas-frequently-asked-questions-about-pediatric-autoimmune-neuropsychiatric-disorders-associated-with-streptococcal-infections.shtml.

Pillemer, K., & Finkelhor, D. (1988). The prevalence of elder abuse: A random sample survey. *The Gerontologist, 28*, 51–58.

Pole, N., Gone, J., & Kulkarni, M. (2008). Posttraumatic stress disorder among ethnoracial minorities in the United States. *Clinical Psychology: Science and Practice, 15*, 35–61.

Reck, C., Struben, K., Backenstrass, M., Stefenelli, U., Reinig, K., Fuchs, T. et al. (2008). Prevalence, onset and comorbidity of postpartum anxiety and depressive disorders. *Acta Psychiatrica Scandinavica, 118* (6), 459–468.

Roy-Byrne, P., Davidson, K., Kessler, R., Asmundson, G., Goodwin, R.D., Kubzansky, L. et al. (2008). Anxiety disorders and comorbid medical illness. *General Hospital Psychiatry, 30*, 208–225.

Sadock, B.J., & Sadock, V.A. (2007). *Kaplan and Sadock's Synopsis of Psychiatry* (2nd ed.). Philadelphia, PA: Lippincott Williams & Wilkins.

Spitzer, R.L., Kroenke, K., Williams, J.B., & Lowe, B. (2006). A brief measure for assessing generalized anxiety disorder: The GAD-7. *Archives of Internal Medicine, 166* (10), 1092–1097.

Stein, M.B., Cox, B.J., Afifi, T., Belik, S., & Sareen, J. (2006). Does comorbid depressive illness magnify the impact of chronic physical illness: A population based perspective. *Psychological Medicine, 36*, 587–596.

Strohle, A. (2009). Physical activity, exercise, depression and anxiety disorders. *Journal of Neural Transmission, 116*, 777–784.

Van Oort, F.V.A., Greaves-Lord, K., Verhulst, F.C., Ormel, J., & Huizink, A.C. (2009). The developmental course of anxiety symptoms during adolescence: The TRAILS study. *Journal of Child Psychology and Psychiatry, 50* (10), 1209–1217.

Varela, R.E., & Hensley-Maloney, L. (2009). The influence of culture on anxiety in Latino youth: A review. *Clinical Child and Family Psychology Review, 12* (3), 217–233.

Wittchen, H.U., Zhao, S., Kessler, R.C., & Eaton, W.W. (1994). DSM-III-R generalized anxiety disorder in the national comorbidity survey. *Archives of General Psychiatry, 51* (5), 355–364.

Wittchen, H.U., Nocon, A., Beesdo, K., Pine, D., Hofler, M., Lieb, R. et al. (2008). Agoraphobia and panic: Prospective-longitudinal relations suggest a rethinking of diagnostic concepts. *Psychotherapy and Psychosomatics, 77*, 147–157.

Woods, M.E., & Hollis, F. (2000). *Casework: A psychosocial therapy* (5th ed.). New York: McGraw-Hill.

Zimmerman, P., Wittchen, H., Hofler, M., Pfistger, H., Kessler, R.C., & Lieb, R. (2003). Primary anxiety disorders and the development of subsequent alcohol use disorders: A 4-year community study of adolescents and young adults. *Psychological Medicine, 33*, 1211–1222.

17 Eating conditions

Danna Bodenheimer and Nina Rovinelli Heller

Eating conditions, traditionally associated with white, middle to upper class Western young women of the twentieth century, are increasingly prevalent among both genders and many socioeconomic, racial and ethnic groups. No longer seen as exclusively conditions of adolescence and early adulthood, eating conditions are recognized as long-term conditions which manifest at points across the life course. Unlike other psychiatric diagnoses, eating conditions "play out" specifically in the body, interacting with social, cultural, and psychological factors. Social workers, with our biopsychosocial perspective, are particularly well situated to understand both the complex etiology and the multimodal approaches required in the work with people with these eating conditions. Deviated eating behaviors, including anorexia nervosa (AN), bulimia nervosa (BN), binge eating disorder (BED), and obesity-related conditions, are both psychiatric and social problems, and increasingly, public health problems (Heller, 2008).

Today, social workers work with clients with eating conditions in a wide variety of settings, including hospitals, schools, outpatient clinics and community settings. Building upon our understanding of the complex transactions between the individual and the environment, we intervene on the levels of primary and secondary prevention, and introduce interventions through groupwork and individual and family work. An understanding of the complex associations among such diverse factors as culture, biology, family, social and physical environments, race/ethnicity, gender and psychological influences provide the foundation for our work with clients who struggle with eating and food issues.

Definitions of eating conditions

Eating conditions can be defined by *social construction theory, by symptom cluster* (as in the American Psychiatric Association's (2000) *Diagnostic and statistical manual*) and through the lenses of *psychodynamic, cognitive-behavioral* or *family systems concepts,* and *genetic/biological theories.* All offer us something useful, but are best utilized together, both in formulating understanding, and in intervening with people with eating conditions. Indeed, having an issue with eating behaviors and attitudes affects all aspects of a person's biopsychosocial functioning. Furthermore, a positive prognosis is almost solely associated with multimodal services (Caparrotta and Ghaffari, 2006; McFarland, 1995; Werne, 1996) and a consideration of the multiple risk factors for developing any of these conditions (Striegel-Moore & Bulik, 2007).

The *social construction* of eating disorder conditions can best be understood by examining the cultural context is which they were first identified. Brumberg (1988) in her study of "fasting girls" noted that anorexia nervosa was first described in the medical literature in the 1870s by a British physician who treated upper middle class women. At the same time, the phenomenon was identified in France and the United States, also among upper middle class young women. This was an illness of affluence, found only among people for whom food was plentiful. Women of this era had tightly constricted social roles and while many were educated, they had few options which allowed any deviation from those traditional gender roles. The first reference to the binge/purge cycle behaviors, now associated with bulimia nervosa was in the late eighteenth century, identified among boarding school girls (Johnson & Connors, 1987). The medical literature contained a few case studies in the 1940s with Binswanger (1944) reporting a case of a woman with chronic symptoms of binge eating and the associated psychological symptoms of a distorted body image and fear of becoming fat. Binge eating as a single symptom was reported by Hilda Bruch (1978), a pioneer in the field, in the literature on obese patients. Selling and Ferraro (1945) observed large numbers of refugee children brought to the United States during the previous decade, and reported gorging behavior in many of these children. This binge eating subsided once the child was placed in a foster home, but was resumed at times of even brief separations from loved ones. This observation was important for many reasons. First, it was the earliest indication that problematic eating behaviors occurred in other than affluent populations. Second, and more importantly, it was one of the first indications that there was a connection between binge eating behavior and the experiences of separation and loss.

The study of eating conditions was continued and brought to the public discourse by Hilda Bruch in the 1950s through the 1970s. While her earlier work focused on obesity in childhood, she is best known for her work about the adolescent female anorectic. Using a psychodynamic framework, she focused primarily on the psychological and family factors associated with anorexia. These girls were described as perfectionistic, bright, and self-sacrificing, with a high rate of suicide attempts and completion. There followed a burgeoning literature in the 1970s and 1980s clinical literature and popular media about bulimia, with *Newsweek Magazine* proclaiming 1981 the "year of the binge-purge syndrome" (Adler, 1982). The influence of the media upon the growing incidence of eating conditions can not be underestimated and has been extensively studied (Drummond, 2002; Fister & Smith, 2004; Stice, Schupack-Neuberg, Shaw, & Stein, 1994). A 1970s icon, the "skinny" supermodel, Twiggy, presented a stark contrast to the "hourglass figure" ideal of the previous decades. Even today, a wait in the supermarket line will bombard one (including impressionable little girls) with images of very thin women on magazine covers, with accompanying stories such as "how to drop six dress sizes in four weeks." Not surprisingly, we have observed the incidence in these eating conditions steadily rise in community populations as well as in clinical populations. Moreover, a wide range of severity exists in eating condition symptoms. For instance, some people have life threatening eating conditions requiring hospitalization while others have similar symptoms but at a lower threshold, which do not impair their functioning to the extent that they require close medical supervision.

This theory holds that eating conditions arise from a confluence of sociocultual factors and influences, including relative affluence, rigid and constricting, or conflicting gender roles, and socially reinforced ideals of "beauty." Pallett, Link, and Lee (2009) report that women with eating conditions are communicating the failure of our society to accept that beauty exists on a continuum rather than on the prescriptive "thin" idea. While girls and women have been most vulnerable to this triad of influences, as social and gender roles evolve (or devolve), some boys and men are increasingly at risk for developing similar food and body image problems (Lewinsohn, Seeley, Moerk, & Striegel-Moore, 2002). The debate about whether an eating condition is in fact an illness or a social construction is in part a misguided one. We should avoid this dichotomy; in developing both assessment and intervention strategies, we must understand how social influences and characteristics of certain individuals and groups of individuals interact to produce social contexts, which can be debilitating and life threatening.

The identification and classification of *symptoms and symptom clusters* is also central in the defining of all of the eating conditions. An individual meets the diagnostic criteria for these conditions when a desire for thinness (central in both anorexia nervosa and bulimia nervosa) becomes critical to one's sense of self, when binging or purging become regular behaviors, when food restriction becomes pervasive or when self-perception of size is distorted by a seemingly unmovable break with reality (Fallon, Katzman, & Wooley, 1994). Because the terms "pervasive," "regular" and "distorted" are largely subjective, diagnostic criteria, which are quite prescriptive, provide clear guidelines for diagnosis.

According to the DSM-IV-TR (APA, 2000) there are four major categories of eating disorders which share some common *symptoms*. These include anorexia nervosa (AN), bulimia nervosa (BN), binge eating disorder (BED), and eating disorder not otherwise specified (NOS). While anorexia nervosa and bulimia are distinct conditions, research indicates that they exist on a continuum; a person with anorexia at one point in her life may suffer with symptoms of bulimia at another time (Bulik, Sullivan, Franz, Fear, & Pickering, 1997; Emmett, 1985; Werne, 1996; Zerbe, 1993). Obesity, not included in the DSM, is nonetheless, because of its increasing incidence among children and within impoverished communities, receiving further attention as a medical condition, with attendant social and psychological problems.

The *symptom criteria* for anorexia (literally lack of appetite) include the refusal to maintain 85 percent or more of normal body weight for age and height; this is the central defining criterion for anorexia without an alternate medically justifiable explanation. People with AN are also characterized by their intense fear of being fat or of gaining weight (although underweight), and their distorted body image. Finally, postmenarcheal women must have had a cessation of their menstrual cycles for three consecutive months.

Some of these criteria have been debated both in clinical practice and in research studies. This last criterion (cessation of menstrual cycles) has been seen as a necessary one in part because it indicates the presence of significant serious endocrinological changes. In a retrospective study of 588 anorexic women, however, Watson and Andersen (2003) found that only 77.4 percent met this diagnostic criterion, the remaining 22.6 percent, some of whom had serious life threatening symptoms, did not technically meet the criteria for the diagnosis. Obviously, this criterion does not apply to men, who are increasingly vulnerable to anorexia (Robb & Dadson, 2002). Neither does it apply to prepubertal children who are also exhibiting, in increasing numbers, symptoms of these eating conditions. When this criterion is used strictly to determine severity of illness or recommended level of treatment, some individuals will not receive the optimal level of specialized care. Additionally, adhering strictly to the threshold of 85 percent of body weight as a cutoff point renders individuals who are just above this, outside of the classification, even if other factors (psychological, behavioral, historical, and cognitive) are present and cause significant distress. This serves as a good reminder to all practitioners of the limitations of any classification system and that multiple means of assessment are critical if we are to determine and secure the proper services for a client.

Bulimia nervosa is characterized by binge eating which is defined as eating in a discrete period of time, quantities of food (which others would definitely see as large) while experiencing a lack of control about the eating. This binge eating is done in concert with a range of compensatory behaviors aimed at mitigating the effects of such large calorie consumption. These may include vomiting, laxative or diuretic use, excessive exercise, and/or fasting. Both the binge eating and the compensatory behaviors must continue on average at least twice per week over a three month period of time. Additionally, one's self-appraisal must be significantly influenced by the individual's weight and body shape. In terms of differential diagnosis, the binge eating does not occur only in instances of anorexia nervosa. The diagnosis of non-purging subtype requires that the individual does not vomit or use laxative like substances, but relies exclusively upon fasting, calorie restriction and excessive exercise to mitigate the effects of the bingeing behaviors. Unlike with AN, there is no weight criteria for BN; in fact, most people with bulimia nervosa are of normal weight.

Binge eating disorder is characterized by recurrent episodes of binge eating, as described above. In addition, these episodes are accompanied by three or more of the following: more rapid eating than usual; eating until physically uncomfortable, eating large amounts when not hungry, eating alone because of embarrassment, feeling disgusted or very guilty about oneself. The binge eating must occur at least twice weekly for six months and the individual must experience distress when the binge eating is present. Finally, to distinguish it from both AN and BN, the binge eating can not be associated with the regular use of the compensatory behaviors described above (APA, 2000). Because of the regular high caloric intake for these individuals without the compensatory behaviors which serve to either eliminate high calorie foods or expend the excess calories, many binge eaters are overweight or obese, conditions which are associated with many acute and chronic health problems.

The DSM-IV-TR (APA, 2000) recognizes that not all individuals who have serious eating condition will exactly meet the criteria for the three diagnoses discussed above. For that reason, the diagnosis of eating disorder not otherwise specified (NOS) is used to classify those individuals who do have problematic eating or restricting of food but may not have the low body weight, associated with anorexia. Likewise, the person who has significant problems with bingeing and purging but does not meet the duration and frequency criteria might be diagnosed with the NOS classification. The use of this diagnosis can be an important step, because it can be conceived of as a harbinger of more serious eating disturbances to come (Devlin et al., 2002). While these subthreshold disturbances may not be as life threatening as full blown conditions, they do indicate difficulty in regulating self-esteem and affect and are often associated with severe trauma histories (Eberly & Heath, 2008).

Obesity, a growing public health concern for children and adults is not classified as a psychiatric, but rather as a medical condition. We include discussion of obesity here, because of its current epidemic proportions and because research suggests that individuals in low income groups and in minority populations – those often served by social workers – may be disproportionately affected (Lopez, 2007). We are also aware that certain sociological, psychological and cohort variables influence the rates of obesity. It is significant that obesity, with its many well-documented long-term medical and psychological complications, has not received nearly as much attention by researchers and clinicians as AN and BN. A fascination with the "thinness ideal" affects all of us, researchers included. It may well be a manifestation of stigma about "fat" that has resulted in this discrepancy. While not traditionally considered a diagnosable eating disorder, obesity ought to be recognized on the continuum of weight and food related struggles. Perhaps the DSM-IV does not classify obesity as a psychological illness because it is classically a medical phenomenon. Despite that fact, there is a definitive psychological toll that obesity inflicts on individual functioning, compromising self-esteem, social identity and an overall sense of wellness. Beyond its impact at the micro-level, obesity is also receiving attention as a public health epidemic, particularly among children. Technically, obesity refers to an excess of body fat in healthy individuals and is measured by calculating the body mass index (BMI). Obesity is measured among children and adolescents as at or above the 95th percentile of the sex-specific BMI for age growth charts. Obesity among adults is defined as a BMI of 30 or higher; extreme obesity is defined as a BMI of 40 or higher (Ogden, Carroll, Curtin, McDowell, Tabak, & Flegal, 2006). Among the general United States population, obesity impacts over 17 percent of children and over 33 percent of adults. Finally, night eating syndrome has been identified in some individuals, precipitated by stressful life circumstances and occurring daily. It is characterized by significant food intake after a normal evening meal and may be related in addition to stress, to the use of sleep sedatives. Specific criteria for this syndrome have not yet been identified.

Psychological symptoms that include affective, behavioral and cognitive components are prevalent across the continuum of eating conditions. As mentioned, for both anorexia and bulimia, these issues revolve particularly around one's body image and the persistent fear of gaining weight. One's self-appraisal is based solely upon weight and body size and shape, along with a persistent denial of the seriousness of the current low weight (APA, 2000). In considering these factors, an understanding of the transactional relationship between psychological and sociocultural forces is critical. Stice (1994) identified three social factors that promote eating conditions. These include: the centrality of appearance to the female gender role; the essential value of appearance in women's social success; and the ideal of the thin body for women. From early on, girls and women (the predominant population with these eating conditions) are bombarded with interpersonal and media content about the value of a stereotypic female ideal. All of us are subject to this exposure; some, for a variety of reasons, seem predisposed to internalize this ideal. The result of the internalization of these images and expectations is the development of both behavioral symptoms and a set of cognitive distortions. People suffering with BN share with their anorectic counterparts the inability to realistically assess their own worth or size, and judgment is severely compromised by a preoccupation with body image. In addition to these body image issues, other psychological motivations have been identified. Many individuals struggle with the management of affect. For anorexics this is accomplished by pervasive denial, of both feelings and food. At the same time, both anorexics and bulimics appear to struggle with the management of affect. Caparrotta and Ghaffari (2006) propose that psychologically, bulimics manage affect by purging and anorectics by restricting. They further note that the restriction of affect in anorexia is not a sustainable way to achieve emotional homeostasis which they seek. The psychological phenomena in bingeing and purging behaviors have also been well documented (Heller, 1990). In many cases individuals report that a "real or perceived disruption of an important object connection precipitated the feelings of mounting tension, anger or despair that eventually led to the purge" (p. 142). Purging behaviors typically occur in isolation as a result of the shame and embarrassment associated with the behavior (Fallon, Katzman, & Wooley, 1994). Certain affective states – disappointment, disgust and self-hatred – often accompany a binge. The binge is often experienced initially as a "high," followed by a "crash," which is both psychological and physiological. This physiological aspect is intensified in the glycemic physical rollercoaster that is induced by a binge (Takii, 1999).

The experience of purging is particularly poignant for the large number of people with bulimia who report histories of either physical or sexual abuse. The activity of purging, whether through self-induced vomiting or laxative abuse, can be understood as an assault upon one's body. It is possible that for this subgroup of bulimics, these behaviors may "represent a reenactment of a passively experienced trauma, whereby she identifies with her aggressor in assaulting her body" (Heller, 1990, p. 172).

In binge eating disorder (BED), psychological factors also play a central role. While binge eating, an individual typically experiences a sense of loss of control, coupled with an inability to track what one has eaten. Any wish to stop eating is trumped by a sense of insatiability or momentum that may not be fully conscious. In other words, the impulse to eat overrides attempts to register one's own sense of satiety or desire to regulate intake.

Earlier theories about the family characteristics of people with these eating conditions evolved during a period of relative "mother-blaming." Minuchin (1970), for instance, believed that anorexia was the by-product of issues of control in the family, specifically failed mother-child attunement. It may be that social forces similar to those implicated in eating conditions themselves, influenced this era of blaming mothers for any "deviance" on the part of their children. However, today there is recognition that eating disorders occur in a variety of family settings. Farber (2008) and Seibold (2008) argue that these eating conditions can be a by-product of family dysfunction and trauma, including sexual, emotional or physical abuse, or forces that are sometimes too latent for us to even detect. This may have particular importance for the subgroup of people with eating disorders who have histories of childhood sexual abuse.

Demographics

According to the National Comorbidity Survey Replication Study, *lifetime prevalence rates* are as follows: anorexia nervosa (0.6 percent); bulimia nervosa (1.0 percent); binge eating disorder (2.8 percent); subthreshold binge eating (1.2 percent); any binge eating (4.5 percent) (Hudson, Hiripe, Pope, & Kessler, 2007). In the cases of the three disorders, AN, BN, and BED, lifetime prevalence was 1.75 to 3.0 times higher for women than men. However, subthreshold binge eating disorders occurred three times more frequently in men than in women and were equal for any binge eating (Hudson et al., 2006). Although these prevalence rates are modest in comparison with those of other major psychiatric conditions, additional data from the survey are important in understanding the scope of the problem for particular groups of people. Average age of onset, persistence of the illness, cohort effects and role impairment all provide a clearer picture of the actual challenges for people with eating conditions and for those who work with them.

The median age of onset for all these eating conditions ranges from 18 to 21 years of age, which is consistent with earlier findings. However, for anorexia nervosa, the earliest onset cases (age 10) were significantly lower than those of the other groups (age 15). Additionally, the period of onset risk was much narrower and there were no cases reported with an onset beyond the mid-twenties. In contrast, cases of the other four conditions occurred in every age range. Another important difference between anorexia nervosa and the other eating conditions emerged; the mean numbers of years with the disorder was low (1.7) compared to bulimia nervosa (8.3); binge eating disorder (8.1); subthreshold binge eating (7.2) and any binge eating (8.7). Figures for 12-month persistence were similar (Hudson et al., 2007). *Cohort effects* are also significant with each successive generational group being at higher risk for all five conditions (Kendler, 1991). This lends credence to the social construction theories and to the popular notion that these eating conditions pose public health challenges at increasing rates. Clinical observations confirm this as well. One of the authors (NH) noted that in the mid 1980s there was an influx of patients with eating disorders on adult inpatient psychiatric units. By the early 1990s college counseling centers were increasingly seeking consultative services for their burgeoning population of students with eating conditions. By the mid 1990s middle school guidance offices were facing the same challenges. It is clear that adolescents, boys as well as girls, are at risk of developing eating disorder conditions (Muise, Stein, & Arbess, 2003; Soban, 2006; Striegel-Moore, Rosselli, Perrin, DeBar, Wilson, May, & Kraemer, 2009) and both screening and interventions services must be available in their natural environments.

Psychosocial functioning is compromised by most psychiatric conditions. In the NCSR study most subjects endorsed some degree of role impairment in work, home, personal life or social life. Additionally, less than half of the respondents reported having received treatment for any of the eating disorders other than anorexia (which was not assessed) (Garfinkel, 1996).

Psychiatric comorbidity is very high for all eating disorder groups (Halmi et al., 2003; Hoek & van Hoeken, 2003; Kaye, 2004). According to the NCS-R (2003) comorbidity with any other psychiatric disorder with anorexia nervosa was 56.2 percent; for bulimia nervosa, 94.5 percent; for binge eating disorder, 78.9 percent; for subthreshold binge eating, 63.6 percent; and for any binge eating 76.5 percent. Virtually all of the most prevalent mood, anxiety, impulse-control and substance abuse conditions were found in association with the eating disorders. This is a very important finding when considered with the data about receiving help for eating conditions. In this study, fewer than half reported having either sought or received treatment for their eating condition, though significantly larger numbers did receive help for other "emotional" problems.

Eating disorders are also comorbid with *post-traumatic stress disorder (PTSD)*. This is an important finding, which provides another explanation for the significant gender disparity in rates of eating disorders. Using data from the National Women's Study, Dansky, Brewerton, Kilpatrick, and O'Neil (1997) reported that the majority of people with bulimia nervosa had been victimized. The study also found that the lifetime prevalence rate of PTSD was three times higher in bulimia nervosa than in a non-eating disorder samples; the current prevalence rate was five times higher in BN than in the non-eating disorder subjects; and the lifetime prevalence rates for BN were nearly twice as high. Importantly, the BN subjects in this study were more likely than binge eaters to have dissociative experiences related to their trauma. Dissociative episodes strongly predict psychiatric comorbidity in this population and it is suggested that purging behaviors, rather than binge eating behaviors are maladaptive behaviors associated with PTSD and major depression (Brewerton, 2007). Clinically, individuals with bulimia nervosa and PTSD will present with numbing, avoidance, and amnesia for traumatic events, all of which complicate both daily life and the processes of clinical interventions.

Brewerton (2007) in an extensive review of the literature also concludes that childhood sexual abuse (and other forms of abuse and neglect) is a non-specific risk factor for eating disorders (Laws & Golding, 1996) and that trauma is more common in bulimia than in the other eating conditions. Furthermore, this holds for adults, children and adolescents and for both genders. He also found that comorbidity with PTSD did not predict severity of eating disorder symptoms. Most importantly, he found that "the trauma and PTSD or its symptoms must be expressly and satisfactorily addressed in order to facilitate full recovery from the ED and all associated comorbidity" (Brewerton, 2007, p. 285). This last finding has significant implications for both assessment and intervention strategies. Seeing the client as a set of bulimic symptoms in need of modification may obscure our understanding of the complexity of the human being, including her history and the meaning of developing a set of behaviors and attitudes which reflect her efforts to manage her experiences of trauma and victimization.

Pedereau, Faucher, Wallier, Vibert, and Godart (2008) in a comprehensive review of the research on *family comorbidity* among people with anorexia found that, first, when mood conditions are considered as a group, they appear more frequently among first degree female relatives of people with anorexia; second, comorbidity of major depressive disorder was higher among first degree female relatives in persons with anorexia nervosa, restricting type; and third, neither dysthymia nor bipolar disorder occur in greater frequency among people with anorexia. They did find, however, that among the anxiety conditions, people with anorexia nervosa were more likely to have a first degree relative with obsessive-compulsive disorder and generalized anxiety disorder than were control subjects. What these data do not tell us are the environmental and transactional effects (rather than or in addition to the genetic effects) of having a first degree relative with a psychiatric disorder. This is particularly salient because many of these studies focused upon maternal psychopathology. In practice, this becomes an important distinction as practitioners attempt to sort out what may be learned behaviors, genetic factors and what might be the effects of living with a highly depressed or anxious parent.

Populations

While there continue to be significant *gender* differences in the occurrence of all eating conditions, the degree of disparity is changing. According to the National Institute of Mental Health, females are far more likely to develop an eating disorder, representing 85–95 percent of cases of anorexia or bulimia, dropping to 65 percent of cases of binge eating disorder. Lifetime prevalence rates for anorexia for women are estimated at between 0.5 percent and 3.7 percent and 1.1 percent to 4.2 percent for bulimia. Binge eating disorder is estimated in community samples to occur between 2 percent and 5 percent. Differences are emerging in relation to specific eating disorder behaviors, however. Striegel-Moore et al. (2009) found that in a random sample of members of a health maintenance organization, men were more likely to report overeating while women reported loss of control while eating. Women were also more likely than men to report behaviors which reflect the influence of social expectations. For example, women were significantly more likely to report "body checking" (checking and inspecting one's body fat or shape) and "body avoidance" (refusing to look in a mirror or weigh oneself, "hiding" in baggy clothing). Men are not immune to the increasing media messages about the ideal male body image (Bordo, 1999; Drummond, 2002). However, the body image precoccupations of men are more apt to be related to body shape than low weight and clothing size, the primary concerns of women (Muise, Stein, & Arbess, 2003). Like women, however, there is an association between eating conditions, victimization, and psychiatric comorbidity (Brewerton, 2007). Kinzl, Mangweth, Traweger, and Biebl (1997) report that chronic adverse family relationships, particularly those that include physical abuse increase the likelihood of boys and men developing these eating conditions.

Like their female counterparts, male athletes are more prone to develop eating conditions (Petrie & Rogers, 2001; Petrie, Greenleaf, Reel, & Carter, 2008). Ray (2004) and Anderson (1995) found that men involved with sports which require lean body mass (such as running, gymnastics, wrestling and swimming) are vulnerable to developing compensatory eating and exercising behaviors. In a non-clinical sample of male college athletes, none met criteria for an eating disorder fully, but 20 percent had sufficient indicators to be considered symptomatic. While 60 percent of the sample expressed satisfaction with their body weight, 66 percent met CDC criteria for overweight or obesity. In addition, a moderate number used exercise (38 percent) and a small number (14.2 percent) used fasting or dieting to control their weight. These findings may represent subclinical or low-threshold variants of eating conditions, particularly when we consider other body related issues of male athletes. For example, Cafri, Thompson, Ricciardelli, McCabe, Smolak, and Yesalis (2005) reported that men may be more likely to develop pathogenic weight behaviors than classic eating conditions. These behaviors might include the use of Creatinine, ephedrine and anabolic steroids. The DSM-IV criterion of cessation of menses clearly does not apply to men; however, some reports suggest that men do experience both drops in testosterone levels and diminshed sexual desire (Crosscope-Happel, Hutchins, Getz & Hayes, 2000). When we consider this along with the psychological dynamics in disordered eating, rather than strictly the diagnostic criteria of DSM-IV, we may obtain a more complete and useful understanding of manifestation of eating conditions in "non-traditional" clients.

While relatively few studies have reported on eating conditions in men, those that have yield interesting information about both *gender and sexual orientation* (Austin et al., 2009). Carlat, Camargo, and Herzog (1997) reported that of 135 men with eating conditions, 46 percent were bulimic, 22 percent were anorexic and 32 percent met criteria for eating disorder NOS. Importantly, diagnostic groups differed significantly by sexual orientation: homosexual or bisexual males were more likely to be bulimic (42 percent) and 58 percent of the anorexic patients were identified as asexual. Russel and Keel (2002) reported that men who identify as having anorexia nervosa are 10–42 percent more likely to be homosexual than their non-anorexic counterparts. Homosexual men (bisexual men were not included in the study) also had higher measures of both body dissatisfaction and anorectic and bulimic symptoms.

The research on eating behaviors and attitudes in lesbian and bisexual women lends credence to the sociocultural theories of eating disorders. While there is some contradictory evidence, most studies (Herzog, Neuman, Yeh, & Warshaw, 1992) have reported that lesbian and bisexual women have lower levels of body dissatisfaction and fewer symptoms of eating disorders than heterosexual women. Possibly, sexual minority women may be *"less* prone to eating disorders because they do not share with heterosexual women the standards of feminine beauty espoused by Western culture" (Feldman & Meyer, 2007, p. 219). Feldman and Meyer (2007) in their study of DSM-IV eating disorder diagnoses in gay, bisexual and heterosexual women found no differences among the three groups and further suggest the importance of seeing all women potentially at risk for developing disordered eating and bona fide eating disorders.

Mental health care disparities

Women of color were once considered to be "protected" from developing eating disorders by their culture's relative acceptance of women with larger shapes (Bordo, 1999; Hesser-Biber, 1996; Williamson, 1998). However, more recent clinical practice and research suggests otherwise (Laws & Golding, 1996; Lester, 1997; Striegel-Moore et al., 2003). Franko (2007) reports that African American and Latina women have lower incidence of anorexia nervosa, but higher rates of bulimia and binge eating disorder. Thompson (1994) found that upwardly mobile Black and Latina women were more likely to be preoccupied with their weight than their lower income counterparts. Hesse-Biber (1996) and Thompson (1994) suggest that poverty can increase vulnerability to a wide range of eating problems, particularly if one considers the role of stress in overeating. A small number of studies have investigated the impact of acculturation, racial identity, internalized racism, and economic deprivation on the incidence and type of eating conditions found in people of color (Franko, 2007).

Worldwide, eating disorders are becoming more prevalent and the issues identified support the sociocultural explanation of the development of these conditions. Ma (2007) reports on ten adolescent females who developed anorexia or bulimia. She found that many of the girls felt that their mothers were powerless in the patriarchal societal structure of their marriages, and used their eating disorders as a point of identification with their mothers. The desire for this identification was largely fueled by a pressure to separate from their mothers, to out-succeed them, to have more. Ma (2007) argues that "these emaciated youths are growing up in a rapidly changing society brought about by modernization and Westernization. On the surface, the society is highly modernized, but beneath this surface, cultural beliefs and values remain traditional" (p. 413). One girl was quoted as saying:

> I find changing people is more difficult than changing oneself. Changing me is easier. I am sensitive to people's responses. I feel that they are not trustworthy . . . Maintaining my strict diet is just like finishing a homework exercise. After finishing it, I have a sense of accomplishment. If I don't do it, I can't feel my being.
>
> (Ma, 2007, p. 412)

Eating conditions, usually associated with adolescents and young adults, can maintain or emerge *at any age*. Among *children*, there are eating behaviors and patterns which may relate to subsequent eating disorders, but this has not been well documented, except for the emerging literature on childhood obesity. Marchi and Cohen (1990), in their longitudinal study of maladaptive eating patterns in children, reported that pica and problem meals in early childhood were predictive of later bulimia nervosa. Picky eating and digestive problems were more likely to be implicated in a later diagnosis of anorexia nervosa. These findings suggest the possibility of an insidious developmental course of eating disorders for a subset of those later diagnosed with anorexia and bulimia.

Far more problematic and widespread is *childhood obesity* which is described as epidemic. In 2008, the National Health and Nutrition Examination Survey (NHANES, 2008) found that childhood obesity among children and adolescents has tripled since 1980. While earlier studies indicated that Latino children had higher rates of obesity (Kimbro, Brooks-Gunn, & McLanahan, 2007), racial and ethnic differences appear to be diminishing, largely because of the rise of rates of obesity in white children (Caprio et al., 2008). However, the age of onset is implicated in the timing of obesity development and Black girls are known to undergo pubertal maturation at earlier ages than white girls. Children who are obese are also at risk for type 2 diabetes, hypertension, dyslipidemia and liver conditions, serious and chronic medical conditions. Further risk factors for obesity include lower socioecomonic status and living in high poverty areas. In fact, in the Harvard Geocoding Study, poverty as measured by census tract, was a more powerful predictor of health outcomes, including obesity, than race or ethnicity (Krieger, Chen, Waterman, Rehkopf, & Subramanian, 2003).

Because of the importance of peer relationships and the pressure to conform, characteristic of *adolescence*, it is not unusual for middle school and high school aged girls to first engage in binge and purge behaviors as part of a group. For example, a group of middle school girls may complain to each other in the cafeteria, that "I ate too much . . . I am such a pig" and then retreat to the girls' room where they vomit. Most of these girls will find this unpleasant and will not repeat it; a few others, vulnerable on other accounts, may find that the ability to regulate weight or manage uncomfortable feelings is useful to them. These girls may be at risk of developing an eating disorder. It is not uncommon, either, on inpatient psychiatric units, group homes, or residential treatment centers, to observe a "contagion" effect for disordered eating behaviors.

For those girls who become anorexic, there are potentially dire consequences. Katzman (2005), in her review of the literature on medical complications of AN for adolescents, finds that cardiovascular complications include sinus bradycardia, orthostatic hypotension, and abnormal electrocardiograms. Additionally, refeeding syndrome, which occurs as a result of oral, enteral or parenteral interventions to restore one's malnourished state, can include cardiovascular, neurologic and hematologic complications. While patients will be treated for these complications by specially trained medical staff, it is critical that social workers who work with these adolescents and their families have a working knowledge of these conditions.

Pregnancy poses particular challenges for women with eating disorders and related concerns. For the individual with a distorted body image, dread of becoming "fat," and any combination of restricting and purging behaviors, the weight gain and bodily changes of pregnancy may be particularly problematic. Certainly, there are concerns for the health and well-being of the mother, but fetal development also requires good nutrition. Eating disorders are most prevalent in the demographic which is of child bearing age. Potential complications are somewhat different for those with anorexia and those with bulimia. Those with a history of anorexia may experience problems with infertility (because of amenorrhea) and with perinatal complications (Bulik et al., 1999). Studies of women with bulimia nervosa have indicated some improvement and some worsening of symptoms (Crow, Peel, Thuras, & Mitchell, 2004) during pregnancy. Crow, Agras, Crosby, Halmi, and Mitchell (2008) in a longitudinal study of women with several eating disorder diagnoses found that while eating disorder symptoms improved during pregnancy, they worsened postpartum. This may indicate a temporary protective function of pregnancy for women, and importantly, for the fetus. However, there may be serious implications in the postpartum period for those women who choose to breastfeed their infants.

Little attention has been paid to traditional eating disorders among *older adults*; the focus being instead upon problems of undernutrition in medically compromised older women (Chapman,

2006). This omission is striking given that we know that many individuals develop a chronic course for anorexia, bulimia nervosa and binge eating disorder. Additionally, Cosford and Arnold (1992) reported that in addition to relapses, older women are reporting new onset eating disorder conditions. The literature that does exist on eating problems among this population focuses on eating difficulties and undernutrition in institutionalized women (Chapman, 2006). However, increasingly, studies indicate that concerns about body image and shape persist across the life cycle (Webster & Tiggermann, 2003). In a study of women 50 years and older, obtained from the Canadian Community Health Survey, Gadalla (2008) reported that 2.6 percent of the women 50–64 years of age and 1.8 percent of women 65 and older reported disordered eating symptoms. Elevated frequencies of dieting behaviors, and preoccupation with food intake and body shape, were predominant among symptoms and were positively associated with stress and negatively with medical problems (Gadalla, 2008, p. 357). Like their younger counterparts, there was high comorbidity with mood and anxiety conditions (Gadalla, 2008).

Individuals, particularly adolescents, who must pay close attention to food intake because of a *chronic medical condition* (e.g. type 1 diabetes, Crohn's disease and cystic fibrosis) may be at increased risk for the development of eating disordered behavior (Smith, Latchford, Hall, & Dickson, 2008). For example, an adolescent girl with diabetes may manipulate her caloric equation by adjusting her insulin dosage. Clinically, such clients may exhibit the same cognitive distortions about body image, weight and shape, that are common among bulimic clients who restrict, binge or purge.

Social work programs and social work roles

Social workers are well positioned and trained to provide help to people with each of these eating conditions in a variety of settings. Given the ample evidence that sociocultural influences are significant in the development of eating conditions and that each generational cohort appears to be at greater risk, preventive strategies are critical. Social workers also provide most of the direct services to people with mental illness and their families and, hence, will be in positions to work with people with these eating conditions. We work in schools, hospitals, outpatient clinics, public and community agencies in a variety of roles. In addition to working as primary practitioners with people with anorexia, bulimia and binge eating conditions, social workers may work with families and groups. One of the most important roles for social workers is that of case manager; even when social workers are functioning as the primary clinician for a client, they will likely coordinate the interdisciplinary team which will usually include a primary care physician or nurse practitioner, a nutritionist and a psychiatrist. On the macro level, social workers can also work toward alleviating some of the sociocultural influences which give rise to the various eating conditions such as constricted or confusing gender roles, poverty (in the case of childhood obesity) and sexism.

Screening for eating conditions is a particularly critical activity. Early assessment, diagnosis and intervention is associated with better prognosis. The screening for these eating conditions will typically occur in clinical settings. In many agencies, screening at intake for eating disorders, is a formal part of the intake assessment, particularly for girls. Given the increased prevalence of eating conditions in populations previously considered not at risk (eg., males, older adults, people of color), social workers must screen a wider range of clients. For example, given that psychiatric comorbidity is high, people with known problems with anxiety, mood conditions, substance abuse or overuse (Hoderness, Brooks-Gunn, & Warren, 1994), and histories of sexual abuse should be asked about problems with eating.

Because eating disorders have their genesis during adolescence and young adulthood, prevention should be aimed at this group, in both clinical and community settings. Yager and

O'Dea (2008) reviewed 27 large-scale controlled prevention programs on university campuses. They concluded that "information based, cognitive-behavioral therapy and psychoeducational interventions had limited success" and recommend instead, "dissonance-media-literacy and self-esteem based educational approaches using some computer-based delivery to improve the body image health behaviors of male and female university students" (Yager & O'Dea, 2008, p. 187). This is similar to findings based on the efficacy of dissonance-media-literacy programs aimed at adolescents. These are important findings for social work; intervening to create dissonance with the media influence implicitly recognizes that the problem lies within the culture and that the *culture* needs changing. Additionally, researchers recommend the development of health promotion activities designed to increase self-esteem, which is a significant risk factor for eating disorders (Croll, Neumark-Sztainer, Story, & Ireland, 2002; Stice et al., 1994). Social workers can develop prevention programs in a variety of natural settings such as schools, youth clubs and church and community groups.

Professional methods and interventions

The research literature on outcomes for eating disorders interventions is interdisciplinary, with a focus upon medical, psychological, cognitive and social factors. Anorexia nervosa has been studied more than the other conditions, perhaps because it poses the most dire consequences for people who are not helped; the mortality among anorectic females ages 15–24 is 12 times higher than the annual death rate for their counterparts in the general population (Keel, Dorer, Eddy, Franko, Charatan, & Herzog, 2003). In their longitudinal study, Keel et al. (2003) also found that significant predictors of mortality from all causes included severity of comorbid substance abuse, poor social adjustment, longer duration of illness, and suicidality related to a comorbid disorder.

Berkman, Lohr, and Bulik (2007) in their extensive review of eating disorder outcome studies concluded that this literature is significantly lacking. They characterize the AN literature as weak and the BN and BED literature as essentially non-existent. This does not bode well for practitioners who turn to the literature for guidance in developing and implementing intervention strategies. However, the literature suggests some general trends that are useful and merit further investigation.

The first treatment goal for people with *anorexia nervosa* is the restoration of normal body weight and for women, menstruation. Steinhausen, Rauss-Mason, and Seidel (1991) reported that that occurs in 50–60 percent of individuals, but that restoration of normal eating behaviors occurs in less than 50 percent of treated anorectics. This is consistent with the finding by Steinhausen et al. (1991) that 30–35 percent of anorexics recover, 30–35 percent improve and 20–25 percent develop a chronic disorder. Furthermore, Zerbe (1993) and Yager et al. (2002) report that multimodal interventions are best, beginning with weight restoration and followed by individual and family interventions. Because of the medical severity of anorexia nervosa, hospitalization is the treatment of choice for medically compromised clients. Those who are treated as outpatients will do best if they meet the following criteria: highly motivated, co-operative families, young age and recent onset of symptoms (Yager, 1989). Though behavioral, cognitive-behavioral and family interventions have been studied for AN, the evidence for any of them as stand alone interventions is inconclusive (Richards, Baldwin, Frost, Clark-Sly, Berrett, & Hardman, 2000). The use of medication to treat the symptoms of anorexia has not been highly successful, although there are some resports that the use of fluoxetine (best known as Prozac) has both reduced the severity of the depression and promoted weight gain in some patients (Hoffman & Halmi, 1993; Johnson, Tsoh, & Varnado, 1996). In practice, medication aimed at alleviating symptoms of comorbid conditions such as depression and anxiety, may help the client restore an euthymic mood, such that her motivation increases, allowing her to engage more fully in attempts to modify eating attitudes and behaviors

Various intervention strategies for patients with bulimia have been investigated. Nearly all studies involve outpatient interventions; nearly all people with bulimia can be treated as outpatients. As many as 70–95 percent of people with BN experience decreases in the frequency of binging and purging behaviors, during outpatient interventions (Mitchell, 1991; Mitchell, Raymond, & Specker, 1993). Gains may not last, however; several studies report that 73 percent continue to binge and purge more than once per month, with nearly 25 percent of those bingeing and purging daily (Mitchell, 1991; Yager, 1988). Importantly, there is evidence that people with bulimia do not improve without treatment, i.e. those on waiting list control groups or no treatment control groups (Fairburn, 1988). Social workers should also be aware that most relapse occurs within six months of the end of the intervention (Yager, 1989); that certainly suggests the need for period follow up and/or a tapered treatment protocol.

The multicausal model of eating disorders – the etiological – includes attention to biological, psychological and social triggers which interact with predisposing genetic, eliciting and maintenance factors (Bloks, van Furth, & Hock, 1999; Brownell & Fairburn, 1995; Gardner, 1997). The model rests on two key assumptions: first, that eating conditions are the by-product of a multitude of factors that vary among individuals; and second, that the same set of factors may not produce the same outcome in two different individuals (Garfinkel, 1996). This approach is certainly consistent with the ecological perspective upon which social work practice is built (Gitterman & Germain, 2008). However, the research literature has focused largely upon identifying singular treatment strategies that produce good outcomes. While this inquiry yields important information, research is needed that considers combination approaches.

While Schmidt (1989) found that there was not consistent evidence favoring one theoretical approach over another, more recent studies suggest that cognitive-behavioral treatment (CBT) is superior. Others (Agras, Telch, Arnow, Eldredge, & Marnell, 1997; Johnson et al., 1996) concur that CBT is more effective than psychodynamic, supportive, and behavior therapies. Typically CBT interventions will be aimed at not only modifying distorted beliefs about food, body weight and shape, but also reducing episodes of binge eating and purging.

The efficacy of a combination of CBT and medication therapy is controversial. However, Agras et al. (1997) report that there may be some evidence that while medication does not cure bulimia, it may have positive effects on the symptoms of binge eating and depression. In addition, there is some evidence that frequency of sessions makes a difference; Mitchell et al. (1993) found that two or three weekly sessions were superior to once weekly. Group therapies are often commonly used in inpatient, outpatient and residential settings. Oesterheld, McKenna and Gould (1987) in their meta-analysis of group therapy outcomes for BN reported average reduction in bulimic symptoms ranging from 52 to 97 percent. The type of group seems to matter; Wilfley and Cohen (1997) found that cognitive-behavioral groups were superior to other forms of group interventions. In a study of group work with female survivors of childhood sexual abuse, Harper, Richter, and Gorey (2009) found that those with histories of childhood sexual abuse had poorer otucomes.

There has been far less study of interventions other than cognitive-behavioral treatments. However, Wilfley and Cohen (1997) and Smith, Marcus and Eldredge (1994) report that interpersonal psychotherapy appears to be effective in both diminishing clients' hyperfocus on shape and weight and in reducing binge eating and purging. It is not clear what the exact mechanism within the CBT intervention is responsible for positive change.

Any interventions with people with these eating conditions must simultaneosly deal with the cognitive distortions (body weight and shape), the behavioral manifestations (bingeing and/or restricting behaviors, and purging behaviors), and their accompanying affects (sadness, rage, and shame). The social worker can utilize food and exercise logs, explore dysfunctional schemas and attributions which maintain cognitive distortions, and co-develop behavioral strategies aimed at modifying dangerous or self-destructive eating behaviors. These strategies and interventions must take place in the context of a therapeutic alliance which honors both the psychological and sociocultural experiences of the individual. For example, bingeing, purging, and restricting behaviors are not simply behaviors. They may represent attempts to communicate distress, fear or rage and unless those affective states are both identified and explored, the client may not be sufficiently engaged in the work to begin enacting some of the behavioral strategies.

Illustration and discussion

One of the authors (DB) provides this account of her work with Erica, a 19-year-old college student who was struggling with anorexia nervosa and parasuicidal behaviors. The case illustrates the challenges in the work with a client with complicated, self-injurious behaviors as well as the complications in working within a problematic service delivery system.

Erica sought services with a social worker at her college counseling center, during her senior year in college. She reported feelings of self-hatred and parasuicidal behaviors. Erica was at an important juncture in her life as she was trying to decide what she wanted to do upon her graduation. She could not decide whether she wanted to live near her boyfriend or stay locally in close proximity to her family. She and her social worker identified this as an important life transition and she was becoming acutely aware of her inability to identify internal resources and make important decisions for herself. Erica reported having been in therapy before. She had seen a therapist in high school to help her with what she described as "intense feelings of sadness." While she generally found this helpful, she also felt that the adjunctive conjoint family therapy sessions were "usurped" by her mother. I took this as a cautionary tale and agreed to focus initially on individual work.

The long-standing feelings of sadness were not easily discerned from observing Erica. While she looked thin, her appearance was perfectly kempt, never a hair out of place. She never looked like she had just rolled out of bed; instead she was always highly presentable. Despite many fluctuations in mood and self-perception, her outside appearance never changed. She was a theatre major and described her happiest moments on stage, the one location where she could completely lose herself. Otherwise, Erica described a life of social isolation. She could not identify one good friend, mentor, teacher or colleague who meant anything to her. The one exception to this was a serious relationship with her boyfriend, the center of her pocket-sized universe. She often described this relationship as akin to "life support," a ventilator of sorts. She was not sincerely engaged in the world beyond her acting. Her life could best be described as one of living minimally, taking up a bare amount of space in the world. She had no job, a small apartment, without a lot of "stuff" and no passions or relationships beyond her "career."

Erica clearly met the diagnostic criteria for anorexia. She was at 85 percent of her body weight and her daily restricting behaviors had become entrenched for more than two years. Erica subsisted on a diet that ranged between 350 and 700 calories per day. These shocking numbers are not uncommon in people struggling with anorexia nervosa; calorie counts are an ever-present part of the anorectic mind (Patton, Selzer, Coffey, Carlin, & Wolfe, 1999). On the rare occasions that Erica exceeded this caloric intake, she became quite dysfunctional, reeling from shame and embarrassment. Complicating the clinical picture and Erica's life were the parasuicidal behaviors which accompanied her eating problems. She would periodically hold fistfuls of pills or a knife to her wrist while looking at her image in a mirror. These behaviors, however, never resulted in actual suicide attempts. Rather, her starvation can be understood as a methodical form of suicide attempt.

As with most clients with eating disorders, the beginning phase with Erica was critical. According to McFarland (1995), "the first and most difficult step in treating any anorexic is to facilitate physiological stabilization" (p. 50). Given her dangerously low weight, I required that Erica agree to regularly seeing a nutritionist, a primary care physician, and a psychiatrist, throughout the course of our work together. Further, we agreed that this team would communicate regularly, both to ensure coordination of treatment and to guard against splitting: this can occur when an individual is struggling with the issues of power and control, which are common in clients with these eating conditions. This sort of "tag teaming" is also essential for ensuring the client's medical and psychological safety. My attempts to develop and coordinate this interdisciplinary team were not exactly seamless, but were possible, given that the initial phases of our work occurred within a university system. This scaffolding of resources allowed Erica to feel "held" and minimized the chances of her precipitously dropping out of the work. Erica's resistance to the work and to the goals of our work was fueled by a fear of gaining weight. This creates a common paradox in the work with people suffering with anorexia; a central goal of the work is to increase one's weight, the very thing that Erica was trying not to do. Progress is in part measured by weight gain and this causes tremendous anxiety and regression. Typically, any weight gain was countered by Erica's increased food restriction. As with many such clients, two steps forward and one step back became the pattern.

Because the stakes were high (her medical and psychiatric fragility) I had established the following ground rules. Erica's being seen as an outpatient was contingent upon the absence of the following criteria: excessive and rapid weight loss, serious metabolic disturbances, increased suicidality or planning for suicide, severe episodes of either binge eating and purging, and psychosis. Continuous assessment for these symptoms and a steady dialogue about weight was central. During the early phase of our work many of our conversations were also about numbers. The facilitation of a therapeutic relationship was tricky; I needed her permission and agreement to engage in a dialogue about her weight – a topic which was typically shrouded in secrecy. This attention to detail mirrored the internal obsession to detail with which people with these eating conditions struggle (Farber, 2008) and importantly, brought it out of hiding. This level of discussion also served two other purposes. It allowed me to join Erica in her wish to remain outside of the hospital, as long as she stayed above a predetermined weight. McFarland (1995) suggests that joining with the patient to stay out of the hospital is an essential part of relationship construction. With Erica, as with many other medically fragile clients, the decision regarding hospitalization needed to be consistently "on the table" as her status fluctuated.

Underlying Erica's considerable resistance to increasing her caloric intake was a sincere fear of change and of loss of control. She, like many people with eating disorders, also had great concerns about any weight gain side effects of medication. Erica saw the psychotropic medication as yet another form of external control and with the agreement of the supervising psychiatrist, we all decided to "hold off" on using any medication. This decision was made based in part on our assessment of her decreasing depressive and suicidal symptoms. Because she was medically stabilized at the time and was making some progress in engaging with her team, we agreed to revisit the issue of medication if necessary, in the future.

This phase of the work was focused upon dealing with Erica's denial about her dangerous weight and restricting behaviors. Vitousek, Daly and Heiser (1991), in their summary of the research literature, write that

Individuals with eating disorders may deny or distort specific behaviors (such as vomiting, laxative abuse and dietary rituals); affective states and beliefs; the objective size and shape of their bodies; the characterization of their attitudes and behaviors as irrational, pathological or dangerous; and the attribution of their symptoms to particular causal factors.

(Vitousek et al., 1991, p. 649)

Typically, this pervasive denial is out of the awareness of the individual and must be addressed in the early phases of the work. Such was the case with Erica. After managing her emotional life by numbing it with hunger and starvation for years, she struggled with managing the range of feelings and emotions which emerged as she began to change her maladaptive coping strategies. This is not uncommon when a person's affective development has been arrested by her single-minded focus on denying herself food. Erica, with her distorted body image, tight control, and resistance to relinquishing her restrictive behaviors, continually overestimated both her actual weight and the appearance of her body. Fortunately, because she was being weighed by two medical professionals on the team with whom I had at least weekly contact, I could carefully counter Erica's denial. This involved challenging some of her schemas about many aspects of herself. This also reinforced the idea that we were a team – all focused on improving her life.

In the course of our initial interviews, the etiology of Erica's problematic eating was not immediately clear. As is necessary in the work with all clients with eating disorders evaluation, intervention planning and goal setting dominated the initial sessions. The goal setting was largely informed by the solution focused model (Berg & Miller, 1992), a variant of cognitive-behavioral work. This approach required that we co-create achievable, efficient and "proximal" goals. This necessitated the recognition that complete alleviation of symptomology is impossible, but that proximal achievements are certainly worth striving for. Berg and Miller (1992) suggest that these goals ought to be characterized by their salience to the client. Solution focused goals are articulated in "situational terms" (i.e. I will make myself lunch to alleviate the stress of fast food calories and to avoid starvation in the middle of the day), and must be based in interactional and interpersonal terms. Further, these goals should be articulated as the presence of something instead of the absence of something and must be realistic. For example, instead of aiming to not worry about her size, Erica would instead aim to recognize one part of her body that she liked. According to Berg and Miller (1992) these goals must all be recognized as difficult and the client and social worker must share the belief that changing long-standing behaviors and thoughts takes diligence. McFarland (1995) describes this technique: "Whatever goal is negotiated, the [social worker] must emphasize that success will require a strong effort on the part of the client." She goes on to say that: "By the same token, when a goal is achieved the [social worker] needs to recognize the hard work that the client has completed" (p. 120). This approach allowed me to "meet the client where the client is" and allowed Erica to "imagine" something different for herself.

Erica identified that she did not want to hate herself any more, wanted to increase her sense of confidence and self-esteem and wanted to have friends. In our discussions, we decided that coming for sessions consistently and constructing a wider social network could help her to begin to confidently make decisions for herself. Each goal was designed to give her a sense of competency and mastery in our work together and outside. Adhering to the calorie count preoccupied Erica to the extent that it was difficult for her to attend to a session. She would take long periods of time to answer questions or would often appear in a fog, clouded by the intensity of her hunger. She was now able to acknowledge the extent of her hunger and her restricting was no longer experienced by her as ego syntonic. This was an important shift for her. She now had a sense of the psychological and physiological sequelae of chronic hunger. The work through this phase was slow and laborious, but she began to be able to connect with me and use the working alliance to explore issues beyond the eating behaviors.

By the fourth or fifth session, I had a clearer understanding of how her anorexia had taken such a strong hold on her. Erica described a tremendous amount of pressure on herself as a young athlete. She joined the swim team at the age of 7 and felt a constant external drive, largely from the community and her family, to "perform." From early on, she heard the message that her performance was largely intertwined with her weight. Preparing for a swim meet required abstinence from "no-sink" foods, those that would presumably have slowed down her swimming. She took these restrictions seriously and no-sink foods quickly became synonymous with foods that were forbidden, in her mind, entirely. Like many dancers, swimmers and gymnasts whose athletic subcultures promote the belief that being thin is essential for success, Erica began to eschew all food. Erica experienced a similar pressure in her family where the relationship between size and success were frequent topics of conversation. She also lived in a small community, largely homogeneous and affluent, that was highly preoccupied with appearance. This small town did not allow for much diversion in how sexuality or gender was expressed. From both her family and her community, she extracted the belief that women and girls were supposed to live diminutively.

Erica was also a twin who described herself, pejoratively, as "the lesser half." She felt that she was "second best" from early on. Her mother had had a difficult labor with her and her sister. Her sister was born first and healthy; Erica's birth was delayed and there was some question of her survival. This story had taken on great meaning for Erica, who felt it served as a template for much of her experience within her family. Attending to family narratives as a matter of course in helping people with eating disorders treatment often frees the client from the jail of their restrictive mind and body (Dallos, 2004). Erica felt she was repeatedly given the message that she was not officially here, an appendage more than an individual who never really asserted her place in the world. She worked to usurp her place in the world by fixating on trying to physically shrink or disappear. During this phase of the work, it was important that we work with this story, because much of the work with patients with eating disorders occurs in the form of metaphor. This is because eating disorder symptoms can be understood as both interpersonal and intrapersonal struggles, which manifest behaviorally. Erica struggled with her own identity as separate from her sister. We used photographs from her childhood as concrete tools to explore her narrative and her early sense of herself. My curiosity and her openness about her earlier life were important in the development of our relationship.

Metaphorically, Erica began to believe that there was indeed "space" for her. As Erica was increasingly able to put words to feelings about both her earlier life and her current relationships and situation, she lessened her hold on her restricting attitudes and behaviors. She not only became less restrictive about her food intake, but also found herself feeling passionate about other things. She was increasingly taking part in activities at school and she no longer felt suicidal. She began to worry, however, about her post-graduation plans. Because she would no longer be within the university system, she needed to find a new psychiatrist and nutritionist, though I would be able to continue with her through another agency. She felt it was important to continue our work together and was aware of her tendency to prematurely sever relationships.

Erica graduated and found an apartment in a neighboring arts community with the intention of launching her acting career. Unfortunately, this was a very competitive industry and she was handed rejection after rejection. The only steady work she could find was as a server in a restaurant. The act of serving food to others was problematic for her and complicated her own struggles with food and eating. Complicating things further, she no longer had health benefits. Fortunately, the agency had a sliding scale, but she was able to attend only one session every other week, down from her customary twice weekly. While we tried to continue the work we had been doing, I also needed to increase my activities as case manager. She needed a new psychiatrist, primary care physician and nutritionist, as well as an eating disorder group. However, because of the lack of health benefits (due in part to her preexisting condition), none were available to her. The lack of a coordinated multidisciplinary team took its toll. Her eating disorder symptoms increased, as did her depressive symptoms. She did not meet the stringent requirements for involuntary hospitalization (the only way her stay would be financed) and she missed several sessions due to traveling. Her boyfriend then called me to report that she had made a suicide attempt. Ironically, this allowed her to access health care with a hospitalization, during which she stabilized medically and psychiatrically. The suicide attempt also served as a wake-up call for her family, who realized that she did need both financial and emotional support from them during this time. As she continued stabilizing, she decided to relocate where she had better career opportunities and social supports.

We had only one session in which to terminate, when she returned to our area to move her things. We reviewed our work together and constructed a list of relapse signs. I also offered to speak with her new worker and psychiatrist. She was very relieved about this and felt that it would help her to feel connected to all of us. In a letter six months following the suicide attempt, Erica reported having made significant strides, although she was not at 100 percent of her ideal weight. However, she indicated that the meaning of how she eats had shifted and that she was eating both regularly and enough. In the process of identifying her passions in life, she found she had a deep affinity for animals. In honor of this Erica became vegan. This was definitely an alternate way of managing her caloric intake. Rather than struggling with feelings of shame and guilt about her food intake, she began to experience feelings of altruism, activism, and empowerment. She also was able to identify many creative elements of her personality through this activism by creating a dog rescue and acting as a midwife for impregnated and orphaned cats. Her eating became part of a larger cause, rather than a general failure.

Erica was not "cured." Under periods of stress she may revert to disordered eating and associated cognitions. She continues to want to succeed in a business that is highly competitive and overvalues thinness and appearance. However, she has become able to talk about feelings rather than suppress them, she has increased her social network and she and her family are making strides in reconnecting with each other. In part, through the use of our working relationship, she was able to give voice to herself and begin to question her firmly held beliefs about what it is to be a woman in this society. Erica is no longer struggling with depression and is clear about what the factors for relapse might be. Having had a positive experience with receiving help, she will seek services again as needed.

Conclusion

Of all the psychiatric diagnoses, the eating disorder conditions most require an understanding of the transactional nature of person and environment; the importance of an appreciation of the conditions of gender, socioeconomics, culture and race; and of the challenges which place individuals at risk over the life course. We discussed from the beginning of the chapter that both sociocultural and "disease/illness" conceptualizations had something to offer us in our work with these clients, but they are best understood in tandem. Eating disorder conditions are sometimes compared to addictions and indeed, the literature suggests that for some people these become chronic conditions. However, while abstinence is an option for people with alcoholism and drug addiction, we all must eat to survive. For the person with anorexia, not eating is an immediate threat; for others, it poses an uneasy challenge; how to use food in a way that supports healthy and social functioning. It is important that we as social workers continue to become familiar with the complexities of differential diagnosis, consider a wide range of multimodal intervention options and continue to follow relevant clinical and research developments.

Furthermore, an awareness and analysis of the evolving sociocultural conditions which shape the shifting demographics and the human face of eating disorder populations can make excellent use of the particular strengths of the social work profession.

Web resources

Alliance for Eating Disorder Awareness
www.eatingdisorderinfo.org

Medline Plus: Eating Disorders
www.nlm.nih.gov/medlineplus/eatingdisorders

National Eating Disorder Association
www.nationaleatingdisorders.org

National Institute of Mental Health Eating Disorders Publications
www.nimh.nih.gov/health/publications/eating-disorders/complete-index.shtml

National Mental Health Information Center, Substance Abuse and Mental Health Service Administration
www.mentalhealth.samhsa.gov/publications

References

Adler, J. (January, 1982). Looking back at 1981. *Newsweek*, 26–52.

Agras, W.S., Telch, C.F., Arnow, B., Eldredge, K., & Marnell, M. (1997). One-year follow-up of cognitive-behavioral therapy for obese individuals with binge eating disorder. *Journal of Consulting and Clinical Psychology*, *65* (2), 343–347.

American Psychiatric Association (APA). (2000). *Diagnostic and statistical manual of mental disorders* (4th ed., text revision). Washington, DC: APA.

Andersen, A.E. (1995). Weight loss, psychological and nutritional patterns in competitive male body builders. *International Journal of Eating Disorders*, *18*, 49–57.

Austin, S., Ziyadeh, H., Corliss, H., Rosario, M., Wypij, D., Haines, J. et al. (2009). Sexual orientation disparities in purging and binge eating from early to late adolescence. *Society for Adolescent Medicine*, *45*, 238–245.

Berg, I.K., & Miller, S. (1992). *Working with the problem drinker*. New York: W.W. Norton.

Berkman, N.D., Lohr, K.N., & Bulik, C.M. (2007). Outcomes of eating disorders: A systematic review of the literature. *International Journal of Eating Disorders*, *40* (4), 293–309.

Binswanger, L. (1944). The case of Ellen West. In R. May (ed.), *Existence* (pp. 237–364). New York: Basic Books.

Bloks, J., van Furth, E., & Hock, H. (1999). *Behandelingsstrategieen bij anorexia nervosa (Treatment strategies of anorexia nervosa)*. Bohn Stafleu van Loghum: Houten/Diegem.

Bordo, S. (1999). *The male body: A new look at men in public and private*. New York: Farrar, Straus & Giroux.

Brewerton, T. (2007). Eating disorders, trauma and comorbidity: Focus on PTSD. *Eating Disorders*, *15*, 285–304.

Brownell, K.D., & Fairburn, C.G. (1995). *Eating disorders and obesity. A comprehensive handbook*. New York: Guilford Press.

Bruch, H. (1978). Obesity and anorexia nervosa. *Psychosomatics*, *19*, 208–212.

Brumberg, J.J. (1988). *Fasting girls: The emergence of anorexia nervosa as a modern disease*. Cambridge, MA: Harvard University Press.

Bulik, C., Sullivan, P., Franz, C.P., Fear, J., & Pickering, A. (1997). Predictors of the development of bulimia nervosa in women with anorexia nervosa. *Journal of Nervous and Mental Disease*, *185* (11), 704–707.

Bulik, C.M., Sullivan, P.F., Fear, J.L., Pickering, A., Dawn, A., & McCullin, M. (1999). Fertility and reproduction in women with anorexia nervosa: A controlled study. *Journal of Clinical Psychiatry, 60* (2), 130–135.

Cafri, G., Thompson, J.K., Ricciardelli, L., McCabe, M., Smolak, L., & Yesalis, C. (2005). Pursuit of the muscular ideal: Physical and psychological consequences and putative risks. *Clinical Psychology Review, 25*, 215–239.

Caparrotta, L., & Ghaffari, K. (2006). A historical overview of the psychodynamic contributions to the understanding of eating disorders. *Psychoanalytic Psychotherapy, 20* (3), 175–196.

Caprio, S., Daniels, S., Drewnowski, A., Kaufman, F., Palinkas, L., Rosenbloom, A., & Schwimmer, J. (2008). Influence of race, ethnicity, and culture on childhood obesity: Implications for prevention and treatment. *Obesity Journal, 16* (12), 2566–2577.

Carlat, D., Camargo, C., & Herzog, D. (1997). Eating disorders in males: A report on 135 patients. *American Journal of Psychiatry, 154* (8), 1127–1132.

Chapman, S.A. (2006). A "new materialist" lens on aging well: Special things in later life. *Journal of Aging Studies, 20* (3), 207–216.

Cosford, P.A., & Arnold, E. (1992). Eating disorders in later life: A review. *International Journal of Geriatric Psychiatry, 7* (7), 491–498.

Croll, J., Neumark-Sztainer, D., Story, M., & Ireland, M. (2002). Prevalence and risk and protective factors related to disordered eating behaviors among adolescents: Relationship to gender and ethnicity. *Journal of Adolescent Health, 31*, 166–175.

Crosscope-Happel, C., Hutchings, D., Getz, H., & Hayes, G. (2000). Male anorexia nervosa: A new focus. *Journal of Mental Health Counseling, 22*, 365–370.

Crow, S., Peel, P.K., Thuras, P., & Mitchell, J.E. (2004). Bulimia symptoms and other risk behaviors during pregnancy in women with bulimia. *International Journal of Eating Disorders, 36*, 220–223.

Crow, S., Agras, W., Crosby, R., Halmi, K., & Mitchell, J. (2008). Eating disorders in pregnancy: A prospective study. *International Journal of Eating Disorders, 41* (3), 277–279.

Dallos, R. (2004). Attachment narrative therapy: Integrating ideas from narrative and attachment theory in systemic family therapy with eating disorders. *Journal of Family Therapy, 26* (1), 40–65.

Dansky, B.S., Brewerton, T.D., Kilpatrick, D.G., & O'Neil, P.M. (1997). The national women's study: Relationship of victimization and posttraumatic stress disorder to bulimia nervosa. *International Journal of Eating Disorders, 21* (3), 213–228.

Devlin, B., Bacanu, S.A., Klump, K., Bulik, C., Fichter, M., Halmi, K. et al. (2002). Linkage analysis of anorexia nervosa incorporating behavioral covariates. *Human Molecular Genetics, 11* (6), 689–696.

Drummond, M. (2002). Men, body image, and eating disorders. *International Journal of Men's Health, 1*, 79–93.

Eberly, M., & Heath, K. (2008). Trauma and eating disorders. In A. Cumell, M. Eberly, & E. Wall (eds). *Eating disorders: A handbook of Christian treatment* (pp. 341–352). Nashville, TN: Remuda Ranch.

Emmett, S.W. (ed.). (1985). *Theory and treatment of anorexia and bulimia: Biomedical, sociocultrual and psychological perspectives*. New York: Brunner/Mazel.

Fairburn, C.G. (1988). The current status of the psychological treatments for bulimia nervosa. *Journal of Psychosomatic Research, 32* (6), 635–645.

Fallon, P., Katzman, M., & Wooley, S. (eds). (1994). *Feminist perspectives on eating disorders*. New York: Guilford Press.

Farber, S. (2008). Dissociation, traumatic attachments, and self-harm: Eating disorders and self-mutilation. *Clinical Social Work Journal, 36*, 63–72.

Feldman, M., & Meyer, I. (2007). Eating disorders in diverse lesbian, gay, and bisexual populations. *International Journal of Eating Disorders, 40*, 218–226.

Fister, S., & Smith, G. (2004). Media effects on expectancies: Exposure to realistic female images as a protective factor. *Psychology of Addictive Behaviors, 18*, 394–397.

Franko, D. (2007). Race, ethnicity, and eating disorders: Considerations for DSM-V. *International Journal of Eating Disorders, 40*, 531–534.

Gadalla, T. (2008). Eating disorders and associated psychiatric comorbidity in elderly Canadian women. *Archives of Women's Mental Health, 11*, 357–362.

Gardner, D.M. (1997). Psychoeducational principles in treatment. In D.M. Garner & P.E. Garfinkel (eds), *Handbook of treatment for eating disorders* (pp. 145–178). New York: Guilford Press.

Garfinkel, P.L. (1996). Should amenorrhea be necessary for the diagnosis of anorexia nervosa? *British Journal of Psychiatry, 168*, 500–506.

Gitterman, A., & Germain, C.B. (2008). *The life model of social work practice: Advances in theory and practice* (3rd ed.). New York: Columbia University Press.

Halmi, K.A., Sunday, S.R., Klump, K.L., Strober, M., Leckman, J.F., Fichter, M. et al. (2003). Obsessions and compulsions in anorexia nervosa subtypes. *International Journal of Eating Disorders, 33* (3), 308–319.

Harper, K., Richter, N., & Gorey, K. (2009). Group work with female survivors of childhood sexual abuse: Evidence of poorer outcomes among those with eating disorders. *Eating Behaviors, 10*, 45–48.

Heller, N.R. (1990). Object relations and symptom choice in bulimics and self-mutilators. Unpublished doctoral dissertation. Smith College, Northampton, MA.

Heller, N.R. (2008). Eating disorders and treatment planning. In A. Roberts & J.M. Watkins, (eds), *Social workers' desk reference* (2nd ed., pp. 531–537). New York: Oxford University Press.

Herzog, D., Neuman, K.L., Yeh, C., & Warshaw, M. (1992). Body image satisfaction in homosexual and heterosexual women. *International Journal of Eating Disorders, 11*, 391–396.

Hesse-Biber, S. (1996). *Am I thin enough yet? The cult of thinness and the commercialization of identity.* New York: Oxford University Press.

Hoderness, C., Brooks-Gunn, J., & Warren, M. (1994). Comorbidity of eating disorders and substance abuse review of the literature. *International Journal of Eating Disorders, 16* (1), 1–34.

Hoek, H.W., & van Hoeken, D. (2003). Review of the prevalence and incidence of eating disorders. *International Journal of Eating Disorders, 34* (4), 383–396.

Hoffman, L., & Halmi, K.A. (1993). Psychopharmacology in the treatment of anorexia nervosa and bulimia nervosa. *Psychiatric Clinics of North America, 16* (4), 767–778.

Hudson, J.I., Lalonde, J.K., Berry, J.M., Pindyck, L.J., Bulik, C.M., Crow, S.J. et al. (2006). Binge-eating disorder as a distinct familial phenotype in obese individuals. *Archives of General Psychiatry, 63* (3), 313–319.

Hudson, J.I., Hiripi, E., Pope, H.G., Jr., & Kessler, R.C. (2007). The prevalence and correlates of eating disorders in the national comorbidity survey replication. *Biological Psychiatry, 61* (3), 348–358.

Johnson, C., & Connors, M.E. (1987). *The etiology and treatment of bulimia nervosa: A biopsychosocial perspective.* New York: Basic Books.

Johnson, W.G., Tsoh, J.Y., & Varnado, P.J. (1996). Eating disorders: Efficacy of pharmacological and psychological interventions. *Clinical Psychology Review, 16* (6), 457–478.

Katzman, D. (2005). Medical complications in adolescents with anorexia nervosa: A review of the literature. *International Journal of Eating Disorders, 37*, 552–559.

Kaye, W.B. (2004). Comorbidity of anxiety disorders with anorexia and bulimia nervosa. *American Journal of Psychiatry, 161*, 2215–2221.

Keel, P.K., Dorer, D.J., Eddy, K.T., Franko, D., Charatan, D.L., & Herzog, D.B. (2003). Predictors of mortality in eating disorders. *Archives of General Psychiatry, 60*, 179–183.

Kendler, K.M. (1991). The genetic epidemiology of eating disorders. *American Journal of Psychiatry, 148*, 1627–1637.

Kessler, R.C., Sonnega, A., Bromet, E., Hughes, M., & Nelson, C.B. (1995). Posttraumatic stress disorder in the National Comorbidity Study. *Archives of General Psychiatry, 52* (12), 1048–1060.

Kimbro, R., Brooks-Gunn, J., & McLanahan, S. (2007). Racial and ethnic differences in overweight and obesity among 3-year-old children. *American Journal of Public Health, 97* (2), 298–305.

Kinzl, J.F., Mangweth, B., Traweger, C.M., & Biebl, W. (1997). Eating-disordered behavior in males: The impact of adverse childhood experiences. *International Journal of Eating Disorders, 22* (2), 131–138.

Krieger, N., Chen, J., Waterman, P., Rehkopf, D., & Subramanian, S.V. (2003). Race/ethnicity, gender, and monitoring socioeconomic gradients in health: A comparison of area-based socioeconomic measures – the public health disparities geocoding project. *American Journal of Public Health, 93*, 1655–1671.

Laws, A., & Golding, J. (1996). Sexual assault history and eating disorder symptoms among White, Hispanic, and African-American women and men. *American Journal of Public Health, 86* (4), 579–583.

Lester, R. (1997). Acculturation in African-American college women and correlates of eating disorders. Unpublished doctoral dissertation. University of Northern Texas, Denton, TX.

Lewinsohn, P.M., Seeley, J.R., Moerk, K.C., & Striegel-Moore, R.H. (2002). Gender differences in eating disorder symptoms in young adults. *International Journal of Eating Disorders, 32*, 426–440.

Lopez, R.P. (2007). Neighborhood risk factors for obesity. *Obesity, 15* (8), 2111–2119.

Ma, J.L.C. (2007). Meanings of eating disorders discerned from family treatment and its implications for family education: The case of Shenzhen. *Child and Family Social Work, 12* (4), 409–416.

Marchi, M., & Cohen, P. (1990). Early childhood eating behaviors and adolescent eating disorders. *Journal of the American Academy of Child and Adolescent Psychiatry, 29* (1), 112–117.

McFarland, B. (1995). *Brief therapy and eating disorders: A practical guide to solution focused work with clients.* San Francisco, CA: Jossey-Bass.

McVey, G., Davis, R., Tweed, S., & Shaw, B. (2004). Evaluation of a school-based program designed to improve body image satisfaction, global self-esteem, and eating attitudes and behaviors: A replication study. *International Journal of Eating Disorders Conditions, 36*, 1–11.

Minuchin, S. (1970). *Psychosomatic families.* Cambridge, MA: Harvard University Press.

Mitchell, J.E. (1991). A review of the controlled trials of psychotherapy for bulimia nervosa. *Journal of Psychosomatic Research, 35*, 23–31.

Mitchell, J.E., Raymond, N., & Specker, S.M. (1993). A review of the controlled trials of pharmacotherapy and psychotherapy in the treatment of bulimia nervosa. *International Journal of Eating Disorders, 14* (3), 229–247.

Muise, A., Stein, D., & Arbess, G. (2003). Eating disorders in adolescent boys: A review of the adolescent and young adult literature. *Journal of Adolescent Health, 33*, 427–435.

National Health and Nutrition Examination Survey (NHANES) (2008). *National Health and Nutrition Examination Survey of the Center for Disease Control.* Retrieved June 19, 2010, from www.cdc.gov/nchs/nhanes/nhanes2007-2008/nhanes07_08.htm

Oesterheld, J.R., McKenna, M.S., & Gould, N.B. (1987). Group psychotherapy of bulimia: A critical review. *International Journal of Group Psychotherapy, 37* (2), 163–184.

Ogden, C.L., Carroll, M.D., Curtin, L.R., McDowell, M.A., Tabak, C.J., & Flegal, K.M. (2006). Prevalence of overweight and obesity in the United States, 1999–2004. *Journal of the American Medical Association, 295* (13), 1549–1555.

Pallett, P.M., Link, S., & Lee, K. (2009). New "golden" ratios for facial beauty. *Vision Research, 50* (2), 149–154.

Patton, G.C., Selzer, R., Coffey, C., Carlin, J.B., & Wolfe, R. (1999). Onset of adolescent eating disorders: population based cohort over 3 years. *British Medical Journal, 328*, 768–768. Retrieved June 19, 2010, from www.bmj.com/cgi/content/full/318/7186/765

Pedereau, F., Faucher, S., Wallier, J., Vibert, S., & Godart, N. (2008). Family history of anxiety and mood disorders in anorexia nervosa: Review of the literature. *Eating Weight Disorders, 13*, 1–13.

Petrie, T., & Rogers, R. (2001). Extending the discussion of eating disorders to include men and athletes. *Counseling Psychologist, 29*, 743–753.

Petrie, T., Greenleaf, C., Reel, J., & Carter, J. (2008). Prevalence of eating disorders and disordered eating behaviors among male collegiate athletes. *Psychology of Men and Masculinity, 9* (4), 267–277.

Ray, S. (2004). Eating disorders in adolescent males. *Professional School Counseling, 8*, 98–101.

Richards, P.S., Baldwin, B.M., Frost, H.A., Clark-Sly, J., Berrett, M.E., & Hardman, R.K. (2000). What works for treating eating disorders? Conclusions of 28 outcome reviews. *Eating Disorders: Journal of Treatment and Prevention, 8* (3), 189–206.

Robb, A.S., & Dadson, M.J. (2002). Eating disorders in males. *Child and Adolescent Psychiatric Clinics of North America, 11* (2), 399–418.

Russel, C., & Keel, P. (2002). Homosexuality as a specific risk factor for eating disorders in men. *International Journal of Eating Disorders, 3*, 300–306.

Schmidt, U. (1989). Behavioral psychotherapy of eating disorders. *International Review of Psychiatry, 1*, 245–256.

Selling, L., & Ferraro, M. (1945). *The psychology of diet and nutrition.* New York: W.W. Norton.

Siebold, C. (2008). Shame, the affective side of secrets: Commentary on Barth's hidden eating disorders. *Clinical Social Work Journal, 36*, 367–371.

Smith, D.E., Marcus, M.D., & Eldredge, K.L. (1994). Binge eating syndromes: A review of assessment and treatment with an emphasis on clinical application. *Behavior Therapy, 25* (4), 635–658.

Smith, F.M., Latchford, G.J., Hall, R.M., & Dickson, R.A. (2008). Do chronic medical conditions increase the risk of eating disorder? A cross-sectional investigation of eating pathology in adolescent females with scoliosis and diabetes. *Journal of Adolescent Health, 42* (1), 58–63.

Soban, C. (2006). What about the boys? Addressing issues of masculinity within male anorexia nervosa in a feminist therapeutic environment. *International Journal of Men's Health, 5,* 251–267.

Steinhausen, H., Rauss-Mason, C., & Seidel, R. (1991). Follow-up studies of anorexia nervosa: A review of four decades of outcome research. *Psychological Medicine, 21* (2), 447–454.

Stice, E. (1994). Review of the evidence for a sociocultural model of bulimia nervosa: An explanation of the mechanisms of action. *Clinical Psychology Review, 14,* 633–661.

Stice, E., Schupack-Neuberg, E., Shaw, H., & Stein, R. (1994). Relations of media exposure to eating disorder symptomatology. *Journal of Abnormal Psychology, 103,* 836–840.

Striegel-Moore, R.H. & Bulik, C.M. (2007). Risk factors for eating disorders. *American Psychologist 62* (3), 181–198.

Striegel-Moore, R., Dohm, F.A., Kraemer, H.C., Taylor, C.B., Daniels, S., Crawford, P.B., & Schreiber, G.B. (2003). Eating disorders in white and black women. *American Journal of Psychiatry, 160* (7), 1326–1331.

Striegel-Moore, R., Rosselli, F., Perrin, N., DeBar, L., Wilson, G., May, A., & Kraemer, H. (2009). Gender difference in the prevalence of eating disorder symptoms. *International Journal of Eating Disorders, 42* (5), 471–474.

Takii, M. (1999). Differences between bulimia nervosa and binge-eating disorder in females with type I diabetes: The important role of insulin omission. *Journal of Psychosomatic Research, 47* (3), 221–231.

Thompson, B. (1994). Food, bodies, and growing up female: Childhood lessons about culture, race, and class. In S.C. Wooley (ed.), *Feminist perspectives on eating disorders* (pp. 355–378). New York: Guilford Press.

Vitousek, K.B., Daly, J. & Heiser, C. (1991). Reconstructing the internal world of the eating disordered individual: Overcoming distortion in self-report. *International Journal of Eating Disorders, 10* (6), 647–666.

Watson, T., & Anderson, A.E. (2003). A critical examination of the amenorrhea and weight criteria for diagnosing anorexia nervosa. *Acta Psychiatrica Scandinavica, 108,* 175–182.

Webster, J., & Tiggemann, M. (2003). The relationship between women's body satisfaction and self-image across the life span: The role of cognitive control. *Journal of Genetic Psychology, 164* (2), 241–252.

Werne, J. (1996). Introduction. In J. Werner (ed.), *Treating eating disorders* (pp. x–xxix). San Francisco, CA: Jossey-Bass.

Wilfley, D.E., & Cohen, L.R. (1997). Psychological treatment of bulimia nervosa and binge eating disorder. *Psychopharmacology Bulletin, 33* (3), 437–454.

Williamson, L. (1998). Eating disorders and the cultural forces behind the drive for thinness: Are African American women really protected? *Social Work in Health Care, 28* (1), 62–73.

Yager, J. (1988). The treatment for eating disorders. *Journal of Clinical Psychiatry, 49* (9), 18–25.

Yager, J. (1989). Psychological treatment for eating disorders. *Psychiatric Annals, 19* (9), 477–482.

Yager, J., Andersen, A., Devlin, M., Egger, H., Herzog, D., Mitchell, J. et al. (2002). Practice guidelines for the treatment of patients with eating disorders (2nd ed.). In APA Steering Committee on Practice Guidelines (eds), *American psychiatric association practice guidelines for the treatment of psychiatric disorders: Compendium 2002* (pp. 697–766). Washington, DC: American Psychiatric Association.

Yager, Z., & O'Dea, J. (2008). Prevention programs for body image and eating disorders on college campuses: A review of large controlled interventions. *Health Promotions International, 23* (2), 173–189.

Zerbe, K. (1993). *The body betrayed: A deeper understanding of women, eating disorders and treatment.* Carlsbad, CA: Gurze.

18 Personality conditions

Terry B. Northcut

We all struggle with our "Ghosts in the nursery" as described by in-home social workers, Fraiberg, Edelson, and Shapiro (1975) that shape our interactions as adults. With insight, behavioral changes, and experience, we hope that we are able to not replay unhealthy inter-personal patterns in our adult relationships. Unfortunately, sometimes through a combination of biological, psychological, and sociological factors, individuals develop rigid patterns of behavior, that while normal on one end of the spectrum of personality traits, have amplified to the extent that pathology results (Paris, 1997). In the profession of social work where we are trained to focus on strengths and the social structures that can impede healthy growth, we are vulnerable to overlooking or minimizing the diagnoses that imply rigid, dysfunctional patterns of coping that "constantly create situations that replay failures" (Millon & Davis, 2000, p. 13). Kirk, Wakefield, Hsieh, and Pottick (1999) studied a group of 250 MSW students and found that despite an assumption that social work students would over-diagnose pathology, respondents were able to distinguish between disordered and non-disordered youth. Of particular interest is the finding that a subset of students displayed bias but in the opposite direction, of under-diagnosing a psychiatric or mental disorder. Social work, while assessing clients via a biopsychosocialspiritual perspective, poses tremendous challenges to keeping a balance of appreciating the bidirectional effects of each of these components in our lives and the lives of our clients. The difficulty is in over-diagnosing or under-diagnosing while maintaining the "start where the client is" maxim of social work practice.

Definitions of personality condition

"All medical illnesses lie on a continuum with normality. The determination of what is a 'case' is in many respects a social construct" (Paris, 1996, p. 1; see also Eisenberger, 1986). As early as the Egyptians, we have been trying to make a connection between emotional problems and problems within the human body. At that time, the theory was that the uterus caused "hysteria" or emotional problems (Alexander & Selesnick, 1966; Magnavita, 2004; Stone, 1997). A Roman physician, Galen, classified temperaments as choleric, sanguine, phlegmatic, and melancholic (Kagan, 1994) each having physiological determinants. It was not, however, until the nineteenth century that clinicians began to divide behavior into "normal" and "abnormal," with abnormal being considered "moral insanity" or an inability to control criminal behavior. (Paris, 1996; Pritchard, 1837, quoted in Livesley, Schroeder, Jackson, & Jang, 1994). Only the most extreme variation of "normal" behavior attracted attention at first, that of psychosis. Kraeplin (1905) was known for the first organized study of what we now call schizophrenia and developed the first method of looking at common patterns of symptoms to be able to classify groupings of psychiatric disorders. Charcot and Freud documented and examined disorders of hysteria, Charcot with the newly invented photography to record in pictures the clients' behavior, and Freud with psychoanalysis utilizing free association to inter- pret dreams and the unconscious (Magnavita, 2004). With the movement from psychiatric hospitals to outpatient practice in mental health clinics in the early twentieth century, clinicians began to examine problems in interpersonal relationships (Paris, 1996). Ironically, while Freud began his research in trying to understand what he later considered neurotic symptomatology, psychoanalysis has done the most to push the study of personality conditions. Perhaps one of the most significant findings of Freud was that certain types of behavior and psychiatric sympto- matology are stable and relatively "egosyntonic" or impervious to analysis of symptoms. The failures of early analysis with certain kinds of clients led later theorists (Reich, 1933) to hypothesize that underlying character must be the focus of clinical work to make the symptoms more unacceptable to the individual so that there would be sufficient anxiety and therefore motivation to change the entrenched patterns of behavior (Paris, 1996).

Certainly, the sociopolitical context of the times, 1930s to 1940s, influenced the push to understand psychopathology. The rugged individualism of Western culture was considered one contributor to psychopathology, as was capitalistic materialism (Horney, 1940; Fromm, 1955; respectively). The influence of a European emphasis on history and its permanency, faced off with the American emphasis on environment and rugged individualism. Prior to World War II, European psychiatry withstood the seductiveness of psychoanalytic theories of etiology and began to focus on how to classify mental disorders believing that they were constitutionally determined and therefore not easily remedied by psychotherapy. Schneider (1950) was responsible for developing the classification system of personality disorders in Europe, while in the United States, Meyer (1957) focused on the reaction patterns of the individuals to their environments that led to rigid patterns of behavioral pathology. The history of mental health classification systems is particularly relevant to our discussion of personality conditions because of the controversies about diagnosing, treating or punishing those individuals who display symptoms of a range of behaviors that are typically seen as "bad" in contemporary society. Those disorders distinguished by externalizing behaviors, such as antisocial and borderline conditions, engender very negative responses from society, practitioners and corrections workers.

The *Diagnostic and statistical manual* (DSM-I) was developed in 1952 by the American Psychiatric Association (APA) and remains the primary diagnostic system in tandem with categories in the International Classification of Diseases (ICD). With the sway of individual idealism, American clinicians moved away from speculating about etiology as an effective classification system, and focused more on the clinical symptoms (an influence of pheno- menology). The spirit of empiricism dictated research and the classification systems to minimize conclusions not based on observable behavior. In the 1970s, Gunderson and his colleagues tried to bridge psychodynamic theories and empiricism in their study of personality disorders (Paris, 1996). This group of clinician researchers took the influence of psychoanalysis and phenom- enology and focused on personality disorders, making important contributions to this field.

Another area of influence on the development of the classification and study of personality disorders is the emphasis on personality traits, which led to study of "dimensions" of per- sonalities. "Psychologists define personality traits as consistent patterns of behavior, emotion, and cognition . . . traits [that] can be identified early in life, and are highly stable over time" (Paris, 1996, p. 18). These traits, such as introversion/extroversion, novelty seeking/harm avoidance, and affiliation/dominance, can be measured quantitatively. Using the polarity of concepts on a continuum led to research that measured traits, or dimensions of personality. When examining the "complex interaction of biogenetic predispositions and environmental experiences that result in an array of possible constellations of adaptive and maladaptive personality traits" (Clark, Livesley, & Morey, 1997), researchers began to recognize the similarities and differences of traits present in personalities. The DSM-III (APA, 1980) began to evaluate individuals on the basis of a multiaxial system grouping information into certain domains (medical problems, highest and lowest level of functioning, clinical syndromes including presenting symptoms, and psychosocial and environmental factors) (Williams, 1985). Personality disorders were classified and grouped as Axis II disorders. Also, the idea of "clusters" was introduced in DSM-III to group personality conditions into clusters of "odd," "impulsive" or "dramatic," and "anxious" (APA, 1980, pp. 309–310) in order to make group-ings based on traits adding additional complexity to the classification system (see DSM-III-TR (APA, 1987) for a complete listing of personality disorders and their criteria).

"Cluster A is characterized by odd or eccentric behavior and includes paranoid, schizoid, and schizotypal personalities. This cluster tends to be the most treatment refractory and is probably the most likely to have underlying biogenetic factors" (Magnavita, 2004, p. 7). Personality conditions in this cluster are often associated with psychotic conditions or symptoms with the assumption that the symptom of psychosis exists on a continuum ranging from most severe, i.e., schizophrenia to "various eccentricities of communication or behavior" (APA, 1980, p. 309). However, when reviewing the research regarding the co-occurrence of Axis I syndromes with Axis II Cluster A personality conditions, the only definitive answer to whether there is a spectrum of psychosis, is that there is a "complex relationship" between Axis I and Axis II disorders (Dolan-Sewell, Krueger, & Shea, 2001, 91).

"Cluster B is characterized by erratic, emotional, and dramatic presentations and includes antisocial, borderline, histrionic, and narcissistic personalities. This cluster includes personality disorders often considered to be severe and that have mixed treatment results" (Magnavita, 2004, p. 7). So far, the majority of research on personality conditions has focused on the borderline and antisocial personalities due to how challenging these clients are to work with and to help, and their probable adverse effects on relationships, and society. Consequently we know more about the outcome of persons with the most severe personality conditions even though they numerically represent a smaller group (Stone, 2001). A common quality among the Cluster B disorders is emotional dysregulation which can lead to suicidal behavior and violence toward others (Newhill, Mulvey, & Pilkonis, 2004). Research on the common characteristics of emo-tional regulation failure, aggression, and violence suggest that these effects stem from abnor-malities in the central serotonergic systems (Coccaro, Siever, Owen, & Davis, 1990; Davidson, Putnam, & Larsen, 2000; Newhill et al., 2004).

"Cluster C is characterized by anxiety and fearfulness and includes avoidant, dependent, and obsessive compulsive personalities. These are generally viewed as the most therapy responsive and have shown the best results with shorter duration therapy protocols" (Beck, Freeman, & Associates, 1990; Magnavita, 2004, p. 7; Winston, Laikin, Pollack, Samstag, McCullough, & Muran, 1994). Research has demonstrated that there is a strong relationship between mood conditions and Cluster C conditions. Individuals experiencing any of the mood conditions are three times as likely to have an anxious/fearful personality disorder (and vice versa) than individuals without a mood condition (Dolan-Sewell et al., 2001). In addition, somatoform symptoms, particularly hypochondriasis, appears to have a strong relationship with Cluster C personality conditions.

The influence of neurobiological research has shaped the study of personality conditions even further. Because the brain encodes our experiences and absorbs genetic, social, and psychological processes as well, it creates a lifelong template for personality development (Elin, 2004). While there is some plasticity in the brain patterns as they are modified by ongoing consistent secure relationships, (Schore, 2003; Schore & Schore, 2008; Siegel, 1999, 2007; Tronick, 2007), the difficulty with persons diagnosed with personality conditions is that the template is rigid and difficult to change. Research by Cloninger (1986, 1987) proposes that there are genetic-neurobiologic trait dispositions such as novelty seeking, harm avoidance, and reward dependence, which are associated with a particular neurotransmitter system. However, that association has yet to be empirically supported. This area of research is on the cutting edge of determining other courses of management as well as further delineation of personality conditions and their continuum.

There are many well-documented controversies surrounding the use of the *Diagnostic and statistical manual*.

> The boundaries between particular disorders, far from being static reflections of some objectively existing and observable behavior, are always being contested, defined, and redefined in light of new theories. In this view, the definition of mental disorder, like the construction of any social problem, is a political process, with the various disciplines of medical psychiatry, psychoanalysis, psychology, and social work participating in an ongoing debate over terms.
>
> (Wirth-Cauchon, 2001, p. 58)

One of the strongest debates about the bias of the classification of personality conditions is the correlation of certain conditions with gender. For example, more women are likely to be diagnosed as borderline, dependent, and histrionic, and more men are likely to be diagnosed as paranoid, schizoid, schizotypal, antisocial, narcissistic, and obsessive compulsive. Several explanations are made for this type of apparent skewed pattern. First, a greater number of women seek out services; however, this does not account for the skewed diagnoses favoring men. Second, diagnostic criteria include both "normal" socially acceptable (even desirable) traits. For example, the histrionic diagnostic category "consistently uses physical appearance to draw attention to self." This is a subjective assessment which in light of persistent societal influences, places a focus on physical appearance, particularly for women (Millon & Davis, 2000, p. 17). Third, the criteria for dependent personality places the emphasis on socially reinforced female ways of relating as pathological (inappropriate sexualization, use of physical appearance to draw attention, and a need to be the center of attention, etc.). However, at the same time, the socially reinforced male pattern of dependency of having someone maintain their home and take care of their children is not considered (Widiger, 1998).

Identifying or labeling someone as having a personality condition does have its political or social control functions. Labeling can marginalize and/or control individuals or groups that the majority group in society finds to be unacceptable or threatening because of their disagreement with the dominant values and rules. Managed care companies usually do not reimburse for working with personality condition diagnoses because they are not viewed as "treatable." As a result clinicians tend to not include the personality disorder diagnosis on treatment plans for their clients, which makes it very difficult to establish reliable data on the prevalence rate of personality conditions (Magnavita, 2004). The multiaxial system developed and included in DSM-III, and continued in the DSM-IV, was designed to provide a more complete picture of the person and include categories such as physical health, psychosocial and environmental stressors and problems, and a global assessment of psychological, social, and occupational functioning. However, when one category, in this case the Axis II personality disorders, is not reimbursable by the health care system, we are reinforcing a system that does not view and value a complete picture of a person. Likewise, due to the negative bias against clients with personality conditions, social workers are reluctant to label someone with this diagnosis. In addition, Bentley, Harrison, and Hudson (1993) remind us of the "staying power" of a diagnosis whether it is supported by research or not. Social workers, like the general public, have been guilty of subscribing to the belief that diagnoses such as borderline exist without adequate proof of their validity.

Fortunately, "the critical thinking movement" has led us to question "the meaning, logic, under-lying assumptions, and behavioral referents of the concepts" (Bentley et al., 1993, p. 469).

In addition to the inequities in helping people with personality conditions, there are problems with our current diagnostic system. While progress has been made, we still struggle with overlapping diagnoses in the DSM model (APA, 1994, 2000). There is also limited empirical support for the efficacy of current categories as predictors of response to therapy. In other words, we are still using a system that has yet to show construct validity (Livesley, 2001; Skodol & Bender, 2009). The "Work Group on Personality Disorders" for the fifth edition of DSM has been considering how to improve the representation of personality conditions to increase reliability and validity of these diagnostic categories. The DSM-V is scheduled to be published in 2013 (www.psych.org/MainMenu/Research/DSMIV/DSMV.aspx). Of particular concern are the major drawbacks to the current DSM in the Axis II category:

> excessive co-occurrence among disorders, extreme heterogeneity among patients receiving the same diagnosis, arbitrary diagnostic thresholds for the boundaries between pathological and "normal" personality functioning, and inadequate coverage of personality psycho-pathology such that the diagnosis of personality disorder not otherwise specified (PDNOS) is the most common.
>
> (Skodol & Bender, 2009)

The debate at this point in time appears to be between two competing types of classification of personality disorders, the "variable-centered" vs. the "person-centered." Rottman, Alin, Sanislow, and Kim (2009) found that clinicians were less able to correctly diagnose personality conditions if they were given variables or traits of the individuals rather than prototypical descriptions using the DSM-IV criteria, for example. The "Personality Disorders Work Group" is trying to establish a core definition of a personality disorder that makes it unique from other clinical syndromes. Also being considered is whether the separate Axis II diagnosis is valuable for determining risk, therapy, prognosis either as stand alone diagnosis or when combined with another Axis I domain related to mood, anxiety, substance use, or eating conditions (Skodol & Bender, 2009).

Theoretical definitions illustrate the struggle with maintaining a balance between "scope and precision" (Millon, Meagher, & Grossman, 2001, p. 41). An emphasis on scope is considered a monotaxic orientation and tries to account for the whole domain of personality pathology. Precision definitions focus on a "single taxonomic unit of analysis" rather than trying to explain all qualities of personality. Theories attempting to provide an explanation for the occurrence of personality disorders are numerous with the major frameworks including intrapsychic, cognitive-behavioral, neurobiological, and diatheses-stress. Trauma theory is often associated with psycho-pathology; however, research demonstrates that trauma is a risk factor for mental conditions rather than a cause of psychiatric conditions (Paris, 1996). While a high statistical association between childhood sexual abuse or childhood physical abuse and the occurrence of psycho-logical symptoms in adulthood exists, the fact remains that many survivors of abuse or trauma do not demonstrate psychopathology. The key factors that seem to affect this apparent discrepancy between childhood trauma and adult psychological problems relate to the parameters of the trauma (identity of the perpetrator, severity and duration of the abuse, and preexisting psycho-logical risks and the presence or absence of post-traumatic mitigating factors) (Paris, 1996). Risk factors will be discussed further in the description of the population affected by personality conditions section.

A number of *intrapsychic* theories, including attachment, have been offered to provide an understanding of the etiology of personality conditions. Historically, psychoanalytic theory focused on character formation as a defensive function against threats from the external or the internal world (Reich, 1933, in Millon et al., 2001). While many of the psychodynamic theories maintained an allegiance to the conflict model of psychoanalysis to include the formation of the intrapsychic world as a result of interpersonal interactions that have been internalized to form "working models" (e.g. Bowlby, 1973, 1980, 1982), others focused more on deficits, e.g., impairment in ego functioning (Blanck & Blanck, 1994; Goldstein, 1984; Hartmann, 1958) or deficiency of the nuclear self (Elson, 1988; Kohut, 1984). However, what is common among the differing models is an emphasis on an imprinting of early relationships that gets reenacted over development and time. These "working models" are a system of expectations and beliefs about the self and others that allow children to predict and interpret an attachment figure's behavior" (Bartholomew, Kwong, & Hart, 2001; Nakash-Eisokovits, Dutra, & Westen, 2002). Once the working models are internalized, they provide a template for the personality to guide interpersonal behavior throughout life (Tronick, 2007). If a child has had secure experiences with attachment figures, the child and subsequent adults expect others to interact in a manner that is consistent with those experiences. However, if a child has anxious or insecure attachment relationships, the template dictates the child to expect others to be unreliable and unavailable (i.e., "ghost in the nursery"). These anxious expectations then translate into a personality that seeks and interprets actions of others as being non-gratifying which leads to differing personality structures that may manifest themselves as disorders. For example, someone with a histrionic personality disorder behaves with excessive emotionality as a desperate need to get attention and reassurance from any potential attachment figures.

Just as the definition of personality conditions in the DSM-IV describes "an enduring pattern of perceiving, relating to, and thinking about the environment and oneself" (Maxmen, Ward, & Kilgus, 2009, p. 547) proponents of *cognitive theory* attempt to understand personality conditions from a cognitive perspective. What are the schemas that seem to guide individuals to act in a consistent manner? From a cognitive perspective, we all have our own unique information processing system, which contains the results of prior experiences. Maladaptive beliefs, attributions, and other appraisal processes form schemas that screen out any experiences that contradict these beliefs. Consequently, the person is susceptible to repeating dysfunctional behaviors that reinforce the "truth" of the maladaptive belief, etc. and demonstrate a persistent and systematic bias.

Strict *behavioral theories* placed emphasis on contextual factors by emphasizing individual situations that contain stimulus properties that lead to unique patterns of behavior ranging from normal to pathological. Effort is made to avoid making inferences about the cognitive or affective level, rather to focus solely on external stimuli and the resulting behaviors. An assumption is made that rigid or repetitive behavior is the result of the tenacity of the behavioral reinforcers. For the most part, a practitioner with a cognitive perspective has distanced him or herself from strict behavioral principles using behavior to make an assessment but employing cognitions to make clinical inquiries. Beck et al. (1990), in their handbook on personality disorders, rooted themselves in evolutionary theory to maintain that personality strategies are attempts to facilitate survival, and attempted to draw a picture of idiosyncratic schemas common to each personality condition. For example, a person with a dependent personality is hypersensitive to the possibility of loss of love from significant others so interprets any kind of behavior that even hints at a potential loss as reality, and reacts accordingly, by becoming more clingy and dependent on the significant other.

Neurobiological theories include a focus on temperament, neurons, and the chemical messengers or neurotransmitters. For example, to a large degree, temperament is determined by the individual's biological constitution. The constitution will exclude some developmental domains and reinforce others, e.g., children with a calm, personal temperament have a greater than average likelihood that they will not develop a histrionic personality disorder. Likewise, the neurobiological activity will prescribe certain kinds of feedback loops. Three behaviors have been found to have a correlation with certain types of activity in the brain: novelty seeking, harm avoidance, and reward dependence. "Specifically, novelty seeking is associated with low basal activity in the dopaminergic system, harm avoidance with high activity in the serotonergic system, and reward dependence with low basal noradrenergic system activity" (Millon et al., 2001, p. 54). Novelty seeking is behavior that would dispose an individual to respond to novel stimuli with exhilaration or excitement, which would then lead to behavior that would result in that same kind of reward and an avoidance of any behavior that would be experienced as monotonous and therefore punishing. Harm avoidance reflects a disposition to react strongly to aversive stimuli which leads an individual to inhibit behaviors to avoid punishment, novelty, and frustration. Reward dependence is seen as a tendency to respond to signals of reward, such as verbal signals of social approval, and consequently seek out situations previously associated with rewards or relief from punishment.

The likelihood of the greatest understanding of personality disorders is inevitably linked to a multidimensional explanation (Paris, 1996). The *diathesis-stress model* was created by Holmes & Rahe (1967), expanded on by Zubin & Spring (1977) and reformulated as the stress–vulnerability–protective factors model, particularly by Dr. Robert P. Liberman and his colleagues (Liberman, 1982, 1987, 2006, 2009; Liberman, Kopelowicz, & Silverstein, 2004) in the field of psychiatric rehabilitation. A diathesis-stress model which specifies that individuals with a biological or genetic vulnerability or predisposition (diathesis) interact with the environment and life events (stressors) to trigger behaviors or psychological disorders is useful and particularly appealing to social workers. The greater the underlying vulnerability, the less stress is needed to trigger the behavior or disorder. Conversely,

> with enough stress even the most resilient people will be at significant risk for the development of symptomatology, although these symptoms will probably be milder than those of the vulnerable person who experiences low to moderate stress and will almost certainly be milder than those of the vulnerable person under significant stress.
>
> (Ingram & Price, 2010, p. 12)

The critical point to remember is that even with a diathesis towards a disorder does not necessarily mean they will ever develop the disorder. Both the diathesis and the stress are required for this to happen.

As social workers we are committed to understanding the biopsychosocialspiritual aspects of our clients and of ourselves. Ethically, we are expected to keep up with current research and clinical wisdom regarding our clients' difficulties. Our difficulty, however, is in understanding a grouping of clients for whom very little research money is invested because of the likelihood of poor outcome as evidenced in clinical experience. It is also difficult to secure accurate data on a population that manifests behavior that consistently makes it difficult to seek and receive help that requires interpersonal relating on some level. Certainly, the behavior evidenced by clients with personality conditions does not "win friends and influence people" (Carnegie, 1936) and requires enormous commitment on the part of clinical social workers. In fact, the converse is more likely to be true; just by hearing a description of a potential client as possibly having a personality disorder increases the likelihood that the clinician will not be expecting positive results and have greater difficulty "meeting the client where the client is." An understanding of the multiple factors that predispose, influence, trigger and maintain consistently maladaptive behaviors will help the social worker understand the client's intrapersonal and interpersonal struggles. Additionally, this understanding can enable the social worker to recognize both the micro and macro influences and solutions to the sometimes very painful struggles of these clients and their families.

Demographics

As discussed earlier, accurate demographic data on incidence and prevalence rates of personality conditions are difficult to acquire. Several factors contribute to this difficulty. First, the nature of personality conditions, their rigidity and long-term duration, means that the behavior is familiar to the individual and less likely to cause the kinds of distress that would lead him or her to initiate therapy. Second, if these individuals do seek help, their social workers are less likely to record their diagnoses as a personality condition due to non-reimbursement from insurance companies and concern about stigmatizing clients. Third, there is a lack of structured instruments for diagnosing the range of personality disorders on Axis II that verifies consistency and reliability of diagnosis (Mattia & Zimmerman, 2001). Consequently, most epidemiological studies avoid looking for and trying to record Axis II diagnoses. An exception is the antisocial disorder whose symptoms include transgressions against person and property, which are grounds for arrest. This places these individuals in contact with institutions, which must keep documentation (Stone, 2001). Fourth, clinical social workers and clinicians of a variety of disciplines rarely contact former clients years after concluding services out of concern for the potential intrusiveness of such inquiries and violation of confidentiality.

Persons with personality conditions that come into contact with mental health providers usually exhibit symptoms on Axis I (major psychiatric diagnosis) as well. This comorbidity of an Axis II diagnosis with an Axis I disorder is often what triggers entering social work services. Consequently the Axis I diagnosis is often the focus of empirical research which focuses on the most pervasive and presenting diagnoses. The prevalence of at least one personality condition (and often there is overlap) is approximately 10–15 percent of the general population. For each diagnostic category of personality disorder, prevalence rates vary from 1 percent to 3 percent of the population at large. Despite clinical and social assumptions mentioned earlier, gender is usually equally distributed among the overall rates of personality conditions, although this varies for each disorder (Arend, 2004; Mattia & Zimmerman, 2001).

The relative lack of research on personality conditions is particularly problematic when we try to understand the incidence among certain minority populations. For example, there are no data on the prevalence of personality conditions according to sexual orientation or physical ability or disability. Because "identity disturbance" is a characteristic of people suffering with borderline personality disorder, there may be some connection with variation in gender of intimate partners, however, there has not been any established correlation between sexual orientation and any of the Axis II conditions (Reich & Zanarini, 2008). However, we do know from existing research (Berkowitz, 2003), that children exposed to violence in the community are more likely to be associated with low school achievement and high levels of anger, anxiety, aggression, antisocial behavior and alcohol use than children not exposed to violence. These children are also more likely to cause more turmoil in their environment and be over-represented in the juvenile justice system. Consequently, we can expect that there will be lingering effects of this experience of violence in the psychological development and neurobiological maturation. Any prolonged disruption of the regulatory aspects of the brain can affect behavioral functioning and psychiatric morbidity creating increased risk and vulnerability to personality disorders. At the very least children exposed to violence are often from minority communities that are severely depressed economically, will react with behavior associated with personality conditions which sets in motion a feedback loop of reinforcements of lowered expectations from their surrounding environment as well as a tracking system that places these children at greater risk for being worked with aggressively by the school and justice system (Berkowitz, 2003).

> The incidence of APD [antisocial personality disorder] is twice as high for inner-city residents than in small towns or rural areas, and five times higher in males than in females. It affects people in all social classes, but if someone with APD is born into a family of wealth and privilege, they will usually manage to eke out a successful business or political career. Poorer people with APD tend to wind up in state prison systems. Since African-Americans are seven times more likely to be represented in state prison systems, it's tempting to speculate the incidence of APD among African-Americans is high. However, there are most likely other causes of crime among African-Americans (like unemployment and racism). The fact is that most of the current prison population, white or black, shares the APD diagnosis. All it takes is a juvenile record, an adult offense career, aggressivity, impulsivity, a checkered work history, and/or lack of demonstrable repentance. These can be easily found in almost any prison inmate's dossier.
>
> (www.apsu.edu/oconnort/crim/crimtheory08.htm)

The results of the National Epidemiologic Survey on Alcohol and Related Conditions (N=43,093) in 2001–2002 revealed that 14.79 percent of adult Americans (approximately 30.8 million) had at least one personality disorder (Grant et al., 2004). The most prevalent disorders in order of occurrence were obsessive compulsive (7.8 percent), paranoid (4.41 percent), antisocial (3.63 percent), schizoid (3.13 percent), avoidant (2.36 percent), histrionic (1.84 percent), and dependent (0.49 percent). The risk factors are greater for women than men for avoidant, dependent, and paranoid personality conditions. Men were more represented in the antisocial personality disorder category. There appeared to be no gender differences in the risk of obsessive compulsive, schizoid or histrionic personality conditions. This is especially interesting considering that the prevailing clinical assumptions are that histrionic diagnoses are more likely given to women. Research from this national study also contrasted somewhat the earlier work by Golomb, Fava, Abraham, and Rosenbaum (1995), which found that men were more likely to meet the criteria for not only narcissistic and antisocial personality disorders but also obsessive compulsiveness. In contrast with other investigations, however, neither research project revealed a higher prevalence of personality disorders in women vs. men.

Some *common risk factors* surfaced for personality conditions: being Native American, black, a young adult, or divorced, separated, widowed or never married. As expected, having low socioeconomic status was also a high risk factor as it usually correlates with cumulative and prolonged stress. In terms of how likely personality conditions are to be associated with emotional disability status, avoidant, dependent, schizoid, paranoid, and antisocial personality disorders ranked highest as leading to unemployability (Grant et al., 2004). As mentioned earlier, assuming the presence of trauma in early childhood is causal for the development of personality conditions in general and borderline personality disorder in specific, is both tempting and controversial (Paris, 1996). However, the relationship appears to be correlational only, as adults with histories of trauma are exposed to many other psychological risk factors as well. For example, the situation of trauma may result from domestic violence, community violence, and/or family "breakdown." Usually the occurrence of one kind of trauma (e.g., divorce) can lead to the occurrence of other changes, such as a marked reduction of income, that can have long-term effects as well and lead to a domino effect of risk factors (Paris, 1996).

Lenzenweger, Lane, Loranger, and Kessler (2007) examined the National Comorbidity Survey Replication Study (NCS-R) to find that the prevalence of personality conditions in the United States is 9.1 percent. They also found that 39 percent of those respondents that measured as having a personality disorder, received mental health and/or substance use treatment within the last year. However, these respondents were likely to make only two visits for treatment and usually were more likely to be seen by general medical providers than by mental health professionals.

Grant et al. (2008) utilized the 2004–2005 National Epidemiological Survey on Alcohol and Related Conditions (N=35,000) and found that those with narcissistic personality disorder have a lifetime prevalence rate of 6 percent with rates greater for men (7.7 percent) than women (4.8 percent). Narcissistic personality disorder was associated with significant disability for men, and co-occurred with a variety of other conditions including substance use, mood and anxiety conditions, and as well as other personality conditions (Stinson et al., 2008).

An interesting finding regarding personality conditions within particular populations found that individuals who volunteer to serve as control subjects for clinical studies show a high prevalence of personality disorders (44 percent) (Bunce, Noblett, McCloskey, & Coccaro, 2005). These results suggest that volunteers with personality conditions may bias a control group sample, particularly because volunteers are rarely screened for anything other than an Axis I disorder. Reliable diagnostic instruments for assessment of personality disorders would be prudent when looking for volunteers for medical and psychiatric research.

Much of the research of personality conditions lies within the United States. Some studies have been done in South Africa (Suliman, Stein, Seedat, & Williams, 2008) and Kenya (Thuo, Ndetei, Maru, & Kuria, 2008), and have found lower prevalence rates in non-clinical and inpatient clinical populations. In South Africa, the study was part of the South African Stress and Health study along with the World Health Organization World Mental Health Survey Initiative. The rate of 7 percent prevalence among people ages 20 or older (in contrast to the approximately 9 percent measured in the United States) examined all clusters diagnosed as personality disordered. One-third of those persons with a personality disorder also show evidence of a substance abuse disorder and/or an anxiety, mood or impulse-control disorder (Suliman et al. 2008). Likewise in the inpatient population in Kenya, prevalence rates were lower than psychiatric patients in the United States or Europe: 20 percent of this inpatient population was found to have personality conditions; 87 percent of those patients were also found to be Cluster B disorders. As with many studies in the United States and in South Africa, there is a strong association between personality diagnoses and Axis I diagnoses (substance abuse/dependence, anxiety, mood, or impulse control problems) (Thuo et al., 2008).

It is commonly accepted knowledge that Western societies have experienced an acceleration of social change leading to changes in social norms (Westen, 1985). This quickly evolving social change suggests that "modernity" may reward, at the very least, the occurrence of certain personality traits, e.g. narcissism as a strong focus on self. It is most likely, however, as with other possible factors contributing to the development of personality conditions (i.e., diathesis-stress model), that there is a feedback loop between biological, psychological, and sociological factors (Paris, 1996). Such a feedback loop reduces the likelihood of a cohort factor playing the primary instigator in the occurrence of personality conditions at this point in history.

Population

One assumption regarding personality conditions is the persistence of the condition given its rigid and pervasive qualities. However, research has begun to indicate that there is a decreasing prevalence of personality conditions across age groups in the general population (using self-reported DSM-IV personality disorder traits) (Ulrich & Coid, 2009). There also does not seem to be increasing stability after age 30, which is usually observed with "normal" personality traits. In fact, the personality condition appears less rigid after the individual's third decade. One possibility or complication in the diagnoses across different age groups is the likelihood that there are not age-appropriate criteria to make that determination (Balsis, Gleason, Woods, & Oltmanns, 2007). Possibly, personality conditions decline with age. However, more likely the pathology does not present itself in the same way in older adults as it does in younger adults. This possibility is considered "heterotypic continuity" (Balsis et al., 2007), which is different than actual change in which the individual would no longer have the disorder at an older age. Heterotypic continuity suggests that the context in which the criteria for the disorders are measured may change (e.g., "problems in occupational functioning" is no longer applicable when the person retires, or the living situation may change in that there are no longer as many opportunities for conflict in daily living such as with driving, working, caring for children, etc.). A trait model suggests that personality stays stable over time; however, the context-dependent model (which may be more similar with the philosophy of social workers and the code of ethics) suggests that personalities may vary in presentation across the life course due to different meaningful contexts (Balsis et al., 2007). Whether personality conditions diminish as one ages, or simply change their presentation due to changing contexts, there are important implication for research, practice, and theories of human behavior across the lifespan.

Professional methods and interventions

Demographic, engagement, and retainment data suggest that the qualities unique to personality conditions – in particular, an individual's lack of awareness of his or her difficulties and projection of blame onto others – would not bode well for successful interventions. Crawford et al. (2009) found that while specialized community-based services for adults with personality disorders could be engaged in therapy (60 percent), out of 1,186 people, 23 percent subsequently dropped out before therapy concluded. Of course, people with the higher levels of personality conditions were less likely to stay in therapy, as were the men and younger persons with personality conditions. This may speak also to how the condition is presented and/or enacted or externalized during young adulthood. For example, if young males are more likely to present with aggressive behavior or are expected to present with aggressive behavior, agencies may respond with very low expectations and covertly or overtly discourage engagement in therapy.

As stated earlier, people suffering with personality conditions are notoriously resistant to behavior change. The very nature of a personality disorder, the fact that they are not defined as such unless they are of lengthy duration, pervasive in scope and rigidity of style, interferes with seeking out and staying with any form of therapy. Persons with personality conditions engender feelings in clinicians of impotence, disinterest, and/or anger and depression (Adler, 1973), which may lead social workers to only reluctantly engage them.

> Moreover, contemporary therapies fail to recognize an intrinsic contradiction between the formal properties of therapy as it is currently practiced and the formal properties of psychotherapy that personality conditions logically require. The premise is simple: Because personality is more than the sum of its parts, therapy must be also.
>
> (Millon, 1999, p. 87)

With the emphasis on efficacy and managed care, brief therapy, a common factors approach (emphasizing the qualities that seem to be present in all successful therapies), and therapeutic eclecticism (in which techniques are borrowed on the basis of whatever works) are emphasized in training and supervision. However, any form of dual diagnosis, particularly if one of the diagnoses is an Axis II or personality disorder, necessitates reconsidering a "one-size-fits-all" approach. Likewise, a therapeutic style that relies on compliance with a particular school of theory, fails to address advances in theory and the strengths that may be present as represented by another school of thought (Livesley, 2008).

In an effort to offer a service model that allows for the complexity and diversity among personality conditions, Millon and Davis (2000) proposed a synergistic psychotherapy which was later combined with "personality-guided" therapy to produce a more "personalized psychotherapy" (Millon & Grossman, 2007) which allows for the "potentiated pairings" of two or more techniques that by themselves would prove futile and or iatrogenic. Determining which pairings of theory and techniques poses significant challenges. However, personality represents biological, cognitive, interpersonal, and intrapsychic aspects, consequently treatment should address each of these areas. The idea of potentiated pairings does suggest some important pairings to be considered when studying personality conditions.

Medications may differentially target symptoms of personality conditions. People with the Cluster B conditions (antisocial, borderline, histrionic, and narcissistic personalities) are usually in significant emotional distress due to their difficulty with affective regulation. Medication sometimes can be helpful for several of these characteristics, depression and impulsivity specifically, however these same qualities make it risky to prescribe medicine that can be easily abused. Likewise, the meaning of these medications and the purpose in prescribing them is influenced by any cognitive distortions that accompany the personality condition. Patients may view the medication as an effort to get rid of them or possibly as justification that they cannot control their behavior or bear no responsibility for their behavior. Generally speaking, pharmacotherapy is best accompanied by some form of psychotherapy to provide a forum for examining intrapsychic and interpersonal issues (Markovitz, 2001) Likewise, different theories are favored for the different subcategories of personality conditions. Several research studies have found that psychodynamic therapy and cognitive therapy or some variation of the two, have been helpful with clients or patients diagnosed with personality disorders (Leichsenring & Leibring, 2003; Livesley, 2008; Vinnars, Thormahlen, Gallop, Noren, & Barber, 2009; Weertman & Arntz, 2007). Understandably there is greater research on the efficacy of treatment for those conditions causing the most difficulty for clinicians e.g., borderline and antisocial. Gunderson (e.g. 2007) for example has published hundreds of articles/reports of his work with colleagues at McLean Hospital in Belmont, MA, Center for the Treatment of Borderline Personality Conditions. Also, Linehan (1993) has published and stimulated much research on dialectical behavioral therapy with clients with the borderline diagnosis. Krampen (2009) has built on the research of many others to examine therapeutic processes and outcomes in outpatient treatment of antisocial behavior. It is beyond the scope of this chapter to examine each condition in depth, and borderline or antisocial in particular. However, readers do have an important source for this kind of therapy research. Many studies of both borderline and antisocial personality conditions are examined in the literature on substance abuse treatment. Suffice it to say, helping approaches vary from inpatient to outpatient, to family work to group work. Services can be provided as a result of the symptoms of the Axis I syndrome and therefore treatment for the Axis II diagnoses enters through the "back door."

Much emphasis has been placed also on *dual diagnoses* as a necessity for treatment focus, which treats a substance abuse addiction in conjunction with a co-occurring mental health condition. Inpatient treatment centers are numerous that focus on dual diagnoses, and serve every population that can afford to pay their prices. Therein lays an important reality with the health care system in the United States. If persons with personality conditions and substance abuse conditions cannot afford inpatient treatment and their health care plan (if they have one) pays only a limited amount, it is very difficult to manage the physical symptomatology that accompanies any kind of withdrawal from substances. With the understanding that higher risk factors include poverty and possible unemployment, it is likely that a population that may have a higher presence of personality disorder and dual diagnoses is the least likely to receive treatment. In addition, social services that provide mental health treatment are often the first systems to be hit when budget deficits are prevalent. Consequently if help is even available, rarely are there sufficient funds to engage in research on helping effectiveness and outcome studies.

Social workers continue to practice in all of the settings mentioned above, whether it is inpatient or outpatient, health care or mental health care with a full range and variety of techniques. We are specifically trained to focus on the whole person ("person curalis") which is less emphasized in other helping professions. The research and clinical literature demonstrates the necessity of seeing personality conditions in all of their complexity, a view that is the core of our profession, viewing the client from the "person-in-the-situation" perspective. This complexity includes the environment that poses unique challenges for personality conditions. Goldstein (1990) argues that while individuals diagnosed with borderline personality disorder have internalized structures that "shape the way the external world is experienced, close interpersonal relationships and the supports or constraints presented by the social environment may nurture or obstruct positive change" (p. 202). Consequently, diagnosis and treatment must be geared to the environmental context of the individual, including work with the family, partners, and other social systems appropriate for the client.

Illustration and discussion

Linda was an extremely thin 45-year-old woman who entered a community mental health center after a suicide attempt. She had seen a social worker at the same community mental health center within the past year but the social worker was on maternity leave when Linda returned to the center. Currently on disability leave from her job in a local factory due to her "mental health issues," Linda was fortunate to have a job in this community. The rural community in which she lived had a high rate of unemployment and poverty despite being in one of the wealthiest counties in the state. Linda lived in a trailer park with occasional friends or relatives living with her during routine crises. Usually they would move out after an extremely loud, often physical altercation with her. The workers at the mental health center were accustomed to being called on a regular basis by either police, the local hospital, or by the school system to evaluate someone from this community. A large percentage of this community did not complete high school while Linda had successfully completed her GED (General Educational Development tests). Linda had one daughter, aged 30, whom she had while a teenager, but was not able to have any more children. This daughter had routine contact with her mother, but was not a usual source of support given that their relationship fluctuated between being "very close" to very contentious. There was no contact with the father of her daughter and no consistent contact with other family members. While a number of "friends" seemed to rotate through her life, there were very few consistent friends. Linda did call a psychic in another state on a routine basis and reported that she had been calling him for a number of years.

Linda seemed distressed somewhat that she could not see her former social worker, but the current crisis was her immediate focus. Mental health center records indicated that Linda had dropped out after a disagreement with her social worker once the social worker announced that she was pregnant. The current crisis seemed to have occurred after a recent rejection by a boyfriend when Linda caught him in bed with another woman. The presenting symptoms included depression and anxiety as well as suicidal thoughts and the recent suicide attempt. Linda's sleeping and eating were erratic. There were several other suicide attempts reported in Linda's case file. Her memories of her own history were sketchy. Her three siblings were older and had moved out of the house by the time Linda was a teenager. Linda described herself as a "late in life" baby. Her earliest memory of her mother was the back of her mother as she stood at the kitchen counter. Linda had learned that she was malnourished as a baby because her mother had not realized Linda wasn't getting milk when she breastfed her. Linda recalled spending a great deal of time outdoors growing up because home life was chaotic and stressed by frequent economic problems and violence. Reportedly, her father was an alcoholic. The details of the family violence were incomplete, but it seemed likely that Linda had been physically abused and possibly sexually abused as well.

During the second session, Linda asked the new social worker if she had any children. However, when the social worker tried to inquire about her question Linda stormed out saying she couldn't trust her, did not want to continue with her, and that the former social worker was much better because she would tell her all kinds of things about herself, etc. Several attempts to reach Linda by phone or by mail were not effective in making contact. Six months later Linda returned to the center requesting the newer social worker by name. She did not have any memory of the "blow-up" but was "ready for therapy" now. Fortunately, the mental health center had the resources to negotiate a fee based on her ability to pay and took into consideration her disability status.

The initial engagement phase included helping Linda manage ongoing crises and answering emergency calls in the middle of the night when Linda hadn't eaten or slept all day and was panicked after an argument with a friend or former co-worker. The social worker did write a letter to the factory on Linda's behalf to extend her leave until the relationship could be more helpful to Linda. Linda's impulsiveness and poor judgment was evident in the numerous arguments she had with others and her tendency to "go where the action was" whenever she heard of a confrontation between people she knew. The worker also facilitated Linda seeing a physician for a checkup since Linda had not had a physical in years. The staff psychiatrist was also consulted to determine if medication might be helpful. While sometimes medication can be helpful for anxiety and depression with clients exhibiting symptoms of borderline personality, a bigger concern for both the social worker and the psychiatrist was Linda's impulsiveness and suicidal thoughts. The decision was made to keep Linda with the worker as often as possible (weekly) but not so often that Linda would be overwhelmed with too much closeness and affect. Consequently, medication was not prescribed at this time. The team of clinicians (clinical social workers, psychiatrist on call, and psychologist available for testing/consultation) believed the most pressing need was to build up Linda's ability to reflect on her actions, thoughts, and feelings as quickly as possible to help her delay acting out any painful feelings or self-destructive thoughts. Linda had agreed already to call the therapist when she felt suicidal.

The middle phase of the work continued the ongoing task of developing and supporting Linda's efforts to think before she acted, and to identify what feelings she had before she reacted. We also worked together to "track the triggers" to some of her more urgent calls to me and gradually she was able to wait until our next session to discuss what had happened. Over the course of time (several years) Linda could say to herself when she started feeling enraged or abandoned "what would T. say?" and hang onto that thought and slow herself down so that she could take care of her immediate physical needs before reacting (e.g., Was she in a safe place? Had she eaten? Was she missing sleep?). We also worked together for Linda to be able to let me know when she felt I had misunderstood her so that she wouldn't have to "show me" by not coming to her appointments. As time passed Linda was able to return to work and was less likely to call in a crisis. She continued to consult with her psychic whenever she felt lonely or disagreed with how her treatment was progressing. During this time of the developing and solidifying of the therapeutic alliance, Linda reported a continuing dream of feeling as if her body was being merged with that of another. The other body, which she could not identify as male or female, was hidden from her and was merging with her from behind. The dream always made her very anxious and woke her up. She said that she didn't know whether this other person was going to hurt her. Linda reported different ideas about

God during this helping phase also, and began to vacillate between seeing God as the traditional male figure of her childhood ("fire and damnation"), and questioning whether God was a woman. She took particular delight in the idea that God might be a Goddess. Linda also talked about being physically attracted to me, but didn't think she was attracted to women in general. When I explored whether she felt this way all of the time or when she felt I understood her, she answered that it seemed to be more about tenderness and closeness then about sex.

During the final helping phase, Linda was working and taking fairly good care of herself, although junk food was still a favorite. She experimented with different hairstyles and colors and even had her daughter "do" her hair. Linda reported less of a need to be in the middle of gossip and conflicts at the factory; however, she was never very far "out of the loop." Linda still called the psychic, which she felt was like talking to a good friend that she had known for years and years. She said she didn't know whether she believed his predictions, but she said, "I just feel good after talking with him." At this point in our work, Linda reported the dream had continued but the danger part of the dream was gone – that the merging part felt good. Ultimately she decided the figure had my face and the dreams stopped. In time, we negotiated a termination date with the understanding that she could return for treatment when needed and how to identify when and how she would know it was time to call for an appointment.

The work with Linda illustrates the essential simultaneous attention to intrapsychic, inter-personal and environmental dynamics required in the work with clients with borderline personality disorder. Linda's style of relating to others – friends, family and work colleagues was mirrored in the work with the social worker. The latter's willingness to work on behalf of the client in her own environment (e.g. writing a letter to her employer, providing for crisis coverage) conveyed to Linda her willingness to "be with her" – a critical stance when working with a client who struggles with issues of trust and fears of abandonment. The work with Linda involved a psychodynamic foundation that attempted to build her "observing ego" and utilize existing ego strengths. Her strengths included motivation to relate to others, motivation to improve how she felt since she felt so bad much of the time, determination and intelligence (as evidenced by her working for and obtaining her GED despite very little encouragement and support from others), curiosity about people and spiritual ideas and experiences, a sense of humor that served to connect her with others when she wasn't feeling so frightened they would leave her or hurt her, reality testing when not in a crisis, and an appreciation of history and staying connected to the community (she enjoyed visiting older cemeteries and working on her family genealogy). Ego defenses included denial, projection, splitting, projective identification, and repression. By utilizing Linda's cognitive strengths, we were able to understand the process of "tracking the triggers" (Demos, 1996) to help her have better control over her own thoughts, feelings, and behavior. Such techniques also enhanced the therapeutic relationship and allowed her to talk with me about any misunderstandings. Understanding about transference was critical for me to stay affectively attuned to Linda and the "shifting affective states" that usually produced self-destructive actions. Also, understanding the transference helped me manage my own frustration and anger at her for being in a crisis so much and calling me, and the discomfort with her intensity and perceptiveness about my feelings and me. By understanding my own reactions and/or countertransference, I became genuinely fond of Linda and supportive of all of her efforts for growth. Many times I was amazed at what she had survived and what internal resources kept her going despite numerous potentially debilitating obstacles. Her resiliency was remarkable. The use of both psychodynamic theory and cognitive-behavioral techniques allowed us to take advantage of her strengths to attend to her vulnerabilities and self-destructiveness. My experience working with Linda is not an atypical one. Many clients like Linda who initially present as both overwhelmed and overwhelming are able to make significant gains when provided with long-term, consistent, and comprehensive interventions. This may include individual work, environmental intervention, medication and crisis stabilization supports.

Conclusion

As the mental health field gradually moves in a direction that builds on interdisciplinary collaboration and a renewed appreciation of holistic approaches, social workers are well positioned to take the lead in treatment with personality conditions. The publication of "Ghosts in the nursery" (Fraiberg et al., 1975) resulted from research conducted when social workers integrated what they had learned from psychodynamic theory and applied it with clients in their home settings. Historically, we have understood the need for viewing the client in his or her own context and as a unique configuration of biology, psychology, sociology, cognitions, and spirit. When we have viewed the dominant risk factors present in the environment, we have advocated for social change to reduce these risks. Likewise, we have helped in clinics that have offered "wrap-around" services for the person-in-their-situation. Research has supported this understanding in terms of utilizing theories and techniques that offer unique "pairings" to accommodate the complexity of personality disorder conditions. Social workers are needed at this critical juncture in history to advocate for better funding for services for this often mistreated population and to publish the results of these holistic interventions.

Web resources

Guilford Press
www.guilford.com/pr/jnpd.htm

Journal of Psychotherapy Practice and Research
www.jppr.psychiatryonline.org

Mayo Clinic
www.mayoclinic.com

Medline Plus
www.medlineplus.com

Mental Help
www.mentalhelp.net

Psychiatry Online
www.psychiatryonline.com

References

Adler, G. (1973). Helplessness in the helper. *British Journal of Medical Psychology, 45*, 315–326.

Alexander, F.G., & Selesnick, S.T. (1966). *The history of psychiatry: An evaluation of psychiatric thought and practice from prehistoric times to the present.* New York: Harper & Row.

American Psychiatric Association (APA). (1980). *Diagnostic and statistical manual of mental disorders* (3rd ed.). Washington, DC: APA.

American Psychiatric Association (APA). (1987). *Diagnostic and statistical manual of mental disorders* (3rd ed., revision). Washington, DC: APA.

American Psychiatric Association (APA). (1994). *Diagnostic and statistical manual of mental disorders* (4th ed.). Washington, DC: APA.

American Psychiatric Association (APA). (2000). *Diagnostic and statistical manual of mental disorders* (4th ed., text revision). Washington, DC: APA.

Arend, P. (2004). Book review: Women and borderline personality disorder. *Critical Sociology, 30* (2), 549–552.

Balsis, S., Gleason, M., Woods, C., & Oltmanns, T. (2007). An item response theory analysis of DSM-IV personality disorder criteria across younger and older age groups. *Psychology and Aging, 22* (1), 171–185.

Bartholomew, K., Kwong, M.J., & Hart, S.D. (2001). Attachment. In W.J. Livesley (ed.) *Handbook of personality disorders: Theory, research, and treatment* (pp. 196–230). New York: Guilford Press.

Beck, A.T., Freeman, A., & Associates. (1990). *Cognitive therapy of personality disorders.* New York: Guilford Press.

Bentley, K.J., Harrison, D.F., & Hudson, W.W. (1993). The impending demise of "designer diagnoses": Implications for the use of concepts in practice. *Research on Social Work Practice, 3* (4), 462–470.

Berkowitz, S.J. (2003). Children exposed to community violence: The rationale for early intervention. *Clinical Child and Family Psychology Review, 6* (4), 293–302.

Blanck, G., & Blanck, R. (1994). *Ego psychology: Theory and practice.* New York: Columbia University Press.

Bowlby, J. (1973). *Attachment and loss: Vol. 2. Separation.* New York: Basic Books.

Bowlby, J. (1980). *Attachment and loss: Vol. 3. Loss.* New York: Basic Books.

Bowlby, J. (1982). *Attachment and loss: Vol. 1. Attachment.* New York: Basic Books.

Bunce, S.C., Noblett, K.L., McCloskey, M.S., & Coccaro, E.F. (2005) High prevalence of personality disorders among healthy volunteers for research: Implications for control group bias. *Journal of Psychiatric Research, 39* (4), 421–430.

Carnegie, D. (1936). *How to win friends and influence people.* New York: Simon & Schuster.

Clark, L.A., Livesley, W.J., & Morey, L. (1997). Personality disorder assessment: The challenge of construct validity. *Journal of Personality Disorders, 11,* 205–231.

Cloninger, C.R. (1986). A unified biosocial theory of personality and its role in the development of anxiety states. *Psychiatric Developments, 3,* 167–226.

Cloninger, C.R. (1987). A systematic method for clinical description and classification of personality variants. *Archives of General Psychiatry, 44,* 573–588.

Coccaro, E.F., Siever, L.J., Owen, K.R., & Davis, K.L. (1990). Serotonin in mood and personality disorders. In E.F. Coccaro & D.L. Murphy (eds), *Serotonin in major psychiatric disorders* (pp. 69–97). Washington, DC: American Psychiatric Press.

Crawford, M.J., Price, K., Gordon, F., Josson, M., Taylor, B., Bateman, A. et al. (2009). Engagement and retention in specialist services for people with personality disorder. *Acta Psychiatrica Scandinavica, 119* (4), 304–311.

Davidson, R.J., Putnam, K., & Larson, C.L. (2000). Dysfunction in the neural circuitry of emotion regulation: A possible prelude to violence. *Science, 289* (5479), 591–594.

Demos, V. (1996). *Affect and the developmental process.* Hillsdale, NJ: Analytic Press.

Dolan-Sewell, R.T., Krueger, R.F., & Shea, M.T. (2001). Co-occurrence with syndrome disorders. In W.J. Livesley (ed.). *Handbook of personality disorders: Theory, research and treatment* (pp. 84–104). New York: Guilford Press.

Eisenberger, L. (1986). When is a case a case? In M. Rutter, C.E. Izard & P.B. Readrd (eds), *Depression in young people* (pp. 469–478). New York: Guilford Press.

Elin, M.R. (2004). The role of trauma, memory, neurobiology, and the self in the formation of personality disorders. In J.J. Magnavita (ed.), *Handbook of personality disorders: Theory and practice* (pp. 443–464). New York: John Wiley & Sons.

Elson, M. (1988). *Self psychology in clinical social work.* New York: Norton.

Fraiberg, S., Edelson, E., & Shapiro, V. (1975). Ghosts in the nursery: A psychoanalytic approach to the problems of impaired infant-mother relationships. *Journal of the American Academy of Child Psychiatry, 14* (3), 387–421.

Fromm, E. (1955). *The sane society.* New York: Holt, Rinehart, & Winston.

Goldstein, E. (1984). *Ego psychology and social work practice.* New York: The Free Press.

Goldstein, E. (1990). *Borderline disorders: Clinical models and techniques.* New York: Guilford Press.

Golomb, M., Fava, M., Abraham, M., & Rosenbaum, J.F. (1995). Gender differences in personality disorders. *American Journal of Psychiatry, 152,* 579–582.

Grant, B.F., Hasin, D.S., Stinson, F.S., Dawson, D.A., Chou, S.P., Ruan, W.J., & Pickering, R.P. (2004). Co-occurrence of 12-month mood and anxiety disorders and personality disorders in the US: Results from the national epidemiologic survey on alcohol and related conditions. *Journal of Clinical Psychiatry, 65* (7), 948–958.

Gunderson, J. (2007). Disturbed relationships as a phenotype for borderline personality disorder: A commentary. *American Journal of Psychiatry, 164* (11), 1637–1640.

Hartmann, H. (1958). *Ego psychology and the problem of adaptation.* New York: Columbia University Press.

Holmes, T.H., & Rahe, R.H. (1967). The Social Readjustment Rating Scale. *Journal of Psychosomatic Research, 11* (2), 213–218.

Horney, K. (1940). *The neurotic personality of our time.* New York: W.W. Norton.

Ingram, R.E., & Price, J.M. (2010). *Vulnerability to psychopathology: Risk across the lifespan.* New York: Guilford Press.

Kagan, J. (1994). *Galen's prophecy.* New York: Basic Books.

Kirk, S., Wakefield, J.C., Hsieh, D.K., & Pottick, K.J. (1999). Social context and social workers' judgment of mental disorder. *Social Service Review, 73* (1), 82–104.

Kohut, H. (1984). *How does analysis cure?* (eds) A. Goldberg & P. Stepansky. Chicago, IL: University of Chicago Press

Kraeplin, E. (1905). *Lectures on clinical psychiatry.* London: Ballière Tindall.

Krampen, G. (2009). Psychotherapeutic processes and outcomes in outpatient treatment of antisocial behavior: An integrative psychotherapy approach. *Journal of Psychotherapy Integration, 19* (3), 213–230.

Leichsenring, F., & Leibring, E. (2003). The effectiveness of psychodynamic therapy and cognitive-behavior therapy in the treatment of personality disorders: A meta-analysis. *American Journal of Psychiatry, 160* (7), 1223–1232.

Lenzenweger, M.F., Lane, M.C., Loranger, A.W., & Kessler, R.C. (2007). DSM-IV personality disorders in the National Comorbidity Survey Replication. *Biological Psychiatry, 62* (6), 553–564.

Liberman, R.P. (1982). Reply: What is schizophrenia? *Schizophrenia Bulletin, 8* (3), 435–437.

Liberman, R.P. (1987). *Psychiatric rehabilitation of chronic mental patients.* Washington, DC: American Psychiatric Publishing.

Liberman, R.P. (2006). Caveats for psychiatric rehabilitation. *World Psychiatry, 5* (3), 158–159.

Liberman, R.P. (2009). *From disability to recovery: Manual of psychiatric rehabilitation.* Washington, DC: American Psychiatric Publishing.

Liberman, R.P., Kopelowicz, A., & Silverstein, S. (2004). Psychiatric rehabilitation. In B.J. Sadock & V.A. Sadock (eds), *Comprehensive textbook of psychiatry* (8th ed., pp. 3884–3930). Baltimore, MD: Lippincott Williams & Wilkins.

Linehan, M. (1993). *Cognitive-behavioral treatment of borderline personality disorder.* New York: Guilford Press.

Livesley, W.J. (2001). Conceptual and taxonomic issues. In W.J., Livesley (ed.) *Handbook of personality disorders: Theory, research, and treatment* (pp. 3–38). New York: Guilford Press.

Livesley, W.J. (2008). Integrated therapy for complex cases of personality disorder. *Journal of Clinical Psychology, 64* (2), 207–221.

Livesley, W.J., Schroeder, M.L., Jackson, D.N., & Jang, K. (1994). Categorical distinctions in the study of personality disorder: Implications for classification. *Journal of Abnormal Psychology, 103*, 6–17.

Magnavita, J.J. (ed.). (2004). *Handbook of personality disorders: Theory and practice.* New York: John Wiley & Sons.

Markovitz, P. (2001). Pharmacotherapy. In W.J. Livesley (ed.) *Handbook of personality disorders: Theory, research, and treatment* (pp. 475–493). New York: Guilford Press.

Mattia, J.I. & Zimmerman, M. (2001). Epidemiology. In W.J. Livesley (ed.) *Handbook of personality disorders: Theory, research, and treatment* (pp. 107–123). New York: Guilford Press.

Maxmen, J.S., Ward, N.G., & Kilgus, M. (2009). *Essential psychopathology and its treatment* (3rd ed.) New York: W.W. Norton.

MegaLinks in Criminal Justice. Retrieved December 19, 2009 from http://www.apsu.edu/oconnort/crim/crimthoery08.htm

Meyer, A. (1957). *Psychobiology.* Springfield, IL: Charles C. Thomas.

Millon, T. (1999). Personality: Guided therapy. In T. Millon, R. Davis, C. Millon, L. Escovar, & S. Meagher (eds), *Personality disorders in modern life.* Hoboken, NJ: John Wiley & Sons.

Millon, T., & Davis, R. (2000). *Personality disorders in modern life.* New York: John Wiley & Sons.

Millon, T., & Grossman, S. (2007). *Moderating severe personality disorders: A personalized psychotherapy approach.* Hoboken, NJ: John Wiley & Sons.

Millon, T., Meagher, S.E., & Grossman, S.D. (2001). Theoretical perspectives. In W.J. Livesley (ed.) *Handbook of personality disorders: Theory, research, and treatment* (pp. 39–59). New York: Guilford Press.

Nakash-Eisikovits, O., Dutra, L., & Westen, D. (2002). Relationship between attachment patterns and personality pathology in adolescents. *Journal of American Academy of Child and Adolescent Psychiatry, 41* (9), 1111–1123.

Newhill, C.E., Mulvey, E.P., & Pilkonis, P.A. (2004). Initial development of a measure of emotional dysregulation for individuals with Cluster B personality disorders. *Research on Social Welfare Practice, 14* (6), 443–449.

Paris, J. (1996). *Social factors in the personality disorders: A biopsychosocial approach to etiology and treatment.* Cambridge: Cambridge University Press.

Paris, J. (1997). Social factors in the personality disorders. *Transcultural Psychiatry, 34* (4), 421–452.

Reich, D.B., & Zanarini, M.C. (2008). Sexual orientation and relationship choice in borderline personality disorder over ten years of prospective follow-up. *Journal of Personality Disorders, 22* (6), 564–572.

Reich, W. (1933, reprinted 1972). *Character analysis.* New York: Farrar, Straus, & Giroux.

Rottman, B.M., Alin, W-K., Sanislow, C.A., & Kim, N.S. (2009). Can clinicians recognize DSM-IV personality disorders from five-factor model descriptions of patient cases? *American Journal of Psychiatry, 166*, 427–433.

Schneider, K. (1950). *Psychopathic personalities* (9th ed.) London: Cassell.

Schore, A.N. (2003). *Affect regulation and disorders of the self.* New York: W.W. Norton.

Schore, A.N., & Schore, J.R. (2008). Modern attachment theory: The central role of affect regulation in development and treatment. *Clinical Social Work Journal, 36*, 9–20.

Siegel, D.J. (1999). *The developing mind: Toward a neurobiology of interpersonal experience.* New York: Guilford Press.

Siegel, D.J. (2007). *The mindful brain: Reflection and attunement in the cultivation of well-being.* New York: Guilford Press.

Skodol, A.E., & Bender, D.S. (2009). The future of personality disorders in DSM-V? *American Journal of Psychiatry, 166*, 388–391.

Stinson, F.S., Dawson, D.A., Goldstein, R.B., Chou, S.P., Huang, B., Smith, S.M. et al. (2008). Prevalence, correlates, disability, and comorbidity of DSM-IV narcissistic personality disorder: Results from the Wave 2 National Epidemiologic survey on alcohol and related conditions. *Journal of Clinical Psychiatry, 69*, 1033–1045.

Stone, M.H. (1997). *Healing the mind: A history of psychiatry from antiquity to the present.* New York: W.W. Norton.

Stone, M.H. (2001). Natural history and long-term outcome. In W.J. Livesley (ed.) *Handbook of personality disorders: Theory, research and treatment* (pp. 259–273). New York: Guilford Press.

Suliman, S., Stein, D.J., Seedat, S., & Williams, D.R. (2008). DSM-IV personality disorders and their Axis I correlates in the South African population. *Psychopathology, 41* (6), 356–364.

Thuo, J., Ndetei, D.M., Maru, H., & Kuria, M. (2008). The prevalence of personality disorders in a Kenyan inpatient sample. *Journal of Personality Disorders, 22* (2), 217–220.

Tronick, E.Z. (2007). *The neurobehavioral and social emotional development of infants and children.* New York: W.W. Norton.

Ulrich, S., & Coid, J. (2009). The age distribution of self-reported personality disorder traits in a household population, *Journal of Personality Disorders 23* (2), 187–200.

Vinnars, B., Thormahlen, B., Gallop, R., Noren, K., & Barber, J.P. (2009). Do personality problems improve during psychodynamic supportive expressive psychotherapy? Secondary outcome results from a RCT for psychiatric outpatients with personality disorders. *Psychotherapy: Theory, Research, Practice, Training, 46* (3), 362–375.

Weertman, A., & Arntz, A. (2007). Effectiveness of treatment of childhood memories in cognitive therapy for personality disorders: A controlled study contrasting methods focusing on the present and methods focusing on childhood memories. *Behaviour Research and Therapy, 45* (9), 2133–2143.

Westen, D. (1985). *Self and society: Narcissism, collectivism and the development of morals.* New York: Cambridge University Press.

Widiger, T.A. (1998). Invited essay: Sex biases in the diagnosis of personality disorders. *Journal of Personality Disorders, 12* (2), 95–118.

Williams, J.W. (1985). The multiaxial system of DSM-III: Where did it come from and where should it go? *Archives of General Psychiatry, 42* (2), 175–180.

Winston, A., Laikin, M., Pollack, J., Samstag, L.W., McCullough, L., & Muran, C. (1994). Short-term psychotherapy of personality disorders. *American Journal of Psychiatry, 15* (2), 190–194.

Wirth-Cauchon, J. (2001). *Women and borderline personality disorder: Symptoms and stories.* New Brunswick, NJ: Rutgers University Press.

Zubin, J., & Spring, B. (1977). Vulnerability: A new view of schizophrenia. *Journal of Abnormal Psychology, 86*, 103–126.

19 Psychotic conditions

Ellen P. Lukens and Lydia P. Ogden

The term psychosis invokes fear and stigma, not surprising given that a dictionary definition is *fundamental mental derangement, characterized by defective or lost contact with reality* (Merriam-Webster Online Dictionary, 2009). Derived from the Latin and Greek word *psychosis*, or *principle of life*, psychosis affects the very core of a person's life, the sense or experience of *self*. Psychotic disorders include a number of mental health conditions ranging from schizophrenia and schizoaffective disorder to psychotic disorders that are relatively brief, substance induced, or due to a general medical condition (American Psychiatric Association (APA), 2000). The overarching description covers several dimensions, including, first, psychotic symptoms, particularly delusions, hallucinations, and disorganized speech that are reflective of a distorted reality; second, interference with ability to function at school, work, at home; and third, documented duration of symptoms (APA, 2000).

The widespread fear and stigma associated with psychosis may also come from the disturbing, and real, images of large inpatient psychiatric institutions where significant numbers of people in the United States with serious psychotic disorders were housed for large parts of their lives until the 1980s (Harvey, 2005; Mechanic, 2008). Although conditions varied among institutions, treatment of the inhabitants was generally ineffective and often abusive. Some developed an institutionalized syndrome, characterized by apathy and limited ability to perform basic tasks of community living even when other symptoms had remitted. Reformers concluded that treatment in institutions had worse effects than the mental illnesses themselves. The deinstitutionalization movement, beginning in full during the 1970s, led to the eventual closing of the vast majority of those hospitals (Mechanic, 2008). Unfortunately, inadequate community care for many of those discharged led to homelessness, substance abuse, and, for their families, instrumental and emotional burden (Mechanic, 2008). However, these failures triggered improved research, interventions, support for and understanding of persons with psychotic disorders, as well as an advocacy movement led by persons with mental illnesses who called themselves *consumers* (Anthony, 1993). This movement, supported now by policies outlined in the President's New Freedom Act, promotes the idea that *recovery* from mental illness is not just a possibility, but a right (Farone, 2006; Mechanic, 2008).

In this chapter, we present a broad overview of how we understand psychotic disorders today, and the evidence-based and promising practices for persons diagnosed with the most severe forms of psychosis. We address the complex hurdles that the psychotic disorders present for persons with illness, their families and other informal caregivers, and for mental health providers and policy makers at both the federal and local level. We discuss the important role for social workers in building, implementing, and advocating for recovery-oriented programs and policies that focus on strengths and opportunities while simultaneously attending to symptoms, challenges, and need.

Definitions of psychotic illnesses

Psychosis can be defined broadly as a schism between person and reality. While most commonly associated with the diagnosis of *schizophrenia*, psychosis can occur in a variety of contexts. In addition to *schizophrenia* and *schizoaffective disorders, brief psychotic disorder, delusional disorder, schizophreniform disorder* and *shared psychotic disorder* also belong to the group of illnesses wherein psychotic symptoms are central to the diagnosis. In this chapter, we particularly focus on schizophrenia and the schizoaffective disorders, the most debilitating of the psychotic disorders.

Although the exact etiology remains unknown, current thought attributes schizophrenia and schizoaffective disorders to the interaction between inherited genetic factors and environmental stressors that activate potentially dormant genes, in what is termed the *stress-diathesis* model (Sadock & Sadock, 2003). Schizophrenia and schizoaffective disorder are often termed *severe and persistent mental illnesses* (SPMI) and in fact are considered the *prototypical* severe mental illnesses (Lehman & Steinwachs, 2003). The severity and recurrence of symptoms as well as the long-held assumption that the impact of the disorder will have enduring and disabling consequences contributes to this conceptualization. However, the severe and persistent nature of schizophrenia and schizoaffective disorders is under increasing scrutiny by researchers, clinicians and mental health consumers alike.

While psychotic disorders cause disruption of functioning in multiple areas, affected individuals are no longer defined by their illnesses through all-encompassing terminology such as the outdated and stigmatizing label *schizophrenic*. Instead, as a group such individuals can be referred to as *people with schizophrenia*, or more broadly, *people with psychotic disorders*, language that represents *personhood* and *humanity* in addition to illness. Using humane language is important since stigma and inaccurate images of people with psychotic disorders pervade society through media, folklore, myth, and even the medical system itself (Deegan, 1996). Erroneous but widespread notions include the idea that schizophrenia can be *caused* by street drug use or poor parenting, particularly mothering, and that people with schizophrenia and other psychotic disorders perpetually display dangerous and out of control behavior. The symptoms of the psychotic disorders do not include *split* or *multiple* personalities, terms more aptly applied to the controversial diagnosis of *dissociative identity disorder* (APA, 2000). False understanding and inhumane terminology, used by both the public and professionals, and reinforced by the media, have led to increased community stigma and internalized stigma among those with psychotic disorders.

Diagnostic terminology divides schizophrenia into two symptom categories: positive and negative. Various biomedical and neurological conditions, such as diabetes and impaired insulin tolerance (Cohn, Remington, Zipursky, Azad, Connolly, & Wolever, 2006; Spelman, Walsh, Sharifi, Collins, & Thakore, 2007), neurological signs and involuntary movements (Whitty, Waddington, & Owoeye, 2009) and immune system abnormalities (Rapaport & Delrahim, 2001) are associated with schizophrenia as well, suggesting that schizophrenia may be a systemic illness rather than purely a disorder of the brain (Kirkpatrick, 2009).

In schizophrenia, *positive* symptoms refer to the presence of psychological features that exist only for people with psychotic disorders: hallucinations, delusions, bizarre behavior, disorganized thoughts, and loose associations. Hallucinations are the sensory perceptions of stimuli that do not exist. They are typically auditory although they can range from olfactory and sensory to, rarely, visual (APA, 2000). Delusions are erroneous beliefs that are maintained despite evidence that proves their faulty nature.

Negative symptoms refer to the various psychological features that are present for those without, but lacking for those with schizophrenia and related psychoses. These include impoverished speech, affective flattening, and avolition. While people more commonly associate schizophrenia with positive symptoms, the limited emotional display of affective flattening, the diminished and constrained conversation of impoverished speech, and the decreased goal-directed behavior of avolition are equally pervasive (APA, 2000). While positive symptoms are targeted increasingly well by antipsychotic medications, negative symptoms are not generally improved by the currently available medications, and can have enduring and disabling consequences. The various combinations of positive and negative symptoms, termed the *symptom structure*, as well as the content of any hallucinations and delusions, contribute to the various subtypes of schizophrenia. These include *paranoid, disorganized, catatonic,* and *undifferentiated* types (APA, 2000). Research suggests that generalized cognitive impairment is also an integral part of schizo-phrenia, since the illness affects such broad areas as cognitive ability, attention, memory, processing speeds and problem solving (Dickinson & Harvey, 2009). Cognitive functioning tends to decrease around the time of onset of illness, affecting particularly areas of memory, attention and organization (Palmer et al., 1997). Some studies suggest that fewer than 30 percent of clinically stable people with schizophrenia have normal cognitive functioning, contributing significantly to ongoing disability (Dickinson & Harvey, 2009; Shad, Tamminga, Cullum, Haas, & Keshavan, 2006).

The convergence of positive and negative symptoms and cognitive impairment typically leads to a loss of functioning in more than one important area, although the APA diagnostic criteria for schizophrenia require only one (APA, 2000). Tasks that people without schizo-phrenia take for granted, such as sustaining adequate housing through regular rent payment and maintenance, and activities of daily living (ADLs), such as bathing, cooking, and cleaning, may require training and assistance to overcome. When such basic life skills are compromised, affected persons are left with lowered self-esteem and self-efficacy, and increased vulnerability to life stressors and stigma (Mueser, Valentiner, & Agresta, 1997).

Those with *schizoaffective disorder* meet criteria for both schizophrenia and an affective disorder, and as such the diagnosis is divided into *depressive* and *bipolar* subtypes (APA, 2000). Differential diagnosis among schizoaffective disorder, mood disorders with psychotic features, and schizophrenia (which may at times include the presentation of both depressed and elevated moods) is difficult and historically unreliable because identical symptoms may appear in each of those illnesses at various points in time (Lake & Hurwitz, 2007). Psychosis can be considered a marker of severity of the mood disorder in some cases; however, the psychotic symptoms usually clear upon mood stabilization (APA, 2000; Austrian, 2005). In schizoaffective disorder and schizophrenia, psychotic symptoms may remain after clearing of the mood symptoms (Walker, Mittal, Tessner, & Trotman, 2008).

Shared psychotic disorder, known more commonly by its French name *folie à deux*, is the only form of mental illness that occurs between two people. According to the DSM-IV, it emerges when a person with an existing psychotic disorder featuring prominent delusions (the *primary* case) develops a close or symbiotic relationship with another. This other is usually in a *subordinate* relationship to the primary person, and comes to share the delusional beliefs of the primary over time. Shared psychotic disorder is only a valid diagnosis when the subordinate person's delusional material is not better accounted for by another psychiatric diagnosis. It is extremely rare, under-studied, and with unknown etiology or course (APA, 2000).

The documentary entitled *Grey gardens* about a mother–daughter duo, both named Edith Beale, and referred to as big Edie and little Edie, movingly portrays this illness (Maysles, Maysles, Hovde, & Meyer, 1976). In this case, the mother is the primary who shows paranoid ideation and agoraphobic behavior with psychotic overtones. The daughter is the subordinate who, for reasons incomprehensible to the viewer, voluntarily joins the mother in isolation and squalor in a large house that they are unable to maintain. As is often the case, it is hard to discern who is subordinate and who is primary, as the daughter appears to have psychotic symptoms as well. Traditionally, treatment has involved separating the duo, resulting in a remission of symptoms in the subordinate (APA, 2000; Austrian, 2005). In the case of the Beales, the daughter sold the home after her mother's death and went on to have a more social and active life, spending time with family and even performing on stage in New York, suggesting a remission of what appeared to be paranoid and phobic symptoms (Martin, 2002; Wilson, 2003).

Other psychotic disorders are more transient and therefore may be somewhat less disruptive. Those who present with the full range of symptoms for less than six months may be diagnosed with *schizophreniform disorder*. After six months, the diagnosis may be changed to schizophrenia (APA, 2000). A diagnosis of *brief psychotic disorder* is determined by the length of symptoms (more than 1 day, less than 30 days) and distinguished by an absence of negative symptoms or cognitive impairment. *Delusional disorder* similarly precludes the presence of negative symptoms or the existence of hallucinations, disorganized speech, grossly disorganized behavior, or catatonic behavior, but is not bounded by time.

A *psychotic disorder due to a general medical condition* is known to coincide with more than 20 medical and neurological illnesses, ranging from Huntington's disease to vitamin B-12 deficiency (Sadock & Sadock, 2003), and can contribute to misdiagnosis or uneven management of the medical illness (Patkar, Mago, & Masand, 2004). These forms of psychosis are often treatable with interventions that target the medical illness. People may experience *substance-induced psychosis* when prescribed medications are incorrectly dosed or mixed with other incompatible drugs. Substance-induced psychosis may also occur when prescription, illicit drugs and/or alcohol are abused. The condition typically subsides once the substance has passed through the system; however, complication occurs when medications that are required to maintain physical health contribute to the psychotic symptoms, such as may happen in Parkinson's disease (Wint, Okun, & Fernandez, 2004). In such cases medications for the physical health condition may be decreased or changed, and/or antipsychotic medications may be introduced (Wint et al., 2004).

Important aspects of psychotic disorders in general and schizophrenia in particular, are not captured within the current diagnostic criteria but are nonetheless central to treatment. Psychotic disorders affect individuals in unique ways. As such, while the symptoms have common modes of expression, the same diagnosis can look very different in different people, with diverse outcomes and functioning at various points over the life course (APA, 2000; U.S. Department of Health and Human Services, 1999). Each individual will have greater or lesser severity of symptoms, diverse content in hallucinatory and delusional material, and will respond to symptoms and diagnoses in ways that are influenced by pre-morbid personality factors (APA, 2000; Birchwood, Iqbal, & Upthegrove, 2005; Bradshaw & Brekke, 1999), social supports and environment, stigmatizing beliefs about mental illness (Lysaker, Daroyanni, Ringer, Beattie, Strasburger, & Davis, 2007a), and cultural and ethnic variation (APA, 2000). As one adult sibling of a person with schizophrenia observed, *the personality customizes the disease* (Lukens, 2001).

People with psychotic disorders also vary greatly in regard to post-psychotic depression. Although not part of the diagnostic criteria, post-psychotic depression is common after first episodes of psychosis and is a leading factor in the high rate of suicides and suicide attempts among this population, particularly within the first year of illness (Addington, Williams, Young, & Addington, 2004). Often symptoms of post-psychotic depression, or of depression concurrent with schizophrenia, are confused with the negative symptoms and thus tend to be under-diagnosed and under-treated (Buckley, Miller, Lehrer, & Castle, 2009; Wittmann & Keshavan, 2007).

Another aspect of psychotic disorders that is highly individuated is that of awareness of illness, the lack of which is termed *anosognosia*. Up to 50 percent of those diagnosed with schizophrenia-type illnesses do not have *insight* into their mental illness (Amador & Paul-Odouard, 2000). The very mechanism with which one might evaluate the veracity of psychic material, the mind, is compromised. The experience of hallucinations and delusions is very real. So it follows that insight, as evaluated through objective measures, could be compromised as well. Although those with better insight have improved functional outcomes, they tend also to have more depressive symptoms, including decreased self-esteem and hopelessness. Since those with less insight experience lower rates of post-psychotic depression and attempt suicide less frequently, lack of or limited insight actually may serve as a form of defense. Yet limited insight is also associated with poor treatment adherence and low rates of recovery (Lysaker, Roe, & Yanos, 2007b).

As scientists develop a better understanding of the lived experience of schizophrenia, the understanding of the role of insight has deepened. Insight is no longer considered dichotomous, wherein one has it or does not, but rather a complex process. In a recent narrative analysis, participants variously accepted their illness but rejected the diagnostic label, rejected the illness entirely and searched for other ways to name their experience (which they typically acknowledged as outside the norm), had passive insight, or actively sought to integrate the diagnosis with their experience in a dynamic way (Roe, Hasson-Ohayon, Kravetz, Yanos, & Lysaker, 2008).

Regardless of level of insight, people generally recognize that their lives have changed dramatically as psychosis evolves or resolves, and struggle to cope with the associated losses (Birchwood et al., 2005; Wittmann & Keshavan, 2007).

Demographics

Men are about 1.42 times more likely to develop schizophrenia than women, and their age of onset is about three to four years earlier (Seeman, 2008). Psychotic disorders are seen cross-culturally and among all *racial and ethnic groupings*, as well as in developing and industrialized countries (Walker et al., 2008). Schizophrenia is estimated to affect 1 percent of the population across racial and ethnic groupings world-wide (APA, 2000; Walker et al., 2008). Schizoaffective disorder appears to have a slightly lower lifetime prevalence rate of 0.5 to 0.8 percent (APA, 2000).

Life course   Onset can occur at any time in the lifespan, although schizophrenia and schizoaffective disorders are generally considered illnesses of late adolescence and young adulthood, with females typically having a slightly later onset than males (APA, 2000). Childhood schizophrenia and onset of schizophrenia after 35 are rare but do occur (Hodgman, 2006; Sadock & Sadock, 2003).

Although *treatment adherence* to medication is associated with improved functional outcomes for the schizophrenia-type illnesses, more than 40 percent discontinue medication during the first nine months of treatment after a first psychotic episode (B. Miller, 2008). In the Clinical Antipsychotic Trials (CATIE) that compared the differential efficacy of antipsychotics, only 26 percent of the sample completed the 18-month drug trial (Manschreck & Boshes, 2007). Discontinuation appeared to be related to intolerability of side effects, fears about drug safety, and questions as to whether the medicines actually improved symptoms (Glazer, Conley, & Citrome, 2006).

Persons with schizophrenia are at an increased risk of *suicide*. Estimates suggest that between 4.9 percent (Palmer, Pankratz, & Bostwick, 2005) and 13 percent (Schwartz & Cohen, 2001a) will commit suicide within the first ten years of illness, while between 17 percent and 50 percent will attempt suicide (Addington et al., 2004; Bromet, Bushra, Fochtmann, Carlson, & Tanenberg-Karant, 2005; Meltzer, 2001). Suicide risk is associated with depressive symptoms and previous suicide attempts, male gender, younger age, earlier onset and stage of illness, good premorbid functioning, and recent experience of traumatic events (Addington et al., 2004; Schwartz & Cohen, 2001b).

Violence has been erroneously over-associated with schizophrenia through media sensationalization. While there is a 7.3 percent lifetime prevalence of violence among members of the general population, people with any form of severe mental illness have a 16.1 percent lifetime prevalence of violence (Swanson, 1994). This contributes to about 3–5 percent of violence in the United States overall, and is considerably lower than the risk of violence from those without psychotic disorders who are abusing or dependent upon illicit drugs or alcohol. For a person with schizophrenia, risk of violence is moderated by personality and symptom factors, and can be significantly decreased by adherence to antipsychotic medications as well as abstinence from street drugs and alcohol (Swanson et al., 2006; Swanson, Van Dorn, Swartz, Smith, Elbogen, & Monahan, 2008).

In the United States, people with severe mental health conditions are more likely to be *incarcerated* than admitted to a psychiatric hospital (Mechanic, 2007). Since people with psychotic disorders are no longer hospitalized for long periods of time, prisons and jails have virtually replaced hospitals as the holding area for many individuals, particularly those labeled as difficult to manage or non-compliant (Lamberti & Weisman, 2004). When effective community programs are minimal or lacking and access to street drugs and alcohol increases, comorbidity psychosis and substance abuse increases, often associated with imprisonment for non-violent and substance abuse related crimes (Mechanic, 2007; Munetz, Grande, & Chambers, 2001).

Housing for persons with mental illness has been a long-standing problem, particularly for those who may not have the skills necessary to maintain an apartment independently and yet do not require inpatient psychiatric care. As many as 42.3 percent of those who are homeless in the United States, Canada and Western Europe meet criteria for a psychotic disorder (Fazel, Khosla, Doll, & Geddes, 2008).

Because onset is typically in late adolescence or early adulthood, many people with schizophrenia do not complete high school or college, and tend to have *high rates of unemployment*. Lack of skills and potential disruptions or disability stemming from psychiatric symptoms, as well as the high rates of physical health comorbidity, contribute to the lower employment rates among this population (Waghorn, Lloyd, Abraham, Silvester, & Chant, 2008). Only 10–30 percent are employed in competitive settings and less than 25 percent receive any kind of vocational support (Bond et al., 2001a; Bond, Resnick, Drake, Xie, McHugo, & Bebout, 2001b). Approximately two-thirds of all persons with serious mental illness receive insurance through Medicare or Medicaid and financial support through Supplemental Security Income (SSI) or Social Security Disability Insurance (SSDI), with costs incurred to the insurances increasing with age and duration of illness (Bartels, Clark, Peacock, Dums, & Pratt, 2003).

Medical comorbidities present a substantial burden for a large proportion of this population, who may have limited access to medical or dental services (Carney, Jones, & Woolson, 2006). Medical conditions not only appear at higher rates than in the general public, but also appear to be more severe and frequently undiagnosed. In the United States, 2.5 percent of *combined* health and mental health expenditures nationwide are for care of persons with schizophrenia, exceeding by far the proportion of the population that they represent (Sadock & Sadock, 2003). Overall, comorbid medical conditions significantly reduce not only the quality of life for people with psychotic disorders and other serious mental illnesses, but also the length of life, on average, by 13 to 20 years (Vreeland, 2007).

Persons with chronic psychotic disorders are more likely than those in the general population to face diabetes, HIV/AIDS, hypertension and heart disease, chronic obstructive pulmonary disease (COPD), and hepatitis B and C (Dixon et al., 2000; Essock et al., 2003; O'Day, Killeen, Sutton, & Iezzoni, 2005). An estimated 75 percent of persons with schizophrenia have at least one co-occurring medical condition, and a significant number have more than one (Rystedt & Bartels, 2008). Risk is further increased because nicotine dependence is significantly more prevalent than among those in the general public (70–90 percent vs. 25 percent), in turn associated with increased risk of emphysema and related pulmonary and cardiac illnesses (Wohlheiter & Dixon, 2008). People with severe mental illness are 22 times as likely to be obese (Dickerson et al., 2006), and incidence of cancer for people with any mental illness, including psychotic disorders, is 2.5 times more than that found in the general population (Pandiani, Boyd, Banks, & Johnson, 2006). At least 15 percent of people with schizophrenia are diabetic, with increased risk among African Americans and Latinos, women, and persons over 55 (Dixon et al., 2000; Kilbourne et al., 2005).

Persons who rely on the antipsychotic medications to control their symptoms also must contend with side effects, creating further health issues (E. Miller, Leslie, & Rosenheck, 2005). For the *first generation* antipsychotics, these can include motor abnormalities such as tardive-dyskinisia (i.e. involuntary movements), and physical reactions that include anticholinergic (e.g. dry membranes, blurred vision, sedation, sexual dysfunction), antiadrenergic (e.g. light-headedness), or extrapyramidal (i.e. slowed movements, shuffling gait, sustained muscle spasms) response patterns (Preston, O'Neal, & Talaga, 2008). Age, duration of treatment with first generation antipsychotics, and substance abuse are among the variables associated with increased risk of tardive-dyskinisia (Cohen et al., 2000; Miller et al., 2005). These side effects can range from minor to debilitating in the extreme and contribute to the fact that non-adherence with medication is a significant factor in relapse of psychosis (Citrome & Stroup, 2006). The more recently developed *second generation* antipsychotics may prove more beneficial for the treatment of psychotic symptoms, but increase risk for diabetes and weight gain.

Schizophrenia also has high rates of *comorbidity with other mental illnesses*, particularly depression and post-traumatic stress syndrome (PTSD). Rates of depressive symptoms during a psychotic episode are about 50 percent (an der Heiden, Konnecke, Maurer, Ropeter, & Hafner, 2005). Psychotic episodes can be traumatic, and in one small study, 61 percent met criteria for PTSD following a first episode of psychosis (Chisholm, Freeman, & Cooke, 2006). For those with additional traumatic experiences beyond the psychosis, such as war veterans, survivors of child abuse, and immigrants from war-torn countries, PTSD rates are increased further, and associated with heightened risk of suicide (Kroll, 2007; Strauss et al., 2006).

For people with schizophrenia, rates of substance abuse or dependence are as high as 47 percent, compared to 16.7 percent for the general population, and for schizophrenia and alcohol abuse or dependence as high as 33.7 percent, compared to 13.5 percent in the general population (Drake, Wallach, Alverson, & Mueser, 2002; Kessler, Nelson, McGonagle, Edlund, Frank, & Leaf, 1996; Regier et al., 1990). Further, alcohol use severity is correlated with severity of medical health issues, particularly pulmonary and cardiovascular illnesses (Batki et al., 2009).

In spite of the multiple challenges faced by persons with psychotic disorders, increased advocacy on the part of persons with mental illnesses and their families, as well as a growing number of clinicians and researchers, has led to the development of what is referred to as the *recovery* model. This forward looking and hopeful model encompasses significantly more than a remission of psychiatric symptoms, and questions to what extent remission is required at all (Anthony, 1993; Bellack, 2006). While schizophrenia and other psychotic disorders are deeply impairing, proponents argue that recovery can occur despite ongoing symptoms and impairment when defined by the values, terms, and goals of the individual (Anthony, 1993; Bellack, 2006; Deegan, 1996).

There is some discordance between the scientific and consumer definitions of recovery (Bellack, 2006). In the consumer recovery model, developing meaningful activity and relation-ships, valued and defined by the person who is affected, are the goals of any pharmacological or psychosocial treatment (Deegan, 2007). From this perspective, recovery involves both managing an illness and *recovering a life* on a person-by-person basis (Padgett, Henwood, Abrams,

& Drake, 2008b), and has less to do with resolution of symptoms (Deegan, 2007; Deegan & Drake, 2006).

In contrast, scientists operationalize recovery in relationship to illness symptoms and their remission. From this standpoint, outcomes are heterogeneous among individuals with psychotic disorders both in the short term and over the life course (APA, 2000; Harrison et al., 2001). In the International Study of Schizophrenia (ISoS), a longitudinal study that included racially, ethnically and globally diverse cohorts, more than half of the study participants were symptomatically recovered 15 years and 25 years after first episode (Harrison et al., 2001). However, when functional capacity was considered, only 37.8 percent of those with schizophrenia met criteria for recovery. In a separate longitudinal study the course of the illness was neither chronic nor continuous for more than 50 percent of participants, with up to 40 percent experiencing episodic periods of symptom relief and improved functioning over time (Harrow, Grossman, Jobe, & Herbener, 2005).

Population

Developmental course and challenges   Since the onset of schizophrenia is typically in early adulthood, individual and familial developmental tasks are interrupted. For the person affected, these include completing education, seeking employment or developing a career, and developing close friendships and romantic relationships with other adults (APA, 2000; McFarlane, Dixon, Lukens, & Lucksted, 2003). Both men and women have lower rates of marriage than the general population, rates consistent with the fact that the illness is characterized by social withdrawal and isolation (APA, 2000; Hutchinson, Bhugra, Mallett, Burnett, Corridan, & Leff, 1999).

Family members play a potentially pivotal role in lives of persons with psychotic disorders when they are able to provide emotional and instrumental care and support (Hall & Purdy, 2000). Although caregiving can be rewarding in some respects, involved families tend to experience psychological and even physical distress (Greenberg, Greenley, McKee, Brown, & Griffin, 1993; Harvey & Burns, 2003; Rossler, Salize, van Os, & Riecher-Rossler, 2005). Burden can be objective, through strained resources and the demands of caregiving, and subjective, through complex emotional response to the illness. Overall burden results from the interaction between the stressful situations and coping strategies of the family members and caretakers, with wide cross-cultural variance in how families and caretakers cope with and experience caregiving responsibilities (Kealey, 2005). Open access to information and support through mental health providers, strong social and community support, and involvement in advocacy organizations such as the National Alliance on Mental Illness (NAMI) can decrease levels of burden and increase resilience among family members (Kealey, 2005; Magliano & et al., 2003).

Approaches to treatment have shifted significantly since the 1960s. While many people benefit from improved psychotropic medications and evidence-based psychosocial interventions, the current cohort of *older adults* with schizophrenia-type illnesses have endured much. Many adults over the age of 55, and perhaps some even younger, survived long-term institutionalization in psychiatric hospitals, with treatments ranging from ineffective to unethical, only to be deinstitutionalized without adequate support or treatment, frequently resulting in homelessness (Harvey, 2005; Mechanic, 2008). Even those who avoided those destinies likely felt more stigma than do today's younger generations, since early etiological theories tended to blame their families, their mothers, or their own self-control. Today, older adults with schizophrenia experience higher rates of disability, in terms of both mental and physical functioning, than do younger persons with schizophrenia or elders in the general population (Sciolla, Patterson, Wetherall, McAdams, & Jeste, 2003).

As many as two-thirds of elderly people with schizophrenia meet criteria for dementia (Arnold, 2001). However, compared to those elders with dementia in the general population who decline at rates of about 10 percent per year, elders with schizophrenia experience cognitive decline at rates of 10 percent per decade, but start at impaired baselines (Harvey, 2005). In post-mortem studies, 30 percent of those with schizophrenia showed evidence of dementia. Thus, cognition and its functional behavioral correlates are of particular concern in this group of seniors.

More than 40 percent of elders with schizophrenia show signs of clinical depression, further linked to poor physical health, low income and decreased social support (Cohen et al., 2000). Rates of diabetes are as high as 29 percent, and in one study, nearly 31 percent of people with schizophrenia over the age of 60 were diagnosed with serious cardiovascular or pulmonary health conditions (Kilbourne et al., 2005). Risk of falls is increased for older people with mental illnesses, including schizophrenia, at rates of 1.5 to 4.5 greater than for those without (Finkelstein, Prabhu, & Chen, 2007).

Limited social functioning and sources of support contribute to ongoing and significant impairment. Among those who are institutionalized, fewer than 10 percent of elders with schizophrenia have ever been married and fewer than 20 percent have ever held a job (Harvey, 2005). A majority lack a close family caregiver (Jeste & Nasrallah, 2003). Of all age-groups of people with schizophrenia, elders are the least likely to receive any form of mental health services (Jin et al., 2003). Persons who are isolated and without proxies may be unable to provide informed consent for treatment, delaying or inhibiting needed services (Dunn, Lindamer, Palmer, Golshan, Schneiderman, & Jeste, 2002; Marson, Savage, & Phillips, 2006).

Mental health care disparities

For a person with psychosis of any age, both assigned diagnosis and access to health care can vary tremendously by circumstance and over time. Diagnoses can fluctuate simply because of impaired cognitive abilities or active psychosis in the person affected, making it difficult for professionals to gather consistent and accurate symptom and psychosocial histories (Royal Australian & New Zealand College of Psychiatrists Clinical Practice Guidelines Team, 2005). When a person is also abusing or using illegal substances or alcohol, accurate diagnosis becomes more challenging (Barnes, 2008). Level of interviewing skill among practitioners also contributes to variability; knowing how to diagnose a person presenting with psychotic symptoms is challenging and can be imprecise, and is further complicated by variation in diagnostic criteria, use of unstructured diagnostic interviews, or cultural or linguistic factors that contribute to distorted assessment (Beauchamp & Gagnon, 2004).

Access to care varies as it does with the general population; those with financial security and a strong network of informal support are more likely to obtain better quality and more consistent services and continuous insurance coverage (Seng, Kohn-Wood, & Odera, 2005; West et al., 2005; Wilk, West, Narrow, Rae, & Regier, 2005). Mental health care access is further limited because parity between health and mental health care services is inconsistent and has only recently emerged as a viable goal for mental health advocates and policy makers (Barry & Ridgely, 2008).

When family members are involved actively in care, the options for the person who is affected are broadened simply because the family can serve as advocate and watchdog (Lukens, 2001; McFarlane et al., 2003). But willingness to access care can be diminished by the stigma attached to the psychotic disorders. Affected persons and their family members may delay or avoid treatment because of fear, stigma, denial, cultural beliefs, or simple lack of information (Schaffner & McGorry, 2001). Such delayed access to treatment is problematic. Duration of untreated psychosis increases the clinical challenges involved in adequately controlling symptoms since those who are acutely psychotic (i.e. *decompensated*) are less able to engage fully in their own treatment and planning (Barnes, Leeson, Mutsatsa, Watt, Hutton, & Joyce, 2008; Royal Australian & New Zealand College of Psychiatrists Clinical Practice Guidelines Team, 2005). In addition, patterns of diagnosis and access to care vary depending on gender, race, ethnicity, cultural perspective, life course, sexual orientation, and position on the continuum between ability and disability.

On average women have higher levels of pre-morbid functioning than men (APA, 2000) and better outcomes in several areas, including overall functioning, longer periods of symptomatic recovery and fewer and shorter hospitalizations (Grossman, Harrow, Rosen, Faull, & Strauss, 2008; Walker et al., 2008). Men with schizophrenia are more likely to carry a diagnosis of comorbid drug or alcohol abuse (Aleman, Kahn, & Selten, 2003), while women are more likely to show increased reactivity to the stresses of daily life (Myin-Germeys, Krabbendam, Delespaul, & van Os, 2004). Women tend to have more symptoms of depression and active hallucinations and delusions associated with their psychoses, while men are more likely to have negative symptoms, particularly social withdrawal and isolation, avolition, and flattened affect (APA, 2000). For women, symptoms may be exacerbated after menopause before leveling off (Myin-Germeys et al., 2004). The long-term prognosis for men and women tends to be about the same.

The over-diagnosis of the psychotic disorders among minority group members in the United States is well documented (Barnes, 2008; Minsky, Vega, Miskimen, Gara, & Escobar, 2003). In the Surgeon General's report *Mental health: culture, race, and ethnicity*, the authors found not only that persons of *non-majority* status use mental health services less than whites, but also when they do use services, these tend to be of poorer quality (U.S. Department of Health and Human Services, 2001). In a large epidemiological study in California, African Americans were approximately three times more likely to be diagnosed with schizophrenia than whites. After controlling for the socioeconomic status of the family at birth, these rates were still about twice as high (Bresnahan et al., 2007). In multiple studies, whites were up to six times more likely than African Americans to be prescribed the currently preferred second-generation antipsychotic medications (Lawson, 2008; Mallinger, Fisher, Brown, & Lamberti, 2006).

An estimated 60 percent of persons of any background and with any form of mental health condition receive no professional help whatsoever. Of those who do receive services, only about 25 percent are treated by specialists in mental health (Kessler et al., 1996). Those of racial or ethnic minority status are among the least likely to be served (Ihara & Takeuchi, 2004; U.S. Department of Health and Human Services, 2001), and once served, less likely to remain in treatment. Adherence further varies by English proficiency among and within ethnic groups (Gilmer et al., 2009).

Multiple factors related to both those in need of services and service providers contribute to limited help-seeking among persons of diverse ethnic and racial background, regardless of diagnosis. For persons affected and their families, these include availability of relevant services, accessibility of care (perceived or actual), stigma, and mistrust of and unfamiliarity with Western approaches to medicine. For providers, they may include cultural biases or limited knowledge, specifically regarding language, traditions, history, religion, values, and beliefs of ethnic group members, and quality and effectiveness of assessment, treatment, and alleviation of symptoms (O'Mahony & Donnelly, 2007; Sue & Sue, 2008).

Issues related to *intimate relationships and sexuality* among persons with psychotic disorders have been overlooked until recently, and minimal information exists on the relationship between the psychotic disorders and sexual orientation. Sexual functioning and sexual risk taking behaviors tend to play out differently for persons with psychotic disorders than for those in the general population, creating unique challenges for intervention. Although sexual activity is comparable (Drescher, 2010; Kopelowicz, Liberman, & Stolar, 2008), sexual functioning generally tends to be diminished among both men and women with schizophrenia, and more so during acute episodes of illness when higher levels of medications are required to treat symptoms (Assalian, Fraser, Tempier, & Cohen, 2000). Because the antipsychotics can interfere with sexual drive, individuals who experience this side effect may be less likely to adhere to a medication regime (Kopelowicz et al., 2008). When treatment adherence rates are low, sexual risk taking tends to increase, associated with high rates of comorbid street drug use and unsafe sexual practices (Koen, Uys, Niehaus, & Emsley, 2007). Simple lack of information may contribute to risk as well. Individuals with schizophrenia are five time more likely to contract hepatitis B and ten times more like to contact hepatitis C than persons in the general population (Cournos, McKinnon, & Sullivan, 2005; Essock et al., 2003).

The picture is more complex for women. They are more likely to have chaotic sexual histories than women in the general population, more sexual partners than men with comparable diagnoses, and sexual experiences characterized more often as non-consensual, violent, unsafe, or sex for trade (Dickerson et al., 2004; Solari, Dickson, & Miller, 2009). They also may have limited knowledge of, or access to, a range of contraceptive options (Solari et al., 2009). In one study, women with schizophrenia had lower rates of pregnancy compared to those without mental illness, but among their pregnancies, higher rates of termination, either due to abortion or miscarriage (Dickerson et al., 2004). When women with psychotic disorders do carry a pregnancy to term, they are faced with the complexities of childbirth, parenthood and childcare that can be challenging under the most ordinary circumstances (L. Miller, 1997). The associated stress may lead to increased symptoms both pre and postpartum (Craig & Bromet, 2004). For mothers with psychotic disorder, estimated loss of child custody ranges from 30 to 70 percent, and few documented services specifically target parenting and childcare (Craig & Bromet, 2004; Hinden, Biebel, Nicholson, Henry, & Katz-Leavy, 2006).

Social work programs and social work roles

To date a series of evidence-based practices (EBPs) that draw on psychosocial intervention strategies have been identified for persons with schizophrenia and the related psychotic disorders. Most involve social workers, either working independently or in collaboration with a cross-disciplinary team. As identified by the Substance Abuse and Mental Health Services Administration (SAMHSA), the six core EBPs include: (1) care coordination, including assertive community treatment (ACT) and intensive case management (ICM), (2) integrated dual-diagnosis treatment (IDDT), (3) family education and psychoeducation, (4) wellness self-management, (5) self-help and peer support services, and (6) supported employment. Medication is also a primary intervention for persons with psychotic disorders. More recently, other programs and interventions have been identified as promising, including housing first programs, supported education, cognitive rehabilitation, shared decision-making, and jail diversion programs.

Assertive community treatment (ACT) is a multifaceted model, including a multidisciplinary team that is on-call 24 hours per day, seven days per week. Social workers typically serve as team leaders or team members, along with nurses, employment specialists, psychiatrists, and more recently, peer educators (Drake, Merrens, & Lynde, 2005). A core element of this model is that each client is known to every staff member, in an effort to ensure ongoing and coordinated care and treatment adherence. Staff members work with ACT clients on every aspect of their lives, from dispensing and monitoring medication to managing finances and diet to securing adequate housing. The ACT teams are open to participants as long as they need the services (Allness & Knoedler, 2003).

Intensive case management (ICM) allows a practitioner to focus on and coordinate the needs and challenges faced by each individual client by building one on one relationships (Pescosolido, Wright, & Sullivan, 1995). Services include advocacy and outreach to promote adherence to treatment and follow-through, assistance with activities of daily living and practical tasks, helping to identify and maintain adequate housing, coordination among providers, and crisis intervention as needed. When the person also carries a dual diagnosis for substance use or medical reasons, or has a history of incarceration and/or trauma, the tasks for the case manager are intensified (Mueser, Torrey, Lynde, Singer, & Drake, 2003).

Because of the large percentage of persons with psychosis who use or abuse illegal substances and/or alcohol, integrated services have increased since the late 1990s (Minkoff, 2001; Mueser et al., 2003). *Integrated dual diagnosis treatment* (IDDT) is an evidence-based practice that addresses the complex needs of those with comorbid mental illness and drug or alcohol abuse.

Traditionally substance abuse and mental health services have been separated, with different agencies setting policy and monitoring care. Services are offered either sequentially or in parallel (Mueser et al., 2003). For multiple reasons this approach is untenable for the clients. Current best practices for integrated dual-diagnosis treatment are stage-wise, broad-based and match the person's stage along the continuum between illness and recovery. They include time unlimited services, motivational strategies that focus on increasing awareness of how substance abuse impinges quality of life, group interventions that focus on both mental health and substance abuse, access to family psychoeducation, pharmacological interventions as appropriate, and participation in self-help and mutual aid groups, such as 12-step programs (Magura, 2008; Mueser et al., 2003). Meticulous monitoring of antipsychotic medications is paramount because alcohol or street drugs can interact with prescription drugs in a counter-productive or dangerous fashion.

Significant attention has been placed on the *role of the family* in the treatment and care of persons with severe psychotic disorders, and how to best serve family members through professional and peer support. Best practices for families highlight the importance of outreach, support, *education*, and *psychoeducation* (Lehman et al., 2004; Resnick, Rosenheck, Dixon, & Lehman, 2005).

Two practices are considered particularly effective for families: professionally led psychoeducational multiple family groups (PEMFG) and peer-led family-to-family programs (Dixon et al., 2001; Pickett-Schenk, Cook, & Laris, 2000). *Psychoeducational multiple family groups* usually are facilitated by social workers or psychologists and follow a carefully defined curriculum. Groups of families, including the person with illness, meet together over a period of up to two years to learn about the psychotic disorders, share and exchange knowledge, and problem solve regarding difficult circumstances facing the individual with illness or the family as a group. Didactic content focuses on such topics as diagnosis and symptoms of the psychotic disorder, medications, stress management, warning signs of relapse, and patterns of illness (Lukens, 2001; McFarlane et al., 2003; Sherman, 2003). The groups enable family members to share experiences and ideas, learn from each other, and extend their social support network. Family members from one family can sometimes communicate more quickly and effectively with someone from another family than they can with each other; this cross-family communication can be very powerful (McFarlane et al., 2003). The PEMFG model is strengths based and recovery oriented.

The second model is peer led and endorsed by the National Alliance on Mental Illness, the highly respected national advocacy group. *Family-to-family programs* also follow a set curriculum and cover educational content comparable to the PEMFG model. Two particular programs have been disseminated widely, including the eight-week Journey of Hope education course and the twelve-week Family-to-Family Education program sponsored by NAMI (Pickett-Schenk,

Lippincott, Bennett, & Steigman, 2008). They usually include caregivers only and not the person with the disorder (Pickett-Schenk et al., 2008). These peer-led programs provide a critical service for family members. They are an important option for serving family members when formal programs are not available, or when families choose not to participate in professionally led groups. In some states, family-to-family programs are more readily available and funded than professionally led family interventions (Dixon, Goldman, & Hirad, 1999). As social workers develop relationships with families facing psychotic disorders, being aware of and suggesting peer-led programs as an option is a vital component of a broad based and comprehensive treatment plan.

Wellness self-management is a curriculum driven group intervention that aims to increase knowledge and insight and improve self and social care skills for persons with psychotic disorders (Drake et al., 2005). Initially referred to as *illness self-management*, the descriptor has shifted as investment in a strengths-based and recovery approach to care had grown. Wellness self-management promotes strategies to improve functioning and coping skills through regular group sessions. Participants learn about mental illness, how to recognize and manage personal symptoms and triggers, build social skills and support, and set and work towards personal goals (Mueser et al., 2002). Facilitators combine cognitive-behavioral, educational, and motivational interviewing strategies embedded in a series of modules that can be adjusted to meet individual needs. Topics may include safe and effective use of medications, building self-awareness, getting needs met through the mental health system, and how to talk to a physician. Groups meet weekly over a period of a year or more (Drake et al., 2005).

Peer support practices can play a significant role for each partner in a mutual help or exchange process. Serving as a guide and support to others who face similar challenges is empowering and can contribute to healing (Ridgway, 2001). In turn, receiving such support allows people to feel understood and encouraged in ways that differ from professional support. The exchange helps people move away from identity based on disability and associated stigma towards increased self-efficacy, self-esteem, and possibility (Ridgway, 2001; Torrey et al., 2001).

Despite underemployment among those with psychotic disorders, as many as 79 percent report that they would prefer to work (Bond et al., 2001a; Gates, Klein, Akabas, Myers, Schwager, & Kaelin-Kee, 2004). As expectations for these individuals have increased, attention has turned to programs that support competitive employment (as opposed to day treatment, sheltered work, or other non-competitive and protected employment programs). Several key parameters guide *supported employment*, including client choice regarding job readiness, preference as to type of job, accommodation in the workplace, and well integrated mental health and vocational supports (Bond, 2004; Mueser et al., 2005). For example, if a person has trouble focusing in the early morning, his or her work schedule might be adjusted accordingly. Or, if a person's antipsychotic medication has a brief sedative effect that interferes with work productivity, the dose scheduling might be adjusted so that the sedation occurs outside of work hours.

To ensure success, employment specialists work with treatment teams to locate appropriate mainstream work settings and identify and reinforce natural supports (i.e. family) and work-related supports (such as supervisors and colleagues) necessary to maintain the job (Gates et al., 2004). Sustained competitive employment is associated with increased community tenure and stability (Bond, 2004; Drake et al., 2005), as captured in the phrase *treatment is working*.

Medications are a critical component of treatment and primarily are used to treat the psychotic symptoms (Austrian, 2005; Bradford, Stroup, & Lieberman, 2002). If social workers are aware of the range, types, effects and side effects of these medications, they can translate complex medical information in a user friendly fashion. The worker can also help the person identify ways to question and work with the prescribing physician, and serve as a go-between as needed (Drake et al., 2005).

Social workers carry no responsibility for prescribing medication and are legally precluded from doing so. Although in some circumstances social workers and other mental health professionals may monitor medication adherence, evaluation and prescription is carried out by a licensed physician, usually a psychiatrist, or a nurse practitioner. Prescription is based on careful assessment of history, stage of illness, diagnosis, symptom configuration, ability to self-monitor medication, race and ethnicity, and potential side effects (D. Miller et al., 2005). Ideally the prescribing professional works closely with the person to adjust dosage and assess effectiveness on an ongoing basis.

The social worker further helps the individual to understand how the antipsychotic medicines work in tandem with psychosocial interventions, or how street drugs or alcohol might interfere with the regimen. When an individual is actively psychotic, he or she may have trouble engaging in educational or employment programs that require some stabilization of symptoms. The goal is to improve adherence with all aspects of treatment by helping the individual understand why the medication is important, how it works, and how to minimize side effects (Austrian, 2005; Bradford et al., 2002). This not only enhances the relationship between client and provider but also empowers the client to take action on his or her own behalf (Deegan & Drake, 2007).

In addition to the EBPs, there are several *promising practices* that have been identified in the literature but are not yet designated as evidence based (Drake et al., 2005). The *housing first model* places significant attention on the dignity afforded to those who are domiciled and who are involved actively in making choices about their treatment. This approach runs counter to the continuum of care strategy endorsed by the Department of Housing and Urban Development, that a client must be in compliance with psychiatric and substance abuse services and drug free and sober to be designated *housing ready* (Drake et al., 2005). In contrast, persons involved in housing first programs reside in permanent and independent housing without requirements for abstinence, sobriety, or treatment adherence (Tsemberis, Gulcur, & Nakae, 2004). ACT teams that are recovery focused and include peer educators provide further support. Evolving research documents the promise of the intervention; participants with comorbid psychosis and substance abuse have been able to reside successfully in permanent housing after long periods of homelessness when compared to a comparable group assigned to traditional continuum of care (Stefancic & Tsemberis, 2007).

Supported education is an emerging practice for persons with psychotic disorders and mirrors some of the principles of the supported employment interventions (Drake et al., 2005). Supported education programs aim to encourage participation in higher education, provide enhanced supports for a range of serious mental health needs, and increase knowledge and reduce stigma regarding mental health conditions among educators and other school personnel. If social workers and others providers recognize stumbling blocks and offer adjunctive services (e.g. tutoring, peer support groups, study and social skills, stress management), then participants can pursue educational goals not otherwise available to them (Gutman, 2008; Sasson, Grinshpoon, Lachman, & Ponizovsky, 2005).

Because cognitive deficits contribute to difficulty with the tasks required to succeed at work, school, or daily living, *cognitive remediation interventions*, offer significant promise (Medalia & Choi, 2009). These range from individualized tasks using paper and pencil or specialized computer exercises to small group programs using some combination of verbal and/or computer-based tasks (Twamley, Jeste, & Bellack, 2003; Velligan, Kern, & Gold, 2006). Graded activities aim to sharpen working memory, attention, organizational, problem-solving, and planning skills (Medalia & Choi, 2009; Revheim & Marcopulos, 2006; Wexler & Bell, 2005). The number of sessions can vary from one to multiple sessions per week and the duration range from several weeks to two years, depending on individual need (Wexler & Bell, 2005). Importantly, the cognitive remediation programs have been well received by the persons who use them. Early findings show improved cognition and acquisition of new skills that are generalizable to daily life activities and work settings (Wykes & Huddy, 2009).

Shared-decision making (SDM) is both an intervention strategy and a communication principle. SDM refers to a working alliance between two partners (i.e. the provider and the consumer) who collaborate on treatment decisions by sharing information about options and acting based on consensus around treatment preferences (Charles, Gafni, & Whelan, 1997; Deegan & Drake, 2006, 2007; Hamann, Leucht, & Kissling, 2006). SDM focuses on empowering the client by decreasing the informational and decisional imbalance in the relationship. The practitioners provide education, information, and discuss options. The affected individual educates the doctor, social worker, or other professional on personal history, experience with side effects, lifestyle choices, values, activities and areas where compromise regarding treatment decisions *is* or *is not* acceptable.

Following the principles of SDM, adherence to a formal treatment plan, including medication, may or may not be part of the desired outcome. Proponents argue that psychopharmacology and any other treatment should not interfere with one's personal recovery plan, since doing so would render such a treatment pointless from the point of view of the care recipient. SDM respects the right of clients to make bad decisions, since client preference should outweigh scientific evidence except in the rare situation of incompetence or immediate danger (Adams & Drake, 2006). Treatment outcomes that are not successful in achieving the goals of the client are considered experiences to be learned from, not as disasters or failures (Deegan & Drake, 2006). An improved provider-client relationship and increased satisfaction with treatment and life are considered important measures of the model's success.

Several forms of intervention show promise in serving the needs of the large sub-group of persons with psychotic disorders who have records of arrest and incarceration. These include *jail diversion programs*, mental health courts, and specialized ACT teams for those recently released through parole or completion of prison term (Morrissey & Cuddeback, 2008). These programs aim to eliminate or reduce time in prison or jail and support involvement of participants in community-based treatment programs that simultaneously address their mental health needs (Baillargeon, Binswanger, Penn, Williams, & Murray, 2009; Redlich, Hoover, Summers, & Steadman, 2008).

Mental health courts have appeared in increasing numbers across the United States since the late 1990s. These focus on problem solving and therapeutic intervention for those facing charges ranging from minor or moderate offenses to violence (Lamb & Weinberger, 2008; Schneider, 2008). Ideally they include ongoing case management and rehabilitation. Judges can mandate treatment, which may include medication, substance abuse programs, assignment to case management, and some form of structured or supported housing (Morrissey & Cuddeback, 2008; Schneider, 2008).

Professional methods and interventions

These evidence-based models and promising practices are consistent with social work values, and all include active roles for social workers. They are enhanced by the ecological systems and life course perspective that social workers bring to their practice, and the readiness to recognize and focus on assets and strengths as well as problems, symptoms, and challenges. They are well-integrated and comprehensive services that are not time limited, use a range of educational, psychotherapeutic and psychoeducational interventions at both the individual and group level, promote active outreach to both the person affected and the family, and focus on hope and recovery in the context of goal attainment and engagement in meaningful activities (Mueser et al., 2002). They emphasize the quality of the relationship between provider and client, the inclusive, continuous, and dynamic nature of these interactions, and individualized treatment planning that attends to the strengths, preference, values and culture of the client, and focuses on outcome and quality of life.

However, in spite of the growing literature on the application and use of the evidence based and promising practices, much of the research on these practices has focused on members of the majority culture (Drake et al., 2005). Cultural competence among providers and practitioners receives significant lip service in the literature on service provision across the mental health professions (President's New Freedom Commission on Mental Health, 2003), and is one of the ethical standards named in the National Association of Social Workers (NASW) Code of Ethics (NASW, 2008). Yet applying these skills effectively is challenging and requires ongoing vigilance and reflection, both at the personal (practitioner) and organizational (provider) levels (Sue & Sue, 2008). Among the core proficiencies involved in this multidimensional and multifaceted construct are knowledge of the prevailing beliefs, customs, norm and values of a particular culture, outreach; personal involvement and interaction with group members; knowledge of culturally specific resources and services; and backing and commitment at the organizational and policy level.

Illustration and discussion

David is a 65-year-old white man with a long-standing diagnosis of schizophrenia. Although initially diagnosed as *paranoid*, he appears now to meet the criteria for the *disorganized* subtype. His current symptoms include auditory hallucinations, flat affect, impoverished speech, and behavioral disorganization.

David was born and raised in a working-class family in the Bronx. In 1963, when David was 20, he experienced his first psychotic break and was hospitalized in a large state psychiatric institution, as was the norm for treatment at the time. He remained there for 17 years.

David no longer remembers (or is unable to report) what led to the initial hospitalization, and his records have long since been lost. Even now he remains shocked that he resided in a state hospital for so long, and expresses concern and surprise that *something must really be wrong with me*. He is rarely willing to speak about the lengthy inpatient stay, usually just shaking his head when the subject is broached. When he does speak of it, he says that long periods of time seemed to blur together. This is possibly due to over-medication, or simply to the mundane, repetitive daily rituals of life in a long-term psychiatric hospital. He reports that *they made me stay in bed for long periods of time*. He does not say whether he was in restraints during those times, but it is possible.

David was discharged from the state hospital in 1980. During his hospitalization he lost contact with most of his family, and upon discharge quickly became homeless. He survived on the streets of New York City for six years, moving into a single-room occupancy (SRO) hotel in 1986.

The conditions of the SRO were poor. The building owner did not perform basic maintenance, and often the plumbing did not work. Broken windows were ignored, and the plaster was crumbling. The building was inhabited by many people who had been homeless, like himself, and like himself, had poor self-care and home-care skills. Many of the other tenants suffered from addiction to street drugs. There was violence in the building related to the drug activity and several deaths resulting from drug overdoses. David says that he stayed in his room for days on end to avoid the mayhem that surrounded him, emerging either to panhandle for the nominal rent money (which was collected only sporadically) or to eat at a nearby soup kitchen. He did not receive psychiatric care at this time, and does not say what he experienced in terms of symptomatology or how he spent his time in his room.

In 1992 the building was deemed uninhabitable by the city, and residents were given the option of moving into what was then a new model of housing, called *supported housing*. David accepted this option and was moved into a single-room apartment, much like the one he had left, but in far superior condition, with more stable neighbors, and perhaps most significantly, with on-site social services. The services consisted of a team of social work case managers and a consulting psychiatrist, who was available to treat the building's tenants.

David received a psychiatric evaluation as part of the housing requirement and the psychiatrist observed that in addition to his negative symptoms, he also appeared to be responding to internal stimuli, probably auditory hallucinations. David denied experiencing auditory hallucinations at that time, but agreed to take medication anyway. Since he tended to smell strongly of urine, his physician prescribed medication to prevent incontinence, despite the fact that the doctor was unable to find any biological reason for the incontinence. David was also diagnosed with high blood pressure and diabetes, and was prescribed medication to manage both conditions. Although he had lost all of his teeth, he refused to consider dentures. The on-site social service team monitored his psychiatric and other medications, by ordering and receiving them from the pharmacy and observing him taking it twice daily.

The social work case manager helped him obtain Supplemental Security Income (SSI) through the Social Security Administration. He agreed to have his monthly checks sent directly to the social services agency, to ensure his rent was paid. The case manager gave him the additional money as a twice monthly allowance. Over time she realized that he was not using the money to buy even basic necessities, such as food and clothing. In fact, David had a cash-store of several thousand dollars in his room because he lacked both the motivation and the organization to bank or spend it.

Prioritizing his nutrition, the case manager determined that David was eligible for meal-delivery services, since he left his apartment so infrequently. He subsequently received one pre-cooked, warm meal delivered daily, from which he would pick out and eat the foods he liked.

Over the course of many years, David has developed a strong rapport with his case manager. She monitors his medication, delivers his allowance, and escorts him to medical and psychiatric appointments, since he lacks the motivation to go on his own, and is too disorganized to manage the subway independently. Although he speaks only in brief sentences, the case manager learned that he is an avid sports fan, and particularly enjoys boxing. She began to read the sports section daily in order to contribute to discussions with him, and eventually their conversations became longer, lasting for several minutes. She arranged to have pay-per-view boxing matches made available to the tenants as important matches arose, and many tenants enjoyed watching these matches with David. Although he remains reclusive and avoids group interactions, he seems to enjoy these events greatly.

Through the course of these interactions, the case manager also learned that his mother was possibly still living and that David would like to get in touch with her. In 2002, David called his mother for the first time in years. His mother, now well into her eighties, was overjoyed to hear from him. He went to see her the same week, showering and putting on clean clothes that he had shopped for (with the assistance of the case manager) for the occasion. Because the subway is overwhelming for David, the case manager arranged for round trip car transportation for him, which he could pay for with his SSI. He now sees his mother weekly, visiting mostly to watch sports events on TV with her, and reports that he enjoys *just being with her again*. Through this reunion, David has also reconnected with his sister and her children.

The family contact has markedly improved David's affect. Although he still speaks very little, he conveys a more optimistic outlook. His daily living skills have improved slightly; upon encourage-ment from his case manager, who helped him buy soap, towels and a shower curtain, he has been willing to shower weekly prior to visiting his mother.

David's primary symptoms continue to be auditory hallucinations, which he experiences on a daily basis, as he now openly acknowledges to his case manager and psychiatrist. Although it is apparent he is attending to something internally, he no longer responds to the voices in a direct manner when in the company of others, suggesting that he has taught himself strategies to cope with his symptoms. He typically does not acknowledge any worsening of symptoms until several months after the fact, when he may tell his case manager that, for example, *during basketball season* he was hearing more voices than usual. This is probably due to extreme reluctance, and fear that he might be forced to return to a psychiatric hospital. While his auditory hallucinations are *command* hallucinations, they do not command him to do anything dangerous. Rather, they tell him to wash his face and clean his room. He says he copes by ignoring the voices; that he finds the voices annoying, but not threatening. He does not want the psychiatrist to increase his medication dosage, and the psychiatrist respects this wish.

Although the social workers in his housing program have a formal *treatment plan* for David, he shows little interest in the goals listed in this plan, which include further improving his daily living skills and continued stabilization of his psychiatric and physical symptoms. David considers himself *retired*, and wishes to spend his time pursuing his interest in sports and visiting with his mother and sister on a regular basis. David probably suffered greatly and unduly in the state hospital system, as well as when he was homeless and living in poor conditions. He did not benefit from second-generation antipsychotics and the recovery movement in the ways that it is hoped the younger generations of people with schizophrenia will. However, he learned to cope with his illness and to maintain a stable living arrangement nonetheless.

In cases like that of David, who has been so disabled by schizophrenia over many years, there may be a feeling of hopelessness on the part of the social work team, or the sense that not much can be done. In this case, David's case manager was particularly diligent in finding ways to relate to him. She was able to reunite him with his family and encourage his participation in a pastime that was important to him.

If a wellness self-management program were available, the social worker might try to convince David to attend. Through the psychoeducational component of those groups, David might develop more trust in psychiatry and be willing to try new medications to address his auditory hallucinations, thus further improving the quality of his life. He might identify additional goals and enjoy socializing with more people in a safe structured environment. If he were opposed to participating in a group intervention, the social worker might consider working on components of the wellness model with him individually.

The social worker must continue to work with David on his physical health problems. She can help monitor his symptoms and navigate the medical system, escorting him to appointments and advocating with doctors if needed. Although David has not complained about his lack of teeth, the social worker might help him obtain and adjust to dentures, if he is interested.

The social worker can also continue to help monitor David's psychiatric symptoms by talking with him and observing his behavior. She can familiarize herself with his baseline functioning, and most importantly, help him recognize and monitor changes in symptoms and functioning for himself. If the nature or intensity of David's auditory hallucinations should change, she would need to evaluate how David is able to cope with them, and whether they present significant challenges to his day-to-day routine. Should difficulties arise, she would work with David and the treating psychiatrist to ensure his medication was adjusted appropriately. A significant departure from baseline that led to suicidal or violent ideation is unlikely, but would require psychiatric hospitalization.

David finds satisfaction in his renewed relationship with his family, and following sports is a meaningful activity for him. While he remains symptomatic, and many aspects of his life are less than ideal, he has learned to manage troubling symptoms of his illness, and has identified and recovered two pieces of his life that are important to him – his family and his hobby. With the support of his family and social worker, he may eventually expand his ideas about his own recovery, or he may remain satisfied with the way he has chosen to spend his *golden years*, as he terms his current situation. This case highlights how recovery can be defined by the consumer, in partnership with a dedicated social worker and shared decision making with a sensitive psychiatrist.

Conclusion

Persons coping with psychotic disorders have long been stigmatized and labeled. As social workers we must continue to humanize our work and collaborate with these individuals through well-conducted EBPs and promising practices that create opportunity and hope and emphasize recovery. We must develop ways to adapt these practices so that they are relevant for individuals and families from a range of cultural backgrounds. We must advocate for comprehensive and broad-based funding and policies at both the local and national level that allow us to implement and continue to build on what we know.

Evidence-based and promising practices for individuals with psychotic disorders and their families highlight the importance of easy-to-access and ongoing services and resources that include comprehensive support, education, and psychoeducation (Drake et al., 2005). Even common sense suggests that such straightforward interventions will lead to improved care coordination for the person who is ill. However, and in spite of significant progress in identifying fine interventions, services for those faced with psychotic disorders are uneven or truncated at best, and vary significantly by state and locale. In a National Report Card on Mental Health Services sponsored by NAMI (2009), entitled *Grading the states, 2009*, both overall services for persons with severe mental health challenges and state supported family services nationwide received a grade of "*D*." For these report cards NAMI identified what it labels as ten *pillars* of a high quality and transformed mental health system, including among these descriptors such as *safe and respectful, integrated, comprehensive, accessible, culturally competent, consumer and family driven*, and *transparent and accountable* (NAMI, 2009).

Not surprisingly, these characteristics represent qualities of what would be considered fine clinical care across the needs of persons and family members faced with a range of health, mental health, and other psychosocial challenges. They are fully consistent with the professional values associated with social work.

As social workers we are trained to identify strengths and build collaborative relationships with our clients. In two recent qualitative studies focusing on recovery and meaning, persons with psychotic disorders describe the immense satisfaction they experienced in relationships with professionals where they felt valued, heard, and respected as individuals. Davidson and his colleagues entitle an article " 'Simply to be let in': Inclusion as a basis for recovery" (Davidson, Stayner, Nickou, Styron, Rowe, & Chinman, 2001). In a study that explored engagement and retention in services by persons with comorbid mental illness, substance abuse and past homelessness, Padgett and colleagues found that participants most valued access to housing, pleasant surroundings, and what the authors movingly refer to as *acts of kindness* (Padgett, Henwood, Abrams, & Davis, 2008a).

In many ways the approach to care for persons with psychotic disorders is at a crossroads. Excellent programs have been identified, and the recovery movement focuses on what individuals with psychotic disorders can do and achieve, in spite of the health and mental health challenges they face. Yet current practices and programs do not consistently support these approaches. As social workers we are on the cusp, charged with promoting and supporting the possibilities for recovery, stability, community tenure and improved quality of life, without minimizing or overlooking the significant hurdles involved.

Web resources

Dartmouth Evidence-based Practice Center
dms.dartmouth.edu/prc/evidence/

Florida International University School of Social Work
www.CriticalThinkRx.org:

National Alliance on Mental Illness
www.nami.org/

National Empowerment Center
www.power2u.org/

SAFE program: Support and Family Education
www.ouhsc.edu/safeprogram/

Social Care Institute for Excellence
www.scie.org.uk

US Psychiatric Rehabilitation Organization
www.uspra.org

References

Adams, J.R., & Drake, R.E. (2006). Shared decision-making and evidence-based practice. *Community Mental Health Journal, 42* (1), 87–105.

Addington, J., Williams, J., Young, J., & Addington, D. (2004). Suicidal behavior in early psychosis. *Acta Psychiatrica Scandinavica, 109*, 116–120.

Aleman, A., Kahn, R.S., & Selten, J.P. (2003). Sex differences in the risk of schizophrenia: Evidence from meta-analysis. *Archives of General Psychiatry, 60* (6), 565–571.

Allness, D.J., & Knoedler, W.H. (2003). *A manual for ACT start-up.* Arlington, VA: National Alliance for the Mentally Ill.

Amador, X.F., & Paul-Odouard, R. (2000). Defending the Unabomber: Anosognoisia in schizophrenia. *Psychiatric Quarterly, 71*, 363–371.

American Psychiatric Association (APA). (2000). *Diagnostic and statistical manual of mental disorders* (4th ed., text revision). Washington, DC: APA.

an der Heiden, W., Konnecke, R., Maurer, K., Ropeter, D., & Hafner, H. (2005). Depression in the long-term course of schizophrenia. *European Archives of Psychiatry and Clinical Neuroscience, 255* (3), 174–184.

Anthony, W.A. (1993). Recovery from mental illness: The guiding vision of the mental health service system in the 1990s. *Psychosocial Rehabilitation Journal, 16* (4), 11–13.

Arnold, S.E. (2001). Contributions of neuropathology to understanding schizophrenia in late life. *Harvard Review of Psychiatry, March-April*, 69–76.

Assalian, P., Fraser, R.R., Tempier, R., & Cohen, D. (2000). Sexuality and quality of life of patients with schizophrenia. *International Journal of Psychiatry in Clinical Practice, 4*, 29–33.

Austrian, S.G. (2005). *Mental disorders, medications, and clinical social work* (3rd ed.). New York: Columbia University Press.

Baillargeon, J., Binswanger, I.A., Penn, J.V., Williams, B.A., & Murray, O.J. (2009). Psychiatric disorders and repeat incarcerations: the revolving prison door. *American Journal of Psychiatry, 166* (1), 103–109.

Barnes, A. (2008). Race and hospital diagnoses of schizophrenia and mood disorders. *Social Work, 53* (1), 77–83.

Barnes, T., Leeson, V., Mutsatsa, S., Watt, H., Hutton, S., & Joyce, E. (2008). Duration of untreated psychosis and social function: One-year follow-up study of first-episode schizophrenia. *British Journal of Psychiatry, 193* (3), 203–209.

Barry, C.L., & Ridgely, M.S. (2008). Mental health and substance abuse insurance parity for federal employees: How did health plans respond? *Journal of Policy Analysis and Management, 27* (1), 155–170.

Bartels, S.J., Clark, R., Peacock, W.J., Dums, A.R., & Pratt, S.I. (2003). Medicare and Medicaid costs for schizophrenia patients by age cohort compared with costs for depression, dementia and medically ill patients. *American Journal of Geriatric Psychiatry, 11* (6), 648–657.

Batki, S.L., Meszaros, Z.S., Strutynski, K., Dimmock, J.A., Leontieva, L., Ploutz-Snyder, R. et al. (2009). Medical comorbidity in patients with schizophrenia and alcohol dependence. *Schizophrenia Research, 107* (2–3), 139–146.

Beauchamp, G., & Gagnon, A. (2004). Influence of diagnostic classification on gender ratio in schizophrenia: A meta-analysis of youths hospitalized for psychosis. *Social Psychiatry and Psychiatric Epidemiology, 39* (12), 1017–1022.

Bellack, A.S. (2006). Scientific and consumer models of recovery in schizophrenia: Concordance, contrasts, and implications. *Schizophrenia Bulletin, 32* (3), 432–442.

Birchwood, M., Iqbal, Z., & Upthegrove, R. (2005). Psychological pathways to depression in schizophrenia: Studies in acute psychosis, post psychotic depression and auditory hallucinations. *European Archives of Psychiatry and Clinical Neuroscience, 255*, 202–212.

Bond, G.R. (2004). Supported employment: Evidence for an evidence-based practice. *Psychiatric Rehabilitation Journal, 27* (4), 345–359.

Bond, G.R., Becker, D.R., Drake, R.E., Rapp, C.A., Meisler, N., Lehman, A.F. et al. (2001a). Implementing supported employment as an evidence-based practice. *Psychiatric Services, 52* (3), 313–322.

Bond, G.R., Resnick, S.G., Drake, R.E., Xie, H., McHugo, G.J., & Bebout, R.R. (2001b). Does competitive employment improve nonvocational outcomes for people with severe mental illness? *Journal of Consulting and Clinical Psychology, 69* (3), 489–501.

Bradford, D., Stroup, S., & Lieberman, J.A. (2002). Pharmocological treatments for schizophrenia. In P.E. Nathan & J.M. Gorman (eds), *A guide to treatments that work* (2nd ed., pp. 169–199). New York: Oxford University Press.

Bradshaw, W., & Brekke, J.S. (1999). Subjective experience in schizophrenia: Factors influencing self-esteem, satisfaction with life, and subjective distress. *American Journal of Orthopsychiatry, 69* (2), 254–260.

Bresnahan, M., Begg, M.D., Brown, A., Schaefer, C., Sohler, N., Insel, B. et al. (2007). Race and risk of schizophrenia in a US birth cohort: Another example of health disparity? *International Journal of Epidemiology, 36* (4), 751–758.

Bromet, E.J., Bushra, N., Fochtmann, L.J., Carlson, G.A., & Tanenberg-Karant, M. (2005). Long-term diagnostic stability and outcome in recent-episode cohort studies of schizophrenia. *Schizophrenia Bulletin, 31* (3), 639–649.

Buckley, P.F., Miller, B.J., Lehrer, D.S., & Castle, D.S. (2009). Psychiatric comorbidities and schizophrenia. *Schizophrenia Bulletin, 35* (2), 383–402.

Carney, C.P., Jones, L., & Woolson, R.F. (2006). Medical comorbidity in women and men with schizophrenia: A population-based controlled study. *Journal of General Internal Medicine, 21* (11), 1133–1137.

Charles, C., Gafni, A., & Whelan, T. (1997). Shared decision making in the medical encounter: What does it mean? (Or, it takes at least two to tango). *Social Science and Medicine, 44* (5), 681–692.

Chisholm, B., Freeman, D., & Cooke, A. (2006). Identifying potential predictors of traumatic reactions to psychotic episodes. *British Journal of Clinical Psychology, 45* (Pt 4), 545–559.

Citrome, L., & Stroup, T.S. (2006). Schizophrenia, Clinical Antipsychotic Trials of Intervention Effectiveness (CATIE) and number needed to treat: How can CATIE inform clinicians? *International Journal of Clinical Practice, 60* (8), 933–940.

Cohen, C.I., Cohen, G.D., Blank, K., Gaitz, C., Katz, I.R., Leychter, A. et al. (2000). Schizophrenia in older adults, an overview: Directions for research and policy. *American Journal of Geriatric Psychiatry, 8* (1), 19–28.

Cohn, T.A., Remington, G., Zipursky, R.B., Azad, A., Connolly, P., & Wolever, T.M. (2006). Insulin resistance and adiponectin levels in drug-free patients with schizophrenia: a preliminary report. *Canadian Journal of Psychiatry, 51*, 382–386.

Cournos, F., McKinnon, K., & Sullivan, G. (2005). Schizophrenia and comorbid human immunodeficiency virus or hepatitis C virus. *Journal of Clinical Psychiatry, 66* (Suppl 6), 27–33.

Craig, T., & Bromet, E.J. (2004). Parents with psychosis. *Annals of Clinical Psychiatry, 16* (1), 35–39.

Davidson, L., Stayner, D.A., Nickou, C., Styron, T.H., Rowe, M., & Chinman, M.L. (2001). "Simply to be let in": Inclusion as a basis for recovery. *Psychiatric Rehabilitation Journal, 24* (4), 375–388.

Deegan, P. (1996). Recovery as a journey of the heart. *Psychiatric Rehabilitation Journal, 19* (3), 91–97.

Deegan, P. (2007). The lived experience of using psychiatric medication in the recovery process and a shared decision-making program to support it. *Psychiatric Rehabilitation Journal, 31* (1), 62–69.

Deegan, P., & Drake, R.E. (2006). Shared decision making and medication management in the recovery process. *Psychiatric Services, 57*, 1636–1639.

Deegan, P., & Drake, R. (2007). Shared decision making: In reply. *Psychiatric Services, 58* (1), 140.

Dickerson, F.B., Brown, C.H., Kreyenbuhl, J., Goldberg, R.W., Fang, L.J., & Dixon, L.B. (2004). Sexual and reproductive behaviors among persons with mental illness. *Psychiatric Services, 55* (11), 1299–1301.

Dickerson, F.B., Brown, C., Daumit, G., LiJuan, F., Goldberg, R., Wohlheiter, K. et al. (2006). Health status of individuals with serious mental illness. *Schizophrenia Bulletin, 32* (3), 584–589.

Dickinson, D., & Harvey, P.D. (2009). Systemic hypothesis for generalized cognitive deficits in schizophrenia: A new take on an old problem. *Schizophrenia Bulletin, 35* (2), 403–414.

Dixon, L., Goldman, H., & Hirad, A. (1999). State policy and funding of services to families of adults with serious and persistent mental illness. *Psychiatric Services, 50* (4), 551–553.

Dixon, L., Weiden, P., Delahanty, J., Goldberg, R., Postrado, L., Lucksted, A. et al. (2000). Prevalence and correlates of diabetes in national schizophrenia samples. *Schizophrenia Bulletin, 26* (4), 903–912.

Dixon, L., McFarlane, W.R., Lefley, H., Lucksted, A., Cohen, M., Falloon, I. et al. (2001). Evidence-based practices for services to families of people with psychiatric disabilities. *Psychiatric Services, 52* (7), 903–910.

Drake, R., Wallach, M., Alverson, H., & Mueser, K. (2002). Psychosocial aspects of substance abuse by clients with severe mental illness. *Journal of Nervous and Mental Disease, 190* (2), 100–106.

Drake, R., Merrens, M., & Lynde, D. (eds). (2005). *Evidence-based mental health practice: A textbook*. New York: W.W. Norton.

Drescher, J. (2010). Gay men. In P. Ruiz & A. Primm (eds), *Disparities in psychiatric care: Clinical and cross-cultural perspectives* (pp. 75–85). Baltimore, MD: Lippincott Williams & Wilkins.

Dunn, L.B., Lindamer, L., Palmer, B.W., Golshan, S., Schneiderman, L.J., & Jeste, D.V. (2002). Improving understanding of research consent in middle-aged and elderly patients with psychotic disorders. *American Journal of Geriatric Psychiatry, 10* (2), 142–150.

Essock, S.M., Dowden, S., Constantine, N.T., Katz, L., Swartz, M.S., Meador, K.G. et al. (2003). Risk factors for HIV, hepatitis B, and hepatitis C among persons with severe mental illness. *Psychiatric Services, 54* (6), 836–841.

Farone, D.W. (2006). Schizophrenia, community integration, and recovery: Implications for social work practice. *Social Work in Mental Health, 4* (4), 21–36.

Fazel, S., Khosla, V., Doll, H., & Geddes, J. (2008). The prevalence of mental disorders among the homeless in western countries: Systematic review and meta-regression analysis. *PLoS Medicine, 5* (12), e225.

Finkelstein, E., Prabhu, M., & Chen, H. (2007). Increased prevalence of falls among elderly individuals with mental health and substance abuse conditions. *American Journal of Geriatric Psychiatry, 15* (7), 611–619.

Gates, L.B., Klein, S.W., Akabas, S.H., Myers, R., Schwager, M., & Kaelin-Kee, J. (2004). Performance-based contracting: Turning vocational policy into jobs. *Administration and Policy in Mental Health, 31* (3), 219–240.

Gilmer, T.P., Ojeda, V.D., Barrio, C., Fuentes, D., Garcia, P., Lanouette, N.M. et al. (2009). Adherence to antipsychotics among Latinos and Asians with schizophrenia and limited English proficiency. *Psychiatric Services, 60* (2), 175–182.

Glazer, W.M., Conley, R.R., & Citrome, L. (2006). Are we treating schizophrenia effectively? Understanding the primary outcomes of the CATIE study. *CNS Spectrums, 11* (9 Suppl. 10), 1–13, quiz 14.

Greenberg, J.S., Greenley, J.R., McKee, D., Brown, R., & Griffin, F.C. (1993). Mothers caring for an adult child with schizophrenia: The effects of subjective burden on maternal health. *Family Relations, 42* (2), 205–211.

Grossman, L.S., Harrow, M., Rosen, C., Faull, R., & Strauss, G.P. (2008). Sex differences in schizophrenia and other psychotic disorders: A 20-year longitudinal study of psychosis and recovery. *Comprehensive Psychiatry, 49* (6), 523–529.

Gutman, S.A. (2008). Supported education for adults with psychiatric disabilities. *Psychiatric Services, 59* (3), 326–327.

Hall, L.L., & Purdy, R. (2000). Recovery and serious brain disorders: The central role of families in nurturing roots and wings. *Community Mental Health Journal, 36* (4), 427–441.

Hamann, J., Leucht, S., & Kissling, W. (2006). Do schizophrenia patients want to be involved in their treatment? Dr. Hamann and colleagues reply. *American Journal of Psychiatry, 163* (5), 937.

Harrison, G., Hopper, K., Craig, T., Laska, E., Siegel, C., Wanderling, J. et al. (2001). Recovery from psychotic illness: A 15- and 25-year international follow-up study. *British Journal of Psychiatry, 178*, 506–517.

Harrow, M., Grossman, L.S., Jobe, T.H., & Herbener, E.S. (2005). Do patients with schizophrenia ever show periods of recovery? A 15-year multi-follow-up study. *Schizophrenia Bulletin, 31* (3), 723–734.

Harvey, P. (2005). *Schizophrenia in late life*. Washington, DC: American Psychological Association.

Harvey, P., & Burns, T. (2003). Relatives of patients with severe mental disorders: Unique traits and experiences of primary, nonprimary and lone caregivers. *American Journal of Orthopsychiatry, 73* (3), 324–333.

Hinden, B.R., Biebel, K., Nicholson, J., Henry, A., & Katz-Leavy, J. (2006). A survey of programs for parents with mental illness and their families: Identifying common elements to build the evidence base. *Journal of Behavioral Health Services and Research, 33*(1), 21–38.

Hodgman, C.H. (2006). Psychosis in adolescence. *Adolescent Medicine Clinics, 17* (1), 131–145.

Hutchinson, G., Bhugra, D., Mallett, R., Burnett, R., Corridan, B., & Leff, J. (1999). Fertility and marital rates in first-onset schizophrenia. *Social Psychiatry and Psychiatric Epidemiology, 34* (12), 617–621.

Ihara, E.S., & Takeuchi, D.T. (2004). Racial and ethnic minorities. In B.L. Levin, J. Petrila & K.D. Hennessy (eds), *Mental health services: A public health perspective* (pp. 310–329). New York: Oxford University Press.

Jeste, D.V., & Nasrallah, H.A. (2003). Schizophrenia and aging: No more dearth of data? *American Journal of Geriatric Psychiatry, 11* (6), 584–588.

Jin, H., Folsom, D.P., Lindamer, L., Bailey, A., Hawthorne, W., Piedad, G. et al. (2003). Patterns of public mental health service use by age in patients with schizophrenia. *American Journal of Geriatric Psychiatry, 11* (5), 525–533.

Kealey, E.M. (2005). Variations in the experience of schizophrenia: a cross-cultural review. *Journal of Social Work Research and Evaluation, 6* (1), 47–56.

Kessler, R.C., Nelson, C.B., McGonagle, K.A., Edlund, M.J., Frank, R.G., & Leaf, P.J. (1996). The epidemiology of co-occurring addictive and mental disorders: implications for prevention and service utilization. *American Journal of Orthopsychiatry, 66* (1), 17–31.

Kilbourne, A., Cornelius, J., Han, X., Haas, G., Salloum, I., Conigliaro, J. et al. (2005). General-medical conditions in older patients with serious mental illness. *American Journal of Geriatric Psychiatry, 13* (3), 250–254.

Kirkpatrick, B. (2009). Schizophrenia as a systemic disease. *Schizophrenia Bulletin, 35* (2), 381–382.

Koen, L., Uys, S., Niehaus, D.J., & Emsley, R.A. (2007). Negative symptoms and HIV/AIDS risk-behavior knowledge in schizophrenia. *Psychosomatics, 48* (2), 128–134.

Kopelowicz, A., Liberman, R.P., & Stolar, D. (2008). Sexuality. In K.T. Mueser & D.V. Jeste (eds), *Clinical handbook of schizophrenia* (pp. 604–615). New York: Guilford Press.

Kroll, J.L. (2007). New directions in the conceptualization of psychotic disorders. *Current Opinion in Psychiatry, 20* (6), 573–577.

Lake, C.R., & Hurwitz, N. (2007). Schizoaffective disorder merges schizophrenia and bipolar disorders as one disease: There is no schizoaffective disorder. *Current Opinion in Psychiatry, 20* (4), 365–379.

Lamb, H.R., & Weinberger, L.E. (2008). Mental health courts as a way to provide treatment to violent persons with severe mental illness. *Journal of the American Medical Association, 300* (6), 722–724.

Lamberti, J.S., & Weisman, R.L. (2004). Persons with severe mental disorders in the criminal justice system: Challenges and opportunities. *Psychiatric Quarterly, 75* (2), 151–164.

Lawson, W.B. (2008). Schizophrenia in African Americans. In K.T. Mueser & D.V. Jeste (eds), *Clinical handbook of schizophrenia* (pp. 616–623). New York: Guilford Press.

Lehman, A.F., & Steinwachs, D.M. (2003). Evidence-based psychosocial treatment practices in schizophrenia: lessons from the patient outcomes research team (PORT) project. *Journal of the American Academy of Psychoanalysis and Dynamic Psychiatry, 31* (1), 141–154.

Lehman, A., Kreyenbuhl, J., Buchanan, R., Dickerson, F., Dixon, L., Goldberg, R. et al. (2004). The schizophrenia patient outcomes research team (PORT): Updated treatment recommendations 2003. *Schizophrenia Bulletin, 30* (2), 193–217.

Lukens, E. (2001). Schizophrenia. In A. Gitterman (ed.), *Handbook of social work practice with vulnerable and resilient populations* (pp. 275–304). New York: Columbia University Press.

Lysaker, P., Daroyanni, P., Ringer, J., Beattie, N., Strasburger, A., & Davis, L. (2007a). Associations of awareness of illness in schizophrenia spectrum disorder with social cognition and cognitive perceptual organization. *Journal of Nervous and Mental Disease, 195* (7), 618–621.

Lysaker, P., Roe, D., & Yanos, P. (2007b). Toward understanding the insight paradox: Internalized stigma moderates the association between insight and social functioning, hope, and self-esteem among people with schizophrenia-spectrum disorders. *Schizophrenia Bulletin, 33* (1), 192–199.

Magliano, L., Fiorilla, A., Malangone, C., Marasco, C., Guarneri, M., Maj, M., & National Mental Health Working Group. (2003). The effect of social network on burden and pessimism in relatives of patients with schizophrenia. *American Journal of Orthopsychiatry, 73* (3), 302.

Magura, S. (2008). Effectiveness of dual focus mutual aid for co-occurring substance use and mental health disorders: A review and synthesis of the "Double Trouble" in Recovery evaluation. *Substance Use and Misuse, 43* (12–13), 1904–1926.

Mallinger, J.B., Fisher, S.G., Brown, T., & Lamberti, J.S. (2006). Racial disparities in the use of second-generation antipsychotics for the treatment of schizophrenia. *Psychiatric Services, 57* (1), 133–136.

Manschreck, T.C., & Boshes, R.A. (2007). The CATIE schizophrenia trial: Results, impact, controversy. *Harvard Review of Psychiatry, 15* (5), 245–258.

Marson, D., Savage, R., & Phillips, J. (2006). Financial capacity in persons with schizophrenia and serious mental illness: Clinical and research ethics aspects. *Schizophrenia Bulletin, 32* (1), 81–91.

Martin, D. (2002, January 25). Edith Bouvier Beale, 84, "Little Edie," Dies. *The New York Times*.

Maysles, A., Maysles, E., Hovde, E. (Directors), & Meyer, M. (Writer) (1976). *Grey gardens*. USA: Criterion Collection.

McFarlane, W.R., Dixon, L., Lukens, E., & Lucksted, A. (2003). Family psychoeducation and schizophrenia: A review of the literature. *Journal of Marital and Family Therapy, 29* (2), 223–245.

Mechanic, D. (2007). Mental health services then and now. *Health Affairs (Millwood), 26* (6), 1548–1550.

Mechanic, D. (2008). *Mental health and social policy: Beyond managed care* (5th ed.). New York: Pearson Education.

Medalia, A., & Choi, J. (2009). Cognitive remediation in schizophrenia. *Neuropsychological Review, 19* (3), 353–364.

Meltzer, N.M. (2001). Treatment of suicidality in schizophrenia. In H. Hendin and J.J. Mann (eds), *The clinical science of suicide prevention* (Vol. 932, pp. 44–60). New York: New York Academy of Sciences.

Merriam-Webster Online Dictionary (2009). Psychosis. Retrieved July 13, 2009, from www.merriam-webster.com/dictionary/psychosis

Miller, B. (2008). A review of second-generation antipsychotic discontinuation in first-episode psychosis. *Journal of Psychiatric Practice, 14* (5), 289–300.

Miller, D., McEvoy, J.P., Davis, S.M., Caroff, S.N., Saltz, B.L., Chakos, M.H. et al. (2005). Clinical correlates of tardive dyskinesia in schizophrenia: Baseline data from the CATIE schizophrenia trial. *Schizophrenia Research, 80* (1), 33–43.

Miller, E., Leslie, D.L., & Rosenheck, R.A. (2005). Incidence of new-onset diabetes mellitus among patients receiving atypical neuroleptics in the treatment of mental illness: Evidence from a privately insured population. *Journal of Nervous and Mental Disease, 193* (6), 387–395.

Miller, L. (1997). Sexuality, reproduction, and family planning in women with schizophrenia. *Schizophrenia Bulletin, 23* (4), 623–635.

Minkoff, K. (2001). Program components of a comprehensive integrated care system for seriously mentally ill patients with substance disorders. *New Directions for Mental Health Services* (50), 13–27.

Minsky, S., Vega, W., Miskimen, T., Gara, M., & Escobar, J. (2003). Diagnostic patterns in Latino, African American, and European American psychiatric patients. *Archives of General Psychiatry, 60* (6), 637–644.

Morrissey, J.P., & Cuddeback, G.S. (2008). Jail diversion. In K.T. Mueser & D.V. Jeste (eds), *Clinical handbook of schizophrenia* (pp. 524–532). New York: Guilford Press.

Mueser, K.T., Valentiner, D.P., & Agresta, J. (1997). Coping with negative symptoms of schizophrenia: Patient and family perspectives. *Schizophrenia Bulletin, 23* (2), 329–339.

Mueser, K.T., Corrigan, P.W., Hilton, D.W., Tanzman, B., Schaub, A., Gingerich, S. et al. (2002). Illness management and recovery: A review of the research. *Psychiatric Services, 53* (10), 1272–1284.

Mueser, K.T., Torrey, W.C., Lynde, D., Singer, P., & Drake, R.E. (2003). Implementing evidence-based practices for people with severe mental illness. *Behaviour Modification, 27* (3), 387–411.

Mueser, K.T., Aalto, S., Becker, D.R., Ogden, J.S., Wolfe, R.S., Schiavo, D. et al. (2005). The effectiveness of skills training for improving outcomes in supported employment. *Psychiatric Services, 56* (10), 1254–1260.

Munetz, M.R., Grande, T.P., & Chambers, M.R. (2001). The incarceration of individuals with severe mental disorders. *Community Mental Health Journal, 37* (4), 361–372.

Myin-Germeys, I., Krabbendam, L., Delespaul, P.A., & van Os, J. (2004). Sex differences in emotional reactivity to daily life stress in psychosis. *Journal of Clinical Psychiatry, 65* (6), 805–809.

National Alliance on Mental Illness (NAMI). (2009). *Grading the states, 2009.* Washington, DC: NAMI.

National Association of Social Workers (NASW). (2008). *Code of Ethics of the national association of social workers* Washington, DC: NASW Press.

O'Day, B., Killeen, M.B., Sutton, J., & Iezzoni, L.I. (2005). Primary care experiences of people with psychiatric disabilities: barriers to care and potential solutions. *Psychiatric Rehabilitation Journal, 28* (4), 339–345.

O'Mahony, J. M., & Donnelly, T.T. (2007). The influence of culture on immigrant women's mental health care experiences from the perspectives of health care providers. *Issues in Mental Health Nursing, 28* (5), 453–471.

Padgett, D.K., Henwood, B., Abrams, C., & Davis, A. (2008a). Engagement and retention in services among formerly homeless adults with co-occurring mental illness and substance abuse: voices from the margins. *Psychiatric Rehabilitation Journal, 31* (3), 226–233.

Padgett, D.K., Henwood, B., Abrams, C., & Drake, R.E. (2008b). Social relationships among persons who have experienced serious mental illness, substance abuse, and homelessness: Implications for recovery. *American Journal of Orthopsychiatry, 78* (3), 333–339.

Palmer, B.A., Pankratz, V.S., & Bostwick, J.W. (2005). The lifetime risk of suicide in schizophrenia: A reexamination. *Archives of General Psychiatry, 62* (3), 247.

Palmer, B.W., Heaton, R.K., Paulsen, J.S., Kuck, J., Braff, D., Harris, M.J. et al. (1997). Is it possible to be schizophrenic and neuropsychologically normal? *Neuropsychology, 11*, 437–447.

Pandiani, J.A., Boyd, M.M., Banks, S.M., & Johnson, A.T. (2006). Elevated cancer incidence among adults with serious mental illness. *Psychiatric Services, 57* (7), 1032–1034.

Patkar, A.A., Mago, R., & Masand, P.S. (2004). Psychotic symptoms in patients with medical disorders. *Current Psychiatry Reports, 6* (3), 216–224.

Pescosolido, B.A., Wright, E.R., & Sullivan, W.P. (1995). Communities of care: A theoretical perspective on case management models in mental health. *Advances in Medical Sociology, 6*, 37–79.

Pickett-Schenk, S.A., Cook, J.A., & Laris, A. (2000). Journey of Hope program outcomes. *Community Mental Health Journal, 36* (4), 413–424.

Pickett-Schenk, S.A., Lippincott, R.C., Bennett, C., & Steigman, P.J. (2008). Improving knowledge about mental illness through family-led education: The journey of hope. *Psychiatric Services, 59* (1), 49–56.

President's New Freedom Commission on Mental Health (PNFCMH). (2003). *Achieving the promise: Transforming mental health care in America.* Rockville, MD: PNFCMH.

Preston, J.D., O'Neal, J.H., & Talaga, M.C. (2008). *Handbook of clinical psychopharmacology for therapists* (5th ed.). Oakland, CA: New Harbinger.

Rapaport, M.H., & Delrahim, K.K. (2001). An abbreviated review of immune abnormalities in schizophrenia. *CNS Spectrums, 6*, 392–397.

Redlich, A.D., Hoover, S., Summers, A., & Steadman, H.J. (2008). Enrollment in mental health courts: Voluntariness, knowingness, and adjudicative competence. *Law and Human Behavior, 34* (2), 91–104.

Regier, D.A., Farmer, M.E., Rae, D.S., Locke, B.Z., Keith, S.J., Judd, L.L. et al. (1990). Comorbidity of mental disorders with alcohol and other drug abuse: Results from the Epidemiologic Catchment Area (ECA) Study. *Journal of the American Medical Association, 264* (19), 2511–2518.

Resnick, S.G., Rosenheck, R.A., Dixon, L., & Lehman, A.F. (2005). Correlates of family contact with the mental health system: Allocation of a scarce resource. *Mental Health Services Research, 7* (2), 113–121.

Revheim, N., & Marcopulos, B. A. (2006). Group treatment approaches to address cognitive deficits. *Psychiatric Rehabilitation Journal, 30* (1), 38–45.

Ridgway, P. (2001). Restorying psychiatric disability: Learning from first person recovery narratives. *Psychiatric Rehabilitation Journal, 24* (4), 335–343.

Roe, D., Hasson-Ohayon, I., Kravetz, S., Yanos, P.T., & Lysaker, P.H. (2008). Call it a monster for lack of anything else: Narrative insight in psychosis. *Journal of Nervous and Mental Disease, 196* (12), 859–865.

Rossler, W., Salize, H.J., van Os, J., & Riecher-Rossler, A. (2005). Size of burden of schizophrenia and psychotic disorders. *European Neuropsychopharmacology, 15* (4), 399–409.

Royal Australian and New Zealand College of Psychiatrists Clinical Practice Guidelines Team (2005). Royal Australian and New Zealand College of Psychiatrists clinical practice guidelines for the treatment of schizophrenia and related disorders. *Australian and New Zealand Journal of Psychiatry, 39* (1–2), 1–30.

Rystedt, I.B., & Bartels, S.J. (2008). Medical comorbidity. In K.T. Mueser & D.V. Jeste (eds), *Clinical handbook of schizophrenia* (pp. 424–436). New York: Guilford Press.

Sadock, B.J., & Sadock, V.A. (2003). *Kaplan and Sadock's synopsis of psychiatry*, (9th ed.). New York: Lippincott Williams & Wilkins.

Sasson, R., Grinshpoon, A., Lachman, M., & Ponizovsky, A. (2005). A program of supported education for adult Israeli students with schizophrenia. *Psychiatric Rehabilitation Journal, 29* (2), 139–141.

Schaffner, K.F., & McGorry, P.D. (2001). Preventing severe mental illnesses: New prospects and ethical challenges. *Schizophrenia Research, 51* (1), 3–15.

Schneider, R.D. (2008). Mental health courts. *Current Opinion in Psychiatry, 21* (5), 510–513.

Schwartz, R.C., & Cohen, B.N. (2001a). Psychosocial correlates of suicidal intent among patients with schizophrenia. *Comprehensive Psychiatry, 42* (2), 118–123.

Schwartz, R.C., & Cohen, B.N. (2001b). Risk factors for suicidality among clients with Schizophrenia. *Journal of Counseling and Development, 79* (3), 314–319.

Sciolla, A., Patterson, T., Wetherall, J., McAdams, L.A., & Jeste, D.V. (2003). Functioning and well-being of middle-aged and older patients with schizophrenia: Measurement with the 36-Item Short-Form (SF-36) Health Survey. *American Journal of Geriatric Psychiatry, 11* (6), 629–637.

Seeman, M.V. (2008). Prevention inherent in services for women with schizophrenia. *Canadian Journal of Psychiatry, 53* (5), 332–341.

Seng, J.S., Kohn-Wood, L.P., & Odera, L.A. (2005). Exploring racial disparity in posttraumatic stress disorder diagnosis: Implications for care of African American women. *Journal of Obstetric, Gynecologic and Neonatal Nursing, 34* (4), 521–530.

Shad, M.U., Tamminga, C.A., Cullum, M., Haas, G.L., & Keshavan, M.S. (2006). Insight and frontal cortical functioning in schizophrenia: A review. *Schizoprenia Research, 86* (1–3), 54–70.

Sherman, M.D. (2003). The Support and Family Education (SAFE) program: Mental health facts for families. *Psychiatric Services, 54* (1), 35–37; discussion 37.

Solari, H., Dickson, K.E., & Miller, L. (2009). Understanding and treating women with schizophrenia during pregnancy and postpartum: Motherisk Update 2008. *Canadian Journal of Clinical Pharmacology, 16* (1), e23–32.

Spelman, L.M., Walsh, P.I., Sharifi, N., Collins, P., & Thakore, J.H. (2007). Impaired glucose tolerance in first-episode drug-naive patients with schizophrenia. *Diabetes Medicine, 24*, 481–485.

Stefancic, A., & Tsemberis, S. (2007). Housing First for long-term shelter dwellers with psychiatric disabilities in a suburban county: A four-year study of housing access and retention. *Journal of Primary Prevention, 28* (3–4), 265–279.

Strauss, J.L., Calhoun, P.S., Marx, C.E., Stechuchak, K.M., Oddone, E.Z., Swartz, M.S. et al. (2006). Comorbid posttraumatic stress disorder is associated with suicidality in male veterans with schizophrenia or schizoaffective disorder. *Schizophrenia Research, 84* (1), 165–169.

Sue, D.W., & Sue, D. (2008). *Counseling the culturally diverse: Theory and practice* (5th ed.). Hoboken, NJ: John Wiley & Sons.

Swanson, J.W. (1994). Mental disorder, substance abuse, and community violence: An epidemiological approach. In J. Monahan & H. Steadman (eds), *Violence and mental disorder: Developments in risk assessment* (pp. 101–136). Chicago, IL: University of Chicago Press.

Swanson, J.W., Swartz, M.S., Van Dorn, R.A., Elbogen, E.B., Wagner, H.R., Rosenheck, R.A. et al. (2006). A national study of violent behavior in persons with schizophrenia. *Archives of General Psychiatry, 63* (5), 490–499.

Swanson, J.W., Van Dorn, R.A., Swartz, M.S., Smith, A., Elbogen, E.B., & Monahan, J. (2008). Alternative pathways to violence in persons with schizophrenia: the role of childhood antisocial behavior problems. *Law and Human Behavior, 32* (3), 228–240.

Torrey, W.C., Drake, R.E., Dixon, L., Burns, B.J., Flynn, L., Rush, A.J. et al. (2001). Implementing evidence-based practices for persons with severe mental illnesses. *Psychiatric Services, 52* (1), 45–50.

Tsemberis, S., Gulcur, L., & Nakae, M. (2004). Housing First, consumer choice, and harm reduction for homeless individuals with a dual diagnosis. *American Journal of Public Health, 94* (4), 651–656.

Twamley, E.W., Jeste, D.V., & Bellack, A.S. (2003). A review of cognitive training in schizophrenia. *Schizophrenia Bulletin, 29* (2), 359–382.

U.S. Department of Health and Human Services (1999). *Mental health: A report of the Surgeon General.* Rockville, MD: U.S. Department of Health and Human Services, Substance Abuse and Mental Health Services Administration, Center for Mental Health Services, National Institutes of Health, National Institute of Mental Health.

U.S. Department of Health and Human Services (2001). *Mental health: Culture, race and ethnicity. A supplement to mental health: A report of the Surgeon General.* Rockville, MD: U.S. Department of Health and Human Services, Substance Abuse and Mental Health Services Administration, Center for Mental Health Services, National Institutes of Health, National Institute of Mental Health.

Velligan, D.I., Kern, R.S., & Gold, J.M. (2006). Cognitive rehabilitation for schizophrenia and the putative role of motivation and expectancies. *Schizophrenia Bulletin, 32* (3), 474–485.

Vreeland, B. (2007). Bridging the gap between mental and physical health: A multidisciplinary approach. *Journal of Clinical Psychiatry, 68* (Suppl 4), 26–33.

Waghorn, G., Lloyd, C., Abraham, B., Silvester, D., & Chant, D. (2008). Comorbid physical health conditions hinder employment among people with psychiatric disabilities. *Psychiatric Rehabilitation Journal, 31* (3), 243–246.

Walker, E., Mittal, V., Tessner, K., & Trotman, H. (2008). Schizophrenia and the psychotic spectrum. In W.E. Craighead, D.J. Miklowitz & L.W. Craighead (eds), *Psychopathology: History, diagnosis, and empirical foundations* (pp. 402–434). Hoboken, NJ: John Wiley & Sons.

West, J.C., Wilk, J.E., Olfson, M., Rae, D.S., Marcus, S., Narrow, W.E. et al. (2005). Patterns and quality of treatment for patients with schizophrenia in routine psychiatric practice. *Psychiatric Services, 56* (3), 283–291.

Wexler, B.E., & Bell, M.D. (2005). Cognitive remediation and vocational rehabilitation for schizophrenia. *Schizophrenia Bulletin, 31* (4), 931–941.

Whitty, P., Waddington, J., & Owoeye, O. (2009). Neurological signs and involuntary movements in schizophrenia: intrinsic to and informative on systems pathology. *Schizophrenia Bulletin, 35* (2), 415–424.

Wilk, J.E., West, J.C., Narrow, W.E., Rae, D.S., & Regier, D.A. (2005). Access to psychiatrists in the public sector and in managed health plans. *Psychiatric Services, 56* (4), 408–410.

Wilson, J.S. (2003, January 12). Edith Bouvier Beale. *The New York Times.*

Wint, D.P., Okun, M.S., & Fernandez, H.H. (2004). Psychosis in Parkinson's disease. *Journal of Geriatric Psychiatry and Neurology, 17* (3), 127–136.

Wittmann, D., & Keshavan, M. (2007). Grief and mourning in schizophrenia. *Psychiatry, 70* (2), 154.

Wohlheiter, K., & Dixon, L. (2008). Assessment of co-occurring disorders. In K.T. Mueser & D.V. Jeste (eds), *Clinical handbook of schizophrenia* (pp. 125–134). New York: Guilford Press.

Wykes, T., & Huddy, V. (2009). Cognitive remediation for schizophrenia: it is even more complicated. *Current Opinion in Psychiatry, 22* (2), 161–167.

20 Substance abuse

Meredith Hanson

Social workers encounter no condition that is more controversial and more perplexing than substance misuse and abuse. Most scholars consider substance use disorders to be social and public health problems, which require extensive intervention and treatment. Yet, experts have competing views about what exactly substance abuse is, how it emerges, and what should be done to prevent its occurrence and to minimize its adverse consequences. Over the years, substance abuse and addictive behavior have been defined as moral defects, diseases, personality disorders, learned behaviors, and mental disorders (Hanson, 2001). Preferred treatments have stressed religious and spiritual conversions, involvement in self-help fellowships, psychosocial counseling, group therapy, family intervention, and medication. Each view of the condition and each treatment have their proponents and opponents who cite persuasive, but often contradictory, evidence to support their respective positions. What all agree on and what is not disputed is that substance abuse and its consequences have profound effects on society, and, although effective interventions are being developed, most people who experience problems associated with substance abuse do not receive professional assistance (Substance Abuse and Mental Health Services Administration (SAMHSA), 2008).

Although social workers are among the helping professionals who are most likely to encounter individuals experiencing difficulties associated with substance abuse, many researchers have discovered that many social workers who are not employed in substance abuse settings are reluctant to take up substance abuse with their clients (Kagle, 1987; Steiker, 2009). Among the reasons cited for not addressing the condition are limited knowledge of substance abuse (Loughran, Hohman, & Finnegan, 2008), poor training (Bliss & Pecukonis, 2009), and doubts about one's right to address substance abuse with particular clients (Loughran et al., 2008). Such factors have led to the development of screening and assessment tools for the rapid identification of substance abuse (Hohman, Clapp, & Carrilio, 2006) and initiatives to improve social workers' competencies in substance abuse assessment and treatment (Bliss & Pecukonis, 2009; Institute of Medicine, 2006; National Association for Children of Alcoholics (NACOA), 2006). Despite these efforts, many people needing treatment for substance abuse-related problems remain unidentified and do not receive effective assistance.

Definitions of substance abuse

Substance abuse has been defined in many different ways. Each descriptive definition of the condition contains an explicit or implicit theory that explains why substance abuse occurs, its variation across population groups, and its developmental course with and without treatment. The theories contain "frameworks of knowledge" and "modes of thinking" that are contestable; they suggest what evidence is relevant, how it should be interpreted, and its implications for practice (Gray & Webb, 2009). How a condition is defined determines in large part where intervention is focused and how it is delivered (Gitterman & Germain, 2008). Over the years substance abuse has been defined in many ways: as immoral activity, as a disease, as a symptom of other problems, as learned behavior, as a product of social arrangements, and as a spiritual disease (Hanson, 2001).

Substance abuse as immoral behavior Historically, the moral view of substance abuse has been prominent in the United States' efforts to address problems associated with addiction (Thombs, 2006). From colonial times to the present, many people have viewed substance abusers as individuals who have made personal choices to break society's laws and misuse and abuse alcohol and other drugs (e.g., Levine, 1978; Thombs, 2006). They have been described as "weak willed" and "criminals;" substance abuse itself has been defined as a "willful indulgence" (Morgan, 1981).

While "moral" views of substance abuse may seem clear-cut, simple, and absolute (e.g., substance abusers are choosing to do something that is wrong and they must "just say no" to drugs), the evidence suggests that morally and legally based drug control efforts have not been very effective (e.g., Prohibition) and that punishment-based initiatives alone rarely change addictive practices (Thombs, 2006). Further, persuasive evidence suggests that moral-legal addiction control efforts have been associated with changes in the characteristics of the substance abusing population (Hanson, 2001; Jonnes, 1995). For example, in the late nineteenth and early twentieth centuries when opium was readily available in over-the-counter medicines, the typical substance abuser was a middle-aged white woman from the middle and upper classes (e.g., Gray, 1998). Currently, now that opiates are less available, opiate addicts are more likely to be men who are marginalized and alienated from many aspects of conventional society – individuals who may be less willing to engage in treatment (Hanson, 2001).

Substance abuse as a disease While a moral perspective of substance abuse still prevails in many legal and control efforts, the most widely accepted view of substance abuse among helping professionals is that it is a manifestation of primary disease processes and possibly genetically and biologically based. Viewing substance abuse as a primary disease suggests that it is a "brain-related" medical condition that is rooted in dispositional and physiological conditions that separate persons with a predisposition toward substance abuse from those who are not pre-disposed (Kissin, 1983; National Consensus Development Panel on Effective Medical Treatment of Opiate Addiction, 1998).

The disease model of addiction has evolved considerably from the classic disease concept of alcoholism that stressed a somewhat linear progression and "loss of control" over alcohol use (Jellinck, 1946, 1960). Considerable biological and genetic research has identified such factors as neurotransmitter adaptations (Julien, 2007), brain wave functions (Almasy et al., 2001), and genetic risks (Dick et al., 2006; Reich et al., 1998) that are associated with the progressive development of addiction. Related research has led to the development of pharmacological interventions, like methadone maintenance and naltrexone treatment for substance abuse (Cohen, Collins, Young, McChargue, Leffingwell, & Cook, 2009).

While little empirical research has supported the classic notions of "progression" and "loss of control" in the development of alcoholism, more recent laboratory research has demonstrated fairly well how alcohol and other drugs can interact with the brain and other bodily organs to disrupt normal biological functions (e. g., Julien, 2007; Koob, 2009). Findings such as these have muted moral views of substance abuse and have legitimized medical and other treatments for addictive behavior and its consequences. Laboratory findings and findings from behavioral genetics studies also have underscored the variability in substance abuse, helping to dispel the notion that addiction is a simple, unitary disorder (Koob, 2009; Ray & Hutchison, 2009). A major limitation of a disease perspective, as it currently is espoused, however, is a tendency toward a "biological reductionism" in which other person-environment factors are ignored or minimized. Consequently, while important pharmacological treatments have been discovered, researchers drawing on a disease perspective have added little to the development of effective psychosocial interventions to prevent substance abuse and minimize its adverse impact.

Substance abuse as a mental disorder and symptom of underlying personality problems   Symptom models of substance abuse draw on psychoanalytic theories of addiction, ranging from classic drive theory in which substance abuse represents a manifestation of oral-dependency and regression to minimize unconscious conflict to more recent formulations that draw on object-relations theory and self-psychology (Yalisove, 1997). Research which draws on object-relations and self-psychological theories has focused on trauma repetition and has illustrated how substance abuse, especially among women, may be related to trauma associated with sexual and physical abuse that occurred in the past and which often continues into the present (e.g., D. Miller & Guidry, 2001).

Another popular explanation for substance abuse that has evolved from psychoanalytic theory is the "self-medication hypothesis," which links substance abuse to deficits in self-care and affect-management (Khantzian & Albanese, 2008; Weegmann, 2006). Research has provided some support for the hypothesis, finding an association between substance use and the diagnosis of mental disorders (Hall & Queener, 2007). Research, however, has not demonstrated a consistent link between negative affective states and increased substance use (Hall & Queener, 2007). The unreliable findings may be explained in part by the way one conceptualizes self-medication. In a study of homeless adults, for example, when self-medication was defined as coping with painful feelings in general, it was a better predictor of substance use than when self-medication referred only to coping with symptoms of mental disorders (Henwood & Padgett, 2007).

A major contribution of symptom perspectives and psychoanalytic theories is the recognition that individuals who are dependent on alcohol and other drugs may have impaired ego functions, which will affect the recovery process. Consequently, intervention efforts must be ego supportive in nature to help them gain increased awareness of the addiction process and to help them strengthen ego functioning. Although this view has heuristic value and makes sense clinically, little empirical research has been conducted to test and refine it.

Substance abuse as learned behavior   The view that addictive behavior is learned and maintained by a combination of antecedent, mediating and consequent factors became more prominent in the latter half of the twentieth century (Leonard & Blane, 1999). Currently, models that draw on cognitive and cognitive-behavioral theories of substance abuse, which highlight how distal factors associated with learning histories and proximal factors associated with life circumstances affect substance use and treatment, guide much of our understanding about substance abuse treatment.

From learning theory perspectives contingent relationships between antecedents, mediators, behaviors, and their consequences explain the existence of substance abuse. Individuals who are vulnerable for substance misuse due to learning histories encounter "triggers" for substance use when they enter high-risk situations (stressful situations; situations in which there are opportunities to use drugs). Whether or not they use drugs in these situations is a function of their mood and cognitions, expectancies about the benefits of drug use, their skill repertoires, their confidence in coping with the situations without using drugs, and other beliefs which mediate the association between antecedent triggers and substance using behaviors. The substance use continues, in turn, due to positively reinforcing (e.g., euphoria) and/or negatively reinforcing (e.g., reduction in feelings of stress; reductions in interpersonal conflict) consequences (Marlatt & Donovan, 2005).

Psychosocial interventions drawing on learning theories have addressed all phases of the therapeutic process from engagement and mobilization, through early recovery, to the maintenance of therapeutic gains (Marlatt & Donovan, 2005; W. Miller & Rollnick, 2002). Learning theories also have informed all modalities of intervention, including group, couple, and family therapies (Hanson, 2009; O'Farrell & Fals-Stewart, 2006; Rowe, Liddle, Dakoff, & Henderson, 2009). A fairly robust empirical literature supports the effectiveness of learning theory-based interventions among diverse population groups (e.g., Magill & Ray, 2009).

Substance abuse as a product of social arrangements Theories that suggest that substance abuse is a product of social arrangements highlight social structural conditions that provide differential opportunities and tension that lead to alcohol and other drug use, and cultural norms that legitimize different patterns of use among different segments of society (Akers, Krohn, Lanza-Kaduce, & Radosevich, 1979; Bourgois, 1995). The social functions of substance abuse include social facilitation, cohesion building and boundary marking among group members, "time-out" or relief from social obligations, and repudiation of conventional societal values (Thombs, 2006).

Substance abuse prevention and intervention initiatives that build on social theories of substance abuse attempt to alter subcultural values among drug users and inculcate values that are more congruent with conventional society and substance-free living. They also attempt to reduce stresses and increase societal resources that will promote drug-free behaviors (Hawkins, Catalano, & Associates, 1992; Rhodes & Jason, 1988). Support for social and cultural views of substance abuse can be found in preventive interventions that have been more effective when they have included "culturally sensitive" components (Botvin, Schinke, Epstein, Diaz, & Botvin, 1995; National Institute on Alcohol Abuse and Alcoholism (NIAAA), 2002).

Substance abuse as a spiritual disease Spiritual perspectives on substance abuse draw attention to values, beliefs, and social connectedness that give meaning to one's life. Spiritual views of substance abuse can trace their origins to Alcoholics Anonymous and other 12-step fellowships that espouse fundamentally spiritual programs of recovery in which a personal transformation must occur before an individual can escape the grips of addiction (Hanson, 2001). According to W. Miller (1998), spirituality can be a protective factor in substance abuse. Persons who are more spiritual, as documented by involvement with religious institutions, seem less likely to develop substance abuse problems and more likely to recover from its effects. Spirituality in Alcoholics Anonymous (AA) membership also has been found to be associated with longer-term abstinence (Galanter, 2008).

Although there have been calls for more systematic research on the association between spirituality and substance abuse, research remains limited (Bliss, 2007). Anecdotal and survey evidence suggest that persons who are "at peace" with themselves and non-judgmentally accept their life circumstances while remaining optimistic about their abilities to survive are more likely to overcome addiction (e.g., Marlatt, 1994). AA involvement, in conjunction with substance abuse treatment, also appears to be associated with recovery (Galanter, 2008), with a vast majority of substance abuse treatment organizations endorsing a 12-step orientation toward recovery (Priester et al., 2009).

The preceding definitions of substance abuse illustrate the range of professional perspectives on addiction. Each is a partial representation of reality. Together, they underscore the complex nature of substance abuse. They suggest that substance abuse is a biopsychosocial condition in which personal lifestyle factors, physiological conditions, social structural arrangements and cultural practices may contribute to the emergence and development of substance abuse. These same factors ought to be assessed and addressed in the recovery process. How the various factors affect particular individuals and how treatment should be designed is a function of a comprehensive, collaborative assessment and service plan. Social workers with their person-environment perspective are uniquely positioned to be responsive to the forces that affect the development of substance abuse and to assist persons suffering from its consequences.

Demographics

As of 2007, national surveys estimated that nearly 20 million U.S. citizens aged 12 or older were current users of illicit drugs (8.0 percent of the population); around 129 million people from the same age group were current users of alcohol (approximately half of that age group). About 20 percent of the population acknowledged current binge drinking and 7 percent reported current heavy drinking (SAMHSA, 2008). These figures have been relatively stable since the late 1990s. They show that substance use and abuse occurs among all population groups, in both genders, and in all socioeconomic strata. Individuals who try alcohol at an earlier age, however, are more likely to develop dependence on alcohol and/or other drugs as they age.

Demographic patterns also reveal that for most people substance use and abuse peaks in early adulthood and declines thereafter. Due to generally heavier substance use among the baby-boom generational cohort, however, some prognosticators project that the number of older adults with substance abuse problems will double by 2020 (Han, Gfroerer, Colliver, & Penne, 2009).

Population

A closer look at the epidemiological data shows, that despite overall trends, substance abuse and its consequences have differential impacts in particular groups. A few examples illustrate this point:

- Serious mental illness is a risk factor for developing substance abuse. People with bipolar disorder, panic disorder, or borderline personality disorder are at high risk for developing substance abuse. Approximately 50 percent of all adults who have been diagnosed with a schizophrenic disorder have met the diagnostic criteria for substance use disorders at some time in their lives. Substance use disorders, on the other hand, do not appear to predict mood or anxiety disorders (Grant et al., 2008) or other serious mental disorders (Mueser, Noordsby, Drake, & Fox, 2003).
- Among the primary ethnic groups in the United States, Whites are more likely to report current alcohol use and to drink more heavily than are African Americans and Latinos. Rates of problem use are highest among Native Hawaiians, Alaska Natives, and American Indians, and lowest among Asian Americans (NIAAA, 2002; SAMHSA, 2008).
- In all ethnic groups, men drink more often and consume larger quantities of alcohol than do women. Women, however, seem to experience disproportionately more drinking-related problems, which progress more quickly in them than in men (Stewart, Gavric, & Collins, 2009).
- Although most self-identified gay, lesbian and bisexual individuals do not develop substance abuse problems, non-heterosexual orientation is associated with greater risk of substance use and abuse. Considerable variation in substance use exists among this population with women appearing to experience more severe outcomes, relative to the general population, than do men (McCabe, Hughes, Bostwick, West, & Boyd, 2009).

Research findings like those reported above support the notion that drugs of all types are readily available in the United States and that substantial numbers of individuals experiment with different substances or use them fairly regularly. Although individuals may be differentially predisposed to developing substance abuse problems, whether or not they develop those problems is a function of their particular life circumstances. While substance abuse occurs in all sociodemographic groups, individuals with other mental health and psychosocial difficulties, as well as people who have experienced discrimination or oppression that has marginalized them seem to be particularly vulnerable to developing problems associated with substance abuse.

Substance abuse is a behavioral disorder that is learned in social contexts. The main contribution of those contexts is to expose people to favorable attitudes, role models and differential reinforcement for drug use. Cultural rituals and practices, as well as social conditions, legitimize and make particular drugs more accessible. Positive attitudes toward drugs like alcohol can emerge in children at an early age (Jahoda & Cramond, 1972). Peers reinforce these attitudes as children grow up, increasing the likelihood that they will view substance use more favorably when they are young adults.

People use drugs because drugs serve adaptive functions: they help people cope with stress, they facilitate peer acceptance, and they allow people to feel "normal" (Hanson, 2001; Thombs, 2006). While the long-term consequences of drug use may be aversive and negative, for persons who develop serious substance abuse problems the immediate positive benefits of drug use outweigh the longer-term costs of use. The meaning of drug use and the role it plays in individuals' lives can be understood only by viewing drug use and abuse in life context. Understanding the role and meaning of drug use for people is essential for preventive and interventive efforts to succeed.

Mental health care disparities

National surveys reveal that people from minority and marginalized racial and cultural groups, not only may be at greater risk for substance abuse, but also may encounter service disparities compared with Whites who are members of majority groups (National Institute of Mental Health (NIMH), 2001; SAMHSA, 2008). In addition, a lack of parity in insurance coverage for mental disorders and substance abuse further limits access to quality care by all people suffering from substance abuse (e.g., Marth, 2009).

Investigators using data from the National Epidemiologic Survey on Alcohol and Related Conditions (NESARC) found that racial and ethnic status was associated with differences in substance abuse treatment utilization. Although Whites were less likely to receive assistance for illicit drug problems than were African Americans, Whites were more likely to use professional services. African Americans were more likely to receive non-professional services like 12-step group involvement and church-related support. Rates of substance abuse rehabilitation services also were higher for African Americans. The authors speculate that these differences may be due to higher rates of drug abuse symptoms among African Americans (Keyes, Hatzenbuehler, Alberti, Narrow, Grant, & Hasin, 2008), and they may indicate lower access to preventive and other substance abuse services, especially culturally relevant services, among African Americans (Perron, Mowbray, Glass, Delva, Vaughn, & Howard, 2009).

These same investigators found no differences in the barriers to service across racial and ethnic groups (Perron et al., 2009). While barriers were present, they seemed to have a similar impact for all people with substance use disorders. The most commonly cited barriers were "internal" ones that kept people from seeking and using assistance (e.g., attitudes and beliefs about the need for treatment or about using treatment; fear of the reactions of others who might discover that they are in treatment; poor peer and family support for treatment). The "external" barrier that respondents cited most often was inadequate or no health care coverage, followed by such barriers as not knowing where to seek help, inconvenient service hours, and no transportation. These findings parallel those reported in other surveys of the general population (e.g., SAMHSA, 2008).

When they examined service utilization among adults with substance use disorders and mental disorders, researchers found that people were more likely to be treated for the mental disorders (mood and anxiety disorders) than for substance abuse. African Americans were less likely than Whites to receive treatment for mood and anxiety disorders; they were equally likely to receive treatment for alcohol-related problems; and they were more likely to receive treatment for the abuse of illicit drugs (Hatzenbuehler, Keyes, Narrow, Grant, & Hasin, 2008).

Research in Hispanic communities found that Hispanics were more likely than Whites to report a need for substance abuse services. Yet, Hispanics were twice as likely as Whites to indicate that they did not receive needed care or that treatment was delayed. They also were more dissatisfied with the care they received than were Whites (Alegria et al., 2006). Several reasons have been offered for these disparities in service utilization and satisfaction. Chief among them are a misunderstanding of substance use and abuse among Hispanics by professionals, non-responsive service delivery models, and poor coordination and integration of substance abuse services with other health and social services.

Similar service disparities are found among other vulnerable or marginalized client groups like older adults and gay, lesbian, and bisexual adults. Historically, the substance abuse service delivery system in the United States has been organized around particular treatment approaches, and practitioners were trained to treat clients from a "one true light perspective" (W. Miller & Hester, 2003) that may not be sensitive to the unique experiences of diverse client groups. Consequently, they are not effective in attracting people to, or retaining them in, treatment. Clients who enter substance abuse treatment generally have multiple, complex problems besides their substance abuse. Although personal factors like attitudes about treatment may keep many people from seeking help, treatment programs that are not responsive to the range of difficulties clients encounter (i.e., that view substance abuse in a vacuum) and which do not individualize service so that it is responsive to the experiences of different client groups are likely to remain ineffective for most people (Alegria et al., 2006; Mathews, Lorah, & Fenton, 2006).

Social work programs and social work roles

Historically, most professionals shunned working with substance abusers or treated the consequences of the condition without ever directly addressing substance use and abuse. Such non-responsive practices were central in the rise of Alcoholics Anonymous in the 1930s and other 12-step fellowships (Kurtz, 1979/1991, 1997). They also influenced the development of treatment enterprises like therapeutic communities, which in their early days were staffed primarily by counselors who were recovering from substance abuse themselves (De Leon, 2000). The 12-step fellowships are composed of people struggling with their own substance abuse. They embrace a spiritual view of recovery, in which substance abusers learn to recognize their addiction and their "powerlessness" over drug use. This is followed by "surrender," acceptance, and other behavioral changes that lead to personal lifestyle transformations that include a new, drug-free existence.

The 12-step fellowships are powerful self-help social networks in which persons struggling with recovery can find nonjudgmental acceptance and support, as well as structured steps and processes, which promote recovery from substance abuse. The group processes embedded in the fellowships encourage bonding and goal direction, they reinforce social activities that do not involve drug use, they provide guiding principles that encourage recovery (e.g., "one day at a time"), and they help participants build self-efficacy and drug-resistant coping skills (Moos, 2008). Alcoholics Anonymous and other 12-step groups reach more substance abusers than do all mental health professionals combined. Approximately 80 percent of all adults seeking help for drinking problems attend AA meetings, and nearly 10 percent of the adult population has been to at least one AA meeting in their lives (more people than have attended alcoholism treatment programs) (Dawson, Grant, Stinson, & Chou, 2006; Room & Greenfield, 1993).

Despite their popularity, little research addresses the effectiveness of self-help fellowships as "stand alone" efforts, and some research questions their value (Ferri, Amato, & Davoli, 2006). However, 12-step fellowship involvement, in particular Alcoholics Anonymous affiliation, has been shown to be useful (especially for persons with more extensive substance use histories), when it is combined with participation in specialized substance abuse treatment programs (Galanter, 2008; Tonigan, Connors, & Miller, 2003). Preparatory assistance that familiarizes individuals with group traditions and norms and teaches them communication skills seems to facilitate participation in 12-step groups and improve the probability that they will benefit from participation (Anderson & Gilbert, 1989; Nowinski, 2003).

The formal service delivery system can be divided into two categories, specialized substance abuse treatment facilities and non-specialized health and social service agencies. As observed earlier, most people who need assistance for substance abuse-related problems do not receive professional treatment. Of those who receive treatment, most receive care in non-specialized settings. Only 10–16 percent of those who need treatment (i.e., meet DSM-IV diagnostic criteria for a substance use disorder) receive assistance in specialized substance abuse treatment facilities (Perron et al., 2009; SAMHSA, 2008).

Specialized substance abuse services exist on a continuum from preventive services, through intensive inpatient detoxification and rehabilitation services, to less intensive outpatient and early intervention services. The settings in which substance abuse treatment is provided include hospitals, freestanding residential programs, therapeutic communities, mental health clinics, other outpatient clinics, schools, prisons, vocational rehabilitation programs, supportive housing programs, and work sites.

The delivery of specialized substance abuse treatment has markedly changed since the mid 1980s. Until the early 1990s much of the treatment was delivered in inpatient and residential care facilities. By 2006, 86 percent of all treatment was delivered on an outpatient basis (McLellan, 2003; SAMHSA, 2007). Although many factors, including the absence of persuasive empirical evidence supporting the value of a continuum of care approach, have contributed to this change, the primary force behind the change seems to be a growing concern with the high economic costs of inpatient and residential care (McLellan, 2003; McLellan, Carise, & Kleber, 2003).

Social work roles vary by the function of the agency in which they are employed. In *non-specialized settings*, the primary professional tasks related to substance abuse are case-finding, early identification and detection, information, referral, coordination of care, and helping clients reconnect with natural support networks as they recover from substance abuse. In these settings, social workers must be able not only to recognize substance abuse-related problems when they are present, but also to form rapidly collaborative therapeutic partnerships with clients. This ability will increase the likelihood that clients will be candid about their substance use, and improve the chances that they will accept referral recommendations.

As observed earlier, many social workers employed in non-specialized settings feel poorly prepared and are reluctant to address substance abuse with their clients. Yet, approximately half of all clients seeking help from mental health professionals experience personal or family problems related to alcohol consumption, and over two-thirds of all social workers encounter clients with drug- and alcohol-related problems (Drake & Mueser, 1996; O'Neil, 2001). Thus, social workers employed in non-specialized settings must remain vigilant and acquire the competencies needed to identify substance abuse and to assist people suffering from its consequences.

Social workers perform a range of functions in specialized substance abuse facilities and efforts. *Education and prevention activities* include policy-level responses like alcohol and cigarette taxes, laws limiting the sale of alcohol and prescription drugs, and community education initiatives. Social workers involved with this level of prevention assist in the development of legislation, analyze the impact of the initiatives, and engage in public education clarifying the need for the initiatives. Some education and prevention responses, like drug-free workplace initiatives, are aimed at the general public. Others, like warnings about the effects of alcohol on fetal development, are designed to reach particular high-risk groups.

Among the most effective prevention programs are group- and classroom-based, skills development initiatives that target children and adolescents. These approaches build on natural group experiences (e.g., in the classroom) to alter norms and to strengthen the preventive message. Programs that are culturally sensitive and which focus on life skills, general and drug-specific coping skills, and social influence, and character development have been especially effective (Beets et al., 2009; Botvin et al., 1995). Social workers in these programs facilitate group processes, identify and develop peer leaders, coordinate the delivery of services, and evaluate service implementation and effectiveness.

The American Society of Addiction Medicine (ASAM) has developed a set of placement rules that specify levels of care for treatment based on the severity of an individual's substance abuse problems (Mee-Lee, Shulman, Fishman, Gastfriend, & Griffith, 2001). These standards, which are widely used in the United States, were developed by a panel of experts in substance abuse treatment, and they have been subjected to a fair amount of research on their clinical utility (Gastfriend & Mee-Lee, 2003). The placement rules define six areas of assessment and several levels of care for adults and adolescents. The guidelines represent a movement away from a linear, unitary view of substance abuse treatment toward multidimensional, person-environment assessment and treatment that is driven by client need rather than program structure.

According to the ASAM placement criteria, the assessment dimensions that should guide a professional's determination about the level of care clients need are: (1) acute intoxication and withdrawal potential, (2) physical condition and concomitant physical health problems, (3) the presence of diagnostic or sub-diagnostic mental health problems, (4) readiness for changing substance use behavior, (5) readiness for relapse prevention services and the potential for continued substance use, and (6) the recovery environment, including the need for family, housing, legal, financial, childcare, educational, vocational, and transportation services (Mee-Lee et al., 2001).

Although research on the ASAM criteria is still incomplete and how uniformly they have been implemented is not certain (Gastfriend & Mee-Lee, 2003; McLellan, 2003), they are a standard part of substance abuse treatment in much of the United States, and they serve as a useful template for discussing specialized substance abuse services. Services for adults include medically supervised care and drug detoxification, residential and inpatient treatment, intensive outpatient and partial hospitalization services, outpatient services, including opioid maintenance, and early intervention. Adolescent services include medically managed and medically monitored inpatient and residential care, intensive outpatient treatment, partial hospitalization, outpatient treatment, and early intervention.

Detoxification services are designed to meet the needs of substance-dependent individuals who suffer from withdrawal symptoms when they stop substance use. Persons whose withdrawal symptoms are so acute and severe that they will experience great distress and potential health risks if they discontinue substance use receive acute inpatient medical detoxification under the care of nurses and physicians. Social workers in these settings work with clients and family members and facilitate discharge planning for continued substance abuse treatment. Individuals who experience less severe withdrawal services and who have social resources and supports available may undergo outpatient detoxification treatment. This type of treatment typically occurs in an outpatient substance abuse facility, where social workers engage clients and their families in ongoing psychosocial care, while monitoring their conditions and coordinating service delivery.

Residential/inpatient services and therapeutic communities are designed to assist adults and adolescents who have severe substance abuse problems, high potential for relapsing behavior, and non-supportive or inadequate environmental resources (Hanson, 2001; Mee-Lee et al., 2001). Clients are physically removed from the environments in which they are at high risk to continue substance use and they are placed in settings where care is provided 24 hours a day. They undergo intensive treatment that educates them about the acute and long-term effects of substance abuse, helps them develop more effective coping skills for handling pressures to use drugs, provides social support, and helps them to develop recovery plans to implement upon discharge. Residential and inpatient programs generally employ group models of treatment that last two to four weeks. Therapeutic communities provide somewhat longer-term treatment; they offer a social therapeutic, group-based approach that attempts to resocialize clients so that they are more resistant to pressures to use drugs (De Leon, 2000). In these settings, social workers partner with counselors, many of whom are themselves recovering substance abusers, to promote a mutual aid system supportive of substance-free living. They provide psychosocial services and they work directly with clients and their family members to prepare them for discharge by helping them to anticipate threats to recovery, develop action plans, and locate professional and community resources that will support recovery.

Partial hospitalization and intensive day treatment services are group and milieu-based programs for clients who do not require inpatient and residential care, but who lack social supports that will encourage abstinence. They offer structured services that may be provided before or after school and work, at night and on weekends. Clients attend these programs from 9 to 20 or more hours per week (Mee-Lee et al., 2001). Essential services include comprehensive assessments, individual, family and group treatment, education, and 24-hour crisis care. Beyond the essential services, many programs offer psychopharmacological assessment and treatment. Partial hospitalization and intensive outpatient programs have been found to be particularly useful for assisting clients, like individuals with severe and persistent coexisting mental disorders, who have other serious life problems besides substance abuse (Mueser et al., 2003). Social workers employed in these settings provide a full range of direct clinical care; they advocate on behalf of clients to locate needed resources; and they coordinate care with other treatment professionals and agencies.

Outpatient care is most appropriate when clients are ready to make changes in their lives, minimal risk exists for symptoms of withdrawal, they have a supportive environment and they have adequate coping mechanisms for handling pressures to use drugs. Some outpatient settings are drug-free; others offer drug substitution chemotherapy or antagonistic drug therapy for opiate, alcohol, or other drug dependence. Chemotherapy may be provided at any level of care. When it is offered it is essential to determine that clients meet the biomedical criteria for drug dependence and that there are no physical or mental health complications that preclude chemotherapy (Mee-Lee et al., 2001).

A primary value of outpatient care is that clients are assisted in their natural environments. With the support of treatment providers they are able to face the situations that triggered substance use in the past, develop effective coping skills and locate alternative support networks that sustain sobriety. As in other levels of care, social workers employed in outpatient settings provide a full range of psychosocial and therapeutic services. In recent years, as cost of care has risen and insurance coverage has become more inadequate, social workers have become more expert in the delivery of time-limited interventions and they have become more proficient in involving clients in 12-step and other self-help groups.

Early intervention programs are targeted at individuals who seem to be developing a substance abuse problem, who are engaging in risky or unsafe actions while under the influence of substances, and/or who may be unaware that they have a problem. These programs may be offered in schools and work sites (e.g., Student Assistance and Employee Assistance programs). They may be available in law enforcement and criminal justice settings (e.g., Drug Courts and Driving Under the Influence programs). The goals of these programs include educating individuals about their substance use and its effects, helping them to recognize the need for treatment, assisting them in developing action plans to address their substance abuse, locating treatment facilities where they can continue their care, and motivating them to follow through with treatment. Social workers in these settings are educators, they mobilize clients to seek additional help, they make referrals, and they follow up to ensure that clients receive the needed assistance.

A philosophy of treatment that stresses complete abstinence from alcohol and other drugs guides treatment in most specialized substance abuse treatment organizations in the United States. While most treatment and policy professionals ascribe to the goal of abstinence, there is disagreement as to how that goal should be achieved, and a growing body of clinicians and advocates have begun to argue that the goal of substance abuse initiatives should be "harm reduction" rather than "use reduction" (Marlatt, 1998; Weatherburn, 2009). Under a harm reduction approach the goal of service is not simply to eliminate substance use, but to minimize the adverse consequences of substance use and associated risk behaviors. How this debate is played out in clinical practice with particular clients depends on the policies and mandates of the treatment organization and the results of comprehensive assessments with the clients.

By the time they enter specialized substance abuse treatment programs, many clients have developed symptoms of substance dependence and have other psychosocial difficulties that affect their abilities to use alcohol or other drugs without encountering problems. Under these circumstances, clinical efforts should be abstinence-oriented and clients should be helped to develop their capacities to resist drug use and to cope with life problems without resorting to drug use. Until clients achieve stable sobriety, however, clinicians can take a "harm reduction" stance and work with them to help them avoid relapses and to minimize the consequences of substance use when lapses and relapses occur. In settings, like early intervention programs, where clinicians encounter clients who may misuse substances but who have not developed a dependence on them, clinicians may work with clients to improve their decision-making and to avoid using alcohol and other drugs at times when use is likely to be problematic. If clients are able to make these changes, they may not need to become totally abstinent from alcohol and other drugs to live adaptive lives.

Improving care   Although not all substance abuse related difficulties are chronic and some persons are able to stop problematic use quickly, substance abuse can be characterized as a chronic condition that shares many features with other chronic disorders and diseases (e.g., hypertension, asthma). First, it seems to be influenced by genetics and other biological factors, as well as personal and environmental factors. Second, it has a prolonged developmental course characterized by periods of remission and relapse. Third, it can be "controlled" or "stabilized" but not "cured." Fourth, acquiring and maintaining stability usually require longer-term care, lifestyle changes, and lifetime vigilance.

While substance abuse may be considered chronic and different levels of specialized care have been established, most treatment services are based upon an "acute care" model of service. They are delivered in discrete units over short periods of time. They are evaluated at single points in time. Little coordination exists between levels of care. Post-treatment relapse and readmission are more likely to be considered individual failures rather than flaws in the service delivery systems (White, 2008). Because of the limitations in an "acute care" approach to service delivery, many experts have argued for service delivery system that is based on a "recovery model" and "sustained recovery management" (White, 2008). To make existing services more "recovery-oriented" social workers and policy makers must strive to improve service coordination across the continuum of care. They must involve other professionals, members of the community, and 12-step fellowship groups in an approach to care that views substance abuse treatment and recovery holistically and as a process. Within a recovery model of care long-term recovery from substance abuse is defined not only by overcoming substance abuse and related difficulties, but also by achieving improved health, and sustaining adaptive functioning in other life areas (Hawkins et al., 1992; Heinrich & Lynn, 2002; White, 2008).

Professional methods and interventions

Many effective practices exist to assist people suffering from substance abuse and its consequences. For the most part, these interventions are based on sound theories of substance abuse and behavioral change and robust empirical, research evidence. They address all phases of the helping process from engagement and assessment to relapse prevention and the maintenance of therapeutic gains.

Assessment Several reliable and valid assessment and screening instruments exist to help clients identify the presence of a substance abuse problem and determine its impact. Screening instruments are particularly useful in non-specialized settings where clients are seeking assistance for difficulties other than substance abuse. These instruments are brief and can be administered rapidly in the form of paper and pencil questionnaires (e.g., the Michigan Alcoholism Screening Test: Selzer, 1971) or questions that may be incorporated into broader assessment interviews. Social workers can use the information obtained from these instruments to help clients recognize the existence of substance abuse and establish its severity. A benefit of using these instruments is that they allow clients to establish the presence of substance abuse problems through their own report.

The CAGE questionnaire is a simple four-question screening tool that is easily integrated into assessment interviews (Mayfield, McLeod, & Hall, 1974). Although it was created to screen for alcohol problems, it can be adapted to screen for other drug problems. Social workers administer the CAGE by asking the client the following questions, either in sequence or embedded into a larger assessment interview:

1   Have you ever thought you should **C**ut down on your drinking (or drug use)?
2   Have you felt **A**nnoyed when people criticize your drinking?
3   Have you ever felt bad or **G**uilty about your drinking?
4   Have you ever had a drink first thing when you wake up to steady your nerves or to get over a hangover (**E**ye-opener)?

Two or more "Yes" answers to these questions suggest that a drinking (or drug) problem exists and should be followed up with further assessment.

More comprehensive substance abuse assessment is necessary to establish how it is manifested in a person's life. The DSM-IV provides the most widely used diagnostic criteria for establishing the presence of a substance use disorder (American Psychiatric Association (APA), 2000). While these criteria are useful for most clients and help to establish treatment parameters, they may not be as useful for individuals whose substance abuse is evident in ways that do not fit readily within the DSM-IV's diagnostic criteria (e.g., older adults, adolescents, people with coexisting mental disorders). Thus, findings from a DSM-IV-based diagnosis should be enhanced by the use of structured clinical interviews like those contained in the Addiction Severity Index (ASI). The ASI is widely used and has established validity for assessing substance abuse and its effects (McLellan et al., 1992). It addresses a range of psychosocial problems including emotional distress, occupational functioning, and family interactions.

A comprehensive assessment is ecological and functional in nature. Substance use and abuse is placed in an environmental context, and both the adaptive and maladaptive functions of substance use and abuse in clients' lives are identified. Among the substance-specific domains that should be covered in a comprehensive assessment are:

- a client's general substance use patterns, including substances used, quantities used, and methods of use
- contexts of use, including triggering events, people presence and their reactions
- thoughts, feelings and expectancies associated with use
- biopsychosocial consequences of use
- the presence of signs of drug dependence and/or withdrawal
- histories of use, including periods of cessation and past treatment attempts
- other life problems that are associated with substance use (e.g., precede use or occur following use)
- available supports and resources (e.g., family, peers, religious institutions, community organizations).

Since most substance abuse is situational in nature, that is, it occurs in some situations and not in others, it is important for social workers to assess the characteristics of those situations in which a person is at "high-risk" for substance abuse, as well as those situations in which there is lower risk. Research has demonstrated, for example, that people are more likely to abuse substances when they experience negative mood states or they encounter social pressures to use drugs. They are also more likely to consume substances if they perceive that they are not able to cope with situational demands without using drugs, they feel like they cannot resist pressures to use drugs, or they believe that they will gain some benefit by using drugs (e.g., will feel better, will be "part of the crowd") (Marlatt & Donovan, 2005).

Information that is gathered through comprehensive screening and assessment should be organized so that it leads logically to service options. The information should describe how substance abuse is manifested in clients' lives. It should help clients and professionals understand the functions of substance use in their lives. It should suggest where intervention efforts should be located and how they should be delivered.

Early intervention   Many substance-involved clients are mandated to seek treatment (e.g., by courts, child protection agencies, work sites) or seek help for problems other than substance abuse (e.g., mental illness, medical conditions, economic difficulties, domestic conflict). Early intervention efforts help them to recognize how substance abuse may be associated with other life problems, come to grips with it, accept that they need help, and seek help.

Motivational interviewing is a client-centered intervention style and strategy that has strong evidence of effectiveness with a wide range of clients (Hanson & El-Bassel, 2004; W. Miller & Rollnick, 2002). It has been found to be particularly useful for clients who are ambivalent about the existence of a substance abuse problem and do not see the need for treatment. Social workers using motivational interviewing adopt an empathic, "not-knowing" stance to inquire about a client's substance use. Through the use of open-ended questioning, reflective listening, affirmation and summarization they encourage clients to discuss their substance use. By helping clients weigh both the benefits and costs of substance use and by pointing out inconsistencies in their statements they help clients to make self-motivational statements that help them move beyond their ambivalence and doubts about substance use to the point where they make a decision to seek treatment and clarify further the effects of substance use in their lives.

Several effective early intervention strategies are aimed at family members of substance abusers who do not recognize the presence of substance abuse or are reluctant to consider treatment (Smith & Meyers, 2004). These strategies attempt to educate family members about substance abuse and help them cope with its presence. They teach interpersonal communication skills and self-care strategies that help family members break free from addiction cycles. The overall goal of these strategies is to disrupt familial patterns that may inadvertently protect substance abusers from the consequences of their substance use and which may "enable" them to continue use. By disrupting these patterns it is hoped that substance abusers will examine further their use patterns and ultimately seek assistance.

Once clients make decisions to seek further assistance, social workers use role induction strategies and preparatory interventions designed to help them understand more about the treatment process, what to expect, and how to act. Such preparatory efforts have been shown to improve the likelihood that clients will follow through on treatment recommendations and engage positively in treatment (W. Miller & Rollnick, 2002).

Intervention practices   Responsive intervention flows from comprehensive assessment and builds on clients' motivations and capacities for recovery. Social workers' efforts involve assisting clients in developing personal and environmental resources and supports for recovery. Traditionally, group-based interventions have been the treatment modalities of choice for substance abuse (Hanson, 2009).

A number of evidence-based practices exist to support clients' recovery efforts. Interventions that draw on cognitive-behavioral practice principles have been found to have efficacy with diverse groups of clients who abuse a variety of substances (Magill & Ray, 2009; W. Miller, Wilbourne, & Hettema, 2003; National Institute on Drug Abuse (NIDA), 1999, 2003). In family, group, and individual treatment modalities, clients are helped to develop cognitive vigilance to increase their awareness of situations in which they are at risk for substance abuse, and they learn more adaptive coping skills to resist pressures to use substances and to better cope without using alcohol and other drugs. Cognitive-behavioral interventions address faulty thinking that may lead to substance abuse; they teach problem-solving skills; and they attempt to improve communication skills. Since many substance abuse-related difficulties occur in interpersonal contexts many cognitive-behavioral interventions focus on marital and family dynamics to help participants better manage conflicts and improve positive interactions (e.g., O'Farrell & Fals-Stewart, 2006).

Supportive-expressive psychotherapy is a time-limited treatment approach that builds on psychodynamic theories of change. Supportive interventions aim to build clients' ego-strengths and self-care capacities while expressive strategy try to help clients gain greater awareness of the reasons they abuse substances and work through intrapsychic and interpersonal conflicts. Research with clients receiving methadone maintenance treatment revealed that supportive-expressive therapy helped them reduce their substance use and maintain therapeutic gains (National Institute on Drug Abuse (NIDA), 1999; Woody, McLellan, Luborsky, & O'Brien, 1995).

Contingency management and comprehensive community-based intervention have long histories of effectiveness with substance abusers. A community reinforcement approach to treatment begins with a functional analysis and assessment of substance abuse to examine the external triggers, cognitive and affective mediators, and the short- and long-term consequences of substance use. This analysis is paired with a client's substance use patterns (e.g., quantity and frequency of use, substances used) to determine the roles alcohol and other drugs play in a person's life. Comprehensive intervention services, including behavioral skills training, job skills preparation, social and recreational counseling, and family/relationship therapy, are then tailored to meet a particular client's needs. Research has revealed that interventions that draw on this treatment approach have been effective with alcohol abusers and with abusers of opiates and cocaine. They have been effective with substance abusers who live with families, and they have had promising outcomes with disaffiliated individuals like adults who are homeless (Meyers & Miller, 2001). Voucher-based, contingency management strategies in which clients receive incentives for reaching therapeutic goals (e.g., having negative drug screening results; establishing continuous abstinence) appear to strengthen this approach with abusers of cocaine (Higgins, Budney, Bickel, Foerg, Donham, & Badger, 1995).

Several effective practices exist for working with adolescent substance abusers. Compared with non-directive supportive therapy, behavioral interventions that helped adolescents learn how to avoid high-risk situations, develop skills to handle urges and pressures to use drugs, and involved family members and other people in treatment were more effective in helping adolescents reduce substance use and maintain therapeutic gains (Azrin et al., 1994; Waldron, Brody, & Slesnick, 2001). Multidimensional family therapy, which addresses adolescent substance use within a family context, has considerable evidence of effectiveness (Rowe et al., 2009). Adolescent substance abuse is viewed developmentally. Teenagers are helped to improve negotiation, decision-making and problem-solving skills. Family members are worked with in parallel sessions and jointly with the adolescents. Parents are encouraged to explore parenting practices, while teens and parents are helped to strengthen their bonds and reduce interpersonal conflict that can lead to substance abuse (Diamond & Liddle, 1996; National Institute on Drug Abuse, 1999).

Although social workers are involved primarily in the psychosocial treatment of substance abusers, pharmacological approaches play important roles in the treatment of substance abuse. Cross-tolerant and other medications are central in the detoxification of clients who are dependent on drugs that produce physical withdrawal symptoms when they are discontinued. Opiate agonists (e. g., methadone) have long been used on an outpatient basis to stabilize and maintain adults addicted to heroin and other opiates. Essentially, treatment involves the administration of a longer acting opioid as a substitute for a shorter acting opiate of abuse. An extensive research literature on methadone maintenance documents its value for retaining clients in treatment, stabilizing their functioning, and reducing criminal activities associated with drug use (Carroll, 2003; National Institute on Drug Abuse, 1999).

Narcotic antagonists (e. g., naltrexone) are non-addicting drugs that have been used successfully to treat adults suffering from opiate and alcohol dependences. The drugs eliminate the reinforcing effects of opiates (e.g., euphoria, feeling "high") and they reduce craving for alcohol (Carroll, 2003). As in the case of agonistic treatment, narcotic antagonists help to stabilize clients. Stabilized clients appear to function normally, hold jobs, avoid crime and violence, and reduce their risks for HIV exposure (National Institute on Drug Abuse, 1999).

Other drugs that have been used in the treatment of problem drinking are disulfiram (Antabuse) and acamprosate. Disulfiram, which has been widely used, interferes with the normal metabolism of alcohol and produces aversive effects like nausea, dizziness, flushing, and irregular heartbeat. Despite disufiram's popularity, medication compliance is a common obstacle and research supporting its effectiveness has not been strong. Acamprosate reduces craving and the side effects of alcohol withdrawal. Research findings on acamprosate's effectiveness come primarily from Europe, and, although results are mixed, they suggest that it affects drinking frequency and abstinence rates (Carroll, 2003; W. Miller et al., 2003).

As observed earlier, pharmacological treatments seem most useful when they are combined with psychosocial interventions. Pharmacological treatment reduces some of the direct physical effects of substances (e.g., withdrawal symptoms and craving), helping clients to stabilize physically. Psychosocial intervention helps clients develop more effective coping skills, supports their efforts and desires to remain substance-free, helps them manage negative affect, assists family members and peers, and helps alter environmental contingencies and processes that lead to substance use.

As the preceding discussion suggests, effective substance abuse prevention and intervention practices are ecological in nature. Since multiple personal and environmental factors affect the emergence and development of substance abuse, social work intervention must be comprehensive. Multiple person-environment domains must be addressed and care must be coordinated and integrated so that treatment is holistic in nature and the chances for recovery are maximized.

Illustration and discussion

Social workers must be responsive to client need, promote autonomy, and use strategies that draw on sound empirical evidence. In recent years, a movement toward evidence-based practice has helped many social workers be both responsive and accountable to their clients by helping them to identify effective practices and to collaborate with clients to fit services to their circumstances. Evidence-based practice is a decision-making strategy in which social workers use their clinical expertise and experience to blend client values and preferences, clinical state and condition, and relevant research evidence to assist clients facing a range of life problems. It involves: (1) collaborative assessments, (2) the transformation of problem statements into searchable questions, (3) literature searches to locate interventions that are effective in addressing particular client concerns, (4) discussions of the findings with clients to clarify intervention options, (5) implementation of the agreed upon interventions, and (6) evaluations of the interventions' effectiveness with the clients (Nock, Goldman, Wang, & Albano, 2004; Shlonsky & Gibbs, 2004). As will be seen in the following practice illustration, an evidence-based practice framework can be useful when working with clients with substance abuse and other life stressors.

Sally George is a 58-year-old, single, white woman who has lived her entire life in a large city.[1] She is a thin, somewhat frail-looking woman. She has had hepatitis B in the past, and she currently suffers from hepatitis C and other health problems. Ms. George lives illegally in an apartment in public housing in the same neighborhood as a senior center where she goes for meals and other services. She sleeps on a couch in the living room of a male friend who she knows from the streets where she buys drugs. According to Ms. George, "I can only be there when he is there because he won't give me a key. So, I spend a lot of time hanging out on the streets." Ms. George's friend abuses alcohol, crack cocaine, and heroin. Ms. George acknowledges that she uses cocaine, heroin, and prescription drugs also, "just to get by. It's not a real problem."

Ms. George has a family history of substance abuse. Her father died several years ago, and she is estranged from her mother. Both parents "had problems" with alcohol and other drugs. She has been separated from her husband, who "had a drinking problem," for ten years. She has two daughters. One died of a heroin overdose four years ago; the other is apparently drug-free and living a successful life with a "wonderful job." She has not seen her living daughter in several years ("She disowned me"). There is an undertone of hopelessness in Ms. George's presentation. She speaks in a monotone and is reluctant to go into details, "because I don't want to upset myself." According to Ms. George, "You live the life you are given, and that's it."

The social worker in the senior center faced several issues: Ms. George is not seeking assistance for substance use, although she seems to be aware that it has caused health problems for her. She is faced with many immediate problems in living. The effort to survive day-to-day may take priority over the consideration of other issues like the long-term consequences of substance abuse. In approaching Ms. George, the social worker asked herself, "What effective strategies exist for engaging older adults in conversations about health and substance abuse-related problems?" A review of the literature reveals that motivational interviewing strategies have proved to be beneficial for engaging older adults with substance abuse and other life problems (Blow, 1998;

Cummings, Cooper, & Cassie, 2009) and that older adults seem to respond to collaborative, informal, and conversational styles of interviewing in which inquiries about substance use are integrated with questions about their other life experiences and concerns (Hanson & Gutheil, 2004).

In conversations with Ms. George, the social worker learned that she had three main areas of concern: her health, her living arrangements, and life on the streets. She acknowledged that she felt sick often and that she "needed to get to the doctor one of these days." She was unhappy not having her own apartment, but she did not know what she could do about this because, "I have no money for rent." She was growing weary spending so much time on the streets. "It's dangerous out there; everyone is trying to take advantage of you. But, what can I do? I have to get out of the apartment when my friend is not there." The social worker, using her practice experience and expertise as well as her familiarity with empirical findings about engaging older adults who have substance-related problems, empathically responded to the client, affirmed the distress she felt, and encouraged the client to elaborate on her immediate concerns. She demonstrated interest in the client, and she explored the issues at the client's pace. As she discussed these issues and sought clarification, she incorporated questions about the client's substance use, following up on the client's own statements that she "used" substances, but they were not "a problem." She integrated questions from the CAGE questionnaire (Mayfield et al., 1974), and she sought information about the circumstances in which Ms. George was likely to use substances and how she felt after she used (exploring situational factors associated with substance use and its consequences: Marlatt & Donovan, 2005). The social worker used summarization, reflection and feedback to raise the client's awareness of the extent of her substance use, and she summarized for the client, using her own words, the apparent benefits and costs of substance use. She was careful never to refer to addiction or alcoholism, since the client never used these terms herself (W. Miller & Rollnick, 2002).

She asked the client what she thought about everything she had told the social worker, and the client responded ambivalently, saying, "I guess it can be a problem, but I have lots of problems. What can I do about it?" The social worker reflected back to the client, that she asked a good question and she asked the client what thoughts she had (encouraging problem-solving in the client and drawing out her solutions). The client focused on housing. So, the social worker agreed and asked her what she thought had to be done to secure housing, knowing that the client had made efforts in this area before. The client acknowledged that if "they" (i.e., the housing authority) thought you had a substance abuse problem they would not help. The social worker used this feedback to help the client understand how substance abuse treatment might be useful then. She added that the client could get medical services at some substance abuse treatment programs and that the treatment activities might help keep her "off the streets."

The social worker was able to make a referral to a hospital-based methadone maintenance program. Since Ms. George was dependent on heroin (as documented by withdrawal symptoms) and she had been unable to stop use in the past ("I get these urges, and I start using again"), methadone treatment was an appropriate service to consider. She was accepted for treatment and was able to get medical services for the hepatitis and other health concerns. Ms. George also was encouraged to "sample" some Alcoholics Anonymous (AA) and Narcotics Anonymous (NA) meetings, partly "as a place to go" to get off the streets. Although she was reluctant, at first, she learned to value the support and benefited from hearing about others' struggles to recover from substance abuse ("I met some good people there, and we help each other. They are not always too keen on me taking methadone – some of the people say I'm still on drugs. Most of them know I'm trying and that I'm taking one day at a time. When I don't need methadone, I'll stop that too.") The social worker also involved Ms. George in group and social activities at the senior center giving her new opportunities to interact in drug-free environments.

A year after referral, Ms. George was still in methadone treatment, attended NA and AA, and participated in senior center activities. She had a few short relapses, but she was abstinent virtually the entire year. She still slept on the couch in her friend's apartment. The social worker sought housing for the client. The client qualified for public assistance, and she was on the waiting list for several apartments. However, a shortage of affordable housing remained a major barrier to acquiring stable housing.

This case illustrates how social workers in non-specialized service settings can use client-centered, motivational strategies to engage substance abusers in treatment and encourage them to take steps to eliminate substance abuse by placing substance abuse in context and linking it to clients' other life problems. It highlights the importance of care management and service co-ordination to avoid fragmentation of service. It also shows how structural problems (e.g., lack of affordable housing) affect the "clinical" process and suggests the need for looking beyond "individual clients" and engaging in class advocacy to expand services and improve "clinical" effectiveness.

Conclusion

From the days of Jane Addams and Mary Richmond, the social work profession has dealt with the consequences of substance abuse (Addams, 1912; Richmond, 1917). In all practice settings social workers must be prepared to assist individuals, families, and communities encountering substance abuse-related problems. This chapter has shown that social workers are uniquely positioned to assist substance-involved clients, that effective practices exist, and that a collaborative, concerned professional practice style can engage clients in treatment and mobilize them for recovery.

Effective social work practice with substance abusers and their families is ecological in nature. Comprehensive assessments identify the situational risks for substance abuse, as well as environmental resources and supports that may reduce the likelihood of abuse and improve chances for recovery. Clients' use of substances is understood in their own words and efforts are made to comprehend how substance use fits into clients' lifestyles. Responsive recovery plans that address not only the substance abuse but also the client's other life problems are developed with clients. Service delivery is coordinated across health and social service settings, and natural support networks are incorporated into assistance plans.

Substance abuse is a pervasive health and social condition. Clients with other health and mental health difficulties are likely to experience difficulties associated with the use of alcohol and other drugs. Generic social work knowledge and skills and specialized substance abuse-related competencies are needed to enable social workers to be responsive to this client population and to deliver effective services.

Note

1   This practice illustration is adapted from a case that was developed with the support of a Gero Innovations Grant from the Council on Social Work Education's (CSWE) Gero-Ed Center's Master's Advanced Curriculum (MAC) Project and the John A. Hartford Foundation (Project #2006-0241). The opinions stated here are the author's and do not necessarily reflect those of CSWE or the John A. Hartford Foundation.

Web resources

National Institute of Alcohol Abuse and Alcoholism
www.niaaa.gov

National Institute of Drug Abuse
www.nida.gov

National Institute of Mental Health
www.nimh.gov

Substance Abuse and Mental Health Services Administration
www.samhsa.gov

References

Addams, J. (1912). *A new conscience and an ancient evil.* New York: Macmillan.

Akers, R.L., Krohn, M., Lanza-Kaduce, L., & Radosevich, M. (1979). Social learning and deviant behavior: A specific test of a general theory. *American Sociological Review, 44,* 636–655.

Alegria, M., Page, J.B., Hansen, H., Cauce, A.M., Robles, R., Blanco, C. et al. (2006). Improving drug treatment services for Hispanics: Research gaps and scientific opportunities. *Drug and Alcohol Dependence, 84S,* S76–S84.

Almasy, L., Blangero, J., Porjesz, B., Chorlian, D.B., Begleiter, H., Goate, A. et al. (2001). Genetics of event-related brain potentials in response to a semantic priming paradigm in families a history of alcoholism. *American Journal of Human Genetics, 68,* 128–135.

American Psychiatric Association (APA). (2000). *Diagnostic and statistical manual of mental disorders* (4th ed., text revision). Washington, DC: APA.

Anderson, J.G., & Gilbert, F.S. (1989). Communication skills training with alcoholics for improving the performance of two of the Alcoholics Anonymous recovery steps. *Journal of Studies on Alcohol, 50,* 361–367.

Azrin, N.H., McMahon, P.T., Donohue, B., Besalei, V.A., Lapinksi, K.J., Kogan, E.S. et al. (1994). Behavior therapy for drug abuse: A controlled treatment outcome study. *Behaviour Research and Therapy, 32,* 857–866.

Beets, M.W., Flay, B.R., Vuchinich, S., Snyder, F.J., Acock, A., Li, K-K. et al. (2009). Use of a social and character development program to prevent substance use, violent behaviors, and sexual activity among elementary-school students in Hawaii. *American Journal of Public Health, 99,* 1438–1445.

Bliss, D.L. (2007). Empirical research on spirituality and alcoholism: A review of the literature. *Journal of Social Work Practice in the Addictions, 7* (4), 5–25.

Bliss, D.L., & Pecukonis, E. (2009). Screening and brief intervention model for social workers in non-substance-abuse practice settings. *Journal of Social Work Practice in the Addictions, 9,* 21–40.

Blow, F.C. (1998). *Substance abuse among older adults.* Treatment Improvement Protocol (TIP) Series 26. Rockville, MD: Center for Substance Abuse Treatment.

Botvin, G., Schinke, S., Epstein, J., Diaz, T., & Botvin, E. (1995). Effectiveness of culturally focused and generic skills training approaches to alcohol and drug abuse prevention among minority adolescents: Two-year follow-up results. *Psychology of Addictive Behaviors, 9* (3), 183–194.

Bourgois, P. (1995). *In search of respect: Selling crack in El Barrio.* New York: Cambridge University Press.

Carroll, K.M. (2003). Integrating psychotherapy and pharmacotherapy in substance abuse treatment. In F. Rotgers, J. Morgenstern, & S.T. Walters (eds), *Treating substance abuse: Theory and technique* (2nd ed., pp. 314–342). New York: Guilford Press.

Cohen, L.M., Collins, Jr., F.L., Young, A., McChargue, D.E., Leffingwell, T.R., & Cook, K.L. (eds). (2009). *Pharmacology and treatment of substance abuse: Evidence- and outcome-based perspectives.* New York: Routledge.

Cummings, S.M., Cooper, R.L., & Cassie, K.M. (2009). Motivational interviewing to affect behavioral change in older adults. *Research on Social Work Practice, 19,* 195–204.

Dawson, D.A., Grant, B.F., Stinson, F.S., & Chou, P.S. (2006). Estimating the effect of help seeking on achieving recovery from alcohol dependence. *Addiction, 101,* 824–834.

De Leon, G. (2000). *The therapeutic community: Theory, model, and method.* New York: Springer.

Diamond, G.S., & Liddle, H.A. (1996). Resolving a therapeutic impasse between parents and adolescents in Multidimensional Family Therapy. *Journal of Consulting and Clinical Psychology, 64,* 481–488.

Dick, D.M., Birut, L., Hinrichs, A., Fox, L., Bucholz, K., Kramer, J. et al. (2006). The role of GABRA2 in risk for conduct disorder and alcohol and drug dependence across developmental stages. *Behavior Genetics, 36*, 577–590.

Drake, R.E., & Mueser, K.T. (1996). Alcohol-use disorders and severe mental illness. *Alcohol Health and Research World, 20* (2), 87–93.

Ferri, M., Amato, L., & Davoli, M. (2006). Alcoholics Anonymous and other 12-step programmes for alcohol dependence. *Cochrane Database Systematic Reviews*, Issue 3, Art. No. CD005032.

Galanter, M.A. (2008). Spirituality, evidence-based medicine, and Alcoholics Anonymous. *American Journal of Psychiatry, 165*, 1514–1517.

Gastfriend, D.R., & Mee-Lee, D. (2003). The ASAM patient placement criteria: Context, concepts, and continuing development. *Journal of Addictive Diseases, 22* (Suppl. 1), 1–8.

Gitterman, A., & Germain, C.B. (2008). *The life model of social work practice: Advances in theory and practice* (3rd ed.). New York: Columbia University Press.

Grant, B.F., Goldstein, R.B., Chou, S.P., Huang, B., Stinson, F.S., Dawson, D.A. et al. (2008, April 22). Sociodemographic and psychopathologic predictors of first incidence of DSM-IV substance use, mood and anxiety disorders: Results from the Wave 2 National Epidemiologic Survey on Alcohol and Related Conditions. *Molecular Psychiatry*, Advanced Online Publication.

Gray, M. (1998). *Drug crazy: How we got into this mess and how we can get out.* New York: Random House.

Gray, M., & Webb, S.A. (2009). Introduction. In M. Gray & S.A. Webb (eds), *Social work theory and methods* (pp. 1–10). Los Angeles, CA: Sage.

Hall, D.H., & Queener, J.E. (2007). Self-medication hypothesis of substance use: Testing Khantzian's updated theory. *Journal of Psychoactive Drugs, 39*, 151–158.

Han, B., Gfroerer, J.C., Colliver, J.D., & Penne, M.A. (2009). Substance use disorder among older adults in the United States in 2010. *Addiction, 104*, 88–96.

Hanson, M. (2001). Alcoholism and other drug addictions. In A. Gitterman (ed.), *Handbook of social work practice with vulnerable and resilient populations* (2nd ed., pp. 64–96). New York: Columbia University Press.

Hanson, M. (2009). People with problematic alcohol use. In A. Gitterman & R. Salmon (eds), *Encyclopedia of social work with groups* (pp. 212–215). New York: Routledge.

Hanson, M., & El-Bassel, N. (2004). Motivating substance-abusing clients through the helping process. In S.L.A. Straussner (ed.), *Clinical work with substance-abusing clients* (2nd ed., pp. 39–64). New York: Guilford Press.

Hanson, M., & Gutheil, I.A. (2004). Motivational strategies with alcohol-involved older adults: Implications for social work practice. *Social Work, 49*, 364–372.

Hatzenbuehler, M.L., Keyes, K.M., Narrow, W.E., Grant, B.F., & Hasin, D.S. (2008). Racial/ethnic disparities in service utilization for individuals with co-occurring mental health and substance use disorders in the general population: Results from the National Epidemiologic Survey on Alcohol and Related Conditions. *Journal of Clinical Psychiatry, 69*, 1112–1121.

Hawkins, J.D., Catalano, Jr., R.F., & Associates. (1992). *Communities that care: Action for drug abuse prevention.* San Francisco, CA: Jossey-Bass.

Heinrich, C.J., & Lynn, Jr., L.E. (2002). Improving the organization, management, and outcomes of substance abuse treatment programs. *American Journal of Drug and Alcohol Abuse, 28*, 601–622.

Henwood, B., & Padgett, D.K. (2007). Reevaluating the self-medication hypothesis among the dually diagnosed. *American Journal on Addictions, 16*, 160–165.

Higgins, S.T., Budney, A.J., Bickel, W.K., Foerg, F.E., Donham, R., & Badger, G.J. (1995). Outpatient behavioral treatment for cocaine dependence: One-year outcome. *Experimental and Clinical Psychpharmacology, 3*, 205–212.

Hohman, M., Clapp, J.D., & Carrilio, T.E. (2006). Development and validation of the alcohol and other drug identification (AODI) scale. *Journal of Social Work Practice in the Addictions, 6* (3), 3–12.

Institute of Medicine. (2006). *Improving the quality of health care for mental and substance-use conditions.* Washington, DC: National Academy Press.

Jahoda, G., & Cramond, J. (1972). *Children and alcohol.* London: Her Majesty's Stationery Office.

Jellinek, E.M. (1946). Phases in the drinking history of alcoholics. *Quarterly Journal of Studies on Alcohol, 7*, 1–88.

Jellinek, E.M. (1960). *The disease concept of alcoholism.* New Haven, CT: College & University Press.

Jonnes, J. (1995). The rise of the modern addict. *American Journal of Public Health, 85,* 1157–1162.

Julien, R.M. (2007). *A primer on drug action* (11th ed.). New York: Worth.

Kagle, J. D. (1987). Secondary prevention of substance abuse. *Social Work, 32,* 446–448.

Keyes, K.M., Hatzenbuehler, M.L., Alberti, P., Narrow, W.E., Grant, B.F., & Hasin, D.S. (2008). Service utilization differences for Axis I psychiatric and substance use disorders between White and Black adults. *Psychiatric Services, 59,* 893–901.

Khantzian, E.J., & Albanese, M.J. (2008). *Understanding addiction as self-medication: Finding hope behind the pain.* Lanham, MD: Jason Aronson.

Kissin, B. (1983). The disease concept of alcoholism. In R.G. Smart, F.B. Glaser, Y. Israel, H. Kalant, R. Popham, & W. Schmidt (eds), *Research advances in alcohol and drug abuse problems* (Vol. 7, pp. 93–126). New York: Plenum.

Koob, G.F. (2009). Neurobiology of addiction. In L.M. Cohen et al. (eds), *Pharmacology and treatment of substance abuse: Evidence- and outcome-based perspectives* (pp. 85–108). New York: Routledge.

Kurtz, E. (1979/1991). *Not God: A history of Alcoholics Anonymous.* Center City, MN: Hazelden.

Kurtz, L.F. (1997). *Self-help and other support groups.* Thousand Oaks, CA: Sage.

Leonard, K.E., & Blane, H.T. (eds). (1999). *Psychological theories of drinking and alcoholism* (2nd ed.). New York: Guilford Press.

Levine, H.G. (1978). The discovery of addiction: Changing conceptions of habitual drunkenness in America. *Journal of Studies on Alcohol, 39,* 143–174.

Loughran, H., Hohman, M., & Finnegan, D. (2008). Predictors of role legitimacy and role adequacy of social workers working with substance-using clients. *British Journal of Social Work, 40* (1), 239–256.

Magill, M. & Ray, L.A. (2009). Cognitive-behavioral treatment with adult alcohol and illicit drug users: A meta-analysis of randomized controlled trials. *Journal of Studies on Alcohol and Drugs, 70,* 516–527.

Marlatt, G.A. (1994). Addiction, mindfulness, and acceptance. In S.C. Hayes, N.S. Jacobson, V.M. Follette, & M.J. Dougher (eds), *Acceptance and change: Content and context in psychotherapy* (pp. 175–197). Reno, NV: Context Press.

Marlatt, G.A. (ed.). (1998). *Harm reduction: Pragmatic strategies for managing high-risk behaviors.* New York: Guilford Press.

Marlatt, G.A., & Donovan, D.M. (eds). (2005). *Relapse prevention: Maintenance strategies in the treatment of addictive behaviors* (2nd ed.). New York: Guilford Press.

Marth, D. (2009). Mental Health Parity Act of 2007: An analysis of proposed changes. *Social Work in Mental Health, 7,* 556–571.

Matthews, C.R., Lorah, P., & Fenton, J. (2006). Treatment experiences of gays and lesbians in recovery from addictions: A qualitative inquiry. *Journal of Mental Health Counseling, 28,* 110–132.

Mayfield, D.G., McLeod, G., & Hall, P. (1974). The CAGE questionnaire: Validation of a new alcoholism screening instrument. *American Journal of Psychiatry, 131,* 1121–1123.

McCabe, S.E., Hughes, T.L., Bostwick, W.B., West, B.T., & Boyd, C.J. (2009). Sexual orientation, substance use behaviors and substance dependence in the United States. *Addiction, 104,* 1333–1345.

McLellan, A.T. (2003). Foreward. *Journal of Addictive Diseases, 22* (Suppl. 1), xv–xviii.

McLellan, A.T., Kushner, H., Metzger, D., Peters, R., Smith, I., Grissom, G. et al. (1992). The fifth edition of the Addictive Severity Index: Historical critique and normative data. *Journal of Substance Abuse Treatment, 9,* 199–213.

McLellan, A.T., Carise, D., & Kleber, H.D. (2003). The national addiction treatment infrastructure: Can it support the public's demand for quality care? *Journal of Substance Abuse Treatment, 25,* 117–121.

Mee-Lee, D., Shulman, G.D., Fishman, M., Gastfriend, D.R., & Griffith, J.H. (eds). (2001). *ASAM patient placement criteria for the treatment of substance-related disorders* (2nd ed. rev., PPC-2R). Chevy Chase, MD: American Society of Addiction Medicine.

Meyers, R.J., & Miller, W.R. (eds). (2001). *A community reinforcement approach to addiction treatment.* New York: Cambridge University Press.

Miller, D., & Guidry, L. (2001). *Addictions and trauma recovery: Healing the body, mind, and spirit.* New York: W.W. Norton.

Miller, W.R. (1998). Researching the spiritual dimensions of alcohol and other drug problems. *Addiction, 93,* 979–990.

Miller, W.R., & Hester, R.K. (2003). Treating alcohol problems: Toward an informed eclecticism. In R.K. Hester & W.R. Miller (eds), *Handbook of alcoholism treatment approaches: Effective alternatives* (3rd ed., pp. 1–12). Boston, MA: Allyn & Bacon.

Miller, W.R., & Rollnick, S. (2002). *Motivational interviewing: Preparing people for change* (2nd ed.). New York: Guilford Press.

Miller, W.R., Wilbourne, P.L., & Hettema, J.E. (2003). What works? A summary of alcohol treatment outcome research. In R.K. Hester & W.R. Miller (eds), *Handbook of alcoholism treatment approaches: Effective alternatives* (3rd ed., pp. 13–63). Boston, MA: Allyn & Bacon.

Moos, R.H. (2008). Active ingredients in substance use-focused self-help groups. *Addiction, 103*, 387–396.

Morgan, H.W. (1981). *Drugs in America: A social history, 1800–1980.* Syracuse, NY: Syracuse University Press.

Mueser, K.T., Noordsby, D.L., Drake, R.E., & Fox, L. (2003). *Integrated treatment for dual disorders: A guide to effective practice.* New York: Guilford.

National Association for Children of Alcoholics (NACOA). (2006). *Core competencies for social workers in addressing the needs of children of alcohol and drug dependent parents.* Rockville, MD: NACOA.

National Consensus Development Panel on Effective Medical Treatment of Opiate Addiction. (1998). Effective medical treatment of opiate addiction. *Journal of the American Medical Association, 280*, 1936–1943.

National Institute of Mental Health (NIMH). (2001). *National Institute of Mental Health five-year strategic plan for reducing health disparities.* Rockville, MD: Office of Special Populations NIMH.

National Institute on Alcohol Abuse and Alcoholism (NIAAA). (2002). Alcohol and minorities: An update. *Alcohol Alert, 55*, 1–4.

National Institute on Drug Abuse (NIDA). (1999). *Principles of drug addiction treatment: A research-based guide.* Rockville, MD: NIDA.

National Institute on Drug Abuse (NIDA). (2003). *Preventing drug use among children and adolescents: A research-based guide for parents, educators, and community leaders* (2nd ed.). Rockville, MD: NIDA.

Nock, M.K., Goldman, J.L., Wang, Y., & Albano, A.M. (2004). From science to practice: The flexible use of evidence-based treatments in clinical settings. *Journal of the American Academy of Child and Adolescent Psychiatry, 43*, 777–780.

Nowinksi, J. (2003). Facilitating 12-step recovery from substance abuse and addiction. In F. Rotgers, J. Morgenstern, & S.T. Walters (eds), *Treating substance abuse: Theory and technique* (2nd ed., pp. 31–66). New York: Guilford Press.

O'Farrell, T.J., & Fals-Stewart, W. (2006). *Behavioral couples therapy for alcoholism and drug abuse.* New York: Guilford Press.

O'Neil, J.V. (2001, January). Expertise in addictions said crucial. *NASW News*, p. 1.

Perron, B.E., Mowbray, O.P., Glass, J.E., Delva, J., Vaughn, M.G., & Howard, M.O. (2009). Differences in service utilization and barriers among Blacks, Hispanics, and Whites with drug use disorders. *Substance Abuse Treatment, Prevention, and Policy, 4* (3). Retrieved from www.substanceabusepolicy.com/content/4/1/3.

Priester, P.E., Scherer, J., Steinfeldt, J.A., Jana-Masri, A., Jashinsky, T., Jones, J.E., & Vang, C. (2009). The frequency of prayer, meditation and holistic interventions in addictions treatment: A national survey. *Pastoral Psychology, 58*, 315–322.

Ray, L.A., & Hutchison, K.E. (2009). Genetics of addiction. In L.M. Cohen et al. (eds), *Pharmacology and treatment of substance abuse: Evidence- and outcome-based perspectives* (pp. 109–126). New York: Routledge.

Reich, T., Edenberg, H.J., Goate, A., Williams, J.T., Rice, J.P., Van Eerdewegh, F.T. et al. (1998) Genome-wide search for genes affecting the risk for alcohol dependence. *American Journal of Medical Genetics, 81*, 207–215.

Rhodes, J.J.E., & Jason, L.A. (1988). *Preventing substance abuse among children and adolescents.* New York: Pergamon.

Richmond, M. (1917). *Social diagnosis.* New York: Russell Sage Foundation.

Room, R., & Greenfield, T. (1993). Alcoholics Anonymous, other 12-step movements, and psychotherapy in the U.S. population. *Addiction, 88*, 555–562.

Rowe, C.L., Liddle, H.A., Dakoff, G.A., & Henderson, C.E. (2009). Development and evolution of an evidence-based practice: Multidimensional family therapy as treatment system. In L.M. Cohen et al.

(eds), *Pharmacology and treatment of substance abuse: Evidence- and outcome-based perspectives* (pp. 441–463). New York: Routledge.

Selzer, M.L. (1971). The Michigan Alcoholism Screening Test: The quest for a new diagnostic instrument. *American Journal of Psychiatry, 127*, 1653–1658.

Shlonsky, A., & Gibbs, L. (2004). Will the real evidence-based practice please stand up? Teaching the process of evidence-based practice to the helping professions. *Brief Treatment and Crisis Intervention, 4*, 137–153.

Smith, J.E., & Meyers, R.J. (2004). *Motivating substance abusers to enter treatment: Working with family members.* New York: Guilford Press.

Steiker, L.K.H. (2009). Motivation interviewing and addiction: An interview with Melinda Hohman. *Journal of Social Work Practice in the Addictions, 9*, 236–239.

Stewart, S.H., Gavric, D., & Collins, P. (2009). Women, girls, and alcohol. In K.T. Brady, S.E. Back, & S.F. Greenfield (eds), *Women and addiction: A comprehensive handbook* (pp. 341–359). New York: Guilford Press.

Substance Abuse and Mental Health Services Administration (SAMHSA) (2007). *National Survey of Substance Abuse Treatment Services (N-SSATS): 2006. Data on substance abuse treatment facilities.* (Office of Applied Studies, DASIS Series: S-39, DHHS Publication No. SMA 07-4296). Rockville, MD: SAMHSA.

Substance Abuse and Mental Health Services Administration (SAMHSA). (2008). *Results from the 2007 National Survey on Drug Use and Health: National findings.* (Office of Applied Studies, NSDUH Series H-34, DHHS Publication No. SMA 084343.) Rockville, MD: SAMHSA.

Thombs, D.L. (2006). *Introduction to addictive behaviors* (3rd ed.). New York: Guilford Press.

Tonigan, J.S., Connors, G.J., & Miller, W.R. (2003). Participation and involvement in Alcoholics Anonymous. In T.F. Babor & F.K. Del Boca (eds), *Treatment matching in alcoholism* (pp. 184–204). New York: Cambridge University Press.

Waldron, H.B., Brody, J.L., & Slesnick, N. (2001). Integrative behavioral and family therapy for adolescent substance abuse. In P.M. Monti, S.M. Colby, & T.A. O'Leary (eds), *Adolescents, alcohol, and substance abuse: Reaching teens through brief interventions* (pp. 216–243). New York: Guilford Press.

Weatherburn, D. (2009). Dilemmas in harm minimization. *Addiction, 104*, 335–339.

Weegmann, M. (2006). Edward Khantzian interview. *Journal of Groups in Addiction and Recovery, 1* (2), 15–32.

White, W.L. (2008). *Recovery management and recovery-oriented systems of care: Scientific rationale and promising practices.* Pittsburgh, PA: Institute for Research, Education, and Training in Addictions.

Woody, G.E., McLellan, A.T., Luborsky, L., & O'Brien, C.P. (1995). Psychotherapy in community methadone programs: A validation study. *American Journal of Psychiatry, 152*, 1302–1308.

Yalisove, D.L. (ed.). (1997). *Essential papers on addiction.* New York: New York University Press.

21 Dementia and related problems in cognition and memory

Sara Sanders and Joelle K. Osterhaus

Alzheimer's disease and related dementia (ADRD) represent a growing crisis among older adults, their families, and the health care system. The number of people with ADRD is rapidly increasing as more individuals reach older adulthood and live longer (Alzheimer's Association, 2009; National Institute on Aging (NIA), 2008). With a definitive cause of and cure for ADRD still unknown, despite great research advances, there is fear that this condition could bankrupt the health care system.

The progressive decline of dementia invariably impacts more than just the diagnosed individual; it also impacts the primary caregiver and the extended family system, as the diagnosed individual evaporates right before their eyes. Families feel little hope as they watch this disease dissolve the past memories, present lives, and future dreams of the diagnosed individual. The most significant of these familial effects takes place within the role of the caregiver. The "caregiving career," as it is commonly referred to, has implications for the caregivers' emotional, psychological, and physical health, as well as putting strain on the larger family system.

As more people reach age 65 and develop ADRD, social workers will be called upon to help the diagnosed individual and caregiver obtain needed community resources, education about the disease, and counseling to assist with the adjustment to the diagnosis and the development of coping strategies. The purpose of this chapter is to provide an overview of dementia and its impact on the diagnosed individual and caregiver. The chapter examines disparities in access to services for the diagnosed individual and caregiver, types of services used by diagnosed individuals and their caregivers, and the roles that social workers assume with this population. For the sake of this chapter, the phrase "Alzheimer's disease and related dementia (ADRD)" will be used to define a broad classification of conditions that lead to progressive memory loss. The authors recognize that there are individual intricacies within each type of dementia; however, all of the conditions generally lead to similar outcomes in diagnosed individuals and produce stress and burden for the caregiver.

Definitions of dementia

Originally discovered in 1906 by Dr. Alois Alzheimer, cognitive impairment in older adults has long been considered a normal part of the aging process, instead of a serious health condition. Terms such as senility, hardening of the arteries, and simply old age, characterized ADRD until the mid 1990s. President Ronald Reagan being diagnosed with Alzheimer's disease brought ADRD into the public domain as it received increased attention, both clinically and empirically. In his letter to the nation following his diagnosis, President Reagan noted the impending impact of the disease on him, as well as his caregiver Nancy. Since this announcement, empirical research on this and related topics, as well as by the growth in public awareness of the organizations and services designed for dementia-related illness, such as the Alzheimer's Association, has grown.

According to the Alzheimer's Association (2009), ADRD includes diseases "of the brain that cause problems with memory, thinking, and behavior" (p. 2). As one ages, changes occur in the brain that result in slowed thinking and difficulty remembering and recalling information. These normal age-related changes in cognitive function are periodic, temporary, and do not impact daily functioning. The cognitive changes that occur with ADRD are not normal aging. These changes are permanent and progressive and eventually prevent a person from functioning independently. As the disease progresses, the diagnosed person eventually fails to recognize that they are experiencing difficulty with their memory (Knopman, Boeve, & Petersen, 2003). Unfortunately, the symptoms of ADRD are still considered a normal part of the aging process by many lay individuals, as well as some professionals (Knopman et al., 2003). This false perception often delays individuals and families from obtaining a diagnosis and accessing needed resources early in the disease process. Individuals diagnosed with ADRD eventually die as a result of the *disease* and the *disease-related changes* that occur in the brain (Alzheimer's Association, 2009). While some individuals with progressive memory loss are cognizant of their cognitive decline, particularly early in the disease process, others may not recognize or accept that cognitive changes are occurring (Knopman et al., 2003). This can create additional challenges to families and friends who are trying to provide assistance and facilitate decision making.

Dementia is a broad term used to describe a group of conditions that cause memory loss. Two criteria commonly define dementia: first, changes in levels of functioning, and second, cognitive impairment (Knopman et al., 2003). Dementia is characterized by changes in memory, language, visuospatial function, and executive function (e.g., ability for abstract thinking, problem resolution, planning, mental focus) (APA, 2000; Knopman et al., 2003). There are over 70 different types of dementia with some being classified as reversible in older adults, for instance depression, confusion from the mismanagement of medications, or secondary infections, and others being identified as non-reversible, including Alzheimer's disease. Historically, the non-reversible forms have been labeled under the broad heading of "dementia." While this is still a common practice, determining the specific type of dementia is important given that the various forms progress in different ways, have some unique characteristics, and respond differently to pharmacological strategies aimed at slowing the disease progression (American Psychiatric Association (APA), 2007).

There are similarities in the symptoms associated with various forms of dementia including progressive memory loss, changes in one's ability to complete routine tasks and activities of daily living (ADLs), and one's ability to function independently (APA, 2007). However, the way in which the disease impacts the brain and the severity of symptoms exhibited varies depending on the individual and the particular disorder (Knopman et al., 2003). For social workers providing services to individuals with ADRD and their caregivers, recognizing distinguishing characteristics of each type of dementia is important in providing treatment, as well as accurate guidance about long-term planning and education.

Mild cognitive impairment is a diagnosis given when the signs of cognitive impairment are apparent, but these symptoms do not significantly impact one's ability to function independently (Knopman et al., 2003). While an individual who has mild cognitive impairment does have some memory loss, the degree of impairment in other areas of functioning, such as disorientation to time, person, or place, changes in one's ability to complete daily tasks, and the significant memory loss that is present in a person with a diagnosed form of ADRD, is not apparent. Obtaining a diagnosis of mild cognitive impairment is important because individuals with this condition are five to ten times more likely to develop ADRD than individuals who have no cognitive impairment (Petersen, 2003; Petersen, Smith, Waring, Ivnik, Tangalos, &

Kokmen, 1999). At the current time, pharmacological treatments are not available for mild cognitive impairment; however, Aricept, a common treatment for Alzheimer's disease, may be considered for individuals with this condition, to assist in slowing any disease progression. Additionally, memory enhancement strategies, such as different types of puzzles, writing down important information, and performing mental checks, may also be employed to help maintain independent functioning. Identifying mild cognitive impairment is also important for families so plans for the future, such as legal and financial planning, can be made should the disease worsen and progress into a form of ADRD (New York University Medical Center, 2008).

The most common form of dementia is *Alzheimer's disease*, which accounts for 60–70 percent of all cases of ADRD (Alzheimer's Association, 2009). Therefore, if a person receives a broad diagnosis of "dementia," they actually have a 60–70 percent chance of having Alzheimer's disease. This is particularly important to consider given that the broad diagnosis of "dementia" is frequently provided by physicians, instead of a diagnosis that identifies the specific form of dementia. This may unintentionally mislead families to believe that the diagnosed individual does not have Alzheimer's disease and thereby creates false hope. Some will argue that a specific diagnosis of Alzheimer's disease cannot be given until death. Thus, the term "dementia" is all that can be provided to concerned individuals and families. However, according to the Alzheimer's Association (2008), a diagnosis of Alzheimer's disease can be provided by physicians with over 90 percent accuracy if a comprehensive diagnosis assessment occurs.

Alzheimer's disease is the result of neuritic plaques and neurofibrillary tangles that develop in the brain. Neuritic plaques are defined as "deposits of a protein fragment called beta-amyloid that builds up in the spaces between the nerve cells" (Alzheimer's Association, 2009, p. 11). Neurofibrillary tangles are "twisted fibers of another protein called tau that build up inside cells" (Alzheimer's Association, 2009, p. 11). All individuals develop plaques and tangles in their brain as they age, but those with Alzheimer's disease develop considerably more of these composites and experience greater damage as a result (Alzheimer's Association, 2009). Plaques and tangles impede the ability for communication to occur between nerve cells, thus leading to the symptoms commonly known as Alzheimer's disease. It is unknown if the entire nerve cell is damaged by the plaques and tangles or if only a portion of the nerve cell is affected. It is known, however, that once a nerve cell becomes damaged, other adjacent cells also become damaged; thereby creating a situation where cells cease to function and eventually die (Alzheimer's Association, 2009). This results in the symptoms commonly seen in Alzheimer's disease. Alzheimer's disease can last between 3 and 20 years, with the course, on average, lasting between 6 and 10 years (Alzheimer's Association, 2007; Wolfson et al., 2007).

Alzheimer's disease is considered a terminal disease from the time of diagnosis because a cure for this condition is not available (Jennings, 2003). Researchers are tirelessly working to determine a conclusive cause for Alzheimer's disease. Research has identified that there is a genetic component of this disease (Alzheimer's Association, 2009; Lautenschlager et al., 1996); however, a genetic predisposition does not equate to a person definitively developing the disorder. According to Knopman et al. (2003), "For most patients with AD, autosomal dominant inheritance . . . is an extreme rarity" (p. 1295). However, genetics do play a significant role in individuals presenting with the disease prior to age 60, usually in their thirties, forties, or fifties. This condition, referred to as early onset Alzheimer's disease, is the result of gene mutations on chromosomes 21, 14, and 1 (National Institute on Aging, 2008). NIA indicated that if one mutated gene passes from a parent to a child, the child will most likely develop Alzheimer's disease. Offspring have over a 50 percent chance of developing early onset Alzheimer's disease if a parent also had this condition (NIA, 2008).

For individuals over age 60, genetics are also being examined. Research has identified that the apolipoprotein E (APOE) found on chromosome 19 increases the risk of developing

Alzheimer's disease (NIA, 2008). Allele 4 of APOE (APOE e4) has been found to exist in 40 percent of individuals who develop Alzheimer's disease after age 60. Fitzpatrick et al. (2004) found that carriers of APOE e4 were twice as likely to develop ADRD as non-carriers. However, not all individuals with Alzheimer's disease have APOE e4 (Farrer et al., 1997; NIA, 2008). More empirical attention needs to be directed to the genetic components of Alzheimer's disease in an attempt to better understand the cause of this condition and determine a cure. In addition to genetic factors, non-genetic factors are also being examined as risk factors for Alzheimer's disease, including brain injury and other health conditions (Alzheimer's Association, 2008; Fleminger, Oliver, Lovestone, Rabe-Hesketh, & Giora, 2003; Itzhaki, 1994; Lopez et al., 2000; Nemetz et al., 1999). An extensive examination of the genetic predisposition of Alzheimer's disease is beyond the scope of this chapter, but can be found on the Alzheimer's Association website. *Vascular dementia*, commonly called multi-infarct dementia, is the second most common form of dementia. It is characterized by mini-strokes, which create symptoms similar to Alzheimer's disease. One of the distinguishing characteristics of vascular dementia versus Alzheimer's disease is the decline or disease progression. For vascular dementia, the decline is not as gradual as is seen in Alzheimer's disease, but instead more like stair steps with periods of decline and then periods of plateaus. Vascular dementia can be distinguished from Alzheimer's disease on CT scans of the brain.

Other forms of dementia, such as *Lewy Body dementia, Parkinson's disease, Huntington's disease*, or *Pick's disease* are also characterized by memory loss, but possess unique characteristics, such as more visual hallucinations, muscle rigidity, greater personality changes, and different patterns of onset (Alzheimer's Association, 2009) that distinguish them from other forms of ADRD. Research into each of these other forms of dementia is also expanding.

Diagnosing the specific type of dementia, as well as ruling out other causes of memory loss, such as depression, secondary infections, and even delirium, is critical for a patient and their caregiver. Identifying the specific type of dementia can impact treatment decisions. In terms of Alzheimer's disease, great strides are being taken in the development of pharmacological interventions designed to slow the progression of the disease (Hansen, Gartlehner, Kaufer, Lohr, & Carey, 2006). While a cure has yet to be found, slowing the progression of the disease helps to maintain the diagnosed individual at a higher level of functioning for a longer period of time. This benefits not only the diagnosed individual and the caregiver, but also the greater health care system because health care dollars are saved. Finally, identifying the specific type of dementia has important consequences in terms of planning for the future given that some forms of ADRD progress more quickly.

Regardless of the type of dementia, ADRD represents many different things to diagnosed individuals, their family systems, and service providers. For the diagnosed individual, the disease creates fear. Older adults have seen friends and relatives progress with ADRD and have heard frightening stories of how this disease changes individuals' personalities and behaviors, and robs the person of their ability to function independently. Phrases, such as "going crazy" and "lost her mind," are commonly associated with ADRD, which exacerbates the fear. Additionally, this disease creates fear because of its association with admission to nursing homes. For most older adults, socialization to nursing homes took place during a period when physical and pharmacological restraints were common and regulations were lacking. While standards for nursing homes have changed since the late 1970s with new policies and regulations (Rehnquist, 2003), the fears are still present and become more pronounced when they consider the impact of being placed in a facility with cognitive impairment.

Coupling fear, ADRD creates stigma for diagnosed individuals. Much of the stigma associated with ADRD is related to the transition from functioning independently to becoming dependent on others to ensure that daily needs are met. Additional stigma is created because of the personality and behavioral changes that occur in diagnosed individuals. As the disease progresses, the essence of their personhood changes, with some individual acting or communicating in ways that were not consistent with their personality pre-diagnosis. Stigmatizing behaviors associated with ADRD, such as incontinence, aggression, behavioral manifestations, communication problems, and losing the ability to speak, walk, and swallow, paint an unsettling picture of a person that is seen as possessing no quality of life and little dignity.

The disease also represents a series of losses for diagnosed individuals. These losses include the loss of one's hopes and dreams for the future, activities, safety and security in their environments, and ultimately control over their own lives Individuals also lose their ability to make decisions, particularly if the diagnosis is not given until after a person is significantly impaired by the disease and is considered no longer competent to make their own choices, such as when selecting their caregiver or their preferred care locations. In addition, individuals lose social networks, as their friends who may not be comfortable with cognitive impairment, slowly withdraw. Individuals also lose their freedom and their ability to be independent because they will eventually reach a point where they require constant supervision. As the disease progresses, they will lose control over their own body and have to rely on others for total care. These losses, while known, may not be addressed or even recognized by formal or informal supports. Caregivers and other family members may shy away from discussing these losses out of "fear of upsetting" the person with ADRD or because of their own emotional and psychological reactions to the ADRD diagnosis. This leaves individuals grieving these losses and many more alone.

Research has extensively examined the impact of ADRD on *caregivers* and the larger family system. With 70 percent of individuals with ADRD being cared for at home for the entire course of the disease (Alzheimer's Association, 2009), familial caregivers are asked to provide substantial amounts of care, often for long durations of time. Providing care for an individual with ADRD includes providing assistance with activities of daily living (ADLs), ensuring safety and constant supervision, planning daily activities and routines, and coping with behavioral and personality changes. Caregivers often struggle with a lack of sleep given that sundowning and confusing days and nights are common behaviors associated with dementia. Providing the degree of care that is required for individuals with ADRD takes a significant toll on the caregivers' emotional, psychological, and physical health status (MetLife Mature Market Institute, 2007; Yaffe et al., 2002). As a result, caregivers are considered to be at risk for depression, anxiety, and other mental health issues (Agronin, 2007), with studies showing that 40 percent of caregivers report high levels of stress (Alzheimer's Association & National Alliance for Caregiving, 2004) and depression impacts almost 30 percent of caregivers (Yaffe et al., 2002). The burden that accompanies caregiving often leads to nursing home placement (Buhr, Kuchibhatla, & Clipp, 2006). Additionally, the demands of caregiving places caregivers at risk of physical health problems (Vitaliano, Zhang, & Scanlan, 2003), including lower immune function and high blood pressure due to stress.

The way that caregivers respond to ADRD varies by race. Compared to Caucasian caregivers, minority caregivers, particularly African American and Latino caregivers, have been found to have better long-term caregiving outcomes. Research has shown that minority caregivers report greater caregiver satisfaction (Lawton, Rajagopal, Brody, & Kleban, 1992), find more positive elements of caregiving (Foley, Tung, & Mutran, 2002), and experience less stress, burden, and depression as compared to their Caucasian counterparts (Aranda & Knight, 1997; Haley et al., 1995; Haley et al., 2004). Haley et al. (2004) found that African American caregivers also used fewer psychotropic medications. These more positive outcomes may be related to coping patterns, such as religion and prayer, which buffer the negative aspects of caregiving for minority caregivers (Dilworth-Anderson, Williams, & Gibson, 2002; Haley et al.,

2004). Minority caregivers provide care within a cultural context, with caregiving being seen as an expectation and part of one's value system (Cox & Monk, 1996).

Research has started to examine the experience of caregiving for a person with ADRD from the standpoint of unrelenting grief and loss. Like the diagnosed individual, caregivers experience a range of losses throughout the course of the disease, including the loss of communication, relationships, roles, future plans and dreams, intimacy, and activities (Collins, Liken, King, & Kokinakis, 1993; Loos & Bowd, 1997). Ultimately, they lose their role as a caregiver when the diagnosed individual dies. This can create many complicated feelings and reactions, particularly if providing care resulted in other losses in their lives, such as careers or social support networks. Research on grief in caregivers of individuals with ADRD has identified that caregiver grief is similar to post-death grief in its intensity and duration (Meuser, Marwit, & Sanders, 2004). Much of the impact of grief on caregivers is associated with the ambiguity that the disease creates for caregivers. Boss (1999) coined the term "ambiguous loss" and identified that the uncertainty or ambiguity, as she states, occurs for dementia caregivers because they are providing care for a person who is physically present, but increasingly psychologically absent as the disease progresses. Thus, the status of their relationship with this person is drawn into question. Feelings of ambiguity are further heightened by elements of disenfranchised grief given that the losses experienced by the caregiver are not recognized and validated by others, many of whom do not have a firm understanding of the disease progression with ADRD and its impact on the caregiver.

ADRD also impacts *service providers*. Like lay people, service providers do not always have the knowledge or an understanding of dementia, which can impact the care that individuals with ADRD receive. Jennings (2003) referred to individuals with dementia as the "hot potato" that no health care setting wants to touch. Research on physicians, nurses, and social workers have identified that these professionals lack the necessary education about the disease, which in turn adversely impacts assessment and treatment (Allen, Ferrier, Sargeant, Loney, Bethune, & Murphy, 2005; Kane, 2003; Kane, Hamlin, & Hawkins, 2004; Meuser, Boise, & Morris, 2004; Pucci et al., 2003; Sanders & Swails, 2009; Turner et al., 2004).

The lack of knowledge observed among these circles is associated with inadequate training. Like family caregivers, caring for an individual with ADRD can cause stress and burden for professionals, particularly if they have not received training in how to manage the symptoms associated with the disease. Research has ventured as far as to argue that providers, particularly in nursing homes, have received "substandard" training (Maas, Specht, Buckwalter, Gittler, & Bechen, 2008), which has resulted in poor care for residents, including those with dementia (Gregory, 2001). Other research has shown similar findings, identifying that nursing home providers have received limited training in issues of depression and dementia (Hughes, Bagley, Reilly, Burns, & Challis, 2008). Brodaty, Draper, and Low (2003) determined that nursing home staff has difficulty coping with the aggressive, resistive, and unpredictability of the behavior of residents with dementia. Staff who are Caucasian, younger, have less experience working at a facility, and have worked in a facility with a special care unit for people with dementia have been found to experience more stress (Zimmerman et al., 2005). These findings demonstrate the need for dementia-specific education for health care staff persons. Zimmerman et al. (2005) determined that staff who are more educated about dementia care tend to be more sensitive to the needs of residents with dementia, which may help with feelings of stress. Additionally, with dementia training being directly related to dementia care (Hughes et al., 2008; Smith, Kerse, & Parsons, 2005), providers should consider if they have had the training necessary to enhance their knowledge of this population so that quality care can be provided.

Demographics

The number of individuals diagnosed with ADRD is rapidly increasing and will continue to grow as more of the Baby Boom generation reaches age 65. Every 72 seconds, someone in the US is diagnosed with ADRD (Alzheimer's Association, 2007). At the current time, there are 5.1 million individuals with a diagnosis of ADRD in the US and this number is expected to climb to between 11 million and 16 million by 2050 (Alzheimer's Association, 2009). Multiple variables are being examined as risk factors for developing ADRD.

Age is one of the primary risk factors for developing ADRD, with the incidence of developing the disease increasing with age. Individuals over age 65 have been found to have a 6–10 percent chance of developing the disease, while individuals over age 85 have a 50 percent chance (Alzheimer's Association, 2009; Hebert, Beckett, Scherr, & Evans, 2001; Hebert, Scherr, Bienias, Bennett, & Evans, 2003; Knopman et al., 2003). Greater attention is being directed to younger individuals (<65) who develop early onset Alzheimer's given that this form of ADRD progresses more quickly than it does in older individuals.

Greater attention is being given to *gender* and the development of ADRD. While research has shown no significant difference in the development of ADRD between men and women (Barnes, Wilson, Schneider, Bienias, Evans, & Bennett, 2003; Kukull et al., 2002), the number of men and women with ADRD differ. Approximately 16 percent of women over age 71 have ADRD, compared to 11 percent of men (Plassman et al., 2007), representing approximately 2.4 million women, compared to one million men (Plassman et al., 2007). Because women have historically lived longer than men, the likelihood of their developing ADRD is greater (Alzheimer's Association, 2007; Plassman et al., 2007). However, this trend may change as the life expectancy rate becomes more balanced between men and women.

Research is examining the differential risk factors among men and women for developing ADRD, particularly regarding early symptom development (Artero et al., 2008). Artero et al. (2008) found that men were at a greater risk of developing ADRD if they had physical health issues, such as diabetes, and were at a high risk for stroke, while women who were more socially isolated, had a disability, and had poorer subjective health status were at a greater risk. Both men and women who had symptoms of depression were at risk. Epidemiological research has identified other risk factors for women developing ADRD. For instance, post-menopausal women have a greater likelihood of developing ADRD than men of the same age cohort (Birge, 1997). In response, research has examined the protective effect of hormone replacement therapy against ADRD in women. The results have been mixed, with some identifying hormone replacement therapy as a protective mechanism against ADRD (Greenfield et al., 2002; Jaffe, Toran-Allerand, Greengard, & Gandy, 1994) and others finding either no effects from the treatment or the treatment actually placing women at greater risk for the development of ADRD (Matthews, Cauley, Yaffe, & Zmuda, 1999; Shumaker et al., 2003). Colucci et al. (2006) found that women who have had more pregnancies were at a greater risk of ADRD, which argues against the notion of hormone replacement therapy as a protective mechanism against ADRD given that the women in this study had increased levels of estrogen, not decreased levels. At the current time, no definitive cause of gender differences in ADRD can be determined; however, research continues to examine the differences between men and women with ADRD.

With the number of older adults from diverse racial groups growing, greater attention is being given to the relationship between *race and ethnicity* and ADRD. Compared to Caucasians, ADRD is under-diagnosed and undertreated among minority groups, particularly African Americans and Latinos (Espino & Lewis, 1998; Perkins, Annegers, Doody, Cooke, Aday, & Vernon, 1997). In 2002, the Alzheimer's Association indicated that the prevalence of African

Americans developing ADRD was between 14 percent and 100 percent. This vast range was the result of differential diagnostic patterns for African Americans. Tang et al. (2001) found that by age 90, African American older adults are four times more likely of developing ADRD than Caucasian elders. While African Americans have continued to show higher prevalence rates than Caucasians, research has found that when factors, such as gender, age, and education are taken into consideration, race plays a less important role in determining ADRD (Fillenbaum et al., 1998; Fitzpatrick et al., 2004; Plassman et al., 2007). Other research has identified that African Americans who have less education possess a greater risk for developing ADRD (Callahan, Hall, Hui, Musick, Unverzagt, & Hendrie, 1996). Health status and preexisting health problems, such as diabetes and high blood pressure, continue to be examined as additional risk factors.

Research on ADRD among the Latino population is also expanding. Hann, Mungas, Gonzalez, Ortiz, Acharya, and Jagust (2003) found that the prevalence of ADRD is 31 percent for those Latinos over age 85. Individuals who had a preexisting health condition, such as diabetes or a history of strokes, were eight times more likely to develop ADRD. Fitten, Ortiz, and Ponton (2001) found that 40 percent of Latinos had undiagnosed cognitive impairment. Of these individuals, almost 39 percent were diagnosed with Alzheimer's disease. As more Latinos immigrate to the United States, more outreach efforts about ADRD need to occur. At present, steps are being taken by many organizations and institutions that serve individuals with ADRD and their caregivers to ensure educational materials are available in both English and Spanish. Additionally, the demand for more Spanish speaking gerontological social workers will also continue to grow.

Greater attention has recently been given to Asians and ADRD. Ferri et al. (2005) reported a rapid expansion in the number of individuals with ADRD in many Asian countries. In fact, in China and neighboring countries, there will be three times more individuals with ADRD by 2040 than most Western European countries combined. One of the challenges in working with individuals who are Asian and experiencing symptoms of ADRD is that the way they define dementia may differ based on their cultural beliefs about aging, disability, and cognitive impairment. Arnsberger (2005) indicated that ADRD is a "relatively recent recognition" among Asians (p. 171), with some reporting to have never heard of the term Alzheimer's disease. As more first generation Asians in the United States age and develop symptoms of ADRD, professionals need to be aware of the lack of recognition of ADRD among this population and subsequently how this will impact diagnosis and treatment, as well as a caregiver's willingness to access assistance.

As aforementioned, *family history* is another important variable in examining the prevalence of ADRD, with individuals who have an immediate relative with ADRD being two to three times more likely to develop ADRD than individuals who do not have a family history with the disease (Alzheimer's Association, 2009). One of the largest areas of federally funded research on ADRD is genetics, with it being recognized that this area of research most likely holds the key to determining the cause of ADRD, as well as the cure.

The *costs* of ADRD are staggering. Researchers estimate that almost $9,300 are spent per year for individuals in the early stages of the disease and almost $20,000 are spent per year for individuals in the more advanced stages (Zhu et al., 2006). The costs are even higher for those who are reside in a long-term care facility (Covinsky & Johnston, 2006), which can cost over $50,000 a year.

In 2002, Koppel conducted an analysis of the cost of ADRD to U.S. businesses. He determined that ADRD costs U.S. businesses more than $61 billion per year (Koppel, 2002). This includes the cost associated with family caregiving, such as absenteeism, productivity losses, and replacement costs, as well as the cost to businesses for the health and long-term care of the diagnosed individual. These dollar amounts were calculated in 2002 when the estimated number of individuals with ADRD was 4 million. As more individuals turn 65 and the number of people with ADRD climbs, it is expected that the total costs of ADRD will significantly increase (Koppel, 2002). With a definitive cause and cure for ADRD unknown, as well as the need to expand the support services for family caregivers, ADRD has the potential to generate great financial costs to businesses as they try to support their workers who are caregivers.

The *mortality* rates for ADRD are difficult to calculate. According to the Alzheimer's Association (2007), ADRD is underreported as the cause of death on death certificates, with physicians reporting a secondary health condition, such as pneumonia, as the primary cause of death. This practice skews death statistics about ADRD and the overall impact of ADRD on society. In 2006, the Centers for Disease Control and Prevention (CDC) estimated Alzheimer's disease as the seventh leading cause of death (CDC, 2006).

Population

ADRD is a disease that progresses through a series of stages, with signs of ADRD being present for several years before an actual diagnosis may be received. Early warning signs, including changes in personality, initiative, difficulty with abstract thinking, problem solving, recall, disorientation to time, place or person, and suspiciousness, are often dismissed by professionals, families, and even the older adults themselves, who label this simply as having a "bad day" or a "senior moment" (Alzheimer's Association, 2007). Overlooking early warning signs can adversely impact the diagnosed individual as they are at a greater risk of losing their voice in long-term planning due to concerns over competency at later points in the disease progression. Overlooking these warning signs can also delay the start of pharmacological interventions designed to slow the disease progression that are most effective in the early stages of the disease (Cummings & Jeste, 1999).

ADRD has been staged in many different ways, from basic staging systems, such as identifying the early, middle, and late stages, to more advanced methods that divide the disease into multiple numeric phases. One of the more popular staging tools, the Functional Assessment Staging Tool (FAST), was developed by Reisberg (Reisberg, 1988; Reisberg, Ferris, & Franssen, 1985). This particular tool has seven stages, each identifying core symptoms associated with disease progression. Stage 1 represents no cognitive impairment. Stage 2 indicates very mild decline. Here, the person may report that they are having cognitive difficulties, but their symptoms cannot be detected by others, including medical personnel with cognitive tests. Even at this stage, it is important for individuals to share their concerns about their memory with their physicians and for family systems to start discussions about long-term planning in case cognitive symptoms worsen.

Stage 3 starts the progression of cognitive impairment with symptoms being obvious to others; this stage represents early stage issues, including a person having difficulty with word recall, remembering names and places, completing familiar tasks, misplacing objects, and experiencing trouble with abstract thinking, such as the planning of events. Stage 4 is identified as moderate cognitive decline and is characterized by frequent memory loss, difficulty with complex tasks, an inability to remember events from one's own life, and changes in personality and initiative. By this stage, diagnosed individual are starting to become unsafe to live alone, manage personal affairs, and operate cars and other machinery. This presents challenges to family systems as they transition into a phase of 24-hour, 7 days a week caregiving. Families do not always recognize that they are this point in the disease process and may need a social worker or other professional to help them recognize and accept that the person with ADRD needs additional assistance.

Stage 5 on the FAST scale (Reisberg, 1988; Reisberg et al., 1985) is defined as moderately severe cognitive decline. Symptoms associated with this stage include disorientation to place and time, continued decline in one's ability to perform ADLs, difficulty in remembering facts about their life and the lives of close friends or family members, and increased difficulty with some abstract thinking. Stage 6 represents severe cognitive decline. Individuals in this stage experience difficulty in identifying familiar people, require significant amounts of assistance with all ADLs, experience changes in sleep patterns, and may experience significant personality changes, including suspiciousness, repetitive behavior, and agitation. Finally, Stage 7 is very severe cognitive decline. At this stage, the individual experiences difficulty walking without assistance and many are bedbound. Individuals also have minimal verbal ability, experience trouble swallowing, lose their ability to smile, and are prone to multiple secondary infections (Reisberg, 1988; Reisberg et al., 1985).

There are other tools available to assist in staging ADRD. For instance, the Global Deterioration Scale (Reisberg, Ferris, de Leon, & Crook, 1982) is also used to determine the stage of disease. Physicians may use the Mini Mental Status Examination (Folstein, Folstein, & McHugh, 1975) to obtain a preliminary diagnosis or determine if cognitive impairment is present. This tool can also be used to determine an approximate stage of the disease. Regardless of the tool being used, staging the disease can be difficult given that the progression of ADRD is not necessarily linear, with a person gradually progressing from one stage to the next. Instead, individuals progress on more of a continuum, with symptoms from more than one stage being apparent. Additional difficulties in using staging tools are related to individuals with ADRD retaining social skills, by following the social cues, such as laughing, smiling, or the gestures of others. This may make them appear more cognitively intact than they actually are. These things can create challenges for service providers as they attempt to determine needs and service eligibility, as well as for caregivers who may be trying to convince others that additional help and support is needed.

Some of the greatest challenges of ADRD are behavioral and personality changes that commonly occur at the end of the early stages of the disease (FAST Stage 3) and then become more pronounced in the later stages. Common behavioral problems of ADRD include paranoia, wandering, sundowning, agitation and aggression, repeating statements/questions, inappropriate sexual behavior and advances, and hallucinations (Alzheimer's Association, 2009). As the disease advances, the ability for the diagnosed person to reason, judge, and perceive also diminishes. This creates additional challenges for caregivers as they are often caring for an individual who does not recognize familiar individuals or even themselves. Additionally, they often misinterpret one's intentions, causing behavioral challenges during personal care as they are not necessarily recognizing that the caregiver is trying to provide assistance instead of harming them. It is not unusual for care providers to take the behavioral problems personally, making caregiving in the later stages of the disease difficult, because the caregiver is unable to reason with the diagnosed individual about why certain types of caregiving assistance is needed.

Identifying the stage of ADRD is critical for service providers who often use this as a guide for the appropriateness of the person for services. For instance, the Medicare guidelines for hospice care indicate that a person needs to be Stage 7 on the FAST scale to be eligible for hospice services (Medicare Hospice Guidelines, 2009). For other services, such as adult day health service, providers may indicate that a person benefits most from the program during the middle stages of the disease or have policies stating that a person is ineligible to attend once they reach the stage of the disease in which they are incontinent. Assisted living facilities may indicate that for a person to receive care they cannot be bedbound or at risk for falls and some states mandate that once a person reaches the advanced stages (e.g. Stages 6 and 7 on the FAST scale) of the disease or exhibit significant behavioral issues, they must be transferred to a nursing home setting. Elder law attorneys or those who engage in estate planning and the development of advance directives are particularly interested in the stage of the disease as they attempt to determine competency of a diagnosed individual to make decisions for their own end-of-life care and other health and financial related decisions (American Psychiatric Association, 2007; Kane, 2001).

Stage of disease is often used to determine the appropriateness of particular interventions for a person with ADRD. For instance, some support groups, particularly early stage support groups, rely on stage of disease to determine if the person with ADRD is appropriate for participation (Zarit, Femia, Watson, Rice-Oeschger, & Kakos, 2004). Early stage interventions are designed to help early stage individuals and their caregivers address their feelings about the disease, as well as engage in important discussions and decision-making about long-term care (Logsdon, McCurry, & Teri, 2006). The ability of the diagnosed person to have insight into their condition is critical for the success of these interventions. Early stage interventions have also been found to benefit caregivers through enhancing their quality of life and reducing family conflict that can result from the diagnosis (Logsdon et al., 2006). By educating families and diagnosed individuals about ADRD and care options early in the disease process, both are better equipped to make plans for their future.

The impact of the middle stages of the disease on caregivers has also been explored. Placement into a nursing home commonly occurs in the middle stages of the disease as caregivers experience more stress and burden originating from behavioral problems common during this phase. Intervention research on caregivers of individuals in the middle stages of the disease has examined the effectiveness of support groups, educational and skill building programs, and case management and counseling programs, which are all designed to address the caregivers' emotional and physical health (Schultz et al., 2003; Thompkins & Bell, 2009). Many of these interventions have been found to delay placement into a facility by assisting caregivers in obtaining respite and developing coping strategies.

Finally, a greater interest is being directed to the end stages of the disease and the types of supports that caregivers need as they prepare for the death of the person with ADRD. Sanders, Butcher, Swails, and Power (2009) found that caregivers' reactions to the end stages of the disease are quite diverse, with some needing more clinical assistance to help with unresolved issues and questions about the disease, while others express readiness for their caregiving careers to be over so that they may engage in other aspects of life. Interventions, such as grief support through hospice programs, can be beneficial during this stage of the disease.

Long and short-term caregiver outcomes have also been linked to stage of disease. A growing area of caregiver research is grief, with multiple studies examining how caregiver grief varies based on the stage of disease. Ponder and Pomeroy (1996) indicated that the intensity of caregiver grief grew over the stages of the disease, with caregiver grief being the highest in the late stages. Marwit and Meuser (2002) and Ott, Sanders, and Kelber (2007) found similar grief patterns, particularly among spouses. Other key caregiving variables, such as depression, burden, and health status, have also been found to be influenced by the stage of the disease. For instance, the *wear and tear hypothesis* for caregivers would suggest that the longer a caregiver remains in a caregiving role and provides care to a person who progresses through the various stages of the disease, the more adverse impact it is likely to have on the caregivers' emotional and physical health (e.g., burden, depression, health status, etc.) (Gaugler, Kane, Kane, Clark & Newcomer, 2005). Conversely, other research has demonstrated that overtime caregivers show improvement in their emotional and psychological outcomes as they relate to caregiving (Townsend, Noelker, Deimling, & Bass, 1989), with Kramer (1997) suggesting that caregivers, particularly men, adapt to caregiving and caregiving roles over the course of the disease.

Mental health care disparities

Like other health conditions, disparities exist in the access to services that can help patients with ADRD and their caregivers. Some of these disparities are historic in nature, while others are complicated by values and beliefs about old age and impairment. These disparities exist across racial groups, geographic locations, and educational levels.

The relationship between *race and ADRD* is complicated by historic patterns of distrust among minorities about health care, cultural values about memory loss and old age, and access to and knowledge about dementia and related services (Manly & Espino, 2004; Williams & Earl, 2007). As stated earlier, minorities have less access to dementia specialists (Snowden, 2001), which may lead to ADRD being under-diagnosed, misdiagnosed, and undertreated among minority populations (Clark et al., 2005; Espino & Lewis, 1998; Perkins et al., 1997). This has ramifications for other aspects of ADRD care, including access to services to support the caregiver, programs for the diagnosed individual, and assistance with long-term planning.

Further complicating the issues of health disparities are the values and perspectives that minority groups have about memory loss. Research has identified that minorities are less likely to use medications aimed at slowing the progression of dementia (Mehta, Yin, Resendez, & Yaffe, 2005; Zuckerman et al., 2008). Research has also found that minority elders use a combination of disease specific information, as well as some folk lore, depending on the cultural group, to define and make sense of ADRD (Hinton, Franz, Yeo, & Levkoff, 2005). Other research has found that many minorities view memory loss as normal aging or as a sign of something negative in the diagnosed person, which decreases their willingness to seek or receive medical assistance. Mahoney, Cloutterbuck, Neary, and Zhan (2005) compared African Americans, Latinos, and Chinese perspectives of ADRD. They found that all three groups viewed ADRD as related to or a part of normal aging. The groups also possessed cultural values about the disease, such as stigma about mental health conditions, including ADRD; fear of public disclosure of ADRD (Chinese); fear of the health care system (African Americans); and the belief that family should be taking care of the person with ADRD instead of a larger outside system (Latino). All three groups expressed displeasure with the treatment they received from the health care system once they pursued a formal diagnosis.

Geographic disparities with ADRD are also prevalent in rural communities where diagnosed individuals and their families do not necessarily have access to specialized medical or social services. Teel (2004) found that rural physicians lacked the ability to consult with other physicians about an ADRD diagnosis given that consultation services were unavailable in many rural communities. The lack of consultation services created challenges for patients should they have wanted to consult with a different provider about the ADRD diagnosis. They often have to travel great distances to these specialists, which in some cases, is not possible. Other research has found that families in rural areas seek a diagnosis of ADRD only when they are in need of assistance to help them manage the patient's other health related concerns (Wackerbarth, Johnson, Markesbery, & Smith, 2001).

Social support is also a concern for diagnosed individuals and their caregivers in rural communities, despite the perception that social networks may be stronger in rural areas (Buettner & Langrish, 2001). In fact, rural caregivers may experience more stress due to the lack of support and resources when compared to their urban caregiver counterparts. Much of this could be related to stigma, which is also prevalent in rural communities. Teel (2004) reported that like minority groups, stigma about ADRD was a concern in rural communities, with some physicians being hesitant to use the words "dementia" or "Alzheimer's." Stigma may also impact the ability of caregivers to receive the emotional support that they need to provide care because they are embarrassed about the diagnosis and concerned about the community response, which prevents them from reaching out for support.

The diagnostic process of ADRD creates additional disparities, particularly for those individuals with lower *educational attainment*. Several of the screening tools for ADRD, such as the Mini Mental State Examination (MMSE) (Folstein et al., 1975) and the Clock Drawing Test have been found to create diagnostic disparities for individuals with lower educational levels (O'Connor, Pollitt, Treasure, & Brook, 1989; Paganini-Hill, Clark, Henderson, & Birge, 2001). Components of the MMSE, such as counting backwards from seven or spelling forwards and backwards, has been identified as creating bias for those individuals who have less education (Jones & Gallo, 2001; Jorm, Scott, Henderson, & Kay, 1988; Shulman et al., 2006). Additionally, components of diagnostic tests, particularly related to comprehension and abstract problem solving may be difficult for individuals with lower educational levels. This, if not addressed, can lead to diagnoses that may be based more on the person's ability to complete the task or their educational level, rather than providing a true representation of the presence or absence of cognitive impairment.

Social work programs and social work roles

Evaluating the work of social workers with individuals diagnosed with ADRD and their caregivers has not received a great deal of empirical attention, despite the growth of evidence-based interventions with this group (McClure & Sanders, 2008; Sanders & Morano, 2008). This may be related to the fact that social workers have not widely embraced work with individuals with ADRD. Kane (1999) was one of the first to identify the views of social workers in providing services to patients with ADRD. Surprisingly, Kane (1999) found that less than 3 percent of social workers were interested in practice with individuals with dementia. Despite this statistic, social workers are increasingly involved in providing services to older adults, with statistics identifying that as many as 78 percent of social workers have older adults on their caseloads (National Association of Social Workers, Center for Workforce Studies, 2006), with some of these older adults having cognitive impairment. With the rates of dementia increasing, social workers will be playing a greater role in the care of individuals with ADRD and their caregivers, which will require them to be better educated about this disease.

Social work roles   The types of roles that social workers play with patients with ADRD and their caregivers are vast and greatly depend on the patient's stage of disease, the social supports available to the caregiver, access to services, and their willingness to accept help. Additionally, the roles that social workers assume with individuals with ADRD and their caregivers will vary depending on the location in which they work. Unlike with other mental health conditions, the role of the social worker in a family affected by ADRD is more commonly focused on the caregivers instead of the diagnosed individual. This is because much of the work of a social worker is designed to address and alleviate the stress and burden associated with providing care to an individual with ADRD, particularly in the middle stages of the disease where the most significant changes occur in the patient.

Social workers assume multiple roles with caregivers that ultimately benefit the quality of life of the diagnosed individual. One of the primary roles of social workers is *case manager*. Case managers can be found in a variety of locations, including county level agencies on aging, area agencies on aging, and non-profits organizations that serve individuals with dementia, such as the Alzheimer's Association. Social workers, as case managers in these settings, assist caregivers in identifying the types of services that may help them with daily caregiving, such as support groups, adult day health programs, in-home assistance, respite, and long-term care. Additionally, case managers guide caregivers to community resources that help with long-term planning, such as elder law attorneys and other specialists, like geriatric psychiatrists, neurologists, and driving specialists. Case managers also assist with financial concerns of caregivers, such as applying for Medicaid/Title 19 to help pay for care. With state-funded community-based waiver programs growing throughout the United States, caregivers are relying on case managers to also assist in managing payment of services through Medicaid dollars. Case management has been credited for reducing many caregiver crises by serving as a contact for the caregiver. In addition to helping with service referrals, case managers also provide emotional support. Research has found that case management services can also help prevent additional health care costs, such as hospitalization (Shelton, Schraeder, Dworak, Fraser, & Sager, 2001).

Another role of social workers with caregivers of individuals diagnosed with ADRD is *educator*. Despite large educational campaigns through the Alzheimer's Association and other community agencies, caregivers still have misinformation about ADRD. Some are unclear about the differences between dementia and Alzheimer's disease, while others are unsure how to manage the behaviors that accompany the disease. Social workers as educators provide caregivers with information about the disease, including the signs and stages, management strategies, and problem solving approaches. Like social workers in case manager roles, social workers as educators also assist caregivers with long-term planning, which is one of the most important functions of social workers in this role. Social workers are able to inform caregivers regarding issues associated with advance directives and other types of legal decisions that need to be made prior to the advance stages of the disease. Finally, social workers as educators can provide caregivers with information for when important, but difficult, decisions need to be made, such as identifying when the diagnosed individual may no longer be able to live alone or drive, when long-term care or hospice care should be considered, and those associated with ethical dilemmas, including the use of feeding tubes and antibiotic treatments.

Social workers frequently assume the role of *facilitator*, particularly support group facilitator, with caregivers of individuals with ADRD. The importance of support groups for caregivers of individuals with ADRD has received a great deal of attention (Pinquart & Sorenson, 2006). The purpose of ADRD support groups is to provide caregivers with both emotional support and education about ADRD, as well as provide caregivers with respite. Support groups can be found in the community, as well as within long-term care facilities. Social workers operate as facilitators also as they conduct family meetings. The purpose of a family meeting depends upon the circumstances occurring within the caregiving situation. Commonly with ADRD, social workers facilitate family meetings to assist families in "getting on the same page" with the condition of the diagnosed individual, addressing potential crises within the caregiving situation, and identifying long-term care needs.

Social workers also assume the role of advocate. Social workers as advocates provide a voice to the individual with ADRD who can often not speak for him/herself. Many times, it is the social worker who has the opportunity to remind other professionals of the personhood that still exists within what looks like a shell of a person. As an advocate, social workers can speak of the wishes of the diagnosed individual and caregiver in situations where care decisions may not be as clear. Also as an advocate, the social worker has the opportunity to work on a more macro level to assure policy decisions are being made that will benefit individuals with ADRD and their caregivers, particularly decisions that are related to service availability and funding.

Finally, social workers also assume the role of *counselors* with caregivers of individuals with ADRD. Caregivers can benefit from counseling throughout the disease process. Counseling revolves around multiple issues including stress and burden, grief and loss, depression, anxiety, coping strategies, and support to name a few. One component of counseling involves responding to caregiver crises through the role of crisis manager. While the goal of social workers is to prevent crises from occurring through careful planning, this may not always occur given the unknowns that accompany ADRD. Crises can develop as a result of a sudden change in the care recipient's condition, a day of challenging behaviors, or from emotional and physical exhaustion. Caregivers who have preexisting mental health conditions or additional stressors in their lives, such as providing care for other individuals in the home (e.g. small children, another individual with physical or cognitive health issues) or trying to maintain a career while providing care, may be more prone to having emotional or psychological crises associated with their caregiving. Crises can also develop due to changes within the condition of the person with ADRD. For instance, a person who has successfully lived alone may have a change in condition, which makes this living arrangement no longer safe. This can trigger a crisis. Likewise, when a person is thought to no longer be safe to drive, crises may also be triggered as options for how to prevent this from occurring are explored. As a crisis manager, social workers intervene in the midst of the crisis to help the caregiver and larger system address immediate needs and then develop a plan to help prevent crises in the future. As a crisis manager, social workers draw upon other roles, including counselors, case manager, educators, facilitators, and advocates, to help the family regain a sense of stability in their situation.

Social work programs   Program and services for individuals with ADRD and their caregivers can be divided into two domains: community-based services and long-term care. While social workers exist within both areas of services, they frequently are not a standalone service. Instead, the services that are provided by the social worker are often part of a larger interdisciplinary team that strives to meet the needs of both the individual with ADRD and the caregiver. Additionally, not all services that are available to individuals with ADRD and their caregivers use social workers. Instead, some services may have individuals with other professional backgrounds providing the aforementioned roles. As more social workers become interested and committed to gerontology, their presence in the care of individuals with ADRD will expand. The services that are noted below are commonly used by individuals with ADRD and their caregivers but not all employ social workers.

Community-based services are available for both the caregiver and the care recipient. For the caregiver, community-based services are designed to provide not only emotional support, but also respite care. For the care recipient, community-based services are designed to provide daily care and assistance, as well as opportunities for socialization. One of the primary community-based services for individuals impacted by ADRD is the adult day service (ADS). ADS combines both social and medical care approaches to individuals with ADRD, while providing respite for the caregiver. A variety of services are available depending on the ADS program, including meals, medication management, assistance with activities of daily living, activity programming, and transportation to and from the center, are available for up to 12 hours a day 5 days a week (MetLife Mature Market Institute, 2007). Nationally, the average daily cost of ADS is $61, which is paid for through private financing, long-term care insurance, or Medicaid waiver programs (MetLife, 2007). Veterans' benefits can also be used for ADS service costs. Depending on the ADS program, individuals with ADRD can participate into the advanced stages of the disease. At the current time, ADS is underdeveloped in many states (Partners in Caregiving, 2002), and this is being addressed at both the state and national levels.

Another community-based service utilized by family systems faced with ADRD is home care. Home care encompasses a range of services, but most importantly, it provides assistance with ADLs and is another form of caregiver respite. This service is provided in the home by paraprofessionals, such as home health aides and nursing assistants. According to MetLife (2007), home care is "appropriate for those with Alzheimer's disease and other forms of dementia who may be physically healthy, but require supervision" (p. 5). The average national cost for a home health aide is $19 per hour, while the rate for a companion (an individual who provides less assistance with ADLs) is $18 per hour (MetLife, 2007). Like ADS, home care can be paid for through personal finances, long-term care insurance, or Medicaid waiver programs.

For end-stage care, the hospice is gaining a great deal of attention as a viable service to assist the diagnosed individual, as well as the family system. Hospice care includes an interdisciplinary team that provides physical and emotional assistance to individuals who have been deemed terminal (e.g. six months or less to live) and their families. Arguments are being made in support of ADRD being considered a terminal condition that requires palliative care (Albinsson & Strang, 2003). Currently 7–10 percent of all hospice patients have some form of ADRD (Jennings, 2003). The National Hospice and Palliative Care Organization (NHPCO) (personal communication, July 19, 2007) reports that approximately 10 percent of patients have a primary diagnosis of dementia at time of admission. With hospices providing services in the community, as well as in long-term care settings, their ability to provide additional support to individuals with ADRD and their families is far reaching. Through the support of hospices, individuals with end-stage dementia are able to receive pain management and other comfort measures as they approach death. Hospices also provide support and respite to the caregiver through their staff, volunteers, and short-term respite programs for patients. Research has found that caregivers emotionally and psychologically respond to the dying process of the individual with ADRD in diverse ways (Sanders, Butcher, Swails, & Power, 2009); thus, the hospice is able to meet the unique needs of caregivers and prepare them for the end of their caregiving tenure.

Other community-based services that can help family systems facing ADRD include community case management, services through the Alzheimer's Association (e.g. National Helpline, support groups, and Safe Return), transportation assistance, meals on wheels, senior centers, and other volunteer programs through churches that may assist in providing respite to caregivers. These services are available through the county-level aging service providers or non-profits and are usually funded through private donations and/or state or federal funds.

Long-term care services are also available to individuals with ADRD and their caregivers. The Alzheimer's Association (2009) estimates that approximately 70 percent of individuals with ADRD reside at home; thus, only 30 percent are receiving services in long-term care. However, within long-term care, approximately 50 percent of residents have some form of ADRD.

Long-term care consists of several types of care, including nursing homes and assisted living facilities. Nursing homes are the best known long-term care service for individuals with ADRD with many diagnosed individuals being moved into nursing home settings because of behavioral manifestations that accompany the disease. The care of individuals with ADRD in nursing homes has greatly improved since 1990 with the passage of the Federal Nursing Home Reform Act of 1987 (Omnibus Reconciliation Act: OBRA). The Omnibus Reconciliation Act created a series of regulations for nursing homes to follow, which enhanced the quality of care for residents (Long-term Care Ombudsman, 2008). The care of individuals with ADRD has greatly evolved since the late 1980s as well. Special care units are frequently seen in nursing homes, which provide individuals with ADRD with specialized activity programming and an environment that is conducive to the behaviors associated with memory impairment. These may include more sensory focused activities, environmental visual cues, alarm systems, and locked areas to create a safe space for wandering. Nursing homes, with the assistance of social workers, have expanded their services to better include the families of individuals with ADRD in the provision of care. Support groups, family educational programs, and individual and family meetings also are provided by social workers in long-term care to assist in adjustment to the facility and preparing for death.

Assisted living is a long-term care option that is growing in popularity. Assisted living facilities gained attention in the late 1980s and early 1990s as older adults and their families were exploring alternative options to nursing home care (Mollica, 2008). Currently, over one million individuals reside in assisted living facilities (Consumer Consortium on Assisted Living, 2009).

Assisted living promotes resident independence and decision making in an environment known for being more "home-like" and less institutional, as was seen in nursing homes (Mollica, 2008). They emphasize the notion of "aging in place;" however the manner in which this occurs varies widely based on the facility (Smith, Buckwalter, Kang, Ellingrod, & Schultz, 2008). Assisted living facilities have faced several challenges as they have grown in popularity, including regulatory changes, funding, documentation of the residents' condition, staffing patterns, and training (Smith et al., 2008). Additionally, there is not a consistent definition of assisted living, which has created diversity in the type of facilities and care provided across the nation. Additionally, social work services in assisted living facilities have not been widely embraced since they are not mandated.

Dementia care in assisted living facilities is gaining attention as research has determined that over 50 percent of all assisted living residents have some form of ADRD (Magsi & Malloy, 2005). Some assisted living facilities are moving to special care units or memory care units for individuals with ADRD with similar programming and environmental adaptations to what has been seen in nursing home special care units. This trend has been well received by those individuals who can afford this care, given that 82 percent of residents privately pay with only some states accepting Medicaid Waiver monies (Assisted Living Federation of America, 2008) to offset portions of the monthly fee. Other individuals may use long-term care insurance to assist with care. Assisted living facilities have received some negative attention as they have been perceived as only an option for financially secure elders. Assisted living facilities have also gained a great deal of attention as debates about regulations and standards have occurred.

Given that individuals with ADRD need more physical assistance as they decline, assisted living may not be the most appropriate level of care for individuals in the most advanced stages of the disease given that staffing patterns are less than is seen in nursing homes. Some states regulate that assisted living residents are not able to have as many physical or cognitive care needs as nursing home residents, unless additional help, such as hospice, can be used in the facility with the resident. This results in a move from assisted living level of care to a nursing home as individuals enter into the final stages of ADRD. Without the assistance of a social worker on staff, families are often left without much needed assistance in identifying and deciding on an alternative facility and addressing their emotions associated with a move. As more individuals with ADRD move into assisted living facilities, continued examination of and revisions to the regulations will need to occur.

Professional methods and interventions

The intervention literature for individuals with ADRD is overflowing with studies associated with medical trials and medication management (Cummings, 2004). This literature is essential as gerontological professionals strive to find a cure for ADRD. However, evidence-based research on psychosocial interventions for individuals with ADRD and their caregivers is equally important and needed. Evidence-based research on interventions for this population is growing; however, the role of the social worker and of social work interventions have not been consistently evaluated. Thus, social workers draw from the evaluation research that has occurred in other fields to help improve their practice.

Since the late 1990s, several large, federally funded intervention studies have been conducted to determine effective interventions for caregivers. These studies have provided a great deal of insight into the types of interventions that are needed to help caregivers reduce their stress, burden, depression, and other symptoms associated with caregiving. Two key studies have been conducted to help enhance the knowledge of professionals about the interventions that are beneficial for caregivers. The New York University (NYU) Spouse Caregiver Intervention

Study (Mittelman, 2002) was implemented to determine if caregiver counseling and support was effective in reducing negative outcomes in caregivers of individuals with ADRD. The NYU study, consisting of over 400 spouse-caregiver dyads, possessed of a four component treatment: (1) Two individual caregiver counseling sessions, (2) Four counseling sessions with the family system, (3) Weekly support group participation, and (4) 24-hour caregiver counseling available to assist with immediate caregiving concerns. The study was designed to provide the first two components of the intervention within the first four months of the study, with the third and fourth components following.

Several key findings emerged from this intervention. Most importantly, this study documented that

> while counseling and support cannot stop the inevitable course of the disease, these interventions can alter its effects on caregivers by improving support and reducing family conflict, decreasing isolation, and directly providing assistance in the form of problem-focused strategies.

(Mittelman, 2002, p. 105)

Additionally, the NYU caregiver study found that this intervention was able to delay placement of individuals into long-term care facilities longer than those caregivers in the control group who received resource referrals and only assistance upon request (Mittelman, 2002). For those caregivers in both the treatment and control groups who did place the person with ADRD into a nursing home, the study found that caregivers in the treatment group reported less burden and depression compared to those in the control condition at the time of placement and following placement (Gaugler, Roth, Haley, & Mittelman, 2008). This intervention was also credited for impacting caregiver health (Mittelman, Roth, Clay, & Haley, 2007). The caregivers in the intervention group reported better self-rating of health compared to those in the control group. The results of this intervention also showed that caregivers who received the interventions compared to those in the control group had lower depression scores before and after the death of the person with dementia (Haley, Bergman, Roth, McVie, Gaugler, & Mittelman, 2008).

A second large federally funded study that has provided insight into interventions effective for caregivers of individuals with ADRD is Resources for Enhancing Alzheimer's Caregivers Health (REACH) (Wisniewski et al., 2003). REACH consisted of nine interventions spread across six different research sites. The interventions were: skills-training, telephone-linked computer, information and referral, behavioral care, enhanced care, family-based structural multisystem in-home intervention, family-based structural multisystem in-home intervention plus computer telephone integration system, coping with caregiving class, environmental skill-building program, and the enhanced support group. These core interventions consist of multiple components, including education and educational resources (e.g. pamphlets and other educational materials), psychoeducational support, support groups, and counseling/therapy (Wisniewski et al., 2003). The control group consisted of information and referral services provided by resource groups in the community (Wisniewski et al., 2003).

The findings from this study have been widespread and have helped enhance the knowledge of caregiver interventions. For instance, Bank, Soledad, Rubert, Eisdorfer, and Czaja (2006) found that the use of a telephone support group was effective for both English and Spanish speaking caregivers. The majority of caregivers reported that the group provided them with both emotional and social support, as well as enhanced knowledge and skill in providing care to the individual with ADRD. Burns, Nichols, Martindale-Adams, Graney, and Lummas (2003) examined the behavior care and enhanced care interventions, which included the behavioral care treatment in addition to material on caregiver well-being. They found that caregivers who received the more intensive enhanced care intervention had better overall well-being and less depression than the caregivers who only received information on managing behavior problems. Burn et al. (2003) concluded that the additional content that the caregivers in the enhanced care group received on coping and self-care assisted them in addressing their well-being and reducing depression. Additional findings from the REACH study can be found on the REACH website.

Other interventions have been examined for caregivers. Beauchamp, Irvine, Seeley, & Johnson (2005) evaluated the use of a support program for caregivers provided via the internet. The intervention consisted of caregivers reading text material and watching videos that provided information on positive caregiving strategies. Beauchamp et al. (2005) found that one month after completing the support program, caregivers had improved levels of depression, anxiety, stress, and strain. Additionally, the caregivers were more apt to seek assistance with caregiving. Gonyea, O'Conner, and Boyle (2006) examined the effectiveness of a behavioral intervention group for caregivers of individuals with ADRD. The intervention, which consisted of teaching specific behavioral management strategies for the home environment to caregivers, showed positive results, with caregivers in the intervention group reporting less caregiver distress. However, overall burden was not impacted by the intervention. Fortinsky, Kulldorff, Kleppinger, and Kenyon-Pesce (2009) evaluated the effectiveness of a consultation program for caregivers that entailed providing primary care physicians with copies of care plans for the caregivers. While the intervention led to a reduced rate of the individual with ADRD being admitted to nursing homes, only about one-quarter of the caregivers in the intervention group discussed their care plans with their physicians during visits.

In looking at this sample of intervention research on caregivers of individuals with ADRD, several key themes exist. First, the effective interventions entailed educating caregivers about ADRD, problematic behaviors, and disease management strategies. Additionally, interventions that were successful also provided an element of caregiver support. Successful interventions were provided to caregivers through a means that was convenient to the caregiver, such as the internet, telephone, or in the caregiver's home. Finally, the interventions were aimed at supporting the caregivers at the various stages of the disease. Thus, the intervention or the knowledge obtained from the intervention could be translated to caregiving throughout their caregiving duration. With the number of individuals being diagnosed with ADRD continuing to grow, more research on caregiver interventions needs to occur. Additionally, it is important for research to begin to highlight the cost effectiveness of many of these interventions to assist agencies who are considering the implementation of the program.

Illustration and discussion

The following case and subsequent discussion highlights many of the struggles that family systems encounter when a person is diagnosed with ADRD. This case, of Sue and Ralph, highlights the role of the social worker with family caregivers and the larger family system, as well as identifies key components of an assessment. Relevant services that would be available are also emphasized.

Sue and Ralph have been married for over 50 years and from how they describe their marriage, it has been and continues to be a very romantic love affair. Sue and Ralph moved from New Jersey to Florida after they retired to be able to participate in many of their hobbies, including golfing and gardening. The couple has one daughter, Sherry, who lives in rural Virginia with her husband, Jim. Sherry and her parents report that they are close; however, Jim has never established a strong relationship with Sue and Ralph, even after knowing them during his 18-year marriage to Sherry. At the age of 76, Sue first showed symptoms of dementia. Ralph reluctantly took her to a doctor in Florida who diagnosed her with Alzheimer's disease and suggested that the couple move to Virginia to be closer to family and support. Eventually, Sue and Ralph moved into the home of Sherry and Jim. At the time they began to receive services Sue was 83 years old and Ralph a year younger.

Sherry and Jim both work full-time so Sue and Ralph are at home alone during the day. Sherry and Jim quickly learn that Sue's condition is much worse than Ralph had described prior to them moving into their home. Sue is unable to dress herself, frequently becomes lost, is unable to recall the names of either Sherry or Jim, refers to Ralph as "that man," experiences difficulty identifying or naming objects, and becomes combative when asserting herself or when she feels challenged, particularly while cooking. She frequently says, "You are the one crazy, not me." Sherry and Jim find having Sue and Ralph living with them to be difficult. Sherry and Jim attempt to get Ralph to read and learn about Alzheimer's disease, but he refuses and frequently becomes upset with what he perceives as their criticism of him. Ralph often lets Sue make her own decisions, even if they are unsafe, such as allowing her to cook unsupervised, going for walks in the neighborhood, and at times driving with Ralph as a passenger in the car. Sherry and Jim, when they are home, try to work with Sue, but they both are often hit by her as she experiences a great deal of agitation. This makes Ralph upset because he feels that they have done something to provoke her.

About six months into this arrangement, these issues reach a climax when Sue becomes incontinent. She refuses to wear protective undergarments and frequently has "accidents" on Sherry and Jim's furniture. Jim becomes angry when these incidents occur and Ralph frequently cries because he feels that he and Sue are being "attacked" for growing old. Jim suggests that Sue move to a nursing home and that Ralph moves into either an independent or assisted living facility. At this point, Sherry decides to contact the Alzheimer's Association for assistance, as well as the Area Agency on Aging for their county, even in the face of Ralph's reluctance.

This case illustrates many of the challenges for caregivers, as well as family systems that are facing ADRD. The challenges involve parents moving in with an adult daughter and her husband, lack of knowledge about ADRD, strained relationships within family system, and no involvement of formal support systems to help the caregiver and family. The following will highlight many of the themes within this case that should be examined upon assessment, as well as the types of interventions and services that could help Ralph, Sherry, and Jim provide the best care for Sue as her disease progresses.

There are multiple factors within this case that should be examined upon *assessment*. First, a social worker should examine the dynamics between Sherry, Jim, Ralph and Sue to determine if this is the best living arrangement or if alternative arrangements should be explored. With the long-standing relational tension between Jim, Sue and Ralph, additional stress may be present that impacts the ability of Sue to obtain the care she needs. Similarly, a social worker needs to assess the values of this family system about formal service usage that may impact their ability to consider alterative living arrangements.

Second, the ability of Ralph to assume a primary caregiver role for Sue should be assessed. From the case, it is clear that Ralph is very committed to Sue and cares for her deeply. However, it is also clear that Ralph is not knowledgeable about ADRD, the behavioral issues associated with the disease, and disease management strategies. This appears to be creating safety concerns as evidenced by Sue getting lost, continuing to take a primary role with cooking, and her driving at times. Additionally, it is not clear if Ralph is able to provide the care that Sue needs as her condition declines, as seen through his reluctance to her wearing undergarments to help with incontinence or learn other strategies for managing this condition.

Third, as seen in the case, Sue's decline is causing a great deal of emotional strain for Ralph. Additionally, the relationship between him and Jim is causing further emotional stress. Ralph's emotional well-being, stress, and coping strategies also need to be evaluated. Similarly, Sherry is under a great deal of stress as she is trying to work full-time, help with Sue's care, provide emotional support to Ralph, and serve as a mediator between Jim and her parents. Her overall mental health also needs to be evaluated, as well as her coping strategies.

Fourth, a social worker should assess the willingness of the entire family system to consider formal support options through both community-based and long-term care options, as well as determine if there is another informal support that could be utilized. It is unclear how willing Ralph is to consider additional assistance; however, both Sherry and Jim believe that additional help is needed at this time. Services for Sue, as well as Ralph, Jim and Sherry should be explored.

Finally, it is evident that Sue's ADRD is progressing. However, it is not clear if any type of long-term plans have been made, including completing advance directives, such as Durable Powers of Attorney for finances and health care. Additionally, it is not clear about the financial status of Ralph and Sue and if they have the ability to pay for any formal services or if Medicaid/Title 19 or other forms of state assistance would be needed. A financial assessment should occur to determine their eligibility for assistance for services.

There are *multiple services* that may be appropriate to help Sue, Ralph, Sherry, and Jim. To begin, Sue, as well as other members of the family, could benefit from using ADS. As previously mentioned, ADS provides social and medical services to individuals with ADRD, as well as provides respite to the caregiver (American Psychiatric Association, 2007). Depending on the program, Sue would be able to attend an ADS program daily, which would ensure that while Sherry and Jim are working, Sue was in a safe environment. She may also be able to receive transportation to and from the center, which would alleviate additional stress for Ralph, Sherry, and Jim. To assist with paying, some ADS providers offer some financial assistance. Depending on the financial status of Ralph and Sue, they may also qualify for assistance through the state Medicaid Waiver programs which would help pay for ADS as a community-based service. Some ADS providers employ social workers who could provide the family with counseling, education, and some case management services.

Second, given the emotional stress of not only Ralph, but also Sherry and Jim, support services for them should also be considered. The Alzheimer's Association provides a range of services for caregivers and family members of persons with ADRD, including support groups, educational programs, and a 24-hour Helpline, which provides educational resources and emotional support. Becoming connected with the services provided through the Alzheimer's Association may be a critical component in educating Ralph about the disease and how best to interact with Sue to ensure that she is safe and her needs are met. Should it be decided that Sue will remain at home, Safe Return would be another program from the Alzheimer's Association that should be explored. Safe Return is a national identification program for individuals with ADRD who wander. Sue would wear an identification bracelet that indicates she is cognitively impaired and provides her with an identification number. In the event that Sue became lost, the family could call the national Safe Return program, which would initiate a search. First responders have been trained in this program and it has been identified as helpful for individuals with ADRD who become lost to return home.

Third, if Ralph decides to keep Sue living in the community, additional community supports should be examined. Many services can be accessed through community-based agencies, such as the Area Agency on Aging and other non-profit organizations that serve older adults, including case management, chore workers, and other forms of in-home assistance. Other community-based agencies may also provide caregiver support and education that would benefit Ralph, Jim, and Sherry. Counseling services may also be available to the family system through some other community-based agencies, such as community mental health centers, non-profits that provide counseling and case management, and other crisis lines. Depending on their finances, the family may also be able to privately hire some assistance through an agency that provides chore workers (homemaker services) or certified nursing assistants to assist with activities of daily living.

Fourth, the option of having Sue move into a special care unit of a nursing facility should be examined, which would ensure her a safe place to reside. A special care unit would be particularly good for Sue because of her wandering. These units are staffed by professionals who have had extra training in ADRD, including the use of redirection and distraction (Kane, 1999), validation therapy (Feil, 1993), activity planning (Kaplan & Hoffman, 1998), and most importantly behavioral modification techniques (Burns et al., 2003). Staff are also trained in how to provide assistance with activities of daily living that will cause the least amount of distress to the resident (Alzheimer's Association, 2008). Additionally, the environment of these units has been specifically designed for individuals with ADRD to include types of amenities that have been empirically examined (Chrisman, Tabar, Whall, & Booth, 1991). Having Sue reside in a nursing home would take substantial pressure off Sherry, Jim, and Ralph, who are struggling to provide care, but would also create a great deal of emotional pain for Ralph given the close relationship that he and Sue have had for over 50 years. Receiving counseling during the transition to a nursing home would be critical for Ralph.

Finally, as Sue's ADRD progresses, the family should be aware of hospice care. While this service is grossly underutilized by individuals with ADRD, steps are being taken to educate the community that hospice care is available for individuals with ADRD (Alzheimer's Association, 2008). Hospice services can be provided in any location that is considered "home" by the patient. Thus, even if Sue moved to a nursing home, she would be eligible to access hospice care. Not only would Sue benefit from the expertise of hospice professionals about end of life care and pain management, but also Ralph, Sherry, and Jim would benefit from the emotional support and education about death that they would receive from the interdisciplinary hospice team.

Conclusion

From the time of diagnosis until death, ADRD causes anguish for families as they watch the diagnosed individual progress from an independent, cognitively intact individual to a state of total dependence. While caregiving has been found to create great rewards and opportunities for caregivers (Sanders, 2005), the stress, burden, and grief associated with this position cannot be ignored. ADRD robs individuals of the essence of their personhood. For the caregiver, they are ultimately caring for a person who they do not know. The losses that are created for the diagnosed individual and caregiver as a result of this disease are significant and require attention.

Social workers have the opportunity to play a significant role with diagnosed individuals and their caregivers throughout all stages of the disease. Social workers' expertise in counseling, case management, resource referral, crisis intervention, and education, combined with their understanding of family systems issues, places them in an excellent position to help diagnosed individuals and their families with coping, planning, and navigating the disease from time of diagnosis until death. Greater attention needs to be directed towards the roles that social workers can play with diagnosed individuals and families. Additionally, more empirical attention needs to be given to how social workers, through their interventions, can help improve the quality of life of this population. With the numbers of individuals with ADRD on the rise, the demand for social workers to provide care to this population will inexorably grow. This places social workers in a critical position to provide leadership in dementia care.

Web resources

Alzheimer's Association
www.alz.org

Alzheimer's Association: Practice guidelines for professionals
www.alz.org/professionals

Alzheimer's Disease Research
www.ahaf.org

American Academy of Neurology: Practice guidelines
www.aan.com/professionals

American Geriatrics Society
www.americangeriatrics.org

American Psychological Association Practice guidelines
www.apa.org.practice/dementia.html

Centers for Disease Control and Prevention
www.cdc.gov

Children of Aging Parents
www.caps4caregivers.org

Eldercare Locator
www.eldercare.gov

Family Caregiving Alliance
www.caregiver.org

Medline Plus
www.nlm.nih.gov/medlineplus

National Institute on Aging
www.nia.nih.gov

REACH study
www.edc.pitt.edu/reach2/

References

Agronin, M.E. (2007). Caring for the dementia caregiver: Ways to identify and reduce burden. *Psychiatric Times, 2*, 15–18.

Albinsson, L., & Strang, P. (2003). Existential concerns of families of late-stage dementia patients: Questions of freedom, choices, isolation, death, and meaning. *Journal of Palliative Medicine, 6*, 225–235.

Allen, M., Ferrier, S., Sargeant, J., Loney, E., Bethune, G. & Murphy, G. (2005). Alzheimer's disease and other dementias: An organizational approach to identifying and addressing practices and learning needs of family physicians. *Educational Gerontology, 31*, 521–539.

Alzheimer's Association. (2002). *African Americans and Alzheimer's disease: The silent epidemic.* Chicago, IL: Alzheimer's Association.

Alzheimer's Association (2007). *Facts and figures.* Retrieved December 30, 2008, from www.alz.org

Alzheimer's Association. (2008). *Facts and figures.* Retrieved December 30, 2008, from www. alz.org

Alzheimer's Association. (2009). *Facts and figures.* Retrieved February 1, 2009, from www.alz.org

Alzheimer's Association and National Alliance for Caregiving. (2004). *Families care: Alzheimer's caregiving in the United States.* Retrieved February 1, 2009, from www.alz.org/national/documents/report_families care.pdf

American Psychiatric Association (APA). (2007). *Practice guidelines for the treatment of patients with Alzheimer's disease and other dementia* (2nd ed.), doi: 10.1176/appi.books.9780890423967.152139

American Psychiatric Association (APA). (2000). *Diagnostic and statistical manual of mental disorders* (4th ed., text revision). Washington, DC: APA.

Aranda, M.P., & Knight, B.G. (1997). The influence of ethnicity and culture of the caregiver stress and coping process: A socio-cultural review and analysis. *Gerontologist, 37*, 342–354.

Arnsberger, P. (2005). Best practices in care management for Asian American elders: The care of Alzheimer's disease. *Care Management Journal, 6,* 171–177.

Artero, S., Ancelin, M.L., Portet, F., Dupuy, A., Berr, C., Dartigues, J.F. et al. (2008). Risk profiles for mild cognitive impairment and progression to dementia are gender specific. *Journal of Neurology, Neurosurgery, and Psychiatry, 79* (9), 979–984.

Assisted Living Federation of America. (2008). *Public policy and regulations.* Retrieved December 5, 2008, from www.alfa.org

Bank, A.D., Soledad, A., Rubert, M., Eisdorfer, C., & Czaja, S.J. (2006). The value of telephone support groups among ethnically diverse caregivers of persons with dementia. *Gerontologist, 46,* 134–138.

Barnes, L.L., Wilson, R.S., Schneider, J.A. Bienias, J.A., Evans, D.A., & Bennett, D.A. (2003). Gender, cognitive decline, and risk of AD in older persons. *Neurology, 60,* 1777–1781.

Beauchamp, N., Irvine, A.B., Seeley, J., & Johnson, B. (2005). Worksite-based internet multimedia program for family caregivers of persons with dementia. *Gerontologist, 45,* 793–801.

Birge, S.J. (1997). The role of estrogen in the treatment and prevention of dementia: Introduction. *American Journal of Medicine, 103,* 1S–2S.

Boss, P. (1999). *Ambiguous loss.* Cambridge, MA: Harvard University Press.

Brodaty, H., Draper, B., & Low, L. (2003). Issues and innovations in nursing practice: Nursing home staff attitudes towards residents with dementia – Strain and satisfaction with work. *Journal of Advanced Nursing, 44,* 583–590.

Buettner, L.L., & Langrish, S. (2001). Rural versus urban caregivers of older adults with probable Alzheimer's disease: Perceptions regarding daily living and recreation needs. *Activities, Adaptation, and Aging, 24,* 51–65.

Buhr, G.T., Kuchibhatla, M., & Clipp, E.C. (2006). Caregivers' reasons for nursing home placement: Clues for improving discussions with families prior to the transition. *Gerontologist, 46,* 52–61.

Burns, R., Nichols, L.O., Martindale-Adams, J., Graney, M.J., & Lummas, A. (2003). Primary care interventions for dementia caregivers: Two-year outcomes from the REACH study. *Gerontologist, 43,* 547–555.

Callahan, D.M., Hall, K.S., Hui, S.L., Musick, B.S., Unverzagt, F.W., & Hendrie, H.C. (1996). Relationship of age, education, and occupation with dementia among a community-based sample of African Americans. *Archives of Neurology, 53,* 134–140.

Centers for Disease Control and Prevention (CDC). (2006). *National statistics report: Death.* Retrieved July 19, 2007, from www.cdc.gov/nchs/deaths.htm

Chrisman, M., Tabar, D., Whall, A.L. & Booth, D.E. (1991). Agitated behavior in the cognitively impaired elderly. *Journal of Geronotological Nursing, 17,* 9–13.

Clark, P.C., Kutner, N.G., Goldstein, F.C., Peterson-Hazen, S., Garner, V., Zhang, R. et al. (2005). Impediments to timely diagnosis of Alzheimer's disease in African Americans. *Journal of the American Geriatrics Society, 53,* 2012–2017.

Collins, C., Liken, M., King, S., & Kokinakis, C. (1993). Loss and grief among family caregivers of relatives with dementia. *Qualitative Health Research, 3,* 236–253.

Colucci, M., Cammarata, S., Assini, A., Croce, R., Clerici, F., Novello, C. et al. (2006). The number of pregnancies is a risk factor for Alzheimer's disease. *European Journal of Neurology, 13* (12), 1374–1377.

Consumer Consortium on Assisted Living. (2009). History and accomplishments. Retrieved April 13, 2009, from www.ccal.org/history_accomplishments.htm

Covinsky, K.E., & Johnston, C.B. (2006). Envisioning better approaches for dementia care. *Annuals of Intern Medicine, 145,* 780–781.

Cox, C., & Monk, A. (1996). Strain among caregivers: Comparing the experiences of African American and Hispanic caregivers of Alzheimer's disease relatives. *International Aging and Human Development, 43,* 93–105.

Cummings, J. (2004). Alzheimer's disease. *New England Journal of Medicine, 351,* 56–67.

Cummings, J., & Jeste, D. (1999). Alzheimer's disease and its management in the year 2010. *Psychiatric Services, 50,* 1173–1177.

Dilworth-Anderson, P., Williams, I.C., & Gibson, B.E. (2002). Issues of race ethnicity, and culture in caregiving research: A 20 year review (1980–2000). *Gerontologist, 42,* 237–272.

Espino, D.V., & Lewis, R. (1998). Dementia in older minority populations: Issues of prevalence, diagnosis, and treatment. *American Journal of Geriatric Psychiatry, 6*, S19–S25.

Farrer, L.A., Cupples, L.A., Haines, J.L., Hyman, B., Kukull, W.A., Mayeux, R. et al. (1997). Effects of aging, sex, and ethnicity on the association between apolipoprotein E genotype and Alzheimer's disease: A meta analysis. *Journal of the American Medical Association, 278* (16), 1349–1356.

Feil, N. (1993). *Validation breakthrough: Simple techniques for communicating with people with Alzheimer's type dementia.* New York: Health Professionals Press.

Ferri, C.P., Prince, M., Brayne, C., Brodaty, H., Fratiglioni, L., Ganguli, M. et al. (2005). Global prevalence of dementia: A Delphi consensus study. *The Lancet, 366* (9503), 2112–2117.

Fillenbaum, G.G., Heyman, A., Huber, M.S., Woodbury, M.A., Leiss, J., Schmader, K.E. et al. (1998). The prevalence and 3 year incidence of dementia in older black and white community residents. *Journal of Clinical Epidemiology, 51* (7), 587–595.

Fitten, L.J., Ortiz, F., & Ponton, M. (2001). Frequency of Alzheimer's disease and other dementias in a community outreach sample of Hispanics. *Journal of the American Geriatrics Society, 49*, 1301–1308.

Fitzpatrick, A.L., Kuller, L., Ives, D.G., Lopez, O.L., Jagust, W., Breitner, J.C.S. et al. (2004). Incidence and prevalence of dementia in the cardiovascular health study. *Journal of the American Geriatrics Society, 52*, 195–204.

Fleminger, S., Oliver, D.L., Lovestone, S., Rabe-Hesketh, S., & Giora, A. (2003). Head injury as a risk factor for Alzheimer's disease: The evidence 10 years on a partial replication. *Journal of Neurology, Neurosurgery, and Psychiatry, 74*, 857–862.

Foley, K.L., Tung, H.J., & Mutran, E.J. (2002). Self-gain and self-loss among African-American and White caregivers. *Journal of Gerontology: Social Sciences, 57B*, S14–S22.

Folstein, M.F., Folstein, S.E., & McHugh, P.R. (1975). "Mini Mental State": A practical method for grading the cognitive state of patients for the clinician. *Journal of Psychiatric Research, 12*, 189–196.

Fortinsky, R.H., Kulldorff, M., Kleppinger, A., & Kenyon-Pesce, L. (2009). Dementia care consultation for family caregivers: Collaborative model linking an Alzheimer's Association chapter with primary care physicians. *Aging and Mental Health, 13*, 162–170.

Gaugler, J.E., Kane, R.L., Kane, R.A., Clark, T., & Newcomer, R.C. (2005). The effects of duration of caregiving on institutionalization. *Gerontologist, 45*, 78–89.

Gaugler, J.E., Roth, D.L., Haley, W.E., & Mittelman, M.S. (2008). Can counseling and support reduce burden and depressive symptoms in caregivers of people with Alzheimer's disease during the transition to institutionalization? Results from the New York University caregiver intervention study. *Journal of the American Geriatrics Society, 56*, 421–428.

Gonyea, J.G., O'Conner, M.K., & Boyle, P.A. (2006). Project CARE: A randomized controlled trial of a behavioral intervention group for Alzheimer's disease caregivers. *Gerontologist, 46*, 827–832.

Greenfield, J.P., Leung, L.W., Cai, D., Kaasik, K., Gross, R.S., Rodriguez-Boulan, E. et al. (2002). Estrogen lowers Alzheimer's beta-amyloid generation by stimulating trans-Golgi network vesicle biogenesis. *Journal of Biological Chemistry, 277*, 12,128–12,136.

Gregory, S. (2001). *The nursing home workforce: Certified nurse assistant's fact sheet.* Retrieved February 10, 2009, from www.aarp.org.research/longtermcare/nursinghomes/aresearch-import-688-FS86.html

Haley, W.E., West, C.A., Wadley, V.G., Ford, G.R., White, F.A., Barrett, J.J. et al. (1995). Psychological, social, and health impact of caregiving: A comparison of black and white dementia caregivers and non-caregivers. *Psychology and Aging, 10*, 540–552.

Haley, W.E., Gitlin, L.N., Wisniewski, S.R., Mahoney, D.F., Coon, D.W., Winter, L. et al. (2004). Well-being, appraisal, and coping in African American and Caucasian dementia caregivers: Findings from the REACH study. *Aging and Mental Health, 8*, 316–329.

Haley, W.E., Bergman, E., Roth, D., McVie, T., Gaugler, J., & Mittelman, M. (2008). Long-term effects of bereavement and caregiver intervention on dementia caregiver depressive symptoms. *Gerontologist, 48* (6), 732–740.

Hann, M.N., Mungas, D.M., Gonzalez, H.M., Ortiz, T.A., Acharya, A., & Jagust, W.J. (2003). Prevalence of dementia in older Latinos: The influence of type 2 diabetes mellitus, stroke, and genetic factors. *Journal of the American Geriatrics Society, 51*, 169–177.

Hansen, R.A., Gartlehner, G., Kaufer, D., Lohr, K., & Carey, T. (2006). *Drug class review of Alzheimer's drugs: Final report.* Retreived April 17, 2009, from www.ohsu.edu/drugeffectiveness/reports/final.cfm

Hebert, L.E., Beckett, L.A., Scherr, P.A. & Evans, D.A. (2001). Annual incidence of Alzheimer's disease in the United States projected to the years 2000 through 2050. *Alzheimer's Disease and Related Disorders, 15*, 169–173.

Hebert, L.E., Scherr, P.A., Bienias, J.L., Bennett, D.A., & Evans, D.A. (2003). Alzheimer disease in the U.S. population: Prevalence estimates using the 2000 Census. *Archives of Neurology, 60*, 1119–1122.

Hinton, L., Franz, C.E., Yeo, G., & Levkoff, S.E. (2005). Conceptions of dementia in a Multi-ethnic sample of family caregivers. *Journal of the American Geriatrics Society, 53*, 1405–1410.

Hughes, J., Bagley, H., Reilly, S., Burns, A., & Challis, D. (2008). Care staff working with people with dementia: Training, knowledge, and confidence. *Dementia, 7*, 227–238.

Itzhaki, R.F. (1994). Possible factors in the etiology of Alzheimer's disease. *Molecular Neurobiology, 9*, 1–13.

Jaffe, A.B., Toran-Allerand, C.D., Greengard, P., & Gandy, S.E. (1994). Estrogen regulates metabolism of Alzheimer's amyloid beta precursor protein. *Journal of Biological Chemistry, 269*, 13,065–13,068.

Jennings, B. (2003). Hospice and Alzheimer's disease: A study in access and simply justice. *The Hasting Center Report, 33*, 24–26.

Jones, R.N., & Gallo, J.J. (2001). Education bias in the Mini Mental Status Examination. *International Psychogeriatrics, 13*, 299–310.

Jorm, A.F., Scott, R., Henderson, A.S., & Kay, D.W. (1988). Educational level differences on the Mini Mental State: The role of test bias. *Psychological Medicine, 18*, 727–731.

Kane, M.N. (1999). Mental health issues and Alzheimer's disease. *American Journal of Alzheimer's Disease and Other Dementias, 14*, 102–110.

Kane, M.N. (2001). Legal guardianship and other alternatives in the care of elders with Alzheimer's disease. *American Journal of Alzheimer's Disease and Other Dementias, 16*, 89–96.

Kane, M.N. (2003). Teaching direct practice techniques for work with elders with Alzheimer's disease: A simulated group experience. *Educational Gerontology, 29*, 777–794.

Kane, M.N., Hamlin, E.R., & Hawkins, W.E. (2004). How adequate do social workers feel to work with elders with Alzheimer's disease. *Social Work in Mental Health, 2*, 63–84.

Kaplan, M., & Hoffman, S. (1998). *Behaviors in dementia: Best practices for successful management.* Baltimore, MD: Health Professions Press.

Knopman, D.S., Boeve, B.F., & Petersen, R.C. (2003). Essentials of the proper diagnoses of mild cognitive impairment, dementia, and major subtypes of dementia. *Mayo Clinic Proceedings, 78*, 1290–1308.

Koppel, R. (2002). *Alzheimer's disease: The costs to U.S. businesses.* Washington, DC: Alzheimer's Association.

Kramer, B.J. (1997). Differential predictors of strain and gain among husbands caring for wives with dementia. *Gerontologist, 37*, 239–249.

Kukull, W.A., Higdon, R., Bowen, J.D., McCormick, W.C., Teri, L., Schellenberg, G.D. et al. (2002). Dementia and Alzheimer's disease incidence: A prospective cohort study. *Archives of Neurology, 59* (11), 1737–1746.

Lautenschlager, N.T., Cupples, L.A., Rao, V.S., Auerbach, S.A., Becker, R., Burke, J. et al. (1996). Risk of dementia among relatives of Alzheimer's disease patients in the MIRAGE study: What is in store for the oldest old? *Neurology, 46* (3), 641–650.

Lawton, M.P., Rajagopal, D., Brody, E., & Kleban, M.H. (1992). The dynamics of caregiving for a demented elder among black and white families. *Journal of Gerontology, 47*, S156–S164.

Logsdon, R., McCurry, S.M., & Teri, L (2006). Time-limited support groups for individuals with early stage dementia and their care partners: Preliminary outcomes from a controlled clinical trial. *Clinical Gerontologist, 30*, 5–19.

Loos, C., & Bowd, A. (1997). Caregivers of persons with Alzheimer's disease: Some neglected implications of the experience of personal loss and grief. *Death Studies, 21*, 501–515.

Long-term Care Ombudsman. (2008). *Federal Nursing Home Reform Act.* Retrieved April 16, 2009, from www.ltcombudsman.org

Lopez, O.T., Becker, J.T., Klunk, W., Saxton, J., Hamilton, R.L., Kaufer, D.I. et al. (2000). Research evaluation and diagnosis of possible Alzheimer's disease over the last two decades: II. *Neurology, 55*, 1863–1869.

Maas, M.L., Specht, J.P., Buckwalter, K.C., Gittler, J., & Bechen, K. (2008). Nursing home staffing and training recommendations for promoting older adults' quality of care and life. *Research in Gerontological Nursing, 1,* 123–133.

Magsi, H., & Malloy, T. (2005). Under recognition of cognitive impairment in assisted living facilities. *Journal of the American Geriatrics Society, 53,* 296–298.

Mahoney, D.F., Cloutterbuck, J., Neary, S., & Zhan, L. (2005). African American, Chinese, Latino family caregivers' impressions of the onset and diagnosis of dementia: Cross-cultural similarities and differences. *Gerontologist, 45,* 783–792.

Manly, J.J., & Espino, D.V. (2004). Cultural influences on dementia recognition and management. *Clinics in Geriatric Medicine, 20,* 93–119.

Matthews, K., Cauley, J., Yaffe, K., & Zmuda, J. (1999). Estrogen replacement therapy and cognitive decline in older community women. *Journal of the American Geriatrics Society, 47* (5), 518–523.

Marwit, S.J., & Meuser, T. (2002). Development and initial validation of an inventory to assess grief in caregivers of persons with Alzheimer's disease. *Gerontologist, 42* (6), 751–765.

McClure, K., & Sanders, S. (2008). Evidenced-based psychosocial treatments for caregivers. In N. Kroft & S. Cummings (eds), *The handbook of psychosocial interventions for older adults: Evidenced-based approaches.* New York: Haworth Press.

Medicare Hospice Guidelines. (2009). *Medicare Hospice Benefits.* Washington, DC: Centers for Medicare and Medicaid Services.

Mehta, K., Yin, M., Resendez, C., & Yaffe, K. (2005). Ethnic differences in acetylcholinesterase inhibitor use for Alzheimer's disease. *Neurology, 65,* 159–162.

MetLife Mature Market Institute (2007). *The MetLife market survey of adult day services and home care costs.* Westport, CT: MetLife Mature Market Institute.

Meuser, T.M., Boise, L., & Morris, J.C. (2004). Clinician's beliefs and practices in dementia care: Implications for health educators. *Educational Gerontology, 30,* 491–516.

Meuser, T.M., Marwit, S.J., & Sanders, S. (2004). Assessing grief in family caregivers. In K. Doka (ed.), *Living with grief: Alzheimer's disease.* Washington, DC: Hospice Foundation of America.

Mittelman, M.S. (2002). Family caregiving for people with Alzheimer's disease: Results of the NYU spouse caregiver intervention study. *Generations, 1,* 104–106.

Mittelman, M.S., Roth, D.L., Clay, O.J., & Haley, W.E. (2007). Preserving health of Alzheimer's caregivers: Impact of a spouse caregiver intervention. *American Journal of Geriatric Psychiatry, 15,* 780–789.

Mollica, R.L. (2008). Trends in state regulation of assisted living. *Generations, 33,* 67–70.

National Association of Social Workers, Center for Workforce Studies. (2006). *Assuring the sufficiency of a frontline workforce: A national study of licensed social workers.* Washington, DC: NASW Press.

National Institute on Aging (NIA) (National Institutes on Health, U.S. Department of Health and Human Services). (2008). *2007 Progress reports on Alzheimer's disease: Discovery and hope.* Retrieved April 2, 2009, from www.nia.nih.gov

Nemetz, P.N., Leibson, C., Naessens, J.M., Beard, M., Kokmen, E., Annegers, J.F., & et al. (1999). Traumatic brain injury and time of onset to Alzheimer's disease: A population based study. *American Journal of Epidemiology, 149,* 32–40.

New York University Medical Center. (2008). *Mild cognitive impairment.* Retrieved February 12, 2009, from www.med.myu.edu/adc/forpatients/cognitiveimpair/html

O'Connor, D., Pollitt, P., Treasure, F., & Brook, C. (1989). The influence of education, social class and sex on Mini-Mental State scores. *Psychological Medicine, 19* (3), 771–776.

Ott, C., Sanders, S. & Kelber, S. (2007). Differences in the grief and personal growth experience of spouses and adult children of persons with Alzheimer's disease. *Gerontologist, 47,* 798–809.

Paganini-Hill, A., Clark, L.J., Henderson, V.W., & Birge, S.J. (2001). Clock drawing: Analysis in a retirement community. *Journal of the American Geriatric Society, 49,* 941–947.

Partners in Caregiving. (2002). *National Study of Adult Day Services.* Winston-Salem, CA: School of Medicine, Wake Forest University.

Perkins, P., Annegers, J.F., Doody, R.S., Cooke, N., Aday, L., & Vernon, S.W. (1997). Incidence and prevalence of dementia in a multiethnic cohort of municipal retirees. *Neurology, 49,* 44–50.

Petersen, R.C. (2003). Conceptual overview. In R.C. Petersen (ed.). *Mild cognitive impairment: Aging to Alzheimer's disease* (pp. 1–14). Oxford: Oxford University Press.

Petersen, R.C., Smith, G.E., Waring, S.C., Ivnik, R.J., Tangalos, E.G., & Kokmen, E. (1999). Mild cognitive impairment: Clinical characterizations and outcomes. *Archives of Neurology, 56*, 303–308.

Pinquart, M., & Sorenson, S. (2006). Helping caregivers of persons with dementia: Which interventions work and how large are their effects? *International Psychogeriatrics, 18*, 577–595.

Plassman, B.L., Langa, K.M., Fisher, G.G., Heeringa, S.G., Weir, D.R., Ofstedal, M.B. et al. (2007). Prevalence of dementia in the United States: The aging, demographics, and memory study. *Neuroepidemiology, 29*, 125–132.

Ponder, R.J., & Pomeroy, E.C. (1996). The grief of caregivers: How pervasive is it? *Journal of Gerontological Social Work, 27*, 3–21.

Pucci, E., Angeleri, F., Borsetti, G., Brizioli, E., Cartechini, E., Giuliani G., & Solari, A. (2003). General practitioners facing dementia: Are they fully prepared? *Neurology Science, 24*, 384–389.

Reisberg B. (1988). Functional assessment staging (FAST). *Psychopharmacology Bulletin, 24*, 653–659.

Reisberg, B., Ferris, S.H., de Leon, M.J., & Crook, T. (1982). The Global Deterioration Scale for assessment of primary degenerative dementia. *American Journal of Psychiatry, 139*, 1136–1139.

Reisberg, B., Ferris, S.H., & Franssen, E. (1985). An ordinal functional assessment tool for Alzheimer's type dementia. *Hospital and Community Psychiatry, 36*, 593–595.

Rehnquist, J. (2003). *Psychosocial services in skilled nursing facilities.* Washington, DC: Office of Inspector General, Department of Health and Human Services. Retrieved April 18, 2009, from www.oig.hhs.gov

Sanders, S. (2005). Is the glass half empty or half full? Reflections of strain and gain in caregivers of individuals with Alzheimer's disease. *Social Work in Health Care, 40*, 57–73.

Sanders, S., & Morano, C. (2008). Evidenced-based psychosocial treatments for individuals with progressive dementia. In N. Kroft & S. Cummings (eds), *The handbook of psychosocial interventions for older adults: Evidenced-based approaches.* New York: Haworth Press.

Sanders, S., & Swails, P. (2009). Caring for patients with end-stage dementia at the end-of-life. *Dementia, 8*, 117–138.

Sanders, S., Butcher, H., Swails, P., & Power, J. (2009). Portraits of caregivers of end-stage dementia patients receiving hospice care. *Death Studies, 33*, 521–556.

Schulz, R., Burgio, L., Burns, R., Eisdorfer, C., Gallagher-Thompson, D., Gitlin, L. & Mahoney, D. (2003). Resources for enhancing Alzheimer's caregiver health (REACH): Overview, site-specific outcomes, and future directions. *Gerontologist, 43* (4), 514–520.

Shelton, P., Schraeder, C., Dworak, D., Fraser, C., & Sager, M.A. (2001). Caregivers' utilization of health services: Results from the Medicare Alzheimer's disease demonstration, Illinois site. *Journal of the American Geriatrics Society, 49*, 1600–1605.

Shumaker, S., Legault, C., Rapp, S., Thal, L., Wallace, R., Ockene, J. et al. (2003). Estrogen plus progestin and the incidence of dementia and mild cognitive impairment in postmenopausal women: The Women's Health Initiative Memory Study: A randomized controlled trial. *Journal of the American Medical Association, 289* (20), 2651–2662.

Shulman, K.I., Herrmann, N., Brodaty, H., Chiu, H., Lawlor, B., Ritchie, K., & Scanlan, J.M. (2006). IPA survey of brief cognitive screening instruments. *International Psychogeriatircs, 18*, 281–294.

Smith, B., Kerse, N., & Parsons, M. (2005). Quality of care for older people: Does education for health care assistants make a different? *New Zealand Medical Journal, 118*, 1214.

Smxith, M., Buckwalter, K.C., Kang, H., Ellingrod, V., & Schultz, S.K. (2008). Dementia care in assisted living: Needs and challenges. *Issues in Mental Health Nursing, 29*, 817–838.

Snowden, L.R. (2001). Barriers to effective mental health services for African Americans. *Mental Health Services Research, 3*, 181–187.

Tang, M.X., Cross, P., Andrews, H., Jacobs, D.M., Small, S., Bell, K. et al. (2001). Incidence of AD in African-Americans, Caribbean Hispanics, and Caucasians in northern Manhattan. *Neurology, 56*, 49–56.

Teel, C.S. (2004). Rural practitioners' experiences in dementia diagnosis and treatment. *Aging and Mental Health, 8*, 422–429.

Thompkins, S.A., & Bell, P.A. (2009). Examination of a psychoeducational intervention and a respite grant in relieving psychosocial stressors associated with being an Alzheimer's caregiver. *Journal of Gerontological Social Work, 52*, 89–104.

Townsend, A., Noelker, L, Deimling, G., & Bass, D. (1989). Longitudinal impact of interhousehold caregiving on adult children's mental health. *Psychology and Aging, 4*, 393–401.

Turner, S., Iliffe, S., Downs, M., Wilcock, J., Bryans, M., Levin, E. et al. (2004). General practitioners' knowledge, confidence and attitude in the diagnosis and management of dementia. *Age and Ageing, 33*, 461–467.

Vitaliano, P.P., Zhang, J., & Scanlan, J.M. (2003). Is caregiving hazardous to one's physical health? A meta analysis. *Psychological Bulletin, 129*, 946–972.

Wackerbarth, S.B., Johnson, M.M., Markesbery, W.R., & Smith, C.D. (2001). Urban-rural differences in a memory disorders clinical population. *Journal of the American Geriatrics Society, 49*, 647–650.

Williams, D.R., & Earl, T.R. (2007). Race and mental health: More questions than answers. *International Journal of Epidemiology, 36*, 758–760.

Wisniewski, S.R., Belle, S.H., Coon, D.W., Marcus, S.M., Ory, M.G., Burgio, L.D. et al. (2003). The Resources for Enhancing Alzheimer's Caregiver Health (REACH): Project design and baseline characteristics. *Psychology and Aging, 18*, 375–384.

Wolfson, C., Wolfson, B.V., Asgharian, M., M'Lan, C.E., Ostbye, T., Rockwood, K., & Hogan, D.B. (2001). Clinical progression of dementia study group: A reevaluation of the duration of survival after the onset of dementia. *New England Journal of Medicine, 344*, 1111–1116.

Yaffe, K., Fox, P., Newcomer, R., Sands, L., Lindquist, K., Dane, K., & Covinsky, K.E. (2002). Patient and caregiver characteristics and nursing home placement in patients with dementia. *Journal of the American Medical Association, 287*, 2090–2097.

Zarit, S.H., Femia, E.E., Watson, J., Rice-Oeschger, L., & Kakos, B. (2004). Memory club: A group intervention for people with early-stage dementia and their care partners. *Gerontologist, 44*, 262–269.

Zhu, C.W., Scarmeas, N., Torgan, R., Albert, M., Brandt, J., Blacker, D. et al. (2006). Longitudinal study of effects of patient characteristics on direct costs in Alzheimer's disease. *Neurology, 67*, 998–1005.

Zimmerman, S., Williams, C.S., Reed, P.S., Boustani, M., Preisser, J.S., Heck, E., & Sloan, P.D. (2005). Attitudes, stress, and satisfaction of staff who care for residents with dementia. *Gerontologist, 45*, 96–105.

Zuckerman, I.H., Ryder, P.T., Simoni-Wastila, L., Shaffer, T., Sato, M., Zhao, L. et al. (2008). Racial and ethnic disparities in the treatment of dementia among Medicare beneficiaries. *Journals of Gerontology: Psychological Sciences and Social Sciences, 63*, S328–S333.

Index

ABC: 'Wonderland' 29
acamprosate 464
Acceptance and Commitment Therapy (ACT) 33
Access to Community Care and Effective Services and Supports (ACCESS) 118
activities of daily living (ADLs) 364, 425, 474, 477
acts of kindness 441
acultural recovery 10
acute care approach to service delivery 460
acute stress disorder (ACD) 124, 358, 360
Adderall 301
Addiction Severity Index (ASI) 461
adjustment disorders 27, 165; with depressed mood 313, 332
adolescents: anxiety in 362, 363; autism spectrum disorders in 270; depression 335, 337, 343; eating conditions 390–1;ODD and CD 314
adult day service (ADS) 487
advocacy groups 28
Affordable Housing Trust Fund 116
Afghanistan war 91
age: bipolar disorder 339; community violence exposure 227; dementia 479; depression 337; eating conditions 390–1
age of onset (AOA) 361
aging in place 489
agoraphobia 358, 359, 361, 367, 371
al-anon 323
al-ateen 323
Alzheimer's disease and related dementia (ADRD) 473–94; brain, disease-related changes 474; definitions 473–8; demographics 479–81; illustration and discussion 491–4; impact on caregivers and the larger family 477; impact on service providers 478; long-term care services 488; mental health care disparities 484–5; population 481–3; professional methods and interventions 489–91; social work programs 485–9; social work roles 485–7: case manager 485–6; educator 486; facilitator 486; advocate 486; counselors 486–7
AMEND (Angry Men Exploring New Directions) program (Colorado) 124

American Psychological Association (APA) Task Force 12 Criteria 269
American Society of Addiction Medicine (ASAM) 458
Americans with Disabilities Act (ADA) 32, 33
anaclitic depression 334–5, 349
anger management, race and 75
anorexia nervosa (AN) 381, 390; onset 386; symptoms 383, treatment goal 392
anosognosia 426
antidepressant medication 342
antipsychotic medication 344, 426; race and 69
antisocial behavior, community violence exposure and 231
antisocial disorder 411
antisocial personality disorder 314, 316, 317, 412, 415
anti-stigma campaigns 28–9, 31
anxiety conditions 337, 356–76; children and adolescents 11, 361, 362; comorbidity 10; cost of 11; community violence exposure 233; 357–60; demographics 360–2; environmental factors 357; genetics 360; illustration and discussion 373–6; lifetime prevalence of 360; medical illness and 363, 364; mental health care disparities 365–9; panic disorder 358; personality, and substance use disorders 23; populations 362–5; postpartum period 363; poverty and 50, 53; prevalence 10, 360, 361; professional methods and interventions 370–3; social work programs and social work roles 369–70; unemployment 25; war and 92
APA diagnostic 425
aphasia 295
applied behavior analysis (ABA) 269, 273, 274
applied relaxation techniques 371
Area Agency on Aging 492
Aricept 475
Asperger's disorder 259, 260, 263, 283; coping interventions 269–70
Assertive Community Treatment (ACT) 14, 433
assisted living 488–9
asymmetrical warfare 87
ataque de nervios 369, 376

at-risk groups 68

attachment 408

attention deficit hyperactivity disorder (ADHD) 11, 133, 270, 285, 291, 313, 314, 338; diagnosis 485; geographic disparities with 484

auditory hallucinations 439, 440

auditory integration therapy 271

autism 259, 283; communication deficits 260; diagnosis 264; *see also* autism spectrum disorders (ASDs)

Autism Diagnostic Interview-Revised 268

Autism Diagnostic Observation Schedule 268

autism spectrum conditions *see* autism spectrum disorders (ASDs)

autism spectrum disorders (ASDs) 259; adolescents, interventions 270; assessment 267; complementary and ; alternative medicines (CAM) 271; comprehensive interventions 268; co-occurring conditions 261; definitions 259–60; demographics 261; etiologies 262; gender 267; illustration and discussion 272–5; medications 270; mental health care disparities 265–7; population 261–4; prenatal or perinatal events 263; programs, culture 266; social skills interventions 270; social work programs and social work roles 267–72

autobiographical memory 298

automatic reinforcement 273

avoidant personality 412

batterer intervention programs 205

Bazelon Center for Mental Health Law 33

behavior disorders 337

behavioral inhibition 287

Behavioral Risk Factor Surveillance System instrument (CDC) 203

behavioral theories 409

behavioral therapy: anxiety conditions 370; mood conditions 344; *see also* cognitive behavioral therapy

benevolence stigma 32

benzodiazepines 373

bereavement 332, 333

biases and etiological assumptions 6, 7

bicultural effectiveness training 168

bicultural recovery 10

binge eating disorder (BED) 381, 382, 383–5, 388

biological model of mental illness 32

biological reductionism 451

biopsychological interview318

biopsychosocial approach 33, 112, 342, 349, 371

biopterin 271

bipolar disorder 22, 335, 338; bipolar disorder I 313, 332, 333, 336, 342; bipolar disorder II 331, 332, 333, 336–7, 342; in children 336; diagnosis 333; employment 27; prisoners with 144; substance abuse 454; suicidal ideation 342; treatment 340, 344 345

bizarre behavior 424

Blueprint for Change: Ending Chronic Homelessness for Persons with Serious Mental Illness and Co-Occurring Substance Use Disorders 112

Board of Education, Better Business Bureau 30

body avoidance 388

body checking 388

body mass index (BMI) 384

borderline personality disorder (BPD) 144, 332, 412, 415; child maltreatment 177, 179–80; dissociation 183; race and 71; substance abuse 454

Bosnian refugees 97

Bowring v. Godwin, 1977 137, 138

brain abnormalities, autism spectrum disorders and 262

brief psychotic disorder 424, 426

Bringing America Home Act (BAHA) 117, 118

bulimia nervosa (BN) 381–3, 385, 387

bullying 226, 234

CAFAS 324

CAGE questionnaire 461, 466

carbamazepine 373

caregiving career 473

casein exclusion 271

catatonic schizophrenia 425

Catholic Charities Refugee Program 167

Celexa 301

Center for Mental Health Services (CMHS) 325

Center for Victims of Torture (CVT) 98

central function 287

behavioral inhibition 287

Charcot, Jean 404

Charity Organization Societies 156, 159

Chicago Cubs 29

Chicago Police Department: Crisis Intervention Team (CIT) in-service training 31

child abuse: physical 408; sexual 387, 408 in war and 93

Child and Adolescent Functional Assessment Scale 323

Child and Adolescent Service System Program (VASSP) 324

child custody rights of parents with mental illness 27

child maltreatment 174–98, 226; adversarial growth and resilience 185; definitions 174–6; illustration and discussion 186–97; individual and group modalities 186–7; mental health/illness 176–; prevalence 176; *see also* child abuse

Child Protective Services 217

child soldiers 96

Childhood Behavior Checklist (CBCL) 166

childhood-onset type conduct disorder 314

children: anxiety disorder in 11, 362; autism spectrum disorders 265; asthma, mothers of 7; bipolar disorder 336, 338; conduct disorder in 11; depression 11, 334, 335, 337, 343; eating disorders in 11; homelessness and 119–20; of immigrants, 161–2; learning disabilities 282; obesity 390; obsessive-compulsive disorder 363; poverty and 50, 53; post-traumatic stress disorder 362; refugee 98; schizophrenia 427; schizophrenic mothers 7; victimization 213; war and 95, 105, 240; welfare, race and 68, 70; *see also* adolescents; child abuse; child maltreatment

choleric temperament 404

chronic obstructive pulmonary disease (COPD) 428

chronically homeless 114

chronotherapy 271

civil rights movement 7

civil war 87, 88, 89, 159

class 2–3

classic drive theory 452

client-run groups 345

Clinical Antipsychotic Trials (CATIE) 427

clomipramine 373

clozapine 271

coexisting disorders 324

cognitive behavioral play therapy (CBPT) 240

cognitive behavioral therapy (CBT) 36, 335, 343, 392, 393, 418, 463; anxiety conditions 371; child maltreatment 192; community violence exposure 240; post-traumatic stress disorder 372; refugees 98; stigma 33

cognitive functions 288

cognitive impairment, mild 474

cognitive remediation interventions 436

cognitive restructuring 372

cognitive symptoms 371

cognitive theory 150, 232, 334, 409

cognitive therapy 370, 371, 415

Cohen Report 141

Cohen, Fred 140, 150

cohort effects 386

cold cognition 289, 290

cold executive abilities 289

Coleman v. Wilson et al., 1995 134, 135

collaborative care model 345, 346

collective efficacy, community violence exposure and 230

collective pathology 230

college students, stigma and 26

color-blind racism 63, 230

command hallucinations 440

Community Action Group 116

community-based services 463, 487

Community Development Block Grant (CDBG) program 116

community factors, community violence exposure 229, 237

community interventions, war and 102

Community Mental Health Services programs 115

Community Support Program (CSP) 115

community violence exposure (CVE) 225–44; academic achievement 233; acculturation level 236; assessment 237; coping skills and appraisal of violence 236; definitions 225–6; externalizing symptoms of 231; home environment and family 235; illustration and discussion 237–44; internalizing and physical symptoms 232, 233; intervention 240; mental health/illness and 226–37; minority youth and criminal behavior 232; normalization 230; outcomes, youth 231, 235; prevention 242; risk factors 227; risk taking behaviors and 232; role of social work 237; social support 236; symptomology and cumulative exposure to stressors 234; type and severity 235; urban settings 229

comorbid disorders 324, 361

compassion fatigue 188

complementary and alternative medicines (CAM) 271

complementary functions 292

complementary moments 294, 296, 308

compliance trials 273

Comprehensive Homeless Assistance Plan (CHAP) 117

Comprehensive Housing Affordability Strategy (CHAS) 117

conceptions of the world 72

concordant moments 294, 308

conduct disorder (CD) *see* oppositional defiant disorders and conduct disorders

conflict model of psychoanalysis 409

conflict resolution skills 344

constructivist self-development theory (CSDT) 184

consumer recovery model 429

contact approaches 30–1

contact conditions 30

contact hypothesis 30, 31

contagion effect: community violence 232; disordered eating behaviors 390

corrections 133–51, 428; definitions 134–7; illustration and discussion 147–51; mental health/illness 137–47

cortisol 233

cost: of Alzheimer's disease and related dementia 480–1; of mental illness 11

countertransference 188, 300

critical thinking movement 408

Crohn's disease 391

culture: child maltreatment 184; recovery 10; as set of norms 365; *see also* race and ethnicity

culture bound syndromes 366, 367, 369

curanderos (faith healers) 164

cystic fibrosis 391

dating violence 210, 211

deep breathing techniques 192

deinstitutionalization movement 14, 423

delayed grief and mourning 303

delusional disorder 359, 424, 426, 427

dementia *see* Alzheimer's disease and related dementia (ADRD)
demographics of mental illness 10–13
Department of Health and Human Services (DHHS) 14
Department of Housing and Urban Development (HUD) 118, 121
dependent depression 334–5
dependent personality 412
depression 333; abuse and 213; attention deficit disorder 332; biological factors 334; child maltreatment 177; children 11; consequences of 331; dependent 334–5; elderly people 337; genetic predisposition 334; immigrants 166; personality traits 334; poverty and 50, 53; prisoners with 144; race, rates of treatment and 340; schizophrenia 24; stressful life events 334; symptoms 334; war and 91, 92
depressive phenomenology, race and 69
detention centers 160
detoxification services 458
developmental disorders 338
developmental variant of executive function disorders 283, 285
diabetes 391, 428
Diagnostic and Statistical Manual (DSM); DSM-I 405; DSM-III 406; DSM-IV 461; DSM-IV-TR 8, 65, 66, 164, 259, 286, 331; 357; criticism of 9, 407; reasons for using 9; DSM-V 408
Diagnostic Interview Schedule 212
diathesis-stress model 410, 413
diet, poverty and 53
Dimarco, Miki Ann 138
Dinosaur School program 320
dirty war tactics 86, 93–4
disability days 11
disaster relief 104
Discrete Trial Teaching (DTT) 274
discrimination 22; against women with disabilities 210; *see also* racism
disease model of addiction 451
disjunction 299
disjunctive moments 294, 299, 308
disorganized personality 425
disorganized thoughts 424
displacement, war and 88, 99
disruptive behavior conditions 313
disservices costs 170
dissociation, child maltreatment 180–1, 182, 183
dissociative identity disorder (DID) 177, 180, 181, 182, 186, 424
dissonance-media-literacy programs 392
disulfiram (Antabuse) 46
diswelfares costs 170
Doe, John 139
domestic abuse *see* intimate partner violence (IPV)
domestic violence programs 210, 217
Doty v. County of Lassen, 1994 138
double-consciousness: 162

drug abuse *see* alcohol abuse; substance abuse
dual diagnosis 324, 415, 416
Dupuis v. Magnusson, 2007 135
dyslexia 287
dysthymia disorder 284, 313, 332; in immigrants 165–6

early onset Alzheimer's disease 475
eating conditions 7, 337, 381–99; adolescence and young adulthood, 391; categories 383; children 11; definitions 381–6; demographics 386–7; illustration and discussion 393–8; mental health care disparities 389–91; multicausal model 393; older adults 390–1; populations 387–9; post-traumatic stress disorder 387; prevalence 389; prevention 391–2; professional methods and interventions 392–4; psychological symptoms 384; screening 391; social work programs and social work roles 391–2; symptoms and symptom clusters 382
eating disorder not otherwise specified (NOS) 383, 384
ecological perspective: child maltreatment 197; community violence exposure 226; IPV 217; migration experience 162, 165
ecological structural family therapy 168
education 434
Effexor 302
ego defenses 418
ego psychology 343
egosyntonic behavior 405
Eighth Amendment, U.S. Constitution 134, 135; violations 137, 138
El Salvador 1980s civil war 99
elderly people *see* age
electroconvulsive therapy (ECT) 342
Emergency Family Assistance Association (EFAA) 124
emotional abuse (EA) 212, 213; adolescents 211; child 176–7; IPV 202, 204
emotional deficit 294
emotional factors 288
empathic listening 344
empathy 293
emphysema 429
employment 27; discrimination 25; stigma and 24, 25; supported 433, 435; *see also* unemployment
empowerment theory 150
entitlement programs 158
environment: anxiety and 357; community violence exposure 235; conduct disorder and ODD 318; homelessness 124–5; mental illness 148; post-traumatic stress disorder and acute stress 359
environmental hazards, poverty and 53, 54
environmental quality 53–4
episodic homelessness 114
episodic memory 297, 298

Estate of Miki Ann Dimarco v. Wyoming Department of Corrections et al., 2007 134, 138
Estelle v. Gamble (1976) 137, 138
ethics of cultural competence 197
ethnic cleansing 88, 159
ethnic conflicts 87
ethnic economies 161
ethnic enclaves 161
ethnic hostility 87
ethnicity *see* race and ethnicity
ethnicization 161
evidence-based practice (EBP) 313, 433, 463, 465; community violence exposure 237; conduct disorder and ODD 319
executive function: behavioral components 286; definition 282; persistent organizational failures in school-age children 286; treatment process and modifying traditional modes of interventions 283
executive function disorders (EFD) 282–308; definitions 285–90; demographics 290; illustration and discussion 300–7; mental health care disparities 291; population 290–1; professional methods and interventions 292–300; role of motivation 289; social work programs and social work roles 291–2
exosystem 225
experience of being a self 292
exposure 371
expressed emotion 335
expressive arts 240
externalizing conditions (disruptive behavior conditions) 313
eye movement desensitization and reprocessing (EMDR) 372

facilitated dialogue model 31
Fair Housing Amendments Act 1988 32, 33
familiarity with persons with mental illness 24
familismo 206
family behavior therapy (FBT) 313, 319, 321, 322; torture and 98
family comorbidity 387
family education 433
Family Environment Scale (FES) 324
family intervention 275, 344; community violence exposure 229, 242
family problem-solving 344
family role in treatment of psychosis 434
Family Strengthening Policy Center (FSPC) 243
family therapy 8, 275, 345; functional family therapy (FFT) 313, 319, 321, 322
Family-to-Family Education program 434
family victimization 215, 233
Farmer v. Kavanagh, 2007; 135
fatalistic beliefs and behaviors 232,
Federal Emergency Management Agency (FEMA) 2, 117
Federal law 94–142 265

Federal Nursing Home Reform Act of 1987 (Omnibus Reconciliation Act: OBRA) 488
fight or flight response, 356
first generation antipsychotics 429
flashbacks 359
fluoxetine (Prozac) 392
folie à deux, 425
food stamps 47, 117
forced migration 159
forward edge concept (Tolpin) 297
free-market 160
Freud, Sigmund 9, 333, 404, 405
frontal lobe dysfunction 285
Frontline 149, 150
Functional Assessment Staging Tool (FAST), 481–2
functional behavior assessment (FBA) 273
functional family therapy (FFT) 313, 319, 321, 322

gacaca trials 98, 99
Gage, Phineas 284
gang violence 226
gay rights movement 6
gays and lesbians 139: anxiety conditions 365; diagnosis as mental illness 6–7; eating disorders 388–9
gender: Alzheimer's disease and related dementia 479; anxiety conditions 364; autism spectrum disorders 267; bipolar conditions 339; community violence exposure 228; depression 337; eating disorders 387, 388–9; homelessnes 120; IPV and 204, 209; ODD and CD 315–16; risk of major depression 335; schizophrenia and 24; violence, war and 93
Gender Identity Disorder 7, 134, 138–9
gendered power differentials, war and 94
generalized anxiety disorder 358, 361, 364, 387; cognitive therapy 372; race and ethnicity 366
Geneva Conventions 88
genital exhibition 136
genocide 87
Geodon 302
George Washington University 33
ghost in the nursery 404, 409
Global Deterioration Scale 482
Global Position System 298
globalization 159
gluten exclusion 271
goal setting 396
Gore, Al 67
Gore, Mrs. Tipper 67
graduated exposure therapy 371
Greason v. Kemp, 1990 138
Great Depression immigration 156
Great Smoky Mountains Study 51–2
Grey Gardens 425–6
grief-based approaches 240
guerilla warfare tactics 88

guided imagery 371
guilt, abuse and 211
Gulf War 87

H.C. by Hewett v. Jarrard, 1986 137
hallucinations 359, 424, 427; auditory 439, 440;
    command 440
harm avoidance 407, 410
harm reduction 460
Harris v. Thigpen, 1991 138
Haudenosaunee 145–6
heart disease 428
heat-or-eat dilemma 53
hepatitis B and C 428
hidden homeless 114
high functioning autism 260
historical deinstitutionalization 116
histrionic personality disorder 376, 410, 412, 415
HIV/AIDS 121, 428; community violence
    exposure and 232; prisoners with 144
homeland 160
Homeless Adults with Serious Mental Illnesses
    program 118
homelessness 110–30; definitions of 112–14;
    dysfunctional interpersonal processes 125;
    illustration and discussion 122–8; mental
    health/illness 114–22; race and 68; rural areas
    120–1; service system components 128–9;
    social, economic, and political factors 114–15;
    state and federal prisoners 144; trauma
    response 111–12
Homes for Heroes Act 117
homicide 227, 228
homophobia 209
homosexuality *see* gays and lesbians
hospice 488
hot cognition 289, 290
hot executive ability 289
housing 25, 117, 428
housing first model 436
housing ready 436
human poverty index 45
Human Rights Watch 146
human trafficking 159
human-created disasters 87
Huntington's disease 426, 476
Hurricane Katrina 2–4
hypertension 428
hypomanic episode 333

I.S.L.E. 238, 239
identity disturbance 411
identity politics 87
identity, race and 71–2
Illegal Immigration Reform and Immigrant
    Responsibility Act (IIRIRA) 159, 160
illness self-management 435
immigration 156–70; children and traumatic stress
    disorders 165; definitions of 158–62;

disenfranchisement and marginalization 160;
    family and community as buffers 160–1; global
    concern 157; homelessness 112; human rights
    160; illustration and discussion 167–9; labor
    and social welfare 159; mental health needs
    166; mental health/illness 163–6; stress 161;
    trauma 160; United States, 1861–2000 156,
    157; urbanization and economic development
    158
Immigration and Nationality Act, amendments
    156
Immigration Reform and Control Act 1986, 160
In Our Own Voice: Living with Mental Illness (IOOV)
    30–1
In re Blodgett, 136–7
In vivo exposure 371
incompetence 23
Incredible Years Child Training Intervention 319
Incredible Years Parent Interventions 319
Incredible Years Parents, Teachers and Children's Training
    319
Incredible Years Teacher Training Intervention 319
Incredible Years training 319
indirect trauma 188
individual stigma 24
individual therapy, torture and 98
individualized education program (IEP) goals 275
Individuals with Disabilities Education Act 265
individuation 292
induced relaxation 371
industrialization 159
infant mortality, conflict and 89
informed consent 183, 197–8
inpatient treatment, race and 68
institutional discrimination 26–7, 32
institutional racism 62– 3, 65, 70, 80, 207
insurance 27, 68, 117, 455
insurgency 88
integrated dual diagnosis treatment (IDDT) 433,
    434
intensive case management (ICM) 433, 434
Intensive Child and Adolescent Psychiatric
    Preventive Services (ICAPPS) 14
intensive outpatient programs 341
Interagency Committee on Disability Research
    (ICDR) 14
interdependence 292
Intermediate Care Program (ICP) 135
internal migration 159
internalization of speech 287
internalized racism 65, 71
internalized stigma 24, 26, 33, 35
Internalized Stigma of Mental Illness (ISMI) scale
    26
internally displaced persons (IDPs) 96–7, 101, 159
International Classification of Diseases (ICD) 405
International Committee of the Red Cross (ICRC)
    88
International Federation of Social Workers 169

international migration 159
International Study of Schizophrenia (ISoS), 430
interpersonal and social rhythm therapy 345
Interpersonal Cognitive Problem Solving (ICPS) 243
interpersonal psychotherapy 343, 394
interpersonal racism 80
intimate partner violence (IPV) 202–17, 226; definitions 202–3; illustration and discussion 215–16; incidence and prevalence 203; *Latino* population 206–7; mental health/illness 203–15; post-traumatic stress disorder 212–13; race and 208; sociocultural risk factors 205; war and 93
intrapsychic theories of personality 408
intrusive thoughts, community violence exposure 233
invisibility syndrome 74
Iowa Department of Corrections 144
Iraq war 91, 97; international trade sanctions 90
isolated mind view 288
isolation, poverty and 55

jail diversion programs, 437
Jessica M. Lewis a/k/a Mark L. Brooks v. Berg et al., 2005 138
Jim Crow era 64
job creation 116
Journey of Hope education course 434
just war theory 88
Juvenile Residential Facility Census (JRFC) 133
juveniles, suicide, detained 143; *see also* adolescents

Kesey, Ken: *One flew over the cuckoo's nest* 284

late life anxiety 364
lay theories 72
Lay v. Norris, 1989 138
Lazarus' Model of behavior medication 150
Learn the Signs, Act Early campaign 266
learning disabilities 286; homelessness and 121; schizophrenia and 8
learning theory 452; refugees and 98
Lesbian, Gay, Bi-Sexual and Transgender (LGBT) community 139
lesbians *see* gays and lesbians
Lewy Body dementia 476
life course research, poverty and 47
Life Model of Social Work Practice 1, 112, 162, 163–4, 343
life stressors 163
life transitions and changes 13
life-modeled practice 124, 126
light therapy, 271
Lithium 349–50,373
livelihoods approach 103
Living with children 318
lobotomies 284

Long v. Nix et al., 1996; 134
loose associations 424
Lord, Ms. Elaine A 135
Luxembourg Income Study (LIS) 45–6

Machismo 206
macrosystem 225
major depressive disorder 313, 331; cost of 11; definition 332; disability days 11; immigrants 165–6; incidence 10, 335; lifetime risk 66; race 66; unemployment 25; *see also* depression
maladaptive anxiety 357
manic episode 332, 333
Mariah Lopez a/k/a Brian Lopez v. The City of New York, 2009 138
marianismo 206
Marshall, Justice 137
mass killings 88
material-spatial disorganization, 286
McKinney Homeless Assistance Act (McKinney-Vento Act) 117–18
Medicaid 5, 8, 27, 47, 115, 117, 265–6; race and 68; Title 19 486; Waiver monies 489
medical comorbidities 428
Medicare 5, 8, 27
Medicine Wheel 146
melancholia 333
melancholic temperament 404
melatonin 271
memory loss in child maltreatment 182, 183
memory recall in child maltreatment 183
mental health care disparities 325, 431–3
mental health courts 437
Mental Health Parity Act, 1996; amended 2010 267
mental health, definition 6–10
Mental health: A report of the Surgeon General 67
Mental health: Culture, race, and ethnicity 67
Mental Illness is a Brain Disease campaign 32
mental illness: definition 6–10; taboo subject 164
Mentally Ill Offender Treatment and Crime Reduction Act 142
mercenaries 88
mesosystems 226
methadone maintenance treatment 463, 464
Michigan Alcoholism Screening Test: 461
microaggressions 62, 73, 74, 78
microinsults 73
microsystems 226
migration *see* immigration
militarization 89
mindsharing 293
Mini Mental State Examination (MMSE) 482, 485
Mitsubishi 29
mixed episode 333
Modified Checklist for Autism in Toddlers (M-CHAT) 268
mood conditions 10, 331–50; comorbidity 332;

definitions 331–5; demographics 335–7;
illustration and discussion 346–9; mental
health care disparities 339–41; population
337–9; professional methods and interventions
342–6; schizophrenia 360; social work
programs and social work roles 341–2
mortality rates: Alzheimer's disease and related
dementia 481; anorectic females 392
mother-blaming 8, 385
motivated forgetting 181
motivational interviewing 462
Moving to Opportunity (MTO) program 51
multidimensional family therapy 464
multiple personality disorder *see* dissociative
identity disorder (DID)
multiple role-plays 323
murder 361
music therapy interventions 271

naïve theories 72
naltrexone 271, 464
narcissistic personality disorder 293, 412, 413,
415
narcotic antagonists 464
Narcotics Anonymous (NA) 466
National Affordable Housing Act 117
National Alliance on Mental Illness (NAMI)
(formerly National Alliance for the Mentally
Ill) 14, 29, 30–1, 35–6, 323, 430; 'Mental
Illness is a Brain Disease' campaign 32;
Stigmabusters 29, 31
National Association for Mental Illness 6
National Association of Social Workers 169; Code
of Ethics 80, 81, 174, 438; Register of Clinical
Social Workers 9
National Center for Health Statistics at the
Centers for Disease Control (CDC) 11
National Coalition for the Homeless 118–19, 121
National Comorbidity Survey Replication Study
(NCRS) 2, 4, 10
National Epidemiologic Survey on Alcohol and
Related Conditions (NESARC) 455
National Health and Nutrition Examination
Survey (NHANES) 11
National Hospice and Palliative Care
Organization (NHPCO) 488
National Housing Trust Fund 116, 117, 118
National Institute of Mental Health (NIMH) 11,
324–5
National Institutes of Health 67
National Longitudinal Survey of Youth (NLSY)46
National Report Card on Mental Health Services
441
National Violence Against Women Survey 203,
207
Native Americans, IPV victimization 208–9
NATO 87–8
natural disasters 2–3, 159
negative mirroring 162

Negro Minstrels 64–5
neighborhood context of poverty 48–9
neurobiological theories 409
Neuropsychiatric Institute (NPI) 29
neuropsychodynamic model 290, 92, 293, 294
neuropsychological deficits 293, 294
neuropsychological testing 268
New Freedom Commission on Mental Health 21
new wars 87, 88
New York University (NYU) Spouse Caregiver
Intervention Study 489
night eating syndrome 384
Nixon-Hughes, Debbie 150
nongovernmental organizations (NGOs) 86
non-traditional conflict 88
nonverbal learning disabilities 283
non-verbal working memory 287
not the only one principle 196
novelty seeking 407, 410

Obama, Barack 63, 116
obesity, 384
obesity-related conditions 381
object relations theory 162, 452
obsessive compulsive disorder (OCD) 2, 285, 358,
360, 368, 387, 412; in children 363; incidence
361; pharmacotherapy in 373
obsessive compulsive personality 412
occupational discrimination, race and 63
Office of Juvenile Justice and Delinquency
Prevention (OJJDP) 133
Office of Mental Health, 135
Ohio Department of Corrections 134
Ohio Department of Youth Services 141–2
olanzapine 271
One flew over the cuckoo's nest 284
opiate agonists 464
opium 451
oppositional defiant disorders (ODD) and conduct
disorders (CD) 313–26; conduct disorder (CD)
11, 313–15, 338; definition 313–15;
demographics 315–16; etiological factors 317;
illustration and discussion 321–5; in children
11; mental health care disparities 318;
parenting and familial factors 317; population
316–17; poverty and 50; prevalence rates 315;
professional methods and interventions
319–21; social work programs and social work
roles 318–19; symptoms of ODD 315
oppositional disorder 313
oppression, definition 11; *see also* stigma
optimal contact interventions 30
outlaw states 89

Panel Study of Income Dynamics (PSID) 46
panic attack (PA) 366
panic disorder (PD) 2, 358, 366, 372; incidence
361; substance abuse 454
paramilitary units 88

paranoia 368
paranoid personality 412, 425
paranoid schizophrenia, cognitive dissonance 148
para-war 91
parent management training (PMT) 313, 319,
    320, 322
Parkinson's disease 426, 476
Parkinsonism 285
partial hospitalization programs, 341
paths of hopelessness 162
Paxil 301
pediatric autoimmune neuropsychiatric disorders
    associated with streptococcal infections
    (PANDAS) 363
peer influence, community violence exposure228
peer mediation 244
peer support 36, 435
people of color *see* race
perceived stigma 25–6
perfectionism 334
peritraumatic dissociation, child maltreatment
    180
Personal Responsibility and Work Opportunity
    Reconciliation Act 158–9
personality conditions 404–19; common risk
    factors 412; customizes the disease 426; decline
    with age 414; definition 404–11; demographics
    411–13; dual diagnoses 416; illustration and
    discussion 416–18; incidence and prevalence
    rates of 411; population 413–14; professional
    methods and interventions 414–16
personality disorder not otherwise specified
    (PDNOS) 408
personality-guided therapy 415
person-in-environment model 237
pervasive developmental disorder (PDD) 259
pervasive developmental disorder not otherwise
    specified (PDD-NOS) (atypical PDD or
    atypical autism) 260
phase of life problems 27
phlegmatic temperament 404
phobias 358, 367
phonological loop 287
physical abuse 211–12; child 174, 175, 176–7
physical disabilities; anxiety and 364;
    homelessness 121; rates of depression 336
physical neglect, child 174–5
physical victimization of women 203
physical violence, IPV 202
physiological hypoarousal and hyperarousal,
    community violence exposure 233
pica 389
Pick's disease 476
pivotal response training (PRT) 269
play therapy 240
polar disorder 331
Positive and Negative Syndrome Scale (PANSS)
    148
positive distancing 215

positive mirroring 162
positive reinforcement 344
postpartum anxiety 363
postpartum depression 335
post-psychotic depression 426
post-traumatic growth, child maltreatment 185
post-traumatic stress disorder (PTSD) 2, 7, 78, 99,
    124, 338, 358, 362, 370, 372, 429; abused
    women 212–13; age and 364; anxiety, and
    depression, war and 86; child maltreatment
    177–9; children, war and 95–6; complex 179;
    community violence exposure 233; diagnosis
    361; homelessness and 112; Hurricane Katrina
    and 2; IPV and 214; lifetime prevalence rate
    387; male war veterans 11, 367; prevalence 10,
    361; racism and 66–7, 76–7; rape 372;
    September 11, 2001 and 100; symptoms 99,
    164–5; war and 91, 92, 93
poverty 44–57; children's mental health 50;
    conceptualization and measurement 44;
    cross-sectional 45–6; community violence
    exposure 229; definitions 44–5; direction of
    causality 50; dynamics 46–7; eating problems
    389; environmental and community context
    53–4; homelessness and 112, 115; Hurricane
    Katrina and 2; illustration and discussion
    54–6; immigration and 160; lack of resources
    52–3; life course risk of 47, 48; longitudinal
    dynamics of 46, 47; mental health/illness
    45–54, 56; neighborhood 48–9; physical
    health 49; prevalence 45, 56; relative
    measure 44; social exclusion and 45;
    socioeconomic status (SES) 49; stress and 53;
    U.S. 44, 45
power, race and 71
precipitating events 334
pregnancy: eating disorders 390; psychosis 433
prejudice 22
premenstrual dysphoric disorder 335
President's New Freedom Act, 423
pre-trauma psychopathology 214
prisons and jails: homelessness and 144; juveniles
    133, 134; mental health services 147; race and
    68, 133; staff, substance abuse system 116;
    suicidal detainees 147; women and 133; *see also*
    corrections
private sector institutional discrimination 27
problem-solving skills training (PSST) 313, 319,
    320, 322
procedural memory 297, 298
procrastination 286, 298
professional stigma 28
Project IMPACT 344
Projects for Assistance in Transition from
    Homelessness (PATH) 118
proportionality 88
prospective retrieval disorganization 286
protest strategies for stigma reduction 28–9,
    31

Providing Alternative Thinking Strategies (PATHS) 243
Prozac 301
psychiatrists, role of 4
psychoanalysis 405
psychoanalytic theory 408
Psychodynamic Diagnostic Manual 289
psychodynamic theories 289, 409, 418
psychodynamic therapy 343, 415
psychodynamics 296; executive function 283
psychoeducation 33, 344–5, 349, 374, 392, 33, 434
Psychoeducational multiple family groups (PEMFG) model 434
psychological abuse 213; adolescents 211; definition 204; IPV 202; women 203
psychological first aid 240
Psychological Maltreatment of Women Inventory 204
psychopathology 2, 405
psychosis *see* psychotic conditions
psychosocial explanations of mental illness 32
psychosocial functioning 386
psychosocial-behavioral factors 228
psychotherapy 290, 350
psychotic conditions 368, 404, 423–41
psychosis 368, 404; definitions 424–7; demographics 427–30; developmental course and challenges 430; general medical condition 426; illustration and discussion 438–41; intimate relationships and sexuality among persons with 432; population 430–1; professional methods and interventions 437–8; racial and ethnic groupings 427; schizophrenia 426; social work programs and social work roles 433–7
psychotic paranoid ideation 148
public stigma 24–6, 32, 35
purging behaviors 385

race and ethnicity 2–3; access to appropriate mental health services 67–9, 340; admission rates to psychiatric hospitals 70; Alzheimer's disease and related dementia 479, 484; anxiety 368; barriers to service 455–6; bipolar disorder 339; CD and ODD 316; community violence exposure and 227; definition 365; depression 335, 338; eating disorders 389; homelessness and 119; IPV and 206; major depressive disorder risk 66; stigma and 24; violent victimization 207–8
racial categories 63–4
racial identity development models 80
racial microaggressions 65
racial profiling 73
racialization 161
racism 62–81; definitions 63–5; illustration and discussion 75–9; mental health/illness 65–75; persistence in the United States 63

rape 203, 20, 361; in war 94–5
rape camps 94
reactive attachment disorder 338
Reagan, Ronald 473
reality therapy 150
reconciliation 98–9
recovered memories, child maltreatment 182
recovery, definitions of 9; styles of 10
recovery model 14, 267, 429, 460
refeeding syndrome 390
reflected images 162
reflected images concept (Winnicott) 162
reflexivity 80
Refugee Act 1980 158
refugees 93, 96–7; in camps 104; definition 158; in third countries 91
reinforcement 273
relational difficulties 27
relaxation techniques 192
Remeron 301
repressed memories, child maltreatment 182
resilience 186
Resisting Internalized Stigma (RIS) 33–4
Resources for Enhancing Alzheimer's Caregivers Health (REACH) 490–1
respeto 206
responsibility for mental illness 23
restraint procedures 274
reward dependence 407, 410
Rice, Thomas (Daddy) 64
Riddle v. Mondragon, 1996 138
risks, politicization 230
risperidone 271
Ritalin SR 301
rogue forces 88
role disability 11
rouge states 89
rubella, congenital 262
Rural Homeless Assistance Act 117, 121
Rush Neurobehavioral Center 291
Rwanda, resolving disputes in 98

S. H. et al. v. Tom Stickrath, 2008 134, 141, 142
Salvation Army 116
sanctions 90
sanguine temperament 404
Satcher, Dr. David 67
Save Our Sons And Daughters (SOSAD) group 242
schizoaffective disorders 424, 425, 427
schizoid personality 412
schizophrenia 4, 6, 285, 404, 424, 427; comorbidity with other mental illnesses 429; criteria 425; depression in 24; diagnosis across race 66; employment 27; gender and 24; incidence 10; learning disability 8; national prevalence rate of 66; onset age 427; prisoners with 144; psychosis 424; race and 68; race, hospitalization and 70; SES and 50; suicide

427; symptom categories: positive and negative 424; treatment adherence 427; unemployment 25

schizophreniform disorder 424, 426

schizophrenogenic mother 7

school community violence exposure 235, 242

school violence226, 244

Scott Company 29

Sears 29

second generation antipsychotics 429

secondary traumatic stress, child maltreatment 187–8

secretin 271

segmented assimilation theory 161

selective mutism 2

selective serotonin re-uptake inhibitors (SSRIs) 270, 273

self psychology 452

self-blame: abuse and 211, 213; IPV 215

self-deficits 287, 292, 293, 295

self-deprecation 162

self-determination, IPV 217

self-doubt 162

self-efficacy 26, 35, 86, 163, 185, 189

self-esteem 26, 392

self-help and peer support services 433

self-identity, race and 73

self-medication hypothesis 452

self-monitoring 286

selfobject deficits 293

selfobject functions 293

self-psychology 293

self-regulation 286, 287

self-regulatory deficit 294

self-statements in problem-solving: 323

self-stigma 24, 25, 26, 33, 35

self-worth 35

sense of self 292

separation anxiety disorder 362

September 11, 2001 88, 91, 99–100

serious mental illness (SMI: cost of 11; homelessness and 121–2; Hurricane Katrina and 2; risk factor for developing substance abuse 454

Settlement House Movement 156, 159

Set-up Program 135

severe and persistent mental illness (SPMI) 5, 424

sex offenders 136–7

sexism 205

sexual abuse 212; child 174–7; homelessness 120; intimate partner 203, 213; in Orthodox Jewish community 184; in war 95

sexual assault 79, 203

sexual dysfunction, IPV and 213

sexual orientation *see* gays and lesbians

sexual victimization *see* sexual abuse

shame: abuse and 211, 213; among families with a mentally ill member 164; poverty and 55–6

shared psychotic disorder 424, 425

shared-decision making (SDM) 437

simpatia 206

situationally homeless 114

slavery 159

sleep 333

Smith, Adam: *Wealth of Nations* 44

smothering mothers 7

social anxiety disorder (social phobia) (SAD) 358, 359, 361, 368, 372

social cognitive models 22

Social Communication Questionnaire 268

social construction model 7, 381

social isolation 205

social mirroring 162

social model of disability *see* recovery model

social phobia (social anxiety disorder) 358, 359, 361, 368, 372

Social Security Act 265

Social Security Administration 27

Social Security Disability Insurance (SSDI) 27, 270, 428

social skills, definition 270

social work programs 13–15, 487

social workers: and mental health 4–6; roles 13–15

social/environmental change agent role model 168–9

socialism 160

socioeconomic status : mental health 49–50; mental illness diagnosis, race and 68; schizophrenia, prevalence of 50

socioeconomic status depression 336

sociotropy 334

Socratic questioning 343

somatic marker hypothesis 288

specific phobias 359, 361

split personalities 424

State Children's Health Insurance Program (SCHIP) 117

stereotypes/stereotyping 22, 23; gender-role, IPV and 205; race, anger and 74–5; racial 65, 72

stigma 21–37, 484; adherence to treatment, perceived stigma 26; Alzheimer's disease and related dementia 476; definition 22; depression 336; illustration and discussion 34–6; psychosis 423; social workers and allied mental health professionals 27; victims of sexual assault and partner violence 205; *see also* stigma reduction

Stigma Busters 31

stigma reduction 28, 67; educational approaches to 29–30, 31, 32; interpersonal contact 30

stigma resistance interventions 26

stress 359; poverty and 53; relaxation techniques 189; war and 92; *see also* post-traumatic stress disorder; trauma

stress-diathesis model 424

stress inoculation 185

stress–vulnerability–protective factors model 410

structural discrimination 26, 27, 33

structural racism 62–3

structural stigma 24, 35
subordinate relationship 425
substance abuse 10, 204, 205, 212, 285, 450–67;
as a disease 451–2; as a mental disorder and
symptom of underlying personality problems
452; as a product of social arrangements 453;
as a spiritual disease 453; as immoral behavior
451; as learned behavior 452; assessment
461–2; community violence exposure and, 232;
definitions 450–3; demographics 454;
dysthymia or anxiety 337; early intervention
459, 462; education and prevention activities
457; homelessness 122; illustration and
discussion 465–7; intervention practices 462–3;
IPV and 213; mental health care disparities
455–6; outpatient care 459; partial
hospitalization and intensive day treatment
services 459; population 454–5; prevention and
intervention initiatives 453; professional
methods and interventions 461–5;
residential/inpatient services and therapeutic
communities 459; social work programs and
social work roles 456–61
Substance Abuse and Mental Health Services
Administration (SAMHSA) 14, 67, 118,
325, 433; report, *Blueprint for change* (2003) 118,
128
substance-induced psychosis 426
suicidal behavior and ideation 342; abuse and
212, 213; homelessness and 122; Hurricane
Katrina and 2
suicide 331; adolescents 143, 232; in adult
corrections 143; American Indians 145; major
depression 342; military personnel 92; U.S.
veterans 92
Summers, Mary 54–6
super-maximum prisons 135–6, 151
Supplemental Nutrition Assistance Program 47
Supplemental Security Disability Income (SSDI)
116
Supplemental Security Income (SSI) 27, 115, 116,
117, 270, 428, 439
Supplemental Security Insurance 266
support groups 345
supported education 436
supported employment 433, 435
supported housing 439
Supported Housing Initiative 118
supportive-expressive psychotherapy 463
Survey of Income and Program Participation
(SIPP) 46
sustained recovery management 460
systematic desensitization 371
systemic-behavioral family therapy 344

Taijin-Kyofusho (TKS) 369
talk therapy 98
tardive dyskinisia 429
tax, homelessness 117

temporal-sequential disorganization 286
temporarily homeless 114
Temporary Assistance to Needy Families (TANF)
program 116, 117
tension trauma 160
terror tactics 89
terrorism 88
Thomas et al. v. McNeil et al., 2009 135
Thresholds Psychiatric Rehabilitation Centers 31
Thresholds Theatre Arts Project 31
timeline follow-back (TLFB) procedure 324
Titanic 2
token economy system 273
Torraco v. Maloney, 1991 138
torture 93–4, 97, 98, 165
transference 296; child maltreatment 186
transgender prisoners 139–40
transitional disorganization 286
transitional justice and reconciliation, war trauma
and 98
transsexuals in prisons 139
trauma: counselling 105; definition 175; migration
160–1; theory 408; Type I 78; Type II 78; *see
also* post-traumatic stress disorder
traumatic brain injury 91, 285
traumatic life event 13
traumatizing, definition 175
tuberculosis, homelessness and 121
Twiggy 382
two-client paradigm 194
two-person psychology perspective 288

U.S. Citizenship and Immigration Services 161
unconditional selfacceptance 33
unemployment 25, 53, 428
unemployment benefits 116
unipolar depression 335
United Nations (UN) 86, 88; Children's Education
Fund 105; Development Fund for Women 95;
guidelines on Mental Health and Psychosocial
Support 104; Security Council resolutions 95
Universal Health Care and a Living Wage 118

valproate 373
variable-centered vs. person-centered 408
vascular dementia 476
verbal working memory 287
Vermont Teddy Bear Company 29
Veterans Administration 116
Veterans Administration Health Services 369
Veterans' Benefits 117
vicarious traumatization 188
victim blaming 205, 206;
victimization 186; child 175; family 215, 233;
women 203 *see also* intimate partner violence;
sexual abuse
videotape modeling 313, 322
Vietnam, post-traumatic stress disorder in 11
violence 428; race and 68; risk of 23, 24; war and

93; *see also* community violence exposure; intimate partner violence
visual-spatial sketchpad 287
vitamin B6 271
voyeurism 136

war 86–105; civilian health and mental health 92; community disruption 94; definitions of 86–91; illustration and discussion 100–3; mental disorders and 93; mental health needs of victims 103–4; mental health/illness 91–100; psychological impact on civilian populations 94; psychosocial approach to impact of 97; stress 92; trauma 92, 93
war on terror 88, 91
war veterans 223
Washington Department of Corrections 134
Way out in left field 29
Way Out in Left Field Society 29
wear and tear hypothesis 483
Webster-Stratton's Videotape Modeling Parent Program 319, 325

welfare use patterns 47
Wellbutrin 301
wellness self-management 433, 435
white gaze 65
White v. Napoleon, 1990 138
Williams's syndrome, 262
withdrawal syndrome 373
women: abuse 203, 209–10, 214, 215; bipolar conditions 339; depression 335, 337; disabilities, abuse and 209–10; homelessness 120; IPV and 205; psychotic disorders 433; war role and 94, 95, 99
work incentives 27
working memory 297
working models 409
World Health Organization 9–10, 91
World War II, women's role, post- 7–8

Youth Risk Behavior Survey 2003 211
Yugoslavia 87–8

zone of proximal development 297

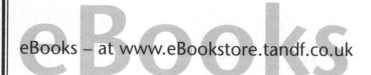